Breastfeeding

A guide for the medical profession

Breastfeeding
A guide for the medical profession

Ruth A. Lawrence, M.D.

Professor of Pediatrics and Obstetrics and Gynecology
University of Rochester School of Medicine
Rochester, New York

THIRD EDITION

With 138 illustrations

The C. V. Mosby Company

ST. LOUIS • BALTIMORE • PHILADELPHIA • TORONTO   1989

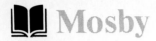

Editor: Stephanie Bircher
Assistant Editor: Anne Gunter
Project Manager: Teri Merchant
Editing and Production: Cracom Corporation
Book Designer: Susan E. Lane

THIRD EDITION

The C. V. Mosby Company
11830 Westline Industrial Drive, St. Louis, Missouri 63146

Library of Congress Cataloging–in–Publication Data

Lawrence, Ruth A.,
    Breastfeeding: a guide for the medical profession/Ruth A.
  Lawrence, 3rd ed.
      p. cm.
  Includes bibliographies and index.
  ISBN 0-8016-2803-2
    1. Breast feeding. 2. Lactation. 3. Milk, Human. I. Title.
  [DNLM: 1. Breast Feeding.]
RJ216.L358 1989
613.2′6—dc20
DNLM/DLC
for Library of Congress

GW/D/D   9 8 7 6 5

Affectionately dedicated to
**Rob, Barbara, Timothy, Kathleen,
David, Mary Alice, Joan, John,** and **Stephen**
for their love and patient understanding
and to **Bob**
for his boundless faith, trust, and inspiration

Foreword

There would have been little need for this book had it been written at the beginning of the century, when more than 50% of the mothers in the United States breastfed infants beyond 1 year, and a wealth of experience, cultural beliefs, and information about breast-feeding was shared by young mothers, their families, and their physicians. There has, however, been so little breastfeeding in the United States for the past 4 decades that the repository of cultural information about lactation has almost disappeared. Fortunately, the feeding of human milk is once again returning to its proper position of preeminence, and the lack of practical information on breastfeeding available to parents-to-be and health-care professionals is being keenly felt.

Dr. Ruth Lawrence, a physician and mother with extensive medical and personal experience in the field, designed this text to fill the gap for physicians, nurses, and other health-care professionals. This detailed and well-written book benefits greatly not only from the author's extensive experience running a normal and sick infant nursery but also from her special and unique personal life, rearing and breastfeeding nine healthy children of her own. Thus the author is a veteran in two areas. She beautifully documents the values of and the simple techniques and procedures for increasing, supporting, and continuing the mother's milk supply.

Health-care professionals in the United States might well ask themselves how and why we stopped the practice of breastfeeding. They might also ask themselves what factors led the educators and leaders of the medical profession to ignore (or discount) the wealth of information regarding the benefits of breastfeeding and the hazards of its discontinuation, information that has been available since early in the twentieth century. The leaders of the medical profession were extremely vocal about these benefits and hazards early in the century, and one wonders where the voices of these medical educators and leaders have been over the past 30 to 40 years. Have these voices been silent because health-care professionals believed (and convinced the general population) that modern medical science could indeed improve on nature?

Medical professionals complain that parents request too many operations, demand too many drugs, and, after medicine's best efforts, are dissatisfied with many aspects of the care provided their children. It would seem that the medical profession has oversold the abilities of modern medical science and undersold the innate wisdom, resources, and responses of the healthy human mother.

Was another of the factors contributing to the trend away from breastfeeding that the "science of nutrition developed a reliance on measurement and analysis that encouraged the impression that prepared foods were superior because they could be measured and calculated to meet precise needs," as Dr. Lawrence suggests in Chapter 1? Working in a neonatal intensive care unit with young physicians, one gets the impression that they with their ever-ready calculators are frustrated because they do not know the precise caloric content or the total volume the breastfeeding mother gives her premature or sick infant. Are their attitudes fundamentally different from those of their paper- and pencil-pushing predecessors of a generation ago?

It does not seem possible that a reader can help but be overwhelmingly impressed by the information presented in this book. For example, Table 1-12 presents data on the difference in mortality and morbidity between artificially fed and breastfed infants and the difference in survivors to age 1 year from the end of the nineteenth century up to 1947 with *always* a marked advantage for the breastfed infant. The data presented on deaths and death rates in seven Punjab villages, show that artificially fed infants had a mortality of 950/1000 in the first 11 months of life in contrast to 120/1000 of the breastfed infants. In this decade in rural New York state the studies of Cunningham showed again the lower incidence of respiratory and gastrointestinal illnesses in breastfed infants compared to those fed cow's milk.

We hope this book will encourage physicians and other health-care personnel to help families realize their own strengths and resources and to adapt their child rearing to the wishes and needs of the infant or child. It will still be some time before we health care professionals can fully readjust our expectations for growth, weight gain, development, and sleeping and feeding behavior to the standard of the breastfed infant rather than make comparisons to the bottle fed infant. We are learning that when an anxious breastfeeding mother asks why her infant does not burp often or loudly enough (or eats too frequently or has bowel movements that are too loose), we should not respond with concern or criticism of the burping technique but should say "great!" and point out that it is wise to use the behavior of the breastfed infant as our standard.

Several studies have suggested that the motor or mental development of breastfed infants may be different from bottle fed infants. There is a great opportunity for careful studies to evaluate this further at the present time. In our own research, filmed observations of mothers bottle feeding their infants have been shocking at times and have reminded us that there can be an enormous difference between the warmth, skin-to-skin contact, and multiple sensory interactions associated with breastfeeding and the situation with some bottle feedings, when the infant may be fed away from any human contact, fed when not hungry, and with an imposed rhythm and schedule that may conflict with the infant's own wishes and rhythms.

Ruth Lawrence points out that "one of the symbols of the emancipation of women that began in the 1920s was bottle feeding." Our present woman's movement is accompanied by an increased interest in breastfeeding. However, are there other features or side effects of the changing life-styles of today that will have a comparable impact on the health and well-being of a generation from now?

We will take this opportunity to comment about the association between breastfeeding and parent-infant attachment. We believe that early mother-infant contact starts a process of mother-infant interaction that gradually builds a strong affectionate tie, first of the mother to her infant and then later on of the infant to the mother. This is most likely to proceed successfully with breastfeeding, in which close contact and interaction occur repeatedly at the times the infant wishes and at a pace that fits the needs and wishes of the mother and the infant, with gratifications for both. Thus breastfeeding provides an optimal model for the development of a strong mother-infant attachment following contact immediately after birth, which in turn has been shown to be a simple maneuver to significantly increase the success of breastfeeding.

Any physician, nurse, or health-care professional who reads this book will be more convinced than ever of the importance of breastfeeding, will have solid data to support this conviction, and will be given a wealth of information about how to help mothers succeed with breastfeeding. Ruth Lawrence points out that there are many reasons why mothers may not be willing to breastfeed, and it will be necessary for us to realize that we cannot produce a change overnight in attitudes that have developed over the last 50 years.

John H. Kennell
Marshall H. Klaus

Preface

In the decade since the first edition of this book was published, the field of human lactation and breastfeeding has changed. Considerable national effort has been made to promote breastfeeding as the norm. In 1984, at the time of the Surgeon General's Workshop on Breastfeeding and Human Lactation, over 62% of women were breastfeeding on discharge from the hospital. The numbers have been gradually declining since then. Of more concern, however, is the fact that the infants who would benefit most—those born to less educated and lower socioeconomic families—are not being breastfed. Public surveys reveal a general knowledge about the value of breastfeeding and support for women who wish to breastfeed among both men and women of all age groups.

Research in the biochemistry and immunology of human milk and the physiology of lactation continues. The medical professional has been overwhelmed with publications on the subject. The task of sorting and sifting the largesse is difficult. This third edition was spawned as a result of efforts to deal with the inundation of information. It is designed to organize and systematize the resources to a form readily accessible for the busy clinician who quickly needs a specific answer to a clinical question. Management problems have shifted as more women breastfeed and return to work. Human milk for the sick and prematurely born infant presents new nutritional issues as more and more infants under 1000 g survive. This edition is a response to the hundreds of physicians who have requested special information or asked puzzling questions.

Search and research have been key. The computerization of library resources has, I hope, made the result more complete, but the task is never finished, since new articles of interest are appearing in the literature daily.

The reorganization of a text is never done alone. Editorial and manuscript preparation would have been impossible without the special talents of Kathryn Cook, Carole Sydelnik, and Heather Brown. The reorganization and expansion of the Appendix on Drugs in Human Milk was skillfully done by Linda Friedman, Ph.D. As with the previous editions, the artwork was created by Anita Mathews of the Medical Illustration Department. The cover art was the work of Rosemary Disney.

Ruth A. Lawrence

Preface to first edition

This book was written in an effort to provide the medical profession with an easily accessible reference for the clinical management of the mother-infant nursing couple. After many decades of championing formula for the newborn and infant, the medical profession has recognized that human milk is preferable for the human infant. The world literature reflects scientists' work on breastfeeding in the fields of nutrition, biochemistry, immunology, psychology, anthropology, and sociology. These researchers have demonstrated what most mothers have long believed: human milk is specifically designed for human infants.

Although reports in dozens of journals have contributed information valuable in the clinical management of lactation, it has remained difficult for the practitioner to gain access to it when an emergency arises. There are other topics, such as the pharmacokinetics of human milk, on which more knowledge and data are needed. This book is intended to provide the information that is available as well as identify areas of deficient information. The first part of this book is basic data on the anatomical, physiological, biochemical, nutritional, immunological, and psychological aspects of human lactation. The remainder centers on the problems of clinical management and, I hope, maximizes scientific data and minimizes anecdotal information. The goal is to provide practical information for managing individual mothers and their infants. It is also hoped that a balance has been struck between basic science, on which rational management should rest, and advice garnered by experience. Through use of the bibliographies interested readers may seek out the original works for details and supporting data.

I recognized some years ago that specific data were accumulating rapidly but remained in scattered, sometimes inaccessible, references. The increasing requests for consultation about breastfeeding sparked the idea for a more formal publication to replace the information sheets and brochures that I had been putting together. My interest in breastfeeding started during internship and residency at Yale–New Haven Hospital where Dr. Edith Jackson, Dr. Grover Powers, and Dr. Milton Senn expressed genuine concern for the declining rate of breastfeeding. Dr. Jackson provided excellent training in the art of breastfeeding for families and professionals in the rooming-in project in New Haven.

This book does not speak to world issues or the political issues of nutrition, since they have been eloquently discussed by Derrick and E.P. Patrice Jelliffe in their many works.

Throughout this book, since a nursing mother is a female, the personal pronoun *she* has been used. In referring to the infant, the choice between *he* or *she* has been made, using the male pronoun only to enhance clarity between reference to mother or child. The physician has been referred to as *he,* although I am thoroughly cognizant of the inordinate injustice perpetrated by this historical usage.

I should like to acknowledge the help and support of the many colleagues who encouraged me to investigate this subject and the hosts of nursing mothers who helped me learn what I am sharing here.

Extensive library research was done by Nancy Hess and Cathy Goodfellow, who worked as professional volunteers. Editing and tracking specific data were done by Timothy Lawrence, whom I also wish to thank. No writing is accomplished without diligent preparation of the manuscript. Loretta H. Anderson prepared many of the rough drafts. Carleen Wilenius was invaluable for her many skills with the manuscripts, not the least of which were final preparation and typing of many of the lengthy charts and bibliographies. I also wish to thank Rosemary E. Disney, who designed the cover art.

Ruth A. Lawrence

Contents

Appendixes

Breastfeeding in modern medicine

There is a reason behind everything in nature.
ARISTOTLE

Until recently, breastfeeding has been a subject considered too imprecise and nonspecific to justify consideration by scientists and clinicians confronted with questions of infant nutrition. Decades have been spent in the laboratory deciphering the nutritional requirements of the growing neonate. A considerably greater investment in time, talent, and money has been put toward the development of an ideal substitute for human milk. On the other hand, artificial feeding has been described as the world's largest experiment without controls.[59] In the veterinary field, a careful study of the science of lactation in other species, especially bovine, has been made because of the commercial significance of a productive herd.

Technology has allowed the gathering of much data about human milk. Unarguably, human milk is for human infants.

Some of the world's finest scientists have turned their interests to human lactation. Time and talent are providing a wealth of resource information about a remarkable fluid—human milk. Old dogmas are being reviewed in the light of new data, and old data are being reworked with newer methods and technology. An interface is developing for the exchange of scientific information worldwide around issues of human lactation, breastfeeding, and human milk. The more detail is deciphered about the specific macro and micro nutrients in human milk, the clearer it becomes that human milk is precisely engineered for the human infant. The clinician should not have to justify the recommendation for breastfeeding, but instead the pediatrician should have to justify the replacement with a cow milk substitute. Harnessing the continuing stream of scientific information into a resource that has clinical application has been encumbered by the need to identify reproducible peer-reviewed scientific information and to cull the uncontrolled, poorly designed studies and reports appearing in print as a result of the widening interest in the clinical field.

The health goals for the nation, first published in 1978 and restated in 1989 for the year 2000, include a statement about breastfeeding to the effect that 75% of women will leave the hospital breastfeeding their infant and at least 35% will continue to nurse for at least 6 months. The Surgeon General of the United States, C. Everett Koop, MD, ScD, took a very firm stand in response to this, saying, "We must identify and reduce the barriers which keep women from beginning or continuing to breastfeed their infants."[46]

A workshop was convened by the Surgeon General in 1984 to address these barriers and to devise a plan to reach the breastfeeding goals.[46] One barrier identified was the lack of training and education of health-care professionals in human milk and the physiology of lactation. A second workshop was convened to bring together representatives of the professional organizations—Academy of Pediatrics, American Academy of Family Practice, American College of Nurse Midwives, American College of Obstetrics and Gynecology, American Dietetic Association, National Association of Pediatric Nurse Practitioners, Nurses Association of American College of Obstetrics and Gynecology—charged with the education and accreditation of their respective members. The organizations have, through individual action of their board of trustees, endorsed a statement supporting breastfeeding and human lactation. The organizations have also devised a plan of ensuring appropriate education for their candidates and the inclusion of the material in the certifying examination for their respective specialties.

Another targeted need for the nation was public education about the subject. Education to put breastfeeding in the mainstream and to classify it as normal behavior has to start with preschoolers and continue through the educational system. Courses in biology, nutrition, health, and human sexuality should all include the breast and its functions. Dolls should not come with bottles. The media should include breastfeeding, not always bottle feeding, in reference to young infants. Public policy should facilitate breastfeeding and provide space in public buildings and in the work place. Of interest were the results of a national survey conducted by professional poll takers for the Surgeon General to explore ideas and feelings about breastfeeding. The pollsters sought out and obtained a statistically representative sample of all age groups from youth to old age, both sexes, married and unmarried, and all socioeconomic and ethnic groups. The majority in all age groups knew breastfeeding was best for infants and would want their child breastfed (75%). Very few people were embarrassed by breastfeeding or thought it should not be done in public.

This commitment to policy for breastfeeding has been part of the Code for Infant Feeding of the World Health Organization (WHO Code) to protect the developing countries from being inundated with formula products discouraging breastfeeding where infant survival depends upon being nourished at the breast.[59] In 1987, the Nutrition Taskforce of the Better Health Commission of Australia[12] set as targets for the year 2000 that 90% of mothers would be breastfeeding on discharge from the hospital and that 80% of babies would still be breastfed at 3 months of age. The rate of breastfeeding in Australia in a survey in 1984–1985 was 80% of mothers exclusively breastfeeding on leaving the hospital. The rate at 3 months was 50%. These rates had been accomplished without public health intervention. The efforts now under way will target high-risk groups with low rates. They plan worksite-based programs that encompass prenatal care, pregnancy-related nutrition and drug education, and preparation for infant feeding during pregnancy.

In general, there are two types of interventions: supply and demand.[4] Supply interventions in relation to breastfeeding are those which increase the availability of breast milk while decreasing the availability of substitutes. Making hospital routines more conducive to breastfeeding is a supply intervention, i.e., early contact, early breastfeeding, rooming-in, or time available at work to breastfeed. Restricting the casual use of substitutes in the hospital or in Women, Infants, and Children (WIC) clinics is a supply intervention. Demand interventions, on the other hand, affect the mother's motivation and attitude about infant feeding. Demand interventions tend to be educational, utilizing facts, such as breast is best; motivations, such as breastfeeding is a great mothering opportunity; or risk messages, such as using substitutes is a health risk.[4]

A summary of interventions as presented at the Surgeon General's workshop appears below and on page 4.

Key elements for promotion of breastfeeding in the continuum of maternal and infant health care

1. Primary-care settings for women of childbearing age should have:
   - a supportive milieu for lactation
   - educational opportunities (including availability of literature, personal counseling, and information about community resources) for learning about lactation and its advantages
   - ready response to requests for further information
   - continuity allowing for the exposure to and development over time of a positive attitude regarding lactation on the part of the recipient of care.
2. Prenatal-care settings should have:
   - a specific assessment at the first prenatal visit of the physical capability and emotional predisposition to lactation. This assessment should include the potential role of the father of the child as well as other significant family members. An educational program about the advantages of and ways of preparing for lactation should continue throughout the pregnancy.
   - resource personnel—such as nutritionists/dietitians, social workers, public health nurses, La Leche League members, childbirth education groups—for assistance in preparing for lactation
   - availability and utilization of culturally suitable patient-education materials
   - an established mechanism for a predelivery visit to the newborn care provider to insure initiation and maintenance of lactation
   - a means of communicating to the in-hospital team the infant feeding plans developed during the prenatal course.
3. In-hospital settings should have:
   - a policy to determine the patient's infant-feeding plan on admission or during labor
   - a family-centered orientation to childbirth including the minimum use of intrapartum medications and anesthesia
   - a medical and nursing staff informed about and supportive of ways to facilitate the initiation and continuation of breastfeeding (including early mother-infant contact and ready access by the mother to her baby throughout the hospital stay)
   - the availability of individualized counseling and education by a specially trained breastfeeding coordinator to facilitate lactation for those planning to breastfeed and to counsel those who have not yet decided about their method of infant feeding
   - on going inservice education about lactation and ways to support it. This program should be conducted by the breastfeeding coordinator for all relevant hospital staff.
   - proper space and equipment for breastfeeding in the postpartum and neonatal units. Attention should be given to the particular needs of women breastfeeding babies with special problems.

From: *Report of the Surgeon General's Workshop on Breastfeeding and Lactation.* Presented by US Department of Health and Human Services, June 11 and 12, 1984, DHHS pub. no. HRS-D-MC 84-2.
Continued.

Key elements for promotion of breastfeeding in the continuum of
maternal and infant health care—cont'd

- the elimination of hospital practices/policies which have the effect of inhibiting the lactation process, e.g., rules separating mother and baby
- the elimination of standing orders that inhibit lactation, e.g., lactation suppressants, fixed feeding schedules, maternal medications
- discharge planning which includes referral to community agencies to aid in the continuing support of the lactating mother. This referral is especially important for patients discharged early.
- a policy to limit the distribution of packages of free formula at discharge only to those mothers who are not lactating
- the development of policies to support lactation throughout the hospital units (e.g., medicine, surgery, pediatrics, emergency room, etc.)
- the provision of continued lactation support for those infants who must remain in the hospital after the mother's discharge.

4. Postpartum ambulatory settings should have:
   - a capacity for telephone assistance to mothers experiencing problems with breastfeeding
   - a policy for telephone follow-up 1–3 days after discharge
   - a plan for an early follow-up visit (within first week after discharge)
   - the availability of lactation counseling as a means of preventing or solving lactation problems
   - access to lay support resources for the mother
   - the presence of a supportive attitude by all staff
   - a policy to encourage bringing the infant to postpartum appointments
   - the availability of public/community-health nurse referral for those having problems with lactation
   - a mechanism for the smooth transition to pediatric care of the infant, including good communication between obstetric and pediatric care providers.

THE HISTORY OF BREASTFEEDING

The world scientific literature, predominantly from countries other than the United States, actually has many tributes to human milk. Early writings on infant care in the 1800s and early 1900s pointed out the hazards of serious infection in bottle fed infants. Mortality charts were clear in the difference in risk of death between breastfed and bottle fed infants.[27,28] Only in recent years have the reasons for this phenomenon been identified in terms comparable to those used to define other anti-infectious properties. The identification of specific immunoglobulins and specific influence of the pH and flora in the intestine of the breastfed infant are examples. It became clear that the infant receives systemic protection transplacentally and local intestinal tract protection orally via the colostrum. It has been further identified that the intestinal tract environment of a breastfed infant continues to afford protection against infection by influencing the bacterial flora until the infant is weaned. Breastfed infants also have fewer respiratory infections.

Refinement in the biochemistry of nutrition has afforded an opportunity to restudy the constituents of human milk. A closer look at the amino acids in human milk has demonstrated clearly that the array is physiologically suited for the human newborn. Forced by legislation mandating mass newborn screening for phenylalanine in all hospitals, physicians were faced with the problem of the newborn who had high phenylalanine or tyrosine levels. It become apparent that many traditional formulas provided an overload of these amino acids, which some infants were unable to handle well.

Although the modern woman may be selectively chastised for abandoning breastfeeding in the past decades because of the ready availability of prepared formulas, paraphernalia of bottles and rubber nipples, and ease of sterilization, it should be pointed out that this is not a new problem. Meticulous combing of civilized history reveals that almost every generation has had to provide alternatives when the mother could not or would not nurse her infant. Blame cannot be placed solely at the feet of an uninformed and unsupportive medical profession or at the feet of the formula manufacturers.

Hammurabi's code from about 1800 BC contained regulations on the practice of wet nursing, that is, nursing another woman's infant, often for hire. Throughout Europe spouted feeding cups have been found in the graves of infants dating from about 2000 BC. Paralleling the information about ancient feeding techniques is the problem of abandoned infants. Well-known biblical stories report such events, as do accounts from Rome during the time of the early popes. In fact, so many infants were abandoned that foundling homes were started. French foundling homes in the 1700s were staffed by wet nurses who were carefully selected and their lives and activities controlled to ensure adequate nourishment for the foundling.

In Spartan times,[53] a woman, even if she was the wife of a king, was required to nurse her eldest son; plebians were to nurse all their children. Plutarch reported that a second son of King Themistes inherited the kingdom of Sparta only because he was nursed with his mother's milk. The eldest son had been nursed by a stranger and therefore was rejected. Hippocrates is said to have written on the subject of nursing, declaring, "One's own milk is beneficial, other's harmful" (Fig. 1-1).

From 1500 to 1700 AD wealthy English women did not nurse their infants according to Fildes,[21] who laboriously and meticulously reviewed infant feeding history in Great Britain. Although breastfeeding was well recognized as a means of delaying another pregnancy, these women preferred to bear anywhere from 12 to 20 babies than to breastfeed them. They had a notion that breastfeeding spoiled their figures and made them old before their time. Husbands had a lot to say about how the infants were fed. Wet nurses were replaced by hand feeding, i.e., feeding a cereal or bread gruel from a spoon became customary. The death rate in foundling homes from this practice approached 100%. Toward the end of the eighteenth century in England the trend to wet nursing and artificial feeding changed, partially because medical writers drew attention to health and well-being and partially because mothers made more decisions about feeding their young.

In eighteenth-century France, both before and during the revolution that swept Louis XVI from the throne and brought Napoleon to power, infant feeding included maternal nursing, wet nursing, artificial feeding with the milk of animals, and feeding of pap and panada. *Panada* is from the French *panade,* bread, and means a food consisting of bread, water or other liquid, and seasoning, boiled to the consistency of pulp (Fig. 1-2). The majority of infants born to wealthy and middle-income women, especially in Paris, were placed out with wet nurses. The reason given for this widespread practice was that maternal nursing was "not the custom." Mothers wished to "guard their beauty and freshness." In 1718, Dionis wrote "today not only ladies of nobility, but yet the rich and the wives of the least of the artisans have lost the custom of nursing their infants." As early as 1705

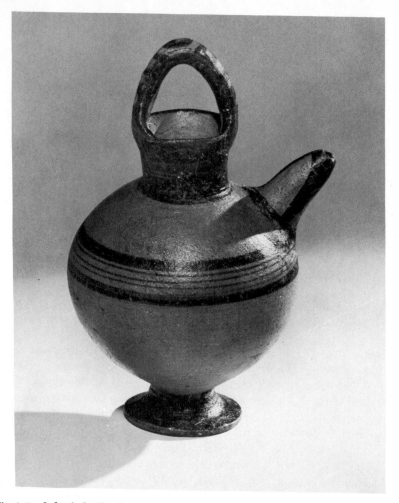

Fig. 1-1.   Infant's feeding bottle from Cyprus. Circa 500 BC. Unglazed pottery. Although ancient Egyptian feeding flasks are almost unknown, specimens of Greek origin are fairly common in infant burials.

there were laws controlling wet nursing. The laws required wet nurses to register, forbade them to nurse more than two infants in addition to their own, and stipulated that there be a crib for each infant to prevent the nurse from taking them to bed and chancing suffocation.*

A more extensive historical review would reveal other examples of social problems in achieving adequate care of infants. Long before our modern society there were women who failed to accept the biologic role as nursing mothers, and society failed to provide adequate support for nursing mothers (Figs. 1-3 and 1-4). Breastfeeding was more common and of longer duration in stable, hard-working eras and rarer in periods of "social dazzle"

---

*It is interesting to note that at the National Convention of France of 1793 laws were passed to provide relief for infants of indigent families. The provisions are quite similar to those in our present-day welfare programs.[17]

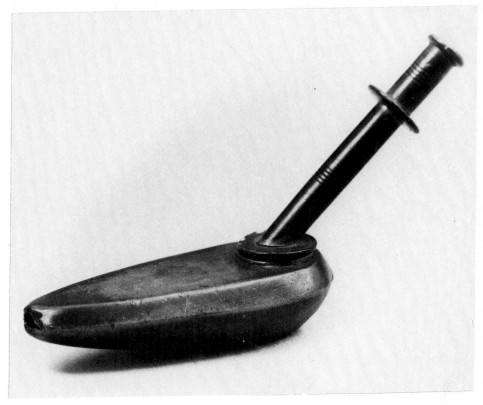

Fig. 1-2. Pewter pap spoon. Circa 1800 AD. Thin pap was placed in bowl. Tip of bowl was placed in child's mouth. Flow could be controlled by placing finger over open end of hollow handle. If contents were not taken as rapidly as desired, one could blow down handle.

and lowered moral standards. Urban mothers have had greater access to alternatives, and rural women have had to continue to breastfeed in greater numbers.

Reasons given for the decrease in breastfeeding in this century have been reviewed by sociologists. Urbanization and technological advances have affected social, medical, and dietary trends throughout the world. The social influences include the changing pattern of family life—smaller, isolated families that are separated from the previous generation. In medicine, the emphasis has been on disease and its treatment, especially as it relates to laboratory study and hospital care. The science of nutrition has developed a reliance on measurement and technology, which has led to the conclusion that prepared foods are superior because they can be measured and calculated to meet precise dietary requirements.

In the 1920s women were encouraged to raise their infants scientifically. "Raising by the book" was commonplace. The US government published a book, *Infant Care,* referred to as the "good book," which was the bible of child rearing read by women from all walks of life. It emphasized cod liver oil, orange juice, and artificial feeding. A quote from *Parents* magazine[10] in 1938 reflects the attitude of women's magazines in general, undermining even the staunchest breastfeeders: "You hope to nurse him, but there is an

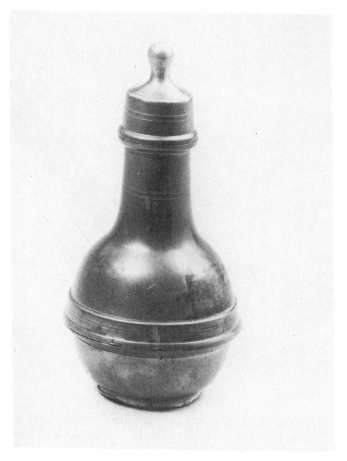

Fig. 1-3. Infant's feeding bottle. English. Circa 1780 AD. This pewter feeder is of type common to England, France, and Holland from 1600 to 1800.

alarming number of young mothers today who are unable to breastfeed their babies and you may be one of them. . . ." A social history of infant feeding from 1890 to 1950, *Mothers & Medicine* by Rima D. Apple,[2] details the transition from breastfeeding to raising children scientifically, by the book, and precisely as the doctor prescribes.

There are encouraging trends, however. The acceptance or rejection of breastfeeding is being influenced in the Western world to a greater degree by the knowledge of the benefits of human lactation. Cultural rejection, negative attitudes, and lack of support from health professionals are being replaced by interest in child rearing and preparation for childbirth. This has created a system that encourages a prospective mother to consider the options for herself and her infant. The attitude in the Western world toward the female breast as a sex object to the exclusion of its ability to nurture has influenced young mothers in particular not to breastfeed. The emancipation of women, which began in the 1920s, was symbolized by short hair, short skirts, contraceptives, cigarettes, and bottle feeding. In the second half of this century, women have sought to be well informed, and many wish the right to choose how they feed their infant. Within the boundaries of medical

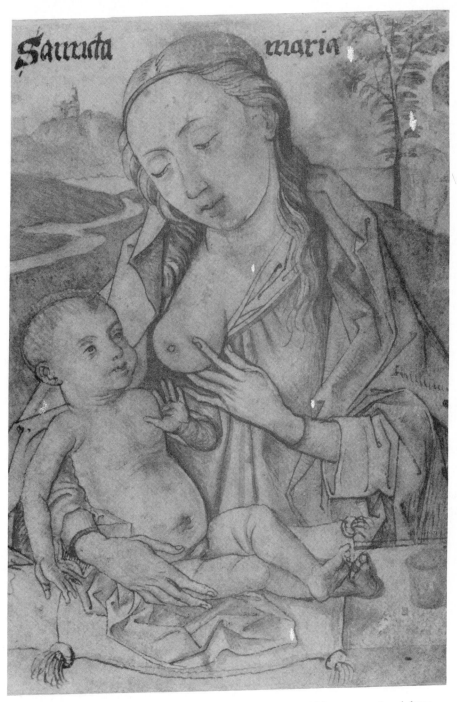

Fig. 1-4. Madonna and Child, School of Burges, Flemish, 15th century colored drawing. (Reproduced with permission from Memorial Art Gallery of the University of Rochester.)

prudence, the medical profession should be prepared with adequate information to support the mother's desire to breastfeed.

The great success of the mother-to-mother program of the LaLeche League and other women's support groups in helping women breastfeed or, as with Childbirth Education (ICEA), in helping women plan and participate in childbirth, is an example of the power of social relationships. Raphael[44] described the *doula* as a key person for lactation support, especially in the first critical days and weeks.

The social networks were explored by Bryant[9] in her study of the impact of kin, friend, and neighbor networks on infant feeding practices in Cuban, Puerto Rican, and Anglo families in Florida. She found that kin, friend, and neighbor networks strongly influenced decisions around breastfeeding, bottle feeding, use of supplements, and introduction of solid foods. Network members' advice and encouragement contributed to a successful lactation experience. The impact of the health-care professional is inversely proportional to the distance of the mother from her network. The health-care worker needs to work within the cultural norms for the network. For individuals isolated from their cultural roots, the health-care system may have to provide more support and encouragement to ensure lactation success and adherence to health-care guidelines.

The trend in infant feeding among mothers who participated in the Women, Infants, and Children (WIC) Program in the late 1970s and early 80s was analyzed separately by Martinez and Stahl[40] from the data collected by questionnaires mailed quarterly. The responses represented 4.8% of the total US births in 1977 and 14.1% of the total US births in 1980 (Table 1-3). WIC participants in 1977, including those who supplemented with formula or cow's milk, were breastfeeding in the hospital in 33.6% of cases. There was a steady and significant increase in the frequency of breastfeeding to 40.4% in 1980 ($p < .05$).

Frequency of breastfeeding

Data collected in the 1970s[39] in the Ross National Mothers Survey MR 77-48, which included 10,000 mothers, revealed a general trend toward breastfeeding. In 1975, 33% of the mothers started out breastfeeding, and 15% were still breastfeeding at 5 to 6 months. In 1977 the figures indicated that 43% of the mothers left the hospital breastfeeding, and 20% were still breastfeeding at 5 to 6 months. Other studies have shown a regional variation, with a higher percentage of mothers breastfeeding on the West Coast than in the East.

A continuation of the study of milk-feeding patterns in 1981 in the United States by Martinez and Dodd[39] showed a sustained trend toward breastfeeding in 55% of the 51,537 new mothers contacted by mail. Although mothers who breastfeed continue to be more highly educated and have a higher income, the greatest increase in breastfeeding occurred among women with less education. From 1971 to 1981, breastfeeding in the hospital more than doubled (from 24.7% to 57.6%), with an average rate of gain of 8.8%. The incidence of breastfeeding at 1 week of age was 56.4%. For infants 2 months old breastfeeding more than tripled (from 13.9% to 44.2%) in the 10-year period (Table 1-1).

The National Natality Surveys (NNS) conducted by the Centers for Disease Control in 1969 and 1980 included questions about infant feeding practices after birth by married women.[23] Questionnaries were mailed at 3 and 6 months postpartum. In 1969 19% of white women and 9% of black women were exclusively breastfeeding. The highest rate was among white women ≤ 34 years old, parity ≤ 3 and >7. In 1980, 51% of white women

Table 1-1. Percentage of infants at 1 week of age receiving different milks and formulas, 1955 to 1987

	Breast milk*	Prepared infant formula	Evaporated milk	Cow's milk	Total*
1955	29.2	23.2	45.9	4.1	102.4
1960	28.4	34.9	40.0	2.8	106.1
1965	26.5	59.0	17.3	1.5	104.3
1970	24.9	74.9	3.0	0.6	103.4
1975	33.4	69.2	0.7	0.3	103.6
1978	45.1	58.6	0.5	0.1	104.3
1979	49.7	54.7	0.3	0.1	104.8
1980	54.0	50.6	0.2	0.1	104.9
1981	56.4	48.5	0.2	0.1	105.2
1985	55.4	49.8	0.1	0.1	105.4
1987	54.1	52.5	<0.1	<0.1	106.7

From Ross National Mothers Survey MR77-48, 1988.
*Includes supplemental bottle feeding, i.e., formula in addition to breastfeeding.

and 25% of black women were exclusively breastfeeding, and they were more highly educated and primiparous.

The social network

Scientific evaluation has established that there is both a theoretical basis and a strong empirical basis for the causal impact of social relationships on health and well-being. The prevailing logic is presented by House, Landis, and Umberson.[32] Scientists have long noted that more socially isolated or less socially integrated individuals are less healthy psychologically and physically. They point out that the unmarried and more socially isolated have more infectious disease, accidents, and mental disorders. Conversely, clinicians have noted health-enhancing qualities of social relationships and contacts. The demographic information indicated that WIC mothers were slightly younger (18.5% <20 years old compared with 5.4% of those not in WIC). WIC respondents did not differ significantly from nonWIC mothers in plans for postpartum employment, although they were less educated. Of infants born to WIC mothers, 7.9% were premature; of infants born to nonWIC mothers, only 4.3% were premature. The national average was 7.1% of births. (Table 1-2).

A study of infants from an urban clinic population in California that served 86% Hispanic, 6.3% white, 4.0% Asian, and 1.8% black clients showed that only 20.8% of babies received any breast milk and only 13.1% were exclusively breastfed in the first 3 months of life.[38] The American Indian populations of Pima and Papago tribes in Arizona were studied retrospectively in 1978 to identify the role of sociodemographic factors in the trends in breastfeeding and bottle feeding.[24] Findings included a significant decline in breastfeeding from 1949 to 1977, with tendency for an increased rate in the last few years among younger women. Bottle feeding was more common among higher-birth order infants and among women of pure tribal background.

In another study, families belonging to a prepaid group practice health care plan in upstate New York were interviewed.[1] Infants were breastfed in 26% of the white, 26% of the black, and 18% of the Hispanic families. Percentages correlated with education and

Table 1-2. Breastfeeding among WIC participants, 1977–1987

	In hospital	At 5 and 6 months of age
1977	33.6	12.5
1978	34.5	11.2
1979	37.0	12.2
1980	40.0	14.4
1985	40.1	12.8
1986	38.0	11.6
1987	37.3	11.5

From Martinez GA and Stahl DA: Am J Pub Health 72:68, 1982; and Martinez GA: Ross mother's survey, unpublished data, 1988.

income levels. The infant feeding practices of middle-class mothers in Seattle, studied by retrospective home interview, revealed that 87% were breastfeeding during the first 5 weeks.

The international trends have also received considerable attention, and data on all countries but Russia are available in *The International Breast Feeding Compendium, 1984.*[58] Because studies vary in methodology, there is no accurate way to generalize. Breastfeeding patterns in low-income countries, as extracted from world fertility surveys and secondary sources, indicate that in all but a few countries most children are breastfed for a few months at least, and in 53% of the 83 countries listed, the incidence is 90% or higher. Most localized trend data in both developed and Third World countries reveal increasing frequency of breastfeeding since the 1970s.

Since 1984, when the incidence of breastfeeding at discharge from the hospital was 61.2%, the rate in the United States has gradually dropped below 60% to 56.7% in 1987.[48] The incidence of breastfeeding in 1988 was 52.4% upon leaving the hospital and 21.8% at 5 to 6 months* (Tables 1-2 and 1-3). The trend among the well-educated, high economic group remains high; the drop is occurring among the high-risk families. Study after study has confirmed the relationship to education, social status, marriage, and other unalterable demographic factors. The well-educated, well-to-do of all races breastfeed. In a study by Wright et al.[60] of 1112 healthy infants in a health maintenance organization (HMO) in Arizona, 70% were breastfed with a mean duration of almost 7 months. Education and marriage were associated with breastfeeding. Maternal employment outside the home and ethnicity (being Hispanic rather than Anglo-American) were related to bottle feeding. The authors suggest that effects of ethnicity are independent of those of education. For newly landed immigrants who would have breastfed in their homeland, the tendency is to bottle feed here because they think it is "American" to bottle feed.

The impoverished mother is choosing to bottle feed not because she is working, as statistics show she is staying home and bottle feeding. When we interviewed mothers about their infant feeding choice in the prenatal clinic at WIC, they knew mother's milk was best.[26] They said it was too hard to breastfeed and there were too many rules. When we listened to the classes on breastfeeding given by the lactation experts, it was obvious. The instructions on preparing the breasts and diet rules were overwhelming. The mothers said

---

*Unpublished data, G.A. Martinez.

Table 1-3. Percentage of infants breastfeeding by selected maternal demographic characteristics, 1971–1987

	1971	1981	1985	1987
Parity				
Primiparous	62.4*	24.2*	59.8	56.8
Multiparous	53.0	25.8	56.2	54.2
Education				
Grade and high school	50.8*	19.7*	48.8	45.9
College	74.0	38.3	76.2	73.2
Employment				
Not employed	59.5*	29.8*	59.0	57.1
Employed	50.9†	10.1†	57.5	54.5
Income				
<$15,000	49.4*	19.2*	44.0	39.8
$15,000-$24,999	61.0	28.0	63.1	59.0
≥$25,000	65.6	30.1	70.6	69.4
TOTAL (all infants)	57.6	25.1	58.0	55.5

From Martinez GA and Dodd DA: Pediatrics 71:166, 1983, Copyright American Academy of Pediatrics 1983; and Ryan AS and Martinez GA: Breastfeeding and the working mother: a profile, Pediatrics 83:524, 1989. Reproduced by permission of Pediatrics.
*Differences within category significant, $p < .01$.
†Refers to employment status at time of survey, i.e., when infants were 6 months of age, employment on a full-time basis. Data are for three quarters of 1981.
‡Refers to employment status at time of survey, i.e., when infants were 12 months of age. Employed represents mothers with full-time employment.

if only their physician would tell them it was important, they would do it for as long as the physician said.[26] Similar data were collected in the Ross Mother's Survey, which also indicated the power of the physician's word. Mothers trusted their physician and were more successful if the physician was supportive.

Duration of breastfeeding

Coupled with concerns about the decreasing number of mothers who breastfeed their infants when they leave the hospital is the concern about duration of breastfeeding. There is a sharp decline by age 6 months; in 1977 this decline was from 43% to 20%. Other studies that have looked at duration more closely have noted an appreciable decline shortly after discharge from the hospital.

In 1984, the duration of breastfeeding in the United States and elsewhere was increasing. The number still breastfeeding at 6 months was 25%. This number, however, has dropped slowly to 21% in 1987[48] (Table 1-4).

Before evaluating the duration of breastfeeding in the industrialized world, it is wise to consider that there are two types of breastfeeding, as Newton[41] points out—unrestricted breastfeeding and token breastfeeding.

Unrestricted breastfeeding usually means that the infant is put to the breast immediately following delivery and breastfed on demand thereafter. The infant is put to the breast without rules or limitations. There may be 10 or 12 feedings a day in the early weeks, with the number gradually decreasing over the first year of life. Breast milk continues to be a major source of nourishment in infancy in these infants.

Table 1-4. Percentage of infants breastfed in hospital and at 6 months and continuance rate by working status and selected demographic characteristics, 1987

Variables	Breastfed in hospital		Breastfed at 6 months		Continuance rate	
	Employed full-time	Not working	Employed full-time	Not working	Employed full-time	Not working
All mothers	54.5	54.5	10.0	24.3	18.3	44.6
Maternal age						
<20 years	38.4	33.4	4.5	7.5	11.7	22.5
20–24 years	47.9	49.6	5.8	17.7	12.1	35.7
25–29 years	57.5	63.2	9.7	31.0	16.9	49.1
30–34 years	61.1	68.4	14.5	39.3	23.7	57.5
35+ years	61.1	66.1	20.0	40.4	32.7	61.1
Family income						
<$7,000	34.3	31.0	5.6	8.3	16.3	26.8
$7,000–$15,000	40.5	49.4	6.4	19.2	15.8	38.9
$15,001–$25,000	49.7	62.4	8.1	29.1	16.3	46.6
>$25,000	63.1	72.9	12.5	38.2	19.8	52.4
Maternal education						
High school or less	43.8	46.0	5.7	17.7	13.0	38.5
College	67.6	75.9	15.3	41.1	22.6	54.2

From Ryan AS and Martinez GA: Breastfeeding and the working mother: a profile, Pediatrics 83:524, 1989. Reproduced by permission of Pediatrics.

Token breastfeeding, in contrast, is characterized by constant restrictions on the time and duration of nursing. Usually the feedings are scheduled. Even the amount of mother-infant contact is limited initially, and the infant is often offered water or glucose water by rubber-nippled bottle. The whole process is inhibited, and a secure milk supply may not be established. If one examines the duration of breastfeeding, there is a difference between unrestricted and token-feeding groups.

There are also cultural differences. In societies that have yet to be caught up in industrialization and continue to maintain ancient cultural patterns of child rearing, the duration is well beyond a year. A study of 46 such societies reported by Ford[22] revealed that weaning at about 2 to 3 years of age occurred in three fourths of them. One fourth of the groups began weaning at 18 months of age, and one culture started at 6 months. A similar anthropologic investigation of primitive child-rearing practices found a distinct correlation between the time of weaning and the behavior of the tribes.[22] Where weaning was delayed, there were peaceful tribes. In contrast, tribes that abruptly weaned their infants at 6 months of age and practiced other rigid disciplinary practices were warlike.

In the United States and Europe at the beginning of this century, over 50% of the infants were breastfed beyond 1 year of age. The Plunket Society of New Zealand conducted three surveys to evaluate the extent and duration of breastfeeding.[16] These showed a progressive decline in the number of nursing mothers and in the duration of nursing (Fig. 1-5).

In 1966, fewer than one in three mothers in the United States were breastfeeding when they left the hospital. Only 5% of the nation's infants are breastfed after 6 months of age.

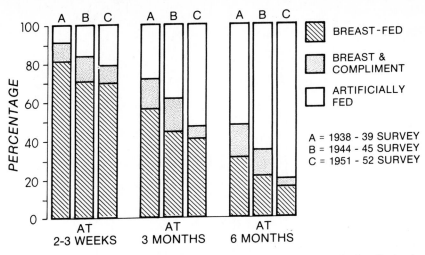

Fig. 1-5. Breastfeeding in New Zealand. Summary of results of Plunket Society's surveys of 1938 to 1939, 1944 to 1945, and 1951 to 1952. (From Deem H and McGeorge M: NZ Med J 57:539, 1958.)

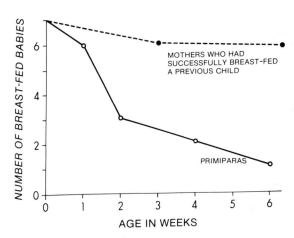

Fig. 1-6. Duration of breastfeeding in primiparas compared with mothers who have successfully breastfed a previous child. (From Fitzpatrick C and Kevany J: J Irish Med Assoc 70:3, 1977.)

A higher rate of success was experienced in mothers who had nursed a previous infant (Fig. 1-6). The rapid decline was attributed to lack of appropriate advice, including the early introduction of solid foods, and lack of psychological support while in the hospital. A study in Boston in 1960 had shown a mean duration of nursing to be 3½ months. Cole[11] conducted a two-part survey in a Boston suburb in 1977 that included 332 pregnant women and 140 new mothers—51% intended to breastfeed, 42% intended to bottle feed, and 1% was undecided. There was a correlation between education of the mother and incidence of breastfeeding, with 44% of high school graduates, 62% of college graduates, and 65% of those with postgraduate education desiring to breastfeed. Other researchers made similar

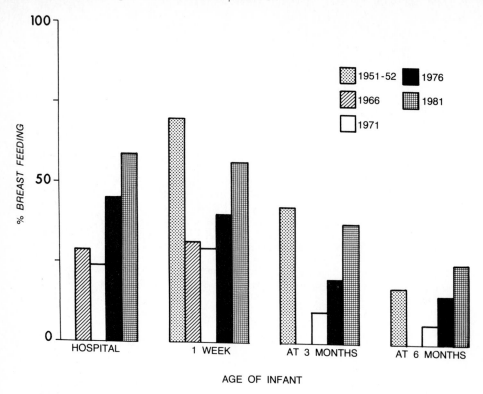

Fig. 1-7. Duration of breastfeeding (1951 to 1981). (Based on data from Woo-Lun M, Gussler J, and Smith N, editors: The international breastfeeding compendium, ed 3, Columbus, Ohio, 1984, Ross Laboratories.)

observations in the 1970s, noting that 40% of the upper- and middle-class mothers breastfeed, compared with 15% in lower classes.

The most frequent reasons given for stopping were (1) not enough milk, (2) felt tired, and (3) infant's physician told mother to stop. This study also pointed out the pivotal role for the pediatrician in the successful maintenance of lactation as well as the importance of the postpartum environment.

The 1981 Milk Feeding Pattern survey by Martinez and Dodd[39] reported on the duration of breastfeeding. The rate of infants breastfed at ages 3 to 4 months was 35.2%, a fourfold increase from 1971; at 5 and 6 months of age the rate was 26.8% in 1981 and only 5.5% in 1971 (Fig. 1-7). Data collected by telephone follow-up further revealed rates of 18% at 8 months, 13% at 10 months, and 9% at 12 months.

The maternal demographic data on duration of breastfeeding in this study further supported the trend of higher educational level and higher income for mothers breastfeeding at 6 and 12 months (Tables 1-3 and 1-4). More multiparas than primiparas continued to breastfeed, but duration was negatively affected by maternal employment. The influence of maternal employment in this survey was significant ($p < .01$). For every 100 mothers employed full time and breastfeeding in the hospital, 19.8% were still breastfeeding at 6 months postpartum, whereas among mothers not employed and breastfeeding in the hospital, 50.1% were still breastfeeding at 6 months postpartum. The employed mothers in most studies tend to be in better-educated, higher socioeconomic groups than those who are

Table 1-5. Comparison of mother's plans for infant feeding expressed during third trimester of pregnancy with practice adopted at birth (study 1)

| | Number (%) of respondents (n = 976) | | |
	Breastfed	Formula fed	Undecided
Plan for infant feeding	504 (52)	421 (43)	51 (5)
Feeding practice in hospital*			
Breastfed	482 (96)	13 (3)	28 (55)
Formula fed	22 (4)	408 (97)	23 (45)

From Sarett HP, Bain KR, and O'Leary JC: Am J Dis Child 137:719, 1983, Copyright 1983, American Medical Association.
*A total of 523 mothers (54%) breastfed their infants, and 453 mothers (46%) formula fed their infants.

Table 1-6. Time of choice of breastfeeding or formula feeding in telephone survey of recent mothers of young infants (study 2)

| | % of Respondents | | | |
Time of decision	Total (n = 200)	Breastfeeding (n = 112)	Formula feeding (n = 84)	Feeding both (n = 4)
Before pregnancy	49	55	43	—
First trimester	29	31	24	75
Second trimester	7	8	7	—
Third trimester	8	5	12	—
After delivery	7	1	14	25

From Sarett HP, Bain KR, and O'Leary JC: Am J Dis Child 137:719, 1983, Copyright 1983, American Medical Association.

unemployed. Thus, it is not necessarily employment alone that deters the lower socioeconomic group from breastfeeding.

A similar study in the United States on infant-feeding trends reported by Sarett et al.[49] in 1983 indicated that 85% to 92% of mothers decide on a feeding method before the end of the second trimester, and 96% to 97% feed their infant as previously planned (Tables 1-5 and 1-6). Between 1976 and 1980 more mothers than in previous years were breastfeeding for 6 months or longer, and solid food was being introduced later. West[56] reported in 1980 that of 239 breastfeeding mothers in Edinburgh, only 5% were breastfeeding at 12 weeks, with the greatest decline in the first 6 weeks, and 46% were breastfeeding at 22 weeks. Duration was influenced by social class but not by the age of the mother. Reasons offered for terminating breastfeeding are noted in Table 1-7. Return to work was a reason for discontinuing in only 5 of the 116 women. One hundred, or 86%, of the mothers who stopped by 22 weeks would have liked to continue but felt they had insufficient milk or other unsurmountable problems. Unrelated to length of breastfeeding, a large percentage of all the survey mothers felt they could have benefited by more assistance from health-care professionals.

The positive and negative emotional and physical experiences of 152 long-term breastfeeding American and Canadian women were reported by Reamer and Sugarman.[45] This sample of mothers was randomly selected from 1,038 women who responded to a 1974 request for volunteers in a La Leche League newsletter. They all answered the eight-

Table 1-7.   Reasons for discontinuing breastfeeding

	Duration of breastfeeding (wk)			
Reason	<6 (n = 49)	6-11 (n = 39)	12-22 (n = 28)	Total (n = 116)
Inadequate milk supply	28	18	12	58
Babt unsettled after breastfeeds	18	11	2	31
Very frequent feeds required	17	8	4	29
Breastfeeding was too tiring	13	5	2	20
Painful nipples	14	2	1	17
Baby refused the breast	9	4	2	15
Unable to go out	6	4	0	10
Too time-consuming	7	2	1	10
Illness of mother	3	6	0	9
Breast abscess	2	3	1	6
Return to work	0	3	2	5
Dislike of breastfeeding	5	0	0	5
Insufficient privacy at home	2	1	0	3
Illness of baby	2	1	0	3
Other factors*				
Anxiety, lack of confidence	6	2	1	9
Breast problems—mastitis, engorgement	1	5	0	6
Older children upset or jealous	3	0	0	3
Contraceptive pill reduced milk supply	0	1	1	2
Anticoagulant therapy	1	0	0	1

From West CP: J Biosoc Sci 12:325, 1980.
*Not listed but volunteered by the mothers.

page, 51 short-answer and 52 free-response questions. All the respondents were older, better educated, predominantly white, and had belonged at some time to the league. The average age was 29.4 years, age at first child was 25, 77% had more than one year of college, and 44% had four or more years of college. Far fewer were employed than the national average (13% full- or part-time vs. 34% nationally). The average weaning age for the 339 children represented by this study was 18 months, with a range of 3 weeks to 5 years for the older children. At the time of the study 136 children were still being breastfed. Two mothers thought there were no positive effects of prolonged nursing on their children, but others gave more than one answer to the question. (See Table 1-8.) Emotional security, happiness, mutual love, and future independence were the key positive outcomes of long-term nursing in the mothers' view. Good health was mentioned by 22%.

When asked to list the negative aspects of nursing past 6 months, 47% of mothers said there were none at 6 months, but only 26% of mothers had no negative feelings about nursing past 12 months. Perceived social hostility was the major negative effect, reported by 24% of mothers at 6 months and by 42% at 12 months. The detailed responses are shown in Table 1-9. Ninety percent felt there were no negative effects for the children. The social stigma has driven many well-educated, caring, dedicated mothers to secret nursing, called "closet nursing," which, unfortunately, leads physicians and the public alike to think that breastfeeding in this country terminates by 6 months of age.[3]

Table 1-8. Positive consequences of long-term nursing as perceived by the mother

Perceived consequences	Mothers (n = 130)	%*
Positive emotional effect on child—child is more secure	65	50.0
Better physical health (fewer allergies)	29	22.3
Child is loving, friendly, cheerier	27	20.8
Child can separate more easily—relative independence achieved with less stress	22	16.9
Enhanced maternal sensitivity	19	14.6
Close relationship of mother and child	18	13.8
Positive influence or education for older siblings	11	8.5
Child easily comforted during crisis, pain, or teething	10	8.0
Broad, all-encompassing positive effect	6	4.6
Incidental positive consequences	13	10.4
No positive effects perceived	2	1.5

From Reamer SB and Sugarman M: J Trop Pediatrics 33:93-97, 1987.
*Mothers could give multiple responses, thus percentages add to more than 100%.

Table 1-9. Mothers' responses to the question: 'What do you think are the negative aspects of nursing past 6 months?' and 'of nursing past 1 year?'

Negative aspects listed by mothers	Past 6 months Total responses = 132 No.	%	Past 12 months Total responses = 133 No.	%
Mother states there are no negative aspects	62	47.1	35	26.4
Social stigma—negative attitudes of others	32	24.3	56	41.9
Mother's activities are restricted	19	14.7	9	6.6
Baby is less discreet—embarrassing in public	3	2.2	13	9.6
Tiredness	7	5.1	3	2.2
Breast-feeding mother has special concerns	1	0.7	5	3.7
Intrudes upon life with husband	1	0.7	4	2.9
Breast discomfort/leaking, soreness	2	1.5	1	0.7
Sex life interrupted—less interest in sex	2	1.5	2	1.5
Mother believes she should ignore negative aspects	2	1.5	1	0.7
Intrudes upon mother's time with siblings	0	—	1	0.7
Baby care, not nursing, causes negative aspects	0	—	1	0.7

From Reamer SB and Sugarman M: J Trop Pediatrics 33:93-97, 1987.
*Mothers could give multiple responses, thus percentages add to more than 100%.

Impact of commercial discharge packs on breastfeeding duration

Whether commercial discharge packs are the cause of diminished breastfeeding duration has been evaluated in several studies. Unfortunately, none of the studies was so well randomized and controlled that the answer was clear. Some studies did not mention use of bottles in the hospital, but those which did noted a stronger correlation with the use of bottles in the hospital and duration of breastfeeding.[8] In New York State regulations regarding breastfeeding support instituted in July 1984, among other things, disallowed discharge packs to breastfeeding women unless they requested them or they were prescribed by the physician. A mother who requests such a pack is usually at high risk for early termination of lactation in most investigators' experience. Certainly giving such a packet to a vulnerable mother (young, less educated, single, poor support system) may be a message not unlike *Parents* magazine circa 1938: "You may be one of them. . . " (i.e., those who fail). In a study in Virginia, Hayden et al.[30] reported that most pediatricians did not know and had never been asked if they approved of the going home packages with samples of powders, creams, baby food, and other baby items that may or may not be appropriate for indiscriminate use. The authors suggest that pediatricians should investigate and review the procedures in their own hospitals. Controlling discharge packs deflects attention from the real problem, which is inadequate counseling about breastfeeding and a system to support the mother who needs it. This point is well illustrated in a study by Feinstein et al.,[19] who found initiating breastfeeding in the first 16 hours and minimizing use of formula in the nursery correlated highly with successful lactation. The negative impact of supplementation could be overcome by frequent breastfeeding at home. A gift packet of breast pads and breastfeeding information of equal monetary value to a formula packet and a special counselor who made five home visits in the first 28 days and three more in the next 6 weeks were found by Frank et al.[25] to result in longer duration of breastfeeding.

In an effort to identify the "real" reason women stopped breastfeeding, Ferris and colleagues[20] followed over 250 women who delivered in Connecticut in 1981. They tried to identify crucial biological sociocultural links in the chain of events that precede the change in feeding from breast to bottle.

Hospital routines influenced the early "failures." Successful breastfeeders experienced letdown a full day sooner than those who discontinued by 2 weeks. They had also fed their infant 5 hours earlier than those who discontinued. Mothers who nursed early had prepared themselves to insist on early feeding. Mothers who were unsure and lacked confidence turned to supplements. Providing just 1 ounce of formula per day led to ultimate discontinuation. A small amount of doubt eroded confidence. The most vulnerable period was the immediate postpartum period. Women who had wanted to lose weight postpartum were disappointed that they did not lose more rapidly. The authors also identified the need for close follow-up by the pediatrician in these critical 2 weeks[20] (see Table 1-10.)

Acute lactation failure

Acute lactation failure has been referred to historically in times of great crisis, fright, or accident when women would abruptly lose their milk. Two such cases have been reported in the literature by Ruvalcaba following the Mexico City earthquake in 1985.[47] Stress-induced lactation is described in a gravida 3 woman, 24 years old, who had been exclusively breastfeeding for 3 months and had fed two previous children for 14 and 18 months. The day of the quake, the building she was in collapsed. She ran home to her children past demolished buildings and could not produce a drop of milk when her infant suckled then or subsequently. Multiple attempts over the next weeks failed to produce a drop. The second woman was 39 weeks pregnant and had been dripping colostrum for several weeks as she had with her previous three pregnancies. The day of the quake, her house collapsed, her husband and two children were missing for several hours, and her sister was killed. She never leaked another drop of colostrum.

Table 1-10. Sources of advice on breastfeeding: Comparison of intent vs. action

Source of advice	Intent: At 1 week postpartum, mothers were asked		Action: At 10 weeks, mothers were asked	
	(1) If you have a problem with nursing, whom will you call? (n = 113)	(2) If you have already had a problem, whom did you call? (n = 19)	(1) If you had a problem with nursing, and continued nursing, whom did you go to for advice? (n = 23)	(2) If you stopped nursing, whom did you go to for advice? (n = 26)
	←		%	→
Pediatrician	36	32	65	46
Support group	24	32	5	0
Family	12	5	4	0
Friends	10	5	0	0
Obstetrician/gynecologist	6	5	0	4
Nurse/midwife	6	21	9	0
No one	0	0	17	50
Do not know	3	0	—	—

From Ferris AM, McCabe LT, Allen LH et al: J Am Dietetic Assoc 87:316-321, 1987.

MORBIDITY AND MORTALITY STUDIES IN BREASTFED AND ARTIFICIALLY FED INFANTS

Assessing the mortality of breastfed compared with bottle fed infants is difficult to do today because many breastfed infants also receive supplements of formula and solid foods. The risk of death in the first year of life has diminished in civilized countries in this century, since the advent of antibiotics and many other advances in pediatric care. Data from previous decades and other nations do show a significant difference, however.[27,28] Knodel[36] presented a complete table, including rates from cities in Germany, France, England, Holland, and the United States (Table 1-11). Mortality among breastfed infants is clearly lower than that among bottle fed infants. Knodel pointed out that early neonatal deaths, in the first week or so of life, were excluded.

In another study in 1922, Woodbury[57] reported mortality of infants by type of feeding. Mortality is lower at all ages for breastfed infants (Fig. 1-8). Overwhelming evidence of the impact of human milk on mortality is displayed in the widely publicized statistics currently available on Third World countries, where infant formulas are rapidly replacing human milk. The death rate is higher, malnutrition starts earlier and is more severe, and the incidence of infection is greater in formula-fed infants (Figs. 1-9 and 1-10). Data from the work of Scrimshaw et al.[51] show mortality of 950/1000 live births in the artificially fed infants and 120/1000 in breastfed infants. The data were collected in Punjab villages from 1955 through 1959. The deaths were predominantly due to diarrheal disease. The Pan American Health Organization has reported similar correlations among malnutrition, infection, and mortality. In Puffer and Serrano's[43] 1973 work in São Paulo, the death rates among breastfed infants were lower and the proportions due to diarrheal disease and malnutrition were also less.

Table 1-11. Mortality rates and survivorship to age 1 year in breastfed and artificially fed infants*

Study area	Date	Mortality (per 1000) Breastfed	Artificially fed	Survivors to age 1 yr (per 1000) Breastfed	Artificially fed	Difference
Berlin, Germany	1895-1896	57	376	943	624	319
Bremen, Germany	1905	68	379	932	621	311
Hanover, Germany	1912	96	296	904	704	200
Boston, Mass.	1911	30	212	970	788	182
Eight U.S. cities†	1911-1916	76	255	924	745	179
Paris, France	1900	140	310	860	690	170
Cologne, Germany	1908-1909	73	241	927	759	168
Amsterdam, Holland	1904	144	304	856	696	160
Liverpool, England	1905	84	134	916	866	144
Eight U.S. cities‡	1911-1916	76	215	924	785	139
Derby, England	1900-1903	70	198	930	802	128
Chicago, Ill.	1924-1929	2	84	998	916	82
Liverpool, England	1936-1942	10	57	990	943	47
Great Britain	1946-1947	9	18	991	982	9

From Knodel J: Science 198:1111, 1977, Copyright 1977 by the American Association for the Advancement of Science.
*Most of these rates do not include deaths in the first few days or weeks of life; mortality is therefore underestimated and survival overestimated. Only the rates for the eight U.S. cities in 1911-1916 represent mortality from birth; deaths that occurred before any feeding are proportionately allocated to the two feeding categories. The rates for Berlin, Bremen, Hanover, Cologne, and the eight U.S. cities were derived by applying life table techniques to mortality given by single months of age.
†Comparison of breastfed infants with infants artificially fed from birth.
‡Comparison of breastfed infants with all infants artificially fed in the period of observation.

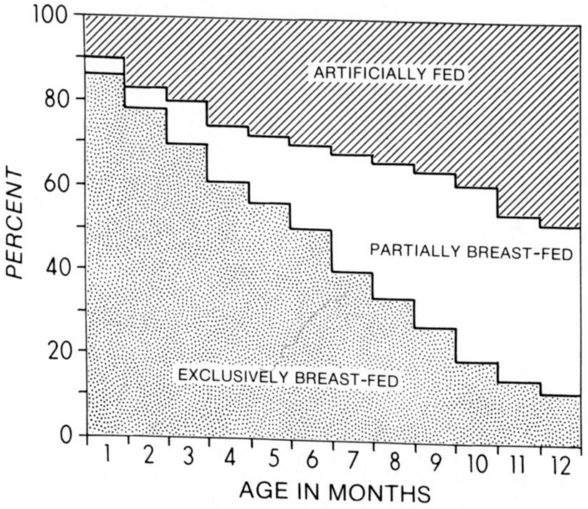

Fig. 1-8. Percentage of infants who are breastfed, partially breastfed, and artificially fed by age in months. (Modified from Woodbury RM: Am J Hyg 2:668, 1922.)

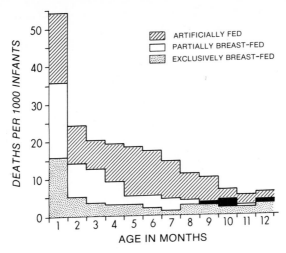

Fig. 1-9. Death rate/1000 infants by type of feeding and age in months. (Modified from Woodbury RM: Am J Hyg 2:668, 1922.)

THE MESSAGE ON BREAST-FEEDING ISN'T NEW

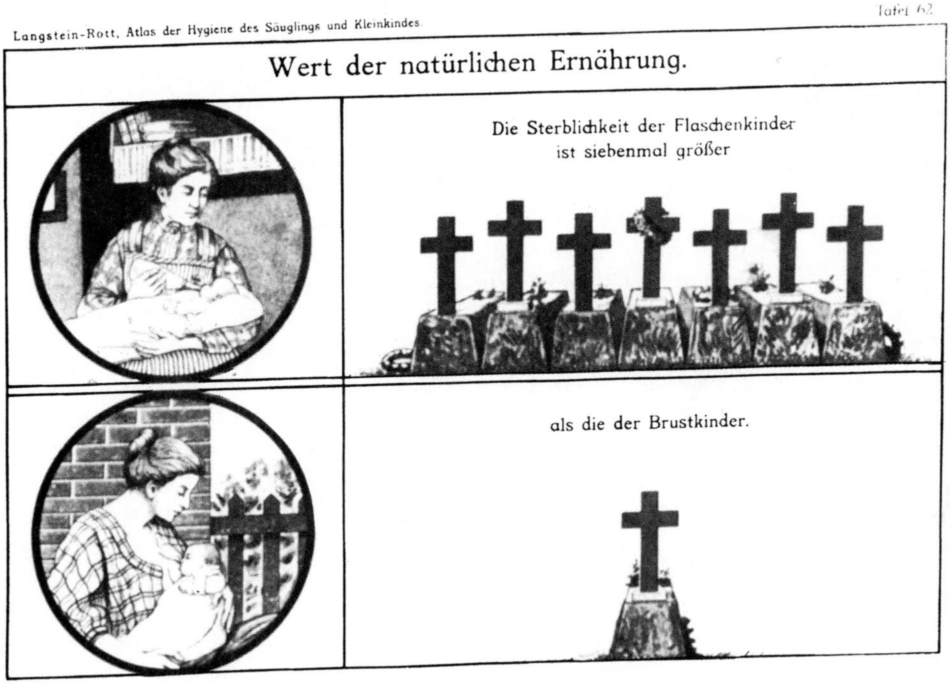

Langstein-Rott, Atlas der Hygiene des Säuglings und Kleinkindes   Tafel 62

Wert der natürlichen Ernährung.

Die Sterblichkeit der Flaschenkinder
ist siebenmal größer

als die der Brustkinder.

Fig. 1-10. Poster used in 1918 to educate parents on value of breastfeeding. Title is *Value of Natural Feeding.* Text explains that mortality of bottle fed infants (Flaschenkinder) is seven times higher than that of breastfed infants (Brustkinder). (From Langstein R: Atlas der Hygiene des Sauglings und Kleinkindes, Berlin, 1918, Julius Springer Verlag.)

The incidence of illness, or morbidity, among artificially fed infants in Third World countries is equally as dramatic as the mortality. Kanaaneh's[34] observations in Arab villages in Israel showed hospitalization rates vary with method of feeding. Only 0.5% of breastfed infants required hospitalization, whereas infants fed more than 3 months but less than 6 months at the breast had a 2.9% hospitalization rate, and infants who were bottle fed had a 24.8% rate. This is a fiftyfold difference.

There is a bias against bottle feeding as sicker, smaller infants are bottle fed. Infants who die are weaned early by death. The benefits of breastfeeding are enhanced by these confounding variables. The authors[29] point out that had there been no breastfeeding in the sample, twice as many infants would have died after the first week of life.

Evidence for protection by breastfeeding against death from infectious diseases in Brazil in infancy in 1987 is even more persuasive in a carefully controlled study by Victora et al.[54] Compared with infants who were breastfed without supplementation, those who were completely bottle fed had a 14.2 greater risk of death from diarrhea and 3.6 greater risk of death from respiratory infection. Partial breastfeeding was less protective. Formula and cow's milk were equally hazardous. The greatest risk from diarrhea was in the first 2 months of life. Barros et al.[6] point out the fact that birthweight influences breastfeeding and small infants tend to be weaned sooner.

Demonstrating the differences in morbidity between infants fed by breast and those fed by bottle has become even more complex in industrialized countries since the resurgence of breastfeeding. Among the confounding variables are the inherent differences between the mothers who choose to breastfeed and those who choose to bottle feed.[50] Although many investigators have recognized the necessity of controlling these variables, none has succeeded totally because there is an unavoidable factor of self-selection that makes random assignment of infants impossible. There is a one-way flow of infants from the breastfed group to the bottle fed group, since a baby may change from breast to bottle but rarely from bottle to breast. Documenting breastfeeding practices is difficult when there is the possibility that some bottle feedings are included or that solid foods have been introduced. Investigators[31,34,43] have reported differences between breastfed and bottle fed infants in the incidence of morbidity associated with diarrhea, respiratory infections, otitis media, and pneumonia; they have also compared breastfed and bottle fed infants seen in clinics and emergency rooms or hospitalized in the first year of life. This extensive material has been reviewed by Cunningham.[13,14,15] The majority of reports demonstrate a significant advantage for the breastfed group. The relationship between breastfeeding or bottle feeding and respiratory illness in the first year of life among nearly 2,000 cohort children was reported by Watkins et al.[55] in England. There was a significant advantage to breastfeeding. Mothers who smoked were less likely to breastfeed, but even when smoking was considered, the breastfeeding advantage remained. Young et al.[61] reported on 1,000 infants in the Yale Harvard Research Project in Tunisia who were followed from birth to 26 months and found breastfed infants had fewer infections, illnesses, and allergies. Correlation of infections in the first postnatal year among 251 babies was made by Holmes et al.[31] with infant-feeding mode, socioeconomic status of the family, maternal educational level, maternal age, and factors including maternal smoking and number of siblings. The education of the mother, not the feeding mode, was the most significant variable.

Cunningham[13,14] undertook a study in rural upstate New York to determine the impact of feeding on the health of the infant. Of 326 infants studied, 162 were fed proprietary formula and 164 were breastfed at birth, with only 4% still breastfed at 1 year. Breastfeeding was associated with significantly less illness during the first year of life. The protection

Table 1-12. Significant episodes of illness according to feeding mode at onset of illness (Cooperstown, 1979)

Illness	Breast	Artificial
Otitis media	3.7*	9.1
Lower respiratory infection	1.1	5.6
Diarrhea, vomiting	3.5	6.9
Hospital admissions	1.0	3.0
Total episodes of illness	8.2	21.1

From Cunningham AS: Breastfeeding and morbidity in industrialized countries: an update. In Jelliffe DB and Jelliffe EFP, editors: Advances in international maternal and child health, vol 1, Oxford, 1981, Oxford University Press.
*Episodes per 1000 patient weeks.

Table 1-13. Significant episodes of illness, regardless of feeding mode at onset of illness (Cooperstown, 1979)

Months of life	Breastfed	Limited breast	Artificially fed
1-2	0.7*	3.8	11.8
3-4	5.9	11.3	16.0
5-6	7.4	20.0	20.5
7-8	18.5	16.3	21.5
9-10	14.1	22.5	21.2
11-12	11.9	20.0	19.8
First year	58.5	93.8	110.8

From Cunningham AS: Breastfeeding and morbidity in industrialized countries: an update. In Jelliffe DB and Jelliffe EFP, editors: Advances in international maternal and child health, vol 1, Oxford, 1981, Oxford University Press.
*Episodes per 100 patients.

was greatest during the early months, increased with the duration of breastfeeding, and appeared more striking for serious illness (Tables 1-12 and 1-13). Breastfeeding was associated with a higher level of parental education, but controlling for that factor, the difference in morbidity is even more significant.

In the United States, diarrheal disease is uncommon in breastfed infants, and the treatment is usually to continue to breastfeed. Similarly, breastfed infants have fewer episodes of respiratory illness and otitis media. When afflicted with such febrile illnesses, the breastfed infant does not become dehydrated and rapidly toxic.

The question is not answered clearly in Western countries because of the associated variables among bottle feeders, i.e., young, low SES, low-educated mother, and the fact that small, sick infants are more likely bottle fed.

Despite the clear-cut data on mortality and morbidity from past generations and from cultures seemingly remote from industrialized and medically sophisticated societies, present-day pediatricians had discounted any but the psychologic advantages of breastfeeding. The current increase in illness in young infants in day care centers is providing a new study group. To date breastfeeding appears to be protective for the few children whose mothers continue to nurse them while in daycare.

REFERENCES

1. Andrew EM, Clancy KL, and Katz MG: Infant feeding practices of families belonging to a prepaid group practice health care plan, Pediatrics 65:978, 1980.
2. Apple RD: Mothers & medicine: a social history of infant feeding 1890–1950, Madison, 1987, The University of Wisconsin Press.
3. Auerbach K: To breastfeed or not to breastfeed, Keeping Abreast J 1:314, 1976.
4. Baer EC: Promoting breastfeeding: a national responsibility, Stud Fam Plan 12:198, 1981.
5. Baghurst KI: Infant feeding—public health perspectives, Med J Aust 148:112, 1988.
6. Barros FC, Victora CG, Vaughn JP et al: Birthweight and duration of breastfeeding: are the beneficial effects of human milk being overestimated? Pediatrics 78:656, 1986.
7. Bauchner H, Leventhal JM, and Shapiro ED: Studies of breastfeeding and infections: how good is the evidence? J Am Med Assoc 256:887, 1986.
8. Bergevin Y, Dougherty C, and Kramer MS: Do formula samples shorten the duration of breastfeeding? Lancet 1:1148, 1983.
9. Bryant CA: The impact of kin, friend, and neighbor networks on infant feeding practices, Soc Sci Med 16:1757, 1982.
10. Carroll EGC: Home from the hospital, Parents 13:22, 52, 1938.
11. Cole JP: Breastfeeding in Boston suburbs in relation to personal-social factors, Clin Pediatr 16:352, 1977.
12. Commonwealth Department of Health: towards better nutrition for Australians, Report of the Nutrition Taskforce of the Better Health Commission, Canberra, AGPS, 1987 (catalogue no. 86-1660).
13. Cunningham AS: Breastfeeding and health, J Pediatr 73:416, 1984.
14. Cunningham AS: Breastfeeding and illness, Pediatrics 73:416, 1984.
15. Cunningham AS: Breastfeeding and morbidity in industrialized countries: an update. In Jelliffe DB and Jelliffe EFP, editors: Advances in international maternal and child health, vol 1, Oxford, 1981, Oxford University Press.
16. Deem H and McGeorge M: Breastfeeding, NZ Med J 57:539, 1958.
17. Drake TGH: Infant welfare laws in France in the 18th century, Ann Med Hist 7:49, 1935.
18. Fallot ME, Boyd JL, and Oski FA: Breastfeeding reduces incidence of hospital admissions for infections in infants, Pediatrics 65:1121, 1980.
19. Feinstein JM, Berkelhamer JE, Gruszka ME et al: Factors related to early termination of breastfeeding in an urban population, Pediatrics 78:210, 1986.
20. Ferris AM, McCabe LT, Allen LH et al: Biological and sociocultural determinants of successful lactation among women in eastern Connecticut, J Am Dietetic Assoc 87:316, 1987.
21. Fildes V: Breast, bottles, and babies, Edinburgh, 1986, Edinburgh University Press.
22. Ford CS: A comparative study of human reproduction, anthropology pub no 32, New Haven, Conn, 1945, Yale University Press.
23. Forman MR, Fetterly K, Graubard BI et al: Exclusive breastfeeding of newborns among married women in the United States: the national natality surveys of 1969 and 1980, Am J Clin Nutr 42:864, 1985.
24. Forman MR, Graubard BI, Hoffman HJ et al: The PIMA infant feeding study: breastfeeding and gastroenteritis in the first year of life, Am J Epidemiol 119:335, 1984.
25. Frank DA, Wirtz SJ, Sorenson JR et al: Commercial discharge packs and breastfeeding counseling: effects on infant-feeding practices in a randomized trial, Pediatrics 80:845, 1987.
26. Gabriele A, Gabriele KR, and Lawrence RA: Cultural values and biomedical knowledge: choices in infant feeding, Soc Sci Med 23:501, 1986.
27. Grulee CG, Sanford HN, and Herron PH: Breast and artificial feeding, JAMA 103:735, 1934.
28. Grulee CG, Sanford HN, and Schwartz H: Breast and artificially fed infants, JAMA 104:1986, 1935.
29. Habicht JP, DaVanzo J, and Butz WP: Does breastfeeding really save lives or are apparent benefits due to biases? Am J Epidemiol 123:279, 1986.
30. Hayden GF, Nowacek GA, Koch W et al: Providing free samples of baby items to newly delivered parents, Clin Pediatr 26:111, 1987.
31. Holmes GE, Hassanein KM, and Miller HC: Factors associated with infections among breast-fed babies and babies fed proprietary milks, Pediatrics 72:300, 1983.
32. House JS, Landis KR, and Umberson D: Social relationships and health, Science 241:540, 1988.
33. Houston MJ: Factors affecting the duration of breastfeeding: early feeding practices and social class, Early Human Dev 8:55, 1983.
34. Kanaaneh H: The relationship of bottle feeding to malnutrition and gastroenteritis in a preindustrial setting, J Trop Pediatr 18:302, 1972.
35. Konner M: The nursing knot, The Sciences 25:10, 1985.
36. Knodel J: Breast feeding and population growth, Science 198:1111, 1977.
37. Loughlin HH, Clappchanning N, Gehlbach S et al: Early termination of breastfeeding: identifying those at risk, Pediatrics 75:508, 1985.

38. Magnus PD and Galindo S: The paucity of breast-feeding in an urban clinic population, Am J Pub Health 70:75, 1980.

39. Martinez GA and Dodd DA: 1981 milk feeding patterns in the United States during the first 12 months of life, Pediatrics 71:166, 1983.

40. Martinez GA and Stahl DA: The recent trend in milk feeding among WIC infants, Am J Pub Health 72:68, 1982.

41. Newton N: Psychologic differences between breast and bottle feeding. In Jelliffe DB and Jelliffe EFP, editors: Symposium, the uniqueness of human milk, Am J Clin Nutr 24:993, 1971.

42. Popkin BM, Bilsborrow RE, and Akin JS: Breast-feeding patterns in low-income countries, Science 218:1088, 1982.

43. Puffer RR and Serrano CV: Patterns of mortality in childhood, scientific pub. no. 262, Washington, DC, 1973, Pan American Health Organization.

44. Raphael D: The tender gift: breast feeding, New York, 1976, Schocken Books, Inc.

45. Reamer SB and Sugarman M: Breastfeeding beyond six months: mothers' perceptions of the positive and negative consequences, J Trop Ped 33:93, 1987.

46. Report of the Surgeon General's workshop on breastfeeding and human lactation, pub no HRS-D-MC 84-2, Dept of Health and Human Services, 1984.

47. Ruvalcaba RHA: Stress-induced cessation of lactation, Western J Med 146:228, 1987.

48. Ryan AS and Martinez GA: Breastfeeding and the working mother: a profile, Pediatrics 83:524, 1989.

49. Sarett HP, Bain KR, and O'Leary JC: Decisions on breast-feeding or formula feeding and trends in infant-feeding practices, Am J Dis Child 137:719, 1983.

50. Sauls HS: Potential effects of demographic and other variables in studies comparing morbidity of breast-fed and bottle-fed infants, Pediatrics 64:523, 1979.

51. Scrimshaw NS, Taylor CE, and Gordon JE: Interaction of nutrition and infection, WHO monograph no. 29, Geneva, 1968, World Health Organization.

52. Sloper K, McKean L, and Baum JD: Patterns of infant feeding in Oxford, Arch Dis Child 49:749, 1974.

53. Taylor J: The duty of nursing children. In Ratner H: The nursing mother: historical insights from art and theology, Child Fam 8(4):19, 1949.

54. Victora CG, Smith PG, Vaughan JP et al: Evidence for protection by breastfeeding against infant deaths from infectious diseases in Brazil, Lancet 2:319, 1987.

55. Watkins CJ, Leeder SR, and Corkhill RT: The relationship between breast and bottle feeding and respiratory illness in the first year of life, J Epidemiol Community Health 33:180, 1979.

56. West CP: Factors influencing the duration of breast-feeding, J Biosoc Sci 12:325, 1980.

57. Woodbury RM: The relation between breast and artificial feeding and infant mortality, Am J Hyg 2:668, 1922.

58. Woo-lun M, Gussler J, and Smith N, editors: The international breast-feeding compendium, ed 3, Columbus Ohio, 1984, Ross Laboratories.

59. World Health Organization: Contemporary patterns of breast-feeding, Report on the WHO collaborative study on breast-feeding, Geneva, 1981, World Health Organization.

60. Wright AL, Holberg C, Taussig LM et al: Infant-feeding practices among middle-class Anglos and Hispanics, Pediatrics 82:496-503, 1988.

61. Young HB et al: Milk and lactation: some social and developmental correlates among 1,000 infants, Pediatrics 69:169, 1982.

Anatomy of the human breast

2

GROSS ANATOMY

The mammary gland, as the breast is medically termed, got its name from *mamma*, the Latin word for breast. Mammary glands begin to develop in the 6-week-old embryo, continuing their proliferation until milk ducts are developed by the time of birth (Table 2-1). Embryologically, the mammary glands develop as ingrowths of the ectoderm into the underlying mesodermal tissue.[11] In the human embryo, a thickened raised area of the ectoderm can be recognized in the region of the future gland at the end of the fourth week of pregnancy. The thickened ectoderm becomes depressed into the underlying mesoderm, and thus the surface of the mammary area soon becomes flat and finally sinks below the level of the surrounding epidermis. The mesoderm in contact with the ingrowth of the ectoderm is compressed, and its elements become arranged in concentric layers, which at a later stage give rise to the stroma of the gland. The ingrowing mass of ectoderm cells soon becomes flask shaped and then grows out into the surrounding mesoderm as a number of solid processes that represent the future ducts of the gland. These processes, by dividing and branching, give rise to the future lobes and lobules and, much later, to the alveoli. The mammary area becomes gradually raised again in its central part to form the nipple. A lumen is formed in each part of the branching system of cellular processes after 32 weeks of gestation, and near term about 15 to 25 mammary ducts form the fetal mammary gland (Fig. 2-1).

The mammary glands of male and female fetuses of 13 to 40 weeks' gestation were studied ultrastructurally by Tobona and Salazar.[16] This work confirms the presence of morphologic developments in the fetal breast tissue in response to hormonal stimuli that is similar to that in the maternal breast. The Golgi system and abundant reticulum with dilated cisternae filled with finely granular material are present in the cellular structure. Abundant mitochondria and lipid droplets are observed. Proliferation and conditioning of the epithelial cells is evident, and in the last trimester there are microvilli along the ductal lumen accompanied by large cytoplasmic protrusions. Study of the ultrastructure of the fetal breast may help understand the functional lactating breast. The secretion of a fluid resembling milk may take place at birth as a result of maternal hormones that have passed across the placenta into the fetal circulation. The lactiferous sinuses appear before birth as

Table 2-1. Embryonic development of the mammary apparatus in humans

Stage	Age of embryo (days)	Crown-rump length (mm) of embryo (mean)
Mammary band	35	6
Mammary streak	36	8
Mammary line	37	10
Mammary crest	40	13
Mammary hillock	42	15
Mammary bud	49	20

Modified from Larson BL, editor: Lactation, Ames, 1985, Iowa State University Press.

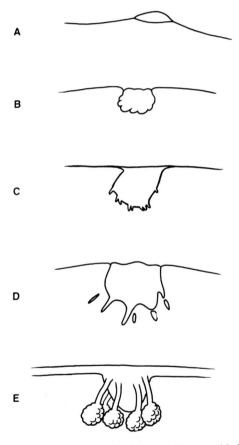

Fig. 2-1. Evolution of nipple. **A,** Thickening of epidermis with formation of primary bud. **B,** Growth of bud into mesenchyme. **C,** Formation of solid secondary buds. **D,** Formation of mammary pit and vacuolation of buds to form epithelial-lined ducts. **E,** Lactiferous ducts proliferate. Areola is formed. Nipple is inverted initially. (Modified from Weatherly-White RCA: Plastic surgery of the female breast, Hagerstown Md, 1980, Harper & Row, Publishers, Inc.)

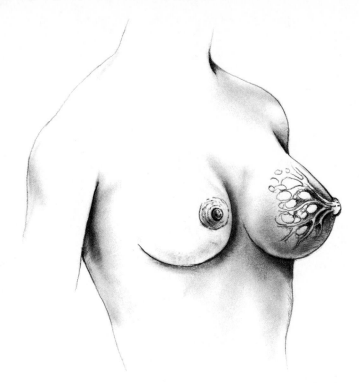

Fig. 2-2.   Mammary gland in longitudinal cross section showing mature nonlactating duct system.

swellings of the developing ducts. In prepuberty these are epithelial-lined ducts that will bud out to form alveoli when stimulated by hormones of menarche (Fig. 2-1).

The breast is made up of glandular tissue, supporting connective tissue, and protective fatty tissue. Right after birth the newborn's breast may even be swollen and secreting a small amount of milk, known as witch's milk. This very common phenomenon among both male and female infants is caused by the stimulation of the infant's mammary glands by the same hormones produced by the placenta to prepare the mother's breast for lactation. This subsides quickly, and from then on the mammary glands are inactive until shortly before the onset of puberty, when hormones begin to stimulate growth again.

The breast is located in the superficial fascia between the second rib and sixth intercostal cartilage and is superficial to the pectoralis major muscle. It tends to overlap this muscle inferiorly to become superficial to the external oblique and serratus anterior muscles. It measures 10 to 12 cm in diameter. It is located horizontally from the parasternal to midaxillary line. The central thickness of the breast is 5 to 7 cm (Fig. 2-2).

At puberty the breasts in the female enlarge to their adult size, one, the left, frequently being slightly larger than the other. In a nonpregnant woman, the mature breast weighs approximately 200 g. During pregnancy there is some increased size and weight; thus near term the breast weighs between 400 and 600 g. During lactation the breast weighs between 600 and 800 g (Fig. 2-3).

The shape of the breast varies from woman to woman, just as do body build and facial characteristics. Racial variations may be associated with discoidal, hemispherical,

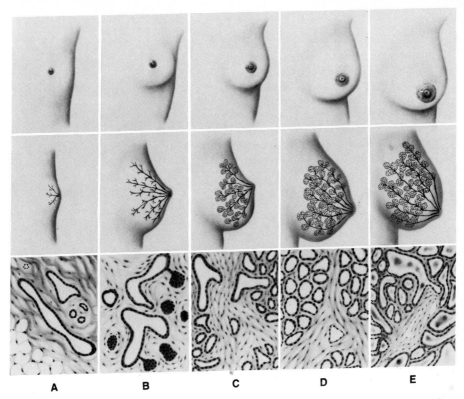

Fig. 2-3. Female breast from infancy to lactation with corresponding cross section and duct structure. **A,B,** and **C,** Gradual development of well-differentiated ductular and peripheral lobular-alevolar system. **D,** Ductular sprouting and intensified peripheral lobular-alevolar development in pregnancy. Glandular luminal cells begin actively synthesizing milk fat and proteins near term; only small amounts are released into lumen. **E,** With postpartum withdrawal of luteal and placental sex steroids and placental lactogen, prolactin is able to induce full secretory activity of alveolar cells and release of milk into alveoli and smaller ducts.

pear-shaped or conical forms. Commonly the breast is dome shaped or conic in adolescence, becoming more hemispheric and finally pendulous in the parous female. There is some projection of mammary glandular tissue into the axillary region. This is known as the tail of Spence. Mammary tissue in the axilla, which is connected to the central duct system, will be more obvious and produce milk during lactation. It has been noted to cause various symptoms during lactation.[1] (See Chapter 8 on Management.)

The three major structures of the breast are skin, subcutaneous tissue, and corpus mammae. The corpus mammae is the breast mass that remains after freeing the breast from the deep attachments and removing the skin, subcutaneous connective tissue, and adipose tissue.

The breasts of the adult female are always paired and develop from a line of glandular tissue, which is found in the fetus, known as the milk lines. This milk streak, or galactic band, develops from axilla to the groin during the fifth week of embryonic fetal life.[14] In the region of the thorax, the band develops into a ridge and the rest regresses. In some

---

Breast abnormalities

Unilateral hypoplasia, contralateral normal
Bilateral hypoplasia with asymmetry
Unilateral hyperplasia, contralateral normal
Bilateral hyperplasia with asymetry
Unilateral hypoplasia, contralateral hyperplasia
Unilateral hypoplasia of breast, thorax, and pectoral muscles (Polands' syndrome)
Acquired abnormalities due to trauma, burns, radiation for hemangioma or intrathoracic
    disease, and chest tube insertion in infancy and preadolescent biopsy

---

Modified from Osbourne MP: Breast development and anatomy. In Harris JR, Hellman S, Henderson IC et al, editors: Breast diseases, Philadelphia, 1986, WB Saunders Co.

women, some additional residual of the galactic band remains as mammary tissue, which can develop anywhere along this line. Hypermastia is the presence of accessory mammary glands, which are phylogenic remnants of the embryonic mammary ridge. Because of this origin, accessory nipples and glandular tissue may be found along these lines, which extend from the clavicular to the inguinal regions. Occasionally, supernumerary glands are found in the urogenital region, on the buttocks, or on the back as well. The glands are derived from the ectoderm, whereas the connective tissue stroma is mesodermal in origin (Fig. 2-4). Other breast abnormalities are noted in the boxed material.

The accessory tissue may involve the corpus mammae, the areola, and the nipple.[18] From 2% to 6% of women have hypermastia. The response of hypermastia to pregnancy and lactation depends on the tissue present. Hyperthelia is the presence of nipple tissue without breast tissue.

A relationship between supernumerary nipple and renal defect has been suggested by some. After careful study of 65 patients with supernumerary nipple, Hersh et al[8] found seven (11%) individuals who had significant renal lesions, somewhat less than the incidence reported originally. In blacks there is apparently no association. Hyperadenia is the presence of mammary tissue without nipples. The swelling and secretion of this tissue may produce pain during lactation. Occasionally, aberrant breast tissue can cause discomfort or embarassment in adolescence and during menses, especially when located in the axilla.[10] Mammographic features of normal accessory axillary breast tissue were reviewed by Adler et al[1] in 13 women who were diagnosed on routine mammography. Seven of these women had a mass or fullness on physical examination; one was seen postpartum because of pain; nine were asymptomatic. They ranged in age from 31 to 67 years. Radiographically, the accessory tissue resembled the rest of the normal glandular tissue but was separate from it. It occurred on the right in 11 of the 13. It was recognized as a normal developmental variant, distinguishable from the frequent axillary tail of Spence, which represents a direct extension from the outer margin of the main mass of glandular tissue. On mammography, the accessory tissue is best visualized on oblique and exaggerated craniocaudal views. In rare cases, it may be appropriate to surgically remove the tissue, a treatment well known to experienced plastic surgeons. If treatment is not initiated before pregnancy and lactation, in these cases, the symptomatology of pain and swelling will be intensified and may progress to mastitis or the necessity to terminate lactation. Apart from physiologic variation, other conditions of abnormal anatomy exist such as hypomastia, (underdeveloped breasts), hypertrophy, and inequality. Amastia is rare (see boxed material). They will be discussed more fully under Management.

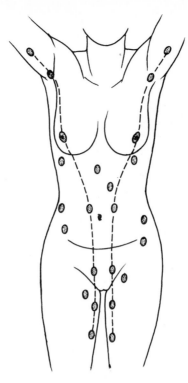

Fig. 2-4. Sites of supernumerary nipples along "milk line." Ectopic nipples, areolae, or breast tissue can develop from the groin to the axilla and upper inner arm. They can lactate or undergo malignant change. (Modified from Weatherly-White RCA: Plastic surgery of the female breast, Hagerstown, Md, 1980, Harper & Row, Publishers, Inc.)

Corpus mammae

The mammary gland is a conglomeration of a variable number of independent glands. Surgical dissection of many postoperative specimens has contributed more precise information about the anatomic structure.[4] The ramifications of the lactiferous ducts and stroma were carefully studied by Hicken, who reported that in 95% of women the ducts ascend into the axilla, occasionally following the brachial plexus and axillary vessels into the apex of the axilla. Ducts are found in the epigastric region in 15% of women. In rare cases, ducts cross the midline (Fig. 2-5).

The morphology of the corpus mammae includes two major divisions, the parenchyma and the stroma.[1] The parenchyma includes the ductular-lobular-alveolar structures. It is composed of the alveolar gland with treelike ductular branching alveoli. The alveoli are approximately 0.12 mm in diameter. The ducts are approximately 2.0 mm in diameter. The lactiferous sinuses are 5 to 8 mm in diameter. The lobi, which are arranged like spokes converging on the central nipple, are 15 to 25 in number. Each lobus is divided again into 20 to 40 lobuli, and each lobulus is again subdivided into 10 to 100 alveoli for tubulosaccular secretory units. The stroma includes the connective tissue, fat tissue, blood vessels, nerves, and lymphatics.

The mass of tissue in the breast consists of the tubuloalveolar glands embedded in fat (the adipose tissue), giving the gland its smooth, rounded contour. The mammary fat

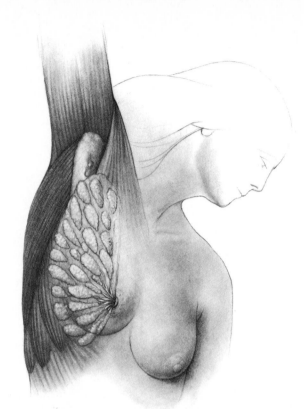

Fig. 2-5.   Ramification of lactiferous ducts and mammary tissue. Ducts extend onto upper medial aspect of arm, to midline, and into epigastrium. Composite drawing from mammographic studies. (Modified from Hicken NF: Arch Surg **40:**6, 1940.)

pad is essential for the proliferation and differentiation of the mammary epithelium, providing the necessary space, support, and local control for duct elongation and, ultimately, lobuloalveolar proliferation. Each gland forms a lobe of the breast, and the lobes are separated by connective tissue septa. These septa attach to the skin. Each tubuloalveolar gland opens into a lactiferous duct, which leads into a more dilated area, the lactiferous sinus; there is a slight constriction before the sinus opens onto the surface of the nipple (Fig. 2-6). Extension of ducts within the fat pad is orderly. There is an inhibitory zone around each duct into which other ducts cannot penetrate, and development does not normally proceed beyond the duct end-bud stage before puberty.

Nipple and areola

The skin of the breast includes the nipple, the areola, and the general skin. The skin is the thin, flexible, elastic cover of the breast adherent to the fat-laden subcutaneous tissue. It contains hair, sebaceous glands, and apocrine sweat glands. The nipple, or papilla mammae, is a conic elevation located in the center of the areola at about the fourth intercostal space, slightly below the midpoint of the breast. Although very different in size, the nipples and areolae of women and men are qualitatively identical.[13] The nipple contains 15 to 25

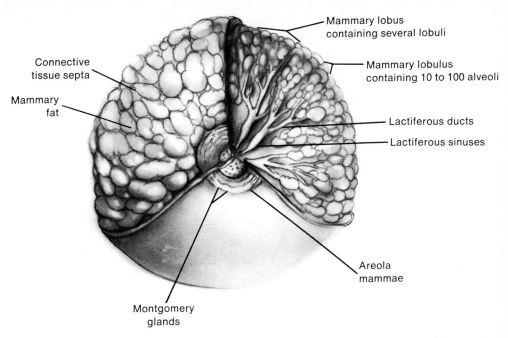

Connective
tissue septa

Mammary
fat

Mammary lobus
containing several lobuli

Mammary lobulus
containing 10 to 100 alveoli

Lactiferous ducts

Lactiferous sinuses

Areola
mammae

Montgomery
glands

Fig. 2-6. Morphology of mature breast with dissection to reveal mammary fat and duct system.

milk ducts. Each of the tubuloalveolar glands that make up the breast opens onto the nipple by a separate opening. The nipple also contains smooth muscle fibers and is richly innervated with sensory nerve endings and Meissner's corpuscles in the dermal papillae and is well supplied with sebaceous and apocrine sweat glands, but no hair. The nipple is surrounded by the areola, or areola mammae, a circular pigmented area. It is usually pink before pregnancy, turning reddish brown during pregnancy, and always maintaining some pigmentation thereafter. The areola measures 15 to 16 mm in diameter, enlarging during pregnancy and lactation. The pigmentation is due to many melanocytes distributed throughout the skin and glands. The understructure of the epidermis of the areola is not as elaborate as that of the nipple but intermediate to that of the surrounding skin.

Little or no true lobuloalveolar development occurs before the first pregnancy. A framework is laid down within which the specialized secretory cells will proliferate. The framework forms a vital part of the gland's overall developmental course, and maldevelopment or trauma during fetal or juvenile life can seriously reduce the size and secretory potential of the mature gland.

Montgomery's tubercles containing the ductular openings of sebaceous and lactiferous glands are present in the areola. Sweat glands and smaller free sebaceous glands are also present in the areola. The corium of the areola lacks fat, but it contains smooth muscle and collagenous and elastic connective tissue fibers in radial and circular arrangements (see Fig. 2-8). The Montgomery glands become enlarged and look like small pimples during pregnancy and lactation. They secrete a substance that lubricates and protects the nipples and areolae during pregnancy and lactation. A small amount of milk is also secreted from these tubercles. After lactation, these glands recede again to their former unobtrusive state. Light microscopy has shown that Morgagni in 1719 was correct when he first described

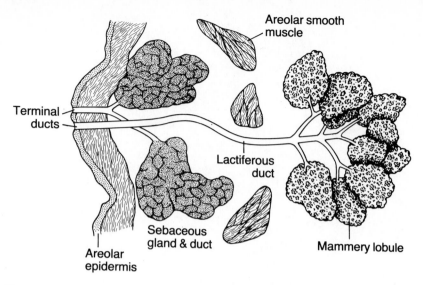

Fig. 2-7. Tubercle of Montgomery and underlying structures. Lactiferous duct may join sebaceous gland ducts and terminate at common opening in areolar epidermis as shown. (Adapted from Smith DM, Peters TG, and Donegan WL: Arch Pathol Lab Med 106:62, 1982.)

the 12 to 20 areolar glands and noted them to be sebaceous and to include lactiferous structure as well. Building on the original work, Montgomery in 1837 prepared a more detailed treatise on the tubercle itself and named it after himself. Serial sections of 35 tubercles also showed that there were lactiferous ducts from the deeper breast parenchyma ascending into the sebaceous glands of the tubercle (Fig. 2-7).[15] The sebaceous gland itself was no different from those of the skin or of those associated with the terminal lactiferous ducts of the nipple. The mammary duct was lined with two layers of cuboidal to columnar cells. They came from the underlying mammary lobules through the subcutaneous tissues and into the region of the sebaceous gland. The terminal portion of the mammary duct in some cases joined the duct to the sebaceous gland and in other cases opened separately but close to it. The ducts appear to be a miniature of the major mammary system. Sebaceous and mammary ductal components underlie the areolar tubercle.

The areola and nipple are darker than the rest of the breast, ranging from light pink in very fair-skinned women to very dark brown in others. The darker color of the areola may be some sort of visual signal to the newborn infant so that he will close his mouth on the areola, not on the nipple alone, to obtain milk. Nipple erection is induced by tactile, sensory, or autonomic sympathetic stimuli. The dermis of the nipple and the areola contains a large number of multibranched free nerve fiber endings. Local venostasis and hyperemia occur to enhance the process of erection of the nipple because the nipple and areola are rich in arterial venous anastomoses. The glabrous skin of the nipple is wrinkled, containing large papillae of the corium.

Each nipple contains 15 to 25 lactiferous ducts surrounded by fibromuscular tissue (Figs. 2-8 to 2-13). These ducts end as small orifices near the tip of the nipple. Within the nipple, the lactiferous ducts may merge. The ductular orifices therefore are sometimes

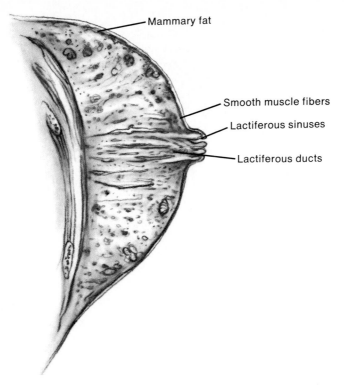

Mammary fat

Smooth muscle fibers

Lactiferous sinuses

Lactiferous ducts

Fig. 2-8. Morphology of mature breast in cross section to reveal lactiferous duct system.

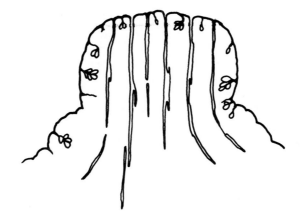

Fig. 2-9. Cross section of nipple. Epidermis has long dermal papillae and is glabrous and heavily pigmented. Sebaceous glands are found near tip and along sides of nipple. Connective tissue stoma and circular muscle bundles are seen in cross section.

fewer in number than the respective breast lobi. The milk ducts within the nipple dilate at the nipple base into the cone-shaped ampullae of milk sinuses. The ampullae function as temporary milk containers during lactation but contain only epithelial debris in the non-lactating state. The lining of the infundibular and ampullar parts of the lactiferous ducts consists of an eight- to ten-cell layered squamous epithelium. The bulk of the nipple is

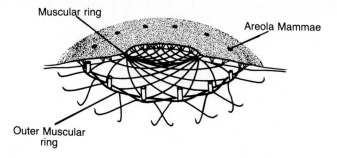

Fig. 2-10.   Nipple and areola with smooth musculature structure.

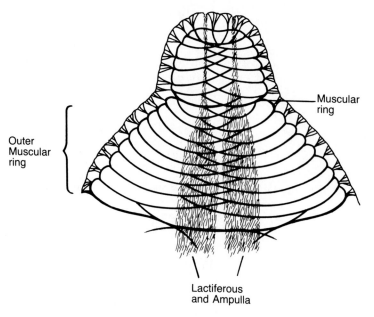

Fig. 2-11.   Smooth musculature of areola and nipple in cross section when contracted to make nipple erect.

composed of smooth musculature, which represents a closing mechanism for the milk ducts and sinuses of the nipple (see Fig. 2-11). The milk ducts in the nipple are embedded in stretchable and mobile connective tissue. The inner longitudinal muscular arrangements and the outer, more circular and radial arrangements do not obstruct the milk ducts. Tangential fibers also branch off from the more circular muscular fibers of the nipple bases to the outer circular muscular range. The functions of the muscular fibroelastic system of the areola and nipple include decreasing the surface area of the areola, producing nipple erection and emptying the lactiferous sinuses and ducts during nursing. When the nipple erects owing to tactile, thermal, or sexual stimulation, the system causes the nipple to become smaller, firmer, and more prominent.

The mammary tissues are enveloped by the superficial pectoral fascia, and the breast

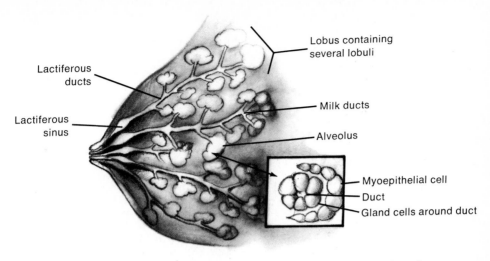

Lobus containing several lobuli

Lactiferous ducts

Milk ducts

Lactiferous sinus

Alveolus

Myoepithelial cell

Duct

Gland cells around duct

Fig. 2-12. Simplified schematic drawing of duct system with cross section of myo-epithelial cells around duct opening. Myoepithelial cells contract to eject milk.

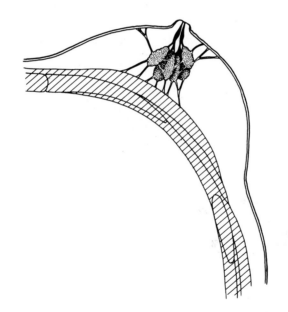

Fig. 2-13. Cross section of ligaments of breast. Ligaments of Cooper suspend 15 to 20 lobes of breast within matrix of fat. They are attached to lobes, skin, and deep fascia.

is fixed by fibrous bands to the overlying skin and the underlying pectoral fascia, which are known as ligaments of Cooper (Fig. 2-13). The glandular part of the breast is surrounded by a fat layer that seldom extends beyond the lower border of the pectoralis major. The breast is supported by the muscles attached to the ribs, the collar bone, and the bones of the upper arm near the shoulder.

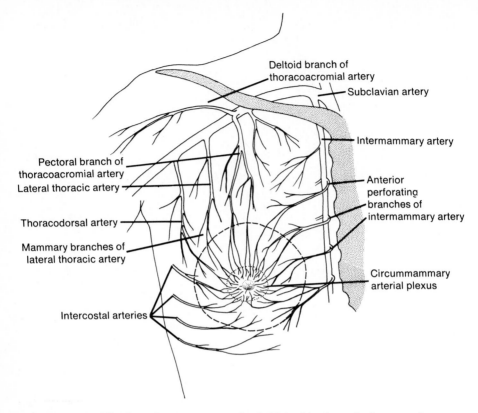

Fig. 2-14.   Blood supply to mammary gland. Major blood supply from anterior per-forating branches of internal mammary artery.

Blood supply

The blood supply to the breast is from branches of the intercostal arteries and the perforating branches of the internal thoracic artery; the third, fourth, and fifth are usually most prominent. The major blood supply to the breast is provided by the internal mammary artery and the lateral thoracic artery. There is a small supply obtained from the intercostal arteries and the arterial branches of the axillary and subclavian arteries, but this contribution is minimal, since 60% of the total breast tissue receives blood from the internal mammary artery. All the mammary branches of this artery lead transversely to the nipple and anas-tomoses, with branches coming from the lateral thoracic artery.[4] Anastomoses with inter-costal arteries are less common, but the blood supply to the nipple is extensive and close to the surface, contributing to the pink color. Many areas of the breast are supplied by two or three different arterial sources. The veins end in the internal thoracic and the axillary veins. Some veins may reach the external jugular vein (Fig. 2-14). The veins create an anastomotic circle around the base of the papilla, called the circulus venosis.[2]

Lymphatic drainage

The lymphatic drainage of the breast has been the subject of considerable study because of the frequency of breast cancer, but it has significance for the lactating breast

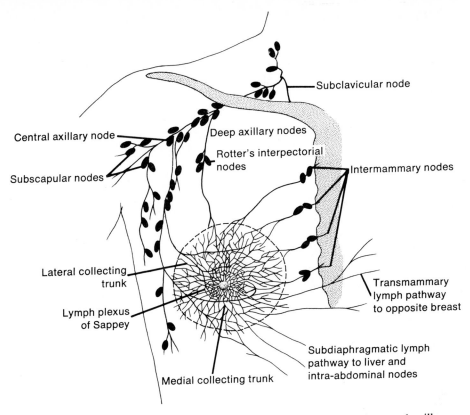

Subclavicular node

Central axillary node

Deep axillary nodes

Rotter's interpectorial nodes

Subscapular nodes

Intermammary nodes

Lateral collecting trunk

Lymph plexus of Sappey

Transmammary lymph pathway to opposite breast

Medial collecting trunk

Subdiaphragmatic lymph pathway to liver and intra-abdominal nodes

Fig. 2-15. Lymphatic drainage of mammary gland. Major drainage is toward axilla.

as well. The lymphatic drainage can be quite extensive. The main drainage is to axillary nodes and to the parasternal nodes along the internal thoracic artery inside the thoracic cavity. The lymphatics of the breast originate in the lymph capillaries of the mammary connective tissue, which surrounds the mammary structures, and drain through the deep substance of the breast. The lymph drainage of the breast consists of the superficial, or cutaneous section, the areola, and the glandular, or deep-tissue section. Other points of drainage are to pectoral nodes between the pectoralis major and minor muscles and to the subclavicular nodes in the neck deep to the clavicle. There is some transmammary lymph drainage to the opposite breast as well as subdiaphragmatic lymphatics that lead ultimately to the liver and intra-abdominal nodes (Fig. 2-15).

Innervation of the mammary gland

The nerves of the breast are from branches of the fourth, fifth, and sixth intercostal nerves and consist of sensory fibers and sympathetic fibers innervating the smooth muscles in the nipple and blood vessels. The sensory innervation of the nipple and areola is extensive and consists of both autonomic and sensory nerves. A detailed anatomic and clinical study of the nipple-areola complex showed that it is from the lateral cutaneous branch of the fourth intercostal nerve, which penetrates the posterior aspect of the breast at the intersection of the fourth intercostal space and the pectoralis major muscle (4 o'clock on the left breast and 8 o'clock on the right breast).[6] The nerve divides into five fasciculi, one central to the nipple, two upper, and two lower branches (always at 5 and 7 o'clock left and right side, respectively) (see Fig. 2-16). The innervation of the corpus mammae is minimal by comparison and predominantly autonomic. There are no parasympathetic or cholinergic fibers supplying any part of the breast. There are no ganglia found in mammary tissue. Norepinephrine-containing nerve fibers are abundant among the smooth muscle cells of the nipple and at the interface between the media and adventitia of the breast arteries. Physiological observations demonstrate that the efferent nerves to these structures are sympathetic adrenergic.

The majority of the mammary nerves follow the arteries and arterioles and supply these structures. A few fibers from the perivascular networks course along the walls of the ducts. They may correspond to sensory fibers for sensing milk pressure. No innervation of mammary myoepithelial cells has been identified. It can therefore be concluded that secretory activities of the acinar epithelium depend on hormonal stimulation, such as that of prolactin, and other hormones and are not stimulated via the nervous system directly.

Stimulation of the sensory nerve fibers or sensory receptors does induce the release of adenohypophyseal prolactin and neurohypohyseal oxytocin via an afferent sensory reflex

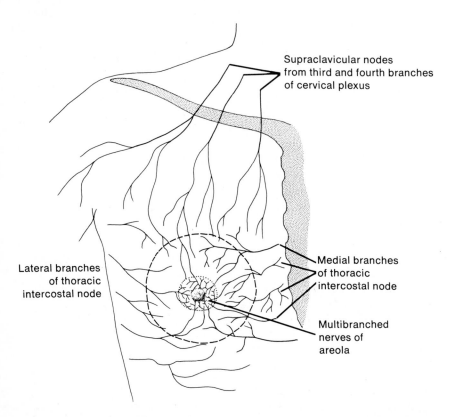

Supraclavicular nodes from third and fourth branches of cervical plexus

Lateral branches of thoracic intercostal node

Medial branches of thoracic intercostal node

Multibranched nerves of areola

Fig. 2-16.   Innervation of mammary gland supraclavicular nerves and lateral and medial branches of intercostal nerves provide sensory innervation. Sympathetic and motor nerves are provided by supracervical and intercostal nerves.

pathway whereby stimuli reach the hypothalamus. Sympathetic mammary stimulation causes the contraction of the small muscles of the areola and the nipple. The locally released norepinephrine induces stimulation of the myoepithelial adrenergic receptors, causing muscular relaxation. In the absence of parasympathetic activity, a minor physiological catamine inhibitory effect on the mammary myoepithelium may exist, which is overcome by oxytocin release during suckling, inducing myoepithelial contraction.

The supraclavicular nerves supply the sensory fibers for innervation of the upper cutaneous parts of the breast. Branches of the intercostal nerves provide the major sensory innervation of the mammary gland. The sympathetic sensory and motor fibers are derived from the supraclavicular and intercostal nerves, respectively. Sympathetic fibers only run along the mammary gland–supplying arteries to innervate the glandular body. There is relatively restricted innervation to the epidermal parts of the nipple and areola, leading to lack of superficial sensory acuity. Breast sensation was measured in a large number of women by Courtiss and Goldwyn using a device that emitted a variable current producing a burning sensation when the threshold was exceeded.[3] The areola was shown to be the most sensitive and the nipple the least sensitive, with the skin of the breast intermediate. Thus the skin in these areas responds only to major stimuli, such as sucking. The relatively large number of dermal nerve endings provides a high mammary responsiveness toward stimuli for elicitation of the sucking reflex. The neuroreflex induces adequate release of both prolactin and oxytocin. It appears that, in addition to the hormonal actions, breast nerves can also influence the mammary blood supply and milk secretion. Abnormalities of sensory or autonomic nerve distributions in the areola and nipple therefore could impair adequate lactation, especially in the functioning of the let-down reflex and the secretion of prolactin and oxytocin.

In summary, the somatic sensory cutaneous nerve supply of the breast includes the

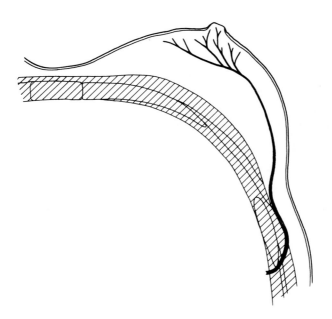

Fig. 2-17. Cross section of nerve supply of breast and nipple. Cutaneous nerves run close to deep fascia before turning outward toward skin.

supraclavicular nerves and the thoracic intercostal nerves. The autonomic motor nerve supply of the breast is derived from the sympathetic fibers of the intercostal nerves, which supply the smooth musculature of the areola and the nipple. The autonomic motor nerve supply of the breast is also derived from sympathetic fibers of the accompanying arteries, which innervate the smooth musculature of the inner glandular blood vessel walls to produce constriction. The nerve supply to the area of the areola and the nipple includes free sensory nerve endings, tactile corpuscles to the papillae of the corium of the nipple and areola, and the fibers around the larger lactiferous duct and in the dermis of the areola and peripheral breast. All cutaneous nerves run radially to the glandular body toward the nipple. The nerve supply to the inner gland is sparse and contains only sympathetic nerves accompanying blood vessels (Fig. 2-17).

MICROSCOPIC ANATOMY

In their structure and mode of development, the mammary glands somewhat resemble the sweat glands. During embryonic life, their differentiation is similar in the two sexes. The male experiences little additional development postnatally. The female, in contrast, experiences extensive structural change paralleling her age and the functional state of the reproductive system.

The greatest development in the female is reached by the twentieth year. Gradual changes are correlated with the menstrual cycle, and major changes accompany pregnancy and lactation.

Resting mammary gland

The mammary gland is a compound tubuloalveolar gland containing 15 to 25 irregular lobes radiating from the nipple. Each lobe has a lactiferous duct (2 to 4 mm in diameter) lined by stratified squamous epithelium. The duct opens on the nipple and has an irregular angular outline. Beneath the areola each duct has a local dilation, the lactiferous sinus, and finally emerges at the end of the nipple as a 0.4 to 0.7 mm opening. Each lobe is subdivided into lobules of various orders; the smallest are elongated tubules, the alveolar ducts, covered by small saccular evaginations, the alveoli. The interlobular connective tissue is dense; however, it is more cellular, has fewer collagenous fibers, and contains almost no fat. Greater distensibility is permitted by the looser connective tissue.

The secretory portions of the gland, the alveolar ducts and the alveoli, have cuboidal or low-columnar secretory cells, resting on basal laminae and myoepithelial cells. These myoepithelial cells enclose the alveoli in a loosely meshed network with their many starlike branchings. The myoepithelial cells are stimulated by prolactin and sex steroids. The presence of myoepithelial cells has been used as evidence that the mammary gland is related to the sweat gland.

In the resting phase, epithelial structures consist of the ducts and their branches. The presence of a few alveoli budded off from the ends of ducts is still under discussion. This variance may be due to the effet of the menstrual cycle. The swelling and engorgement accompanying the menstrual cycle are associated with hyperemia and some edema of the connective tissue. Most significant is the fact that the gland does not have a single duct but many. Each lobe is a separate compound alveolar gland whose primary ducts join into larger and larger ducts. These ducts drain into a lactiferous duct. Each lactiferous duct drains separately at the tip of the nipple.

The epidermis of the nipple and areola is invaded by unusually long dermal papillae whose capillaries richly vascularize the surface and impart the pinkish hue. Bundles of smooth muscle, placed longitudinally along the lactiferous ducts and circumferentially within the nipple and at its base, permit the erection of the nipple. In the areola are the areolar Montgomery glands, which are intermediate in their microscopic structure between sweat glands and true mammary glands. The periphery of the areola also has sweat glands and sebaceous glands (see Figs. 2-7 and 2-8).

Mammary gland in pregnancy

Changes in levels of circulating hormones result in profound changes in the ductular-lobular-alveolar growth during pregnancy. During the first trimester there is rapid growth and branching from the terminal portion of the duct system. As the epithelial structures proliferate, the adipose tissue seems to diminish. During this time there is increasing infiltration of the interstitial tissue with lymphocytes, plasma cells, and eosinophils. The rate of hyperplasia levels off. In the last trimester, any enlargement is the result of enlargement of the parenchymal cells and the distention of the alveoli with early colostrum, which is rich in protein and relatively low in lipid. There is a gradual accumulation of fat droplets in the secretory alveolar cells. The interlobular connective tissue is noticeably decreased and alveolar proliferation extensive. The histologic appearance of the gland is quite variable. The functional state appears to vary from dilated, thin-walled lumen to narrow-lumened, thick-walled glandular tissue. Epithelial cells vary, being flat to low columnar in shape with indistinct boundaries. Some cells protrude into the lumen of the alveoli; others are short and smooth. The lumen of the alveoli is crowded with fine granular material and lipid droplets similar to those protruding from the cells.

The former concepts of mammary gland secretion indicated that the mode of release was apocrine secretion. Apocrine secretion is the process by which the cell undergoes partial disintegration. A fat-filled portion projects into the lumen; the fat globule constricts at the base, and the cell replaces itself. Electron microscopy has shown that the cell has two distinct secretory products, formed and released by different mechanisms. The protein constituents of milk are formed and released identically to those of other protein-secreting glands, classed as merocrine glands. Secretory materials are passed out through the cell apex without appreciable loss of cytoplasm in merocrine glands. The fatty components of milk arise as lipid droplets free in the cytoplasmic matrix. The droplets increase in size and move into the apex of the cell. They project into the lumen, covered by a thin layer of cytoplasm. The droplets are ultimately cast off, enveloped by a detached portion of the cell membrane and a thin rim of subjacent cytoplasm. This process is referred to as apocrine, since it involves the loss of some cytoplasm (Fig. 2-3).

Lactating mammary gland

The lactating mammary gland is characterized by a large number of alveoli. The alveoli of the lactating gland are made up of cuboidal epithelial and myoepithelial cells. Only a small amount of connective tissue separates the neighboring alveoli. Under special preparations, lipid can be seen as small droplets within the cells. These droplets become larger and are discharged into the lumen.

The functioning of the mammary gland depends on the interplay of multiple and complex nervous and endocrine factors. Some factors are involved in the development of the mammary glands to a functional state (mammogenesis), others in the establishment of milk secretion (lactogenesis), and others in responsibility for the maintenance of lactation (galactopoiesis).

The division and differentiation of mammary epithelial cells and presecretory alveolar cells into secretory milk-releasing alveolar cells takes place in the third trimester. Stimulation of RNA synthesis promotes galactopoiesis and apocrine milk secretion into the alveoli. The DNA and RNA content of the cellular nuclei increases during pregnancy and is highest at lactation (see Fig. 2-3).

The ultrastructure of the human mammary gland during lactogenesis was studied by Tobon and Salazar,[17] who reviewed surgical specimens from seven lactating women, 1 day to 5½ months postpartum. They noted widespread hypertrophy and hyperplasia of the acini accompanied by dilatation and engorgement of the lumen by milk. The vascular channels were engorged. The lactogenic epithelial cells had rich cytoplasm, prominent layers of reticulum, and enlarged oval mitochondria. The Golgi apparatus was hypertrophied. The myoepithelium was stretched and thinned to contain the filled acini.

Postlactation regression of the mammary gland

If milk is not removed from the breast, the glands become greatly distended and milk production gradually ceases. Part of the decrease is due to the lack of stimulation of sucking, which initiates the neurohormonal reflex for maintenance of prolactin secretion. Perhaps a stronger effect is the engorgement of the breast with compression of blood vessels, causing diminished flow. The diminished flow results in decreased oxytocin to the myoepithelium. The alveoli are greatly distended and the epithelium flattened. The secretion remaining in the alveolar spaces and ducts is absorbed. There is a gradual collapse of the alveoli and an increase in perialveolar connective tissue. The glandular elements gradually return to the resting state. Adipose tissue increases. There are increased macrophages. The gland does not return completely to the prepregnancy state in that the alveoli formed do not totally involute. Some appear as scattered, solid cord of epithelial cells.

Microscopically, there are increased autophagic and heterophagic processes in the first few days after weaning. Lysosomal enzymes increase, whereas nonlysosomal enzymes decrease.

Although the process of regression has been studied carefully in animals, little study has been done in the human. It is probable that slow weaning, which usually takes 3 months, has a very different timetable from abrupt weaning, in which marked involution has been intense and rapid over a matter of days or weeks.

REFERENCES

1. Adler DD, Rebner M, and Pennes, DR: Accessory breast tissue in the axilla: mammographic appearance, Radiology 163:709, 1987.
2. Clemente CD, editor: Gray's anatomy of the human body, Philadelphia, 1985, Lea and Febiger.
3. Courtiss EH and Goldwyn RM: Breast sensation before and after plastic surgery, Plast Reconstr Surg 58:1, 1976.
4. Crafts RC: A textbook of human anatomy, New York, 1966, Ronald Press Co.
5. Egan RL: Breast embryology, anatomy, and physiology. In Breast imaging diagnosis and morphology of breast diseases, Philadelphia, 1988, WB Saunders Co.
6. Farina MA, Newby GG, and Alani HM: Innervation of the nipple-areolar complex, Plast Reconstr Surg 66:497, 1980.
7. Fawcett DW: Bloom and Fawcett: a textbook on histology, ed 11, Philadelphia, 1986, WB Saunders, Co.
8. Hersh JH, Bloom AS, Cromer AO et al: Does a supernumerary nipple/renal field defect exist? Am J Dis Child 141:989, 1987.

9. Hicken NF: Mastectomy: a clinical pathologic study demonstrating why most mastectomies result in incomplete removal of the mammary gland, Arch Surg 40:6, 1940.
10. Kaye BL: Axillary breasts: a significant esthetic deformity, Plast Reconstr Surg 53:61, 1974.
11. Knight CH and Peaker M: Development of the mammary gland: symposium report no. 19, Lactation, J Reprod 65:521, 1982.
12. Larson BL, editor: Lactation, Ames, 1985, Iowa State University Press.
13. Montagna W and Macpherson EE: Some neglected aspects of the anatomy of human breasts, J Invest Dermatol 63:10, 1974.
14. Osbourne MP: Breast development and anatomy. In Harris JR, Hellman S, Henderson IC, and Kinne DW, editors: Breast diseases, Philadelphia, 1986, WB Saunders Co.
15. Smith DM, Peters TG, and Donegan WL: Montgomery's areolar tubercle, Arch Pathol Lab Med 106:60, 1982.
16. Tobon H and Salazar H: Ultrastructure of the human mammary gland. I. Development of the fetal gland throughout gestation, J Clin Endocrin Metab 39:443, 1974.
17. Tobon H and Salazar H: Ultrastructure of the human mammary gland. II. Postpartum lactogenesis, J Clin Endocrin Metab 40:834, 1975.
18. Vorherr H: The breast: morphology, physiology, and lactation, New York, 1974, Academic Press, Inc.
19. Weatherly-White RCA: Plastic surgery of the female breast, Hagerstown Md, 1980, Harper & Row, Publishers, Inc.

Physiology of lactation

3

Lactation is the physiologic completion of the reproductive cycle. The human infant at birth is the most immature and dependent of all mammals except for marsupials. The marsupial joey is promptly attached to the teat of a mammary gland in an external pouch. The gland changes as the offspring develops, and the joey remains there until able to survive outside the pouch. In the human throughout pregnancy the breast develops and prepares to take over the role of fully nourishing the infant when the placental connection is severed. The breast is prepared for full lactation without any active intervention from the mother from 16 weeks. It is kept inactive by a balance of inhibiting hormones that suppress target cell response. In the first few hours and days postpartum, the breast responds to changes in the hormonal milieu and the newborn infant's suckling to produce and release milk. This chapter provides a review of the physiologic adaption of the mammary gland to its role in infant survival. Several major reviews are referenced that include substantial bibliographies for readers who need the detailed reports of the original investigators.[7,21,24,27] Newer scientific techniques have been applied in the study of human lactation providing more precise, more detailed, and more integrated data upon which the clinician can base a physiologic approach to lactation management.

HORMONAL CONTROL OF LACTATION

Lactation is an integral part of the reproductive cycle of all mammals, including humans. The hormonal control of lactation can be described under three main headings: mammogenesis, or mammary growth; lactogenesis, or initiation of milk secretion; and galactopoiesis, or the maintenance of established milk secretion.

Under the influence of sex steroids, especially the estrogens, the mammary glandular epithelium proliferates, becoming multilayered. Buds and papillae then form. The growth of the mammary gland is a gradual process that starts during puberty. It has been shown to depend on pituitary hormones. Lobuloalveolar development and ductal proliferation also depend on an intact pituitary gland.

Mammogenesis: mammary growth
Prepubertal growth

The primary and secondary ducts that develop in the fetus in utero continue to grow in both the male and the female in proportion to growth in general. Shortly before puberty, a more rapid expansion of the duct system begins in the female. The growth of the duct system seems to depend predominantly on estrogen and does not occur in the absence of ovaries. The complete growth of the alveoli requires stimulation by progesterone as well.

Studies of hypophysectomized animals have shown failure of full mammary growth even with adequate estrogen and progesterone. It has been shown that the secretion of prolactin and somatotropin by the pituitary gland effects mammary growth. Adrenocorticotropic hormone (ACTH) and thyroid-stimulating hormone (TSH) acting on the adrenal gland and the thyroid gland also play a minor role in growth of the mammary gland.

Pubertal growth

When the hypophyseal-ovarian-uterine cycle is established, a new phase of mammary growth begins, which includes extensive branching of the system of ducts and proliferation and canalization of the lobuloalveolar units at the distal tips of the branches. Organization of the stromal connective tissue forms the interlobular septa. The ducts, ductules (terminal intralobular ducts), and alveolar structures are all formed by double layers of cells. One layer, the epithelial cells, circumscribes the lumen. The second layer, the myoepithelial cells, surrounds the inner epithelial cells and is bordered by a basement lamina.

Menstrual cycle growth

The cyclical changes of the adult mammary gland can be associated with the menstrual cycle and the hormonal changes that control that cycle. Estrogens stimulate parenchymal proliferation, with formation of epithelial sprouts. This hyperplasia continues into the secretory phase of the cycle. Anatomically, when the corpus luteum provides increased amounts of estrogens and progesterone, there is lobular edema, thickening of the epithelial basal membrane, and secretory material in the alveolar lumen. Lymphoid and plasma cells infiltrate the stroma. Clinically, there is increased mammary blood flow in this luteal phase. This is experienced by women as fullness, heaviness, and turgescence. The breast may become nodular because of interlobular edema and ductular-acinar growth.

After the onset of menstruation and the reduction of sex steroid levels, there is limited milk-secretory prolactin action. Postmenstrual changes occur rapidly, with degeneration of glandular cells and proliferation tissue, loss of edema, and decrease in breast size. The ovulatory cycle actually enhances mammary growth in the early years of menstruation (until about age 30) because the postmenstrual regression of the glandular-alveolar growth after each cycle is not complete. These changes of ductal and lobular proliferation, which occur during the follicular phase before ovulation, continue in the luteal phase and regress after the menstrual phase, exemplifying the sensitivity of this target organ to variations in the balance of hormones.

Growth during pregnancy

Hormonal influences on the breast cause profound changes during pregnancy (Fig. 3-1). Early in pregnancy a marked increase in ductular sprouting, branching, and lobular formation is evoked by luteal and placental hormones. Placental lactogen, prolactin, and chorionic gonadotropin have been identified as contributors to the accelerated growth. The dichorionic ductular sprouting has been attributed to estrogen, and lobular formation has been attributed to progesterone.

From the third month of gestation, secretory material that resembles colostrum appears in the acini. Prolactin from the anterior pituitary gland stimulates the glandular production of colostrum. By the second trimester, placental lactogen begins to stimulate the secretion of colostrum. The effectiveness of hormonal stimulation on lactation has been demonstrated by the fact that a mother who delivers after 16 weeks of gestation will secrete colostrum, even though she has had a nonviable infant.

GESTATION

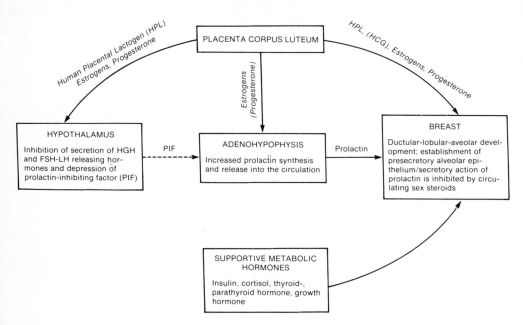

Fig. 3-1. Hormonal preparation during pregnancy of breast for lactation. (Modified from Vorherr H: The breast, morphology, physiology and lactation, New York, 1974, Academic Press, Inc.)

An estrogen-mediated increase in prolactin secretion in pregnancy may produce as much as a tenfold to twentyfold increase in plasma prolactin. This effect may be partially controlled by lactogen from the placenta, which inhibits the production of prolactin. Hormonal regulation of the growth and proliferation of the mammary gland cells has been carefully studied in many species.

A complex sequence of events, governed by hormonal action, prepares the breast for lactation (Fig. 3-1). Estradiol 17β stimulates the ductal system of epithelial cells to elongate during pregnancy. In contrast to puberty, however, when estrogens appear to directly and indirectly stimulate breast development, there is no indispensable role for estrogens in mammary development in pregnancy except as a prolactin potentiator according to Neville;[26] when estrogen levels are low in pregnancy, the breast still develops. Estrogen levels are normally high in pregnancy, but not for mammogenesis. Induced lactation in the cow is dependably reproduced with 7 days of estrogen and progesterone treatment. Progesterone, in turn, induces the specific epithelial cells of the tubular invaginations to produce distinct ducts, which branch from the main tubules. The end result of the combined actions of estrogen and progesterone is a richly branched arborization of the gland. Highly differentiated secretory alveolar cells develop at the ends of these ducts under the influence of prolactin.

Serum growth factor, which is present in normal human serum, and insulin can stimulate the stem cells of the gland to proliferate. These dividing cells are further directed to the formation of alveoli by corticosteroid hormones. There are at least two types of cells

POSTPARTUM

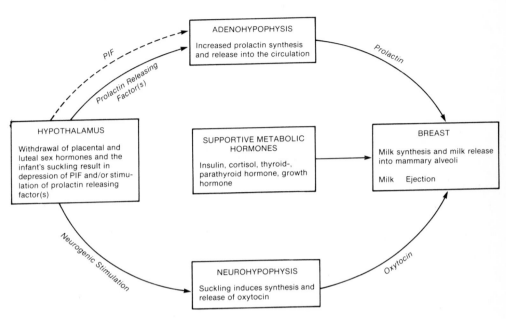

Fig. 3-2. Hormonal preparation of breast postpartum for lactation. (Modified from Vorherr H: The breast, morphology, physiology and lactation, New York, 1974, Academic Press, Inc.)

identified in the epithelial layer of the gland: stem cells and secretory alveolar cells. At this point in the pregnancy, prolactin influences the production of the constituents of milk.

That the high circulating levels of prolactin are not associated with milk production is due in part to the progesterone antagonism of the stimulatory action of prolactin on casein messenger *(m)* RNA synthesis. During late pregnancy the lactogenic receptors, which have similar affinities for both prolactin and human placental lactogen (HPL), are predominantly occupied by HPL. High doses of estradiol impair the incorporation of prolactin into milk secretory cells.

Lactogenesis: initiation of milk secretion

The two stages of lactogenesis have been described by Hartman.[12] Stage I starts about 12 weeks before parturition and is heralded by significant increases in lactose, total proteins, and immunoglobulin and by decreases in sodium and chloride, the gathering of substrate for milk production. The composition of prepartum secretion is fairly constant until delivery as monitored by milk protein α-lactalbumin. Stage II includes the increase in blood flow and oxygen and glucose uptake as well as the sharp increase in citrate concentration, considered a reliable marker for lactogenesis stage II. Stage II at 2 to 3 days postpartum begins clinically when the secretion of milk is copious and biochemically when plasma α-lactalbumin levels peak (paralleling the period when "the milk comes in"). The major changes in milk composition continue for 10 days, when "mature milk" is established.

The breast, one of the most complex endocrine target organs, has been prepared during pregnancy and responds to the release of prolactin by producing the constituents of milk (Fig. 3-2). The lactogenic effects of prolactin are modulated by the complex interplay of pituitary, ovarian, thyroid, adrenal, and pancreatic hormones.

Prolactin

Human prolactin is a significant hormone in pregnancy and lactation.[9] Prolactin also has a range of actions in various species that is greater than any other known hormone. Prolactin has been identified in many animal species whether they nurse their young or not. Because of the original association with lactation, the term describes its action, "support or stimulation of lactation." Prolactin, however, has been shown to control nonlactating responses in other species and has been identified with over 80 different physiological processes. Study of prolactin was hampered until 1970, when it became possible to separate prolactin from human growth hormone (HGH) and to isolate and characterize prolactin from human pituitary glands.[36]

Before 1971, HGH and prolactin in humans were considered the same hormone. Until 1971, in fact, it was thought that prolactin did not exist in humans. HGH, however, is present in the human pituitary gland in an amount 100 times that of prolactin.

In vitro, prolactin stimulates the synthesis of the *m* RNAs of specific milk proteins by binding to membrane receptors of the mammary epithelial cells. Prolactin has been demonstrated to penetrate the cytoplasm of these cells and even their nuclei. These specific actions in the gland require the presence of extracellular calcium ions. Some prolactin actually appears in the milk substrate itself, the functional significance of which is uncertain, although it is thought to influence fluid and ion absorption from the neonatal jejunum.

The effect of the stimulation of protein synthesis by allowing the expression of milk protein genes is not a direct effect of the hormone but rather the consequence of the activation of the Na/K ATPase in the plasma membrane. The intracellular concentration of potassium is kept high and sodium low compared with the concentrations in extracellular fluid. As a result, the Na/K ratio is high both in the milk and in the intracellular fluid. Further action of prolactin has been identified in the development of the immune system in the mammary gland and, possibly more directly, in the lymphoid tissue. In conjunction

Table 3-1. Prolactin levels

	Range (ng/ml)	Average (ng/ml)
Males and prepuberty and postmenopausal females	2-8	
Females' menstrual life	8-14	10
Term pregnancy	200-500	200
Amniotic fluid	up to 10,000	
Lactating women		
First 10 days	Baseline 200	Rise to 400
10–90 days	60–110	70–220
90–180 days	50	100
180–1 year	30–40	45–80

Collation of values from multiple studies and sources.

with estrogen and progesterone, prolactin attracts and retains IgA immunoblasts from the gut-associated lymphoid tissue for the development of the immune system for the mammary gland. A very sensitive bioassay has been developed using the in vitro biologic effect of prolactin to stimulate the growth of cell cultures for malignant Nb rat lymphomas.

The baseline levels of prolactin are essentially the same in the normal human male and female (Table 3-1). Moreover, both male and female experience a rise in prolactin levels during sleep. At puberty, the increase in estrogens causes a slight but measurable increase in prolactin. There is an increase in prolactin during the proliferative phase of the menstrual cycle but not during the secretory phase. There is also a normal diurnal variation in levels in both male and female. A number of factors, including some that are significant for the nursing mother, increase prolactin levels. Psychogenic influence and stress increase prolactin levels. Anesthesia, surgery, exercise, nipple stimulation, and sexual intercourse also produce increased amounts in both lactating and nonlactating female. Prolactin levels increase as serum osmolality increases.

Prolactin-inhibiting factor

The prolactin-inhibiting factor (PIF) controls the secretion of prolactin from the hypothalamus. Prolactin thus is unusual among the pituitary hormones, since it is inhibited by a hypothalamic substance. Catecholamine levels in the hypothalamus control the inhibiting factor. The inhibiting factor is poured into the circulation as a result of dopaminergic impulses. Drugs and events that decrease catecholamines also decrease the inhibiting factor, causing a rise in prolactin. Dopamine itself can act directly on the pituitary gland to decrease prolactin secretion. Agents that increase prolactin by decreasing catecholamines and thus the PIF level include the phenothiazines and reserpine. Thyrotropin-releasing hormone (TRH) is a strong stimulator of prolactin secretion, but its physiological role is not clear, since thyrotropin levels do not rise during normal nursing. In the postpartum period a dose of TRH will cause a marked increase in prolactin. Even the nonnursing postpartum mother will experience engorgement and milk release when stimulated with TRH. Ergot, which is frequently prescribed for the postpartum patient, inhibits prolactin secretion either by direct inhibition or by its effect on the hypothalamus.

Prolactin response to breast stimulation in lactating women is not mediated by endogenous opioids. Neither baseline nor stimulated prolactin values were affected by Naloxone.[4]

Following are factors affecting prolactin release in normal humans:

Physiologic stimuli
  Nursing in postpartum women—breast stimulation
  Sleep
  Stress
  Sexual intercourse
  Pregnancy
Pharmacologic stimuli
  Neuroleptic drugs
  TRH
  Metoclopramide (procainamide derivative)
  Estrogens
  Hypoglycemia
  Phenothiazines

Pharmacologic suppressors
  L-dopa
  Ergot preparations (2-Br-α-ergocryptine)
  Clomiphene citrate
  Large amounts of pyridoxine
  Monoamine oxidase inhibitors
  Prostaglandins E and $F_{2\alpha}$

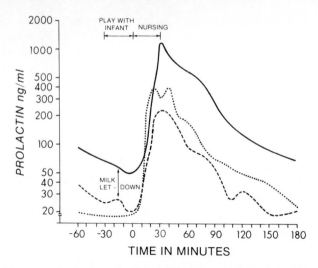

Fig. 3-3. Plasma prolactin measured by radioimmunoassay before, during, and after period of nursing in three mothers, 22 to 26 days postpartum. Prolactin rose with suckling and not with infant contact. (Modified from Josimovich JB, Reynolds M, and Cobo E: Lactogenic hormones, fetal nutrition, and lactation. In Josimovich JB, Reynolds M, and Cobo E: Problems of human reproduction, vol 2, New York, 1974, John Wiley & Sons.)

In pregnancy prolactin levels begin to rise in the first trimester and continue to rise throughout gestation. In the nonnursing mother prolactin levels drop to normal in 2 to 3 weeks, independent of therapy to suppress lactation.

At delivery, with the expulsion of the placenta, there is an abrupt decline in placental lactogen, estrogens, and progesterone.

Placental lactogen disappears within hours.[27] Progesterone drops over several days, and estrogens fall to baseline levels in 5 to 6 days (see Figs. 18-2 to 18-4). Prolactin in nonlactating women requires 14 days to reach baseline. Progesterone is considered the key inhibiting hormone and decline in plasma progesterone levels is considered the lactogenic trigger for stage II lactogenesis according to Neville. Progesterone, on the other hand, does not inhibit established lactation, as breast tissue does not contain progesterone binding sites. Estrogens enhance the effect of prolactin on mammogenesis but antagonize prolactin by inhibiting secretion of milk. After delivery, there are low estrogen and high prolactin levels. Suckling provides a continued stimulus for prolactin release. If prolactin, essential for lactation, is diminished by hypophysectomy or medication, lactation ceases. Baseline prolactin levels do eventually diminish to more normal levels months after parturition, although lactation may continue. Suckling stimulates the release of adenohypophyseal prolactin and neurohypophyseal oxytocin. These hormones stimulate milk synthesis and production of milk-ejection metabolic hormones, which are also necessary in the process of milk synthesis. Thus suckling, emptying the breast, and receiving adequate precursor nutrients are essential to effective lactation (Fig. 3-3).

The most effective and specific stimulus to prolactin release is nursing. The stimulation is a result of nipple or breast manipulation, especially suckling, not a psychological effect of the presence of the infant (Fig. 3-3). The prolactin-release reflex during nipple stimulation is suppressed in some adult women, being evidenced only during pregnancy and lactation.

During human pregnancy, when serum prolactin rises steadily to 150 to 200 ng/ml at term, there is a brief drop in levels hours before delivery and then a rise again in 3 to 4 hours or as soon as the neonate is suckled.[19,24] In the nonlactator, levels gradually drop over 2 to 3 weeks, when they return to prepregnancy levels. The response to nipple stimulation can be abolished by applying local anesthetic. On the other hand, trauma or surgery to the chest wall can initiate a prolactin rise and, in some reported cases, milk production.

Although it had initially been reported that the high levels of prolactin measured in the first days and weeks of lactation dwindled to normal baseline by 6 months and showed no response to suckling stimulus, newer studies clearly show a different picture with more sensitive assays.[19] Baseline does not drop to normal, but further stimulus causes a doubling of levels at all stages of lactation through the second year (Table 3-1).

Eight fully lactating women were followed through the first 6 months postpartum at 10, 40, 80, 120, and 180 days recording serum prolactin, luteinizing hormone, follicle-stimulating hormone, and estradiol (zero time only) obtained just before the initiation of suckling and during the next 120 minutes.[6] Samples were obtained at 0, +15, +30, +60, +120 every minute. Prolactin levels were high the first 10 days (90.1 ng/ml) but slowly declined over 180 days (44.3 ng/ml). The stimulus of suckling doubled the baseline values. Mean estradiol levels were low at 10 days (7.2 pg/ml), then gradually rose to a mean of 47.3 pg/ml at 180 days postpartum in the subjects whose menses had resumed. In the amenorrheic subjects the estradiol levels remained low (4.25 pg/ml), while baseline prolactin remained high (63.6 ng/ml). The subjects were breastfeeding on demand, averaging 11 feedings (range 8 to 16) per day at 10 days and 8 feedings (range 5 to 12) at 120 and 180 days. All infants had dropped one night feeding, and two infants had started some solids between the third and fourth months (Figs. 3-4 and 3-5).

The effort to relate the prolactin level to the volume of milk has not produced consistent findings. It is clear, however, that stimulating both breasts simultaneously either by feeding two babies or "double pumping" (attachment to both breasts to pump via a Y-tube) does produce higher prolactin surge and a greater volume of milk totally as well as per unit of time. The relationship between suckling-induced prolactin response and production of milk was reported by Howie et al.[14] as imprecise, as they found no close temporal correlation between prolactin concentrations and milk yield. Milk yield was measured by electronic scale weighings before and after feeds. They calculated not only the peak prolactin level but the area under the curve, and it was this latter value that was consistent within the same individual mother. Aono et al[1] had reported significant differences in prolactin level between "good" and "poor" feeders but had measured milk production by postfeed pumping, which may have influenced lactogenesis, but also is dependent on let-down reflex while pumping. Complete breast emptying also plays a role in milk production.

When specific binding was looked for in the tammar wallaby, many sites were demonstrated in the lactating mammary gland but not the inactive gland.[21] Mammary prolactin receptors were also identified in the rabbit. Perry and Jacobs[28] noted that the binding capacity increased over time in lactation. Thus the increased binding capacity would enhance tissue responsiveness, which may explain the maintenance of full lactation in the face of falling concentrations of prolactin.

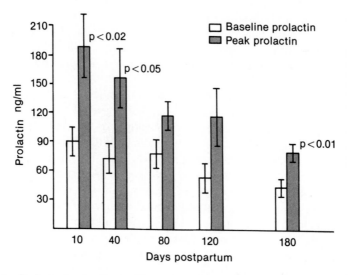

Fig. 3-4. Prolactin levels after suckling. (From Battin DA, Marrs RP, Fleiss PM et al: Obstet Gynecol 65: 785, 1985.)

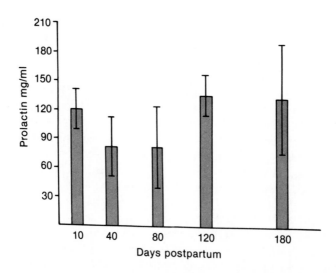

Fig. 3-5. Percent increase in prolactin after suckling. (From Battin DA, Marrs RP, Fleiss PM et al: Obstet Gynecol 65:785, 1985.)

Human placental lactogen and human growth hormone

Three main hormones are recognized in the lactogenic process: HPL, HGH, and prolactin. The progressive rise in prolactin during pregnancy parallels the rise in HPL, becoming measurable at 6 weeks' gestation and increasing to 6000 ng/ml at term. This parallel action contributed to the belief that prolactin and HPL were the same. Although the principal function of HPL and prolactin in the human is a lactogenic one, no lactation appears prior to delivery.[33]

First described in 1962, HPL has been studied more than lactogens from any other species.[25] There is extensive immunologic and structural homology between HGH and HPL, which probably explains their similar biologic activities. Concentrations of HPL increase steadily during gestation and decrease abruptly with the delivery of the placenta. A large-molecular-weight substance, HPL is derived from the chorion. Receptor sites that bind lactogen also bind protein and HGH.[39] HPL has been associated with mobilization of free fatty acid and inhibition of peripheral glucose utilization and lactogenic action.

HGH is secreted from the anterior pituitary eosinophilic cells. These cells have been identified by staining techniques that distinguish them from those which produce prolactin. Toward the end of pregnancy, the cells that produce prolactin are noticeably more numerous, whereas those which produce HGH are "crowded out." The role of HGH in the maintenance of lactation is poorly defined and may be synergistic with prolactin and glucocorticords. It has been demonstrated that normal lactation is possible in ateliotic dwarf women in the absence of detectable quantities of HGH.[30] For any hormone to exert its biologic effects, however, specific receptors for the hormone must be present in the target tissue. Changes in serum concentration are without effect if receptors are not present in the mammary gland to bind the hormone.

Galactopoiesis: maintenance of established lactation

The maintenance of established milk secretion is called galactopoiesis. An intact hypothalamic-pituitary axis regulating prolactin and oxytocin levels is essential to the initiation and maintenance of lactation.[16] The process of lactation requires milk synthesis and milk release into the alveoli and the lactiferous sinuses. When the milk is not removed, effecting the diminution of capillary blood flow, the lactation process can be inhibited. Lack of sucking stimulation means lack of prolactin release from the pituitary gland. Basal prolactin levels that are enhanced by the spurts that result from sucking are necessary to maintain lactation in the first weeks postpartum. Without oxytocin, however, a pregnancy can be carried to term, but the female will fail to lactate because she will fail to let-down.

Sensory nerve endings, located mainly in the areola and nipple, are stimulated by suckling. The afferent neural reflex pathway, via the spinal cord to the mesencephalon and then to the hypothalamus, produces secretion and release of prolactin and oxytocin. Hypothalamic suppression of PIF secretion causes adrenohypophyseal prolactin release. When prolactin is released into the circulation, it stimulates milk synthesis and secretion. A conditioned milk ejection can occur in lactating women without a concomitant release of prolactin so that indeed the releases are independent, which may be significant in treating apparent lactation failure (Fig. 3-6).

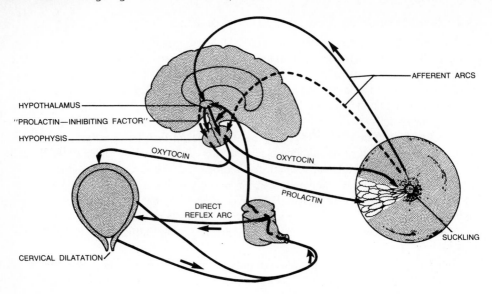

Fig. 3-6.   Neuroendocrine control of milk ejection. (Modified from Vorherr H: The breast, morphology, physiology and lactation, New York, 1974, Academic Press, Inc.)

Hormonal regulation of prolactin and oxytocin

The release of prolactin is inhibited by PIF.[17] The PIF has not been described, but it is closely associated with dopamine. There is also evidence of either serotonin release of prolactin or catecholamine-serotonin control of prolactin release. TSH has also been shown to simulate the release of prolactin. In addition, the release of prolactin is related to stress and sleep states. The amount of prolactin is proportional to the amount of nipple stimulation during early stages of lactation.

When suckling occurs, oxytocin is released. It enters the circulation and rapidly causes ejection of milk from alveoli and smaller milk ducts into larger lactiferous ducts and sinuses. This is the pathway of the let-down, or ejection, reflex. Oxytocin also causes contraction of the myometrium and involution of the uterus.

The human pituitary has an excessive storage capacity and contains 3000–9000 mU oxytocin, but the reflex milk ejection only involves the release of 50 to 100 mU. Except in extreme cases (Sheenan's syndrome), hormone depletion is rarely an issue, but hormone release and target-organ sensitivity are. Opiate and B-endorphin released during stress are known to block stimulus-secretion coupling by dissociating electrical activity at the terminal. This inhibition is Naloxone reversible.

The mammary gland from the platypus to the human has identical fine structure consisting of alveolar tissue that has increased its surface area 10,000 fold during gestation compared to the size of the gland.[22] It continuously produces milk throughout lactation, but the most complex issue is the release of milk. Due to the substantial surface tension forces opposing the movement of fluid in the small ducts, simple suction applied by suckling is relatively ineffective, especially in early lactation. Thus the alveolus is enveloped in a basket-like network of myoepithelial cells that respond to oxytocin by contracting and expelling the milk into larger and larger ductules until it can be removed by the infant.

This is a classic example of a neuroendocrine reflex, a process that is remarkably uniform in all mammals.

Neuroendocrine control of milk ejection

Milk ejection involves both neural and endocrinologic stimulation and response. A neural afferent pathway and an endocrinologic efferent pathway are required.[25]

The ejection reflex depends on receptors located in the canalicular system of the breast. When the canalicules are dilated or stretched, the reflex release of oxytocin is triggered. Tactile receptors for both oxytocin and reflex prolactin release are in the nipple. Neither the negative and postive pressures exerted by suckling nor thermal changes trigger the milk-ejection reflex. There is some minor effect of negative pressures, but tactile stimulation is the most important factor.

Studies in tactile stimulation show changes in sensitivity at puberty, during the menstrual cycle, and at parturition.[31] There is no difference in sensitivity between the sexes before puberty. In the female, tactile sensitivity increases after puberty and is increased at midcycle and during menstruation. (Midcycle peak is absent in women taking oral contraceptives.) Dramatic changes occur within 24 hours of delivery after several weeks of complete insensitivity. The nipple is the more sensitive area to both touch and pain, followed by the areola; the least sensitive area is the cutaneous breast tissue. The increased sensitivity of the breast continues several days postpartum, even when the woman does not breastfeed. Estrogen treatment suppresses the induction of prolactin release on nipple stimulation, whereas on withdrawal of estrogen the prolactin response returns. Increased tactile sensitivity may be the key event activating the suckling-induced release of oxytocin and prolactin at delivery (Fig. 3-7).

The oxytocin binding sites are located within the basement membrane of the mammary alveolus and along the interlobular ducts. There is a gradual 10-fold increase in the concentration of oxytocin receptor sites in the mammary gland during pregnancy.[20] This contrasts sharply with the sudden 40-fold increase in oxytocin receptors in the uterus in the hours before delivery that then rapidly disappear. These changes in receptor availability may be why copious milk does not occur until shortly after delivery, since oxytocin first facilitates delivery and then promotes milk ejection sequentially. When the increase in intramammary pressure obtained with varying doses of oxytocin in nonpregnant, pregnant, and lactating women was recorded by Caldeyro-Barcia,[3] the amount of oxytocin required for a response dropped from 1000 mU in nonpregnancy to about 1 mU in late pregnancy and further to 0.5 mU in lactation.[26] The maximum intramammary pressure that could be evoked increased from 1 mm Hg to a peak of 10 mm Hg 5 days postpartum. It appears that not only the sensitivity of the myoepithelial cells but the number of receptor sites increases as well during pregnancy (Fig. 3-8).

Conflicting information has been available as to the exact nature of the release of oxytocin from the pituitary. The dose-response curve of the mammary gland has a very limited dynamic range, so that a bolus of 0.1 mU oxytocin (0.2 mg) given intravenously to a lactating rat fails to change intramammary pressure. An injection of 1.0 mU evokes an increase in pressure that begins after a delay of 10 seconds and peaks in 15 seconds at 8 to 10 mm Hg. A bolus has greater effect than a slow push, suggesting that a pulsatile pattern of hormone release would be the most effective way of utilizing oxytocin to produce milk ejection.

Plasma oxytocin levels measured by Lucas et al[22] with continuous sampling every

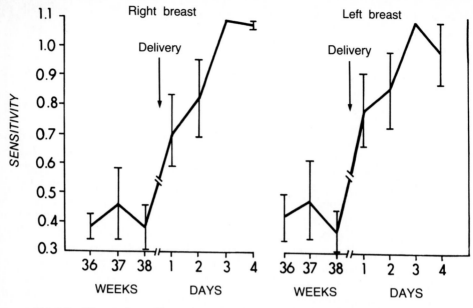

Fig. 3-7. Changes in tactile sensitivity of cutaneous breast tissue in perinatal period. Sensitivity was calculated from two-point discrimination according to formula $K\text{-log}^e$. K is an arbitrary figure employed to portray low two-point discrimination values as peaks of sensitivity. (From Robinson JE and Short RV: Br Med J 1:1188, 1977.)

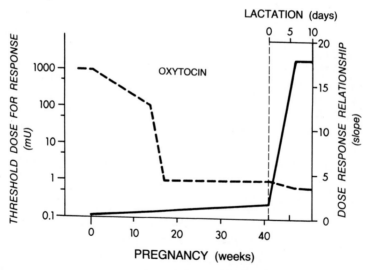

Fig. 3-8. Sensitivity of human mammary epithelium to oxytocin during pregnancy and lactation. Right-hand scale shows threshold dose necessary to evoke increase in intra-mammary pressure; left-hand scale shows maximum intramammary pressure obtained. (Adapted from Caldyro-Barcia R: Milk ejection in women. In Reynolds M and Folley SJ, editors: Lactogenesis, the invitation of milk secretion of parturition, Philadelphia, 1969, University of Pennsylvania Press.

20 seconds revealed the hormone was released in surges and persisted in the circulation for less than 1 minute. The multiparas had a greater total response, but there was no difference between early (1 to 3 days postpartum) and late (5 to 7 days). When a similar study was done by Dawood et al[6] collecting samples only every 3 minutes, no pulsing was identified. Oxytocin was measurable within 2 minutes of suckling, peaked at 10 minutes, and had a bimodal curve dropping to a mean at 20 minutes comparable to that before suckling which followed the burping and changing breasts at about 15 minutes. A secondary peak occurred at 25 minutes. They found maximum response of intramammary pressures at the fifth to seventh day. McNeilly et al[24] measured release of oxytocin in response to suckling in early and established lactation, drawing samples every 30 seconds. A catheter was placed in the forearm 40 minutes before lactation. Oxytocin levels increased 3 to 10 minutes before suckling in response to the baby crying or becoming restless or the mother preparing herself to feed. There was no prolactin response until suckling began.

Most results clearly showed response before tactile stimuli and then a second surge in response to suckling. The levels were pulsatile in nature during suckling and not related to milk volume, prolactin response, or parity of the mother. When oxytocin levels were measured after initiating breast stimulation with mechanical breast pump in early lactation (10 to 90 days), midlactation (90 to 190 days), and late (180 days to 12 months), baseline levels were similar in all three periods. The stimulated plasma oxytocin levels were greater in early than late lactation, but there was always a response. Thus the oxytocin secretory reflex appears to continue for the first year of lactation.

The release of oxytocin by neurohypophyseal responses during lactation has been evoked both by infant's suckling and by mechanical dilation of the mammary ducts. This release of oxytocin was demonstrated to be independent of vasopressin release. Conversely, further study[16,17] demonstrated that there could be stimulation of vasopressin release independent of oxytocin release.*

When the levels of HGH, vasopressin, prolactin, calcitonin, gastrin, insulin, epinephrine, norepinephine, and dopamine were measured by Widstrom et al[44] in six lactating women during breastfeeding, they confirmed the rise in prolactin and demonstrated the progressive increase in insulin that may be secondary to prolactin rise and may participate in stimulating milk production. There was no increase in gastrin but a decline, and there were no consistent findings for calcitonin, HGH, norepinephrine, or epinephrine and no change in dopamine and vasopressin. Vagally stimulated release of insulin and gastrin is antagonized when the tone of the sympathetic nervous system is increased, such as during stress, pain, or anxiety. Increased insulin also is known to stimulate the synthesis of casein and lactalbumin and thus secondarily milk production. It should be advantageous to breastfeed after a meal rather than before (practically, many mothers eat while feeding the infant).

Human myoepithelium, the effector tissue, is specifically stimulated by oxytocin, and this sensitivity and specificity increase throughout pregnancy. Suckling can induce milk secretion, which is under control of the adenohypophysis. In this case, oxytocin released by the neurohypophysis because of the suckling stimulus would cause both milk ejection and release of the anterior pituitary hormones responsible for milk secretion as well. This is probably the mechanism behind relactation and induced lactation in the woman who has never been pregnant. Mammary growth and lactogenesis may be induced by suckling, massage, and breast stimulation in many species.[8]

---

*It has been shown that alcohol has an effect on the CNS in inhibiting milk ejection. This effect is dose related.

Suckling brings about functional changes in the offspring. An infant who sucks on an artificial nipple quickly decreases the amount of body movement, increases mouth activity, and decreases crying. The suckling experience may affect infant behavior and mother-infant interaction. Nonnutritive sucking is observed in many species. In the human infant, nutritive sucking is shown to be a continuous stream of regular sucks with few, if any, pauses. Nonnutritive sucking has bursts of activity alternating with no sucking. Suckling can be altered by extraneous aural, visual, or olfactory stimuli.

Effects of suckling on the mother include the stimulation of afferent nerves for the removal of milk.[18] Reduction in sucking stimulus produces a reduction in prolactin and in milk synthesis. The lactating glands are good at adjusting the milk supply to demand, probably because of both a local and an endocrinologic mechanism. Variations in milk secretion are rapidly reflected in anatomic changes in the mammary gland. Mammary tissue shows regression after the first week or so, if unstimulated. Tissue regression proceeds at a rate parallel to the demand for secretory tissue. Thus, when a suckling infant signals needs, the breast will respond.

There are effects on maternal behavior that have been attributed to lactation. Maternal behavior is more easily defined in many other species, in which early nursing is initiated by the mother, who stimulates the neonate to suckle by grooming. She then presents her mammary gland to the offspring so that the nipple is located with minimal effort. It has been shown that lactating females have a lessened response to stress. In the human, however, there is a strong voluntary nature to nursing behavior.

Investigations of the agile wallaby, *Macropus agilis,* have revealed the let-down reflex as this species displays concurrent asynchronous lactation.[21] The young, weighing 35 g, attach to the teat at birth. The lactating gland continues to grow for 200 days, increasing 10-fold in size. At 200 to 220 days, weighing 2500 g, the young first leave the pouch. Twenty-six days later a second young is born, although the older one continues to suckle intermittently for another 160 days at the original teat. The second young attaches to an unused nipple, which begins to develop, displaying complete autonomy. Measurements of oxytocin over the time of the initial lactation show an increase in intraductal pressure response with a decline in sensitivity over time. This permits milk ejection in response to a small release of oxytocin to be confined to the mammary gland to which the neonate is continuously attached. The release of large quantities of oxytocin in response to the suckling of the juvenile would cause release in both gland.[21] Mammals have thus evolved diverse strategies for survival. Tandem nursing in the human has not been so carefully studied, but there is no known change in let-down, although the milk reverts to colostrum at the birth of the new infant.

If one explores the possible spinal and brain stem pathways by which the suckling stimulus reaches the forebrain, the spinothalamic tract is the most likely. The areas of the forebrain influenced by the sucking stimulus include the hypothalamic structures that mediate oxytocin and prolactin release. The inhibition of milk ejection by visual and auditory stimuli, pinealectomy, and ventrolateral midbrain lesions in lactating rats has been studied to define further the neurohormonal pathways. In these experiments, the pineal gland appeared to mediate an inhibitory visual reflex on both oxytocin release and milk ejection.[11,29]

A mechanism consisting of smooth muscle and elastic fibers acting as a sphincter at the end of the ducts in the nipple appears to prevent most unwanted loss of milk. Sympathetic control does not appear to be present in humans, although it is demonstrable in most other species.

Concentrations of oxytocin in milk

Human milk samples obtained by manual expression daily from the first to the fifth postpartum day were collected immediately before and after a feeding as well as 2 hours post nursing.[35] The baseline mean oxytocin concentrations were 3.3 to 4.7 mg/ml, increasing significantly with nursing. Oxytocin in milk is fairly stable compared to that in maternal serum, which is inactivated by oxytocinase in plasma, liver, and kidney. When H-oxytocin was administered to rat dams, it was also found in the suckling offspring's gastric contents, where it is stable in acid. Some is absorbed into the neonatal blood, where it is unstable. Levels of oxytocin in neonatal serum are produced predominantly by the neonate itself. Whether oxytocin has a physiologic role on the gut or other hormones is unknown.

The role of prostaglandins as milk ejectors

Since prostaglandins have a multitude of physiologic effects and they are known to increase mammary duct pressure, the role of prostaglandins as milk ejectors was investigated.[37] Comparison was made among three treatments: intravenous injections of oxytocin, PGE_2, and 16-phenoxy-PGE_2 given to one group of women on the third to sixth day postpartum; IV oxytocin, 15-methyl-$PGF_{2\alpha}$, and $PGF_{2\alpha}$ tromethamine salt to a second group; and oxytocin and PGF intranasally to a third group. All combinations had some effect, with the intravenous route having a shorter latency period than the intranasal. $PGF_{2\alpha}$, the more potent of the prostaglandin preparations, was more potent via the nasal route than oxytocin nasally. The response lasted 25 minutes after intranasal instillation of 400 µg. Prostaglandin E_2 and $F_{2\alpha}$ orally reduce prolactin levels and appear to be successful in suppressing lactation in the immediate postpartum when given in large doses of 2 to 4 mg or in multiple doses up to 10 times greater. Although they are produced in larger quantities by the mammary gland in vitro and in vivo, the role of prostaglandins is still not clear, as these studies by Toppozada et al[37] are in conflict with previous results by Vorherr.[42] The practical application of this in lactation failure has not been reported.

SYNTHESIS OF HUMAN MILK

The function of the mammary gland is unique in that it produces a material that makes tremendous demands on the maternal system without producing any physiologic advantage to the maternal organism. Because lactation is anticipated, the body prepares the breast anatomically and physiologically.[34] When lactation begins, there is a marked alteration in the metabolism of the mother. There is a redistribution of the blood supply and an increased demand for nutrients, which requires an increased metabolic rate to accommodate the production. The mammary gland may have to produce milk at the metabolic expense of other organs. The supply of materials to the lactating breast for milk production and energy metabolism requires extensive cardiovascular changes in the mother. There is increased mammary blood flow, increased blood flow into the gastrointestinal tract and liver, and a high cardiac output. The mammary blood flow, cardiac output, and milk secretion are suckling dependent. Suckling induces the release of anterior pituitary hormones that act directly on breast tissue.

Milk is isosmotic with plasma in all species. Human milk differs from many other milks in that the concentration of major monovalent ions is lower and of lactose is higher.

If one looks at other milks, the higher the ions, the lower the lactose, and vice versa. Many of the disparities in the intermediary metabolism among species of animals can be linked to evolutionary adaptions involving the digestive process. Nonruminants rely on glucose, derived from carbohydrate in the diet. Ruminants, because of extensive fermentation in the rumen, absorb little glucose. The microbial fermentation products, which include acetate, propionate, and butyrate, play a significant part as energy and carbon sources for tissue metabolism. Amino acids are primary substitutes for glucose in ruminants.

The biosynthesis of milk involves a cellular site where the metabolic processes occur. The epithelial cells of the gland contain stem cells and highly differentiated secretory alveolar cells at the terminal ducts. The stem cells are stimulated by HGH and insulin. Prolactin synergizes the insulin effect to stimulate the cells to secretory activity.

The cells of the acini and smaller milk ducts are active in milk synthesis and the secretion of the milk into the alveoli and smaller milk ducts. Most milk is synthesized during the process of suckling; its production is stimulated by prolactin. Cortisol plasma levels are increased during suckling as well. The secretory cells are cuboidal, changing to a cylindrical shape just before milk secretion, while cellular water uptake is increased. The cell's single nucleus is at the base in the dormant cell but migrates to the apex just prior to milk secretion.

The differentiated structure of the functional cell is acquired gradually during pregnancy, differing little from species to species. Very early in lactation mammary cells show active synthesis and secretion of proteins and fat. The cells are polarized with abundant rough endoplasmic reticulum, Golgi dictyosomes above the nucleus, which is smooth and rounded with many mitochondria. The apical surface has microvilli, and the basal surface

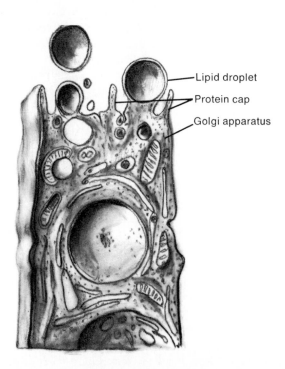

Lipid droplet

Protein cap

Golgi apparatus

Fig. 3-9. Apocrine secretory mechanism for lipids, proteins, and lactose in milk.

is extensively convoluted for the active transport of materials from the bloodstream into the cell. Fat droplets are in the cytoplasm and bulging at the membrane. Proteins, lactose, calcium, phosphate, and citrate are packaged into secretory vesicles and pass into the lumen of the alveolus by exocytosis.

The cytoplasm is finely granular in the resting phase but striated as milk secretion begins. As secretion commences, the enlarged cell with its thickened apical membrane becomes clublike in shape. The tip pinches off, leaving the cell intact. The protein is thus free in the secreted solution, retaining a cap of membrane (Fig. 3-9).

Function of the cellular components of the lactating breast

The schema of the mammary secretory cell is represented in Figs. 3-10 and 3-11.

Nucleus

The nucleus is essential to the duplication of genetic material and the transcription of the genetic code. The nucleus is also considered a regulatory organelle in cell metabolism, transmitting the design of the enzymatic profile of the cell. The DNA and RNA content of the cellular nuclei increases during pregnancy and is highest at the time of lactation.

Cytosol

The cytosol, which consists of the cytoplasm minus the mitochondrial and microsomal fractions, is also called the particle-free supernatant. The cytosol contains enzymes that involve key intermediates and cofactors essential to the process of milk synthesis.

Mitochondrial proliferation

The alveolar cell population of the mammary gland must have a greatly expanded oxidative capacity during lactation. It is supplied by an increase in size and function of the mitochondrial population of the cell.[15] Mitochondria are increased in the epithelial cell at the onset of the lactation process. Mitochondrial proliferation has been observed in all cells with a high metabolic rate and high oxygen utilization.

During the presecretory differentiation phase in late pregnancy and early lactation, each mitochondrion undergoes a type of differentiation in which the inner membrane and matrix expand greatly. As with other cells, the mitochondria are key to the respiratory

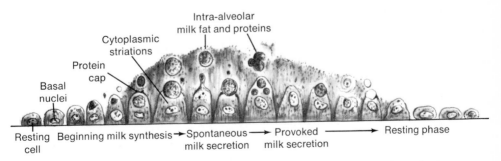

Fig. 3-10.   Diagram of cycle of secretory cells from resting stage to secretion and return to resting stage. (Modified from Vorherr H: The breast, morphology, physiology and lactation, New York, 1974, Academic Press, Inc.)

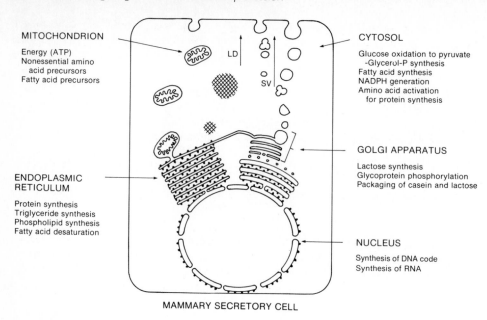

Fig. 3-11.   Schema of cytologic and biochemical interrelationships of secretory cell of mammary gland; *LD*, Lipid droplet; *SV*, secretory vesicle.

activity of the cell. Mitochondria control some cellular metabolism through differential permeability to certain anions. The citrate in the mitochondria is a major source of carbon for fatty acid biosynthesis. Mitochondria also supply the carbon for synthesis of nonessential amino acids.

Microsomal fraction

The microsomal fraction of the cell, which includes the Golgi apparatus, the endoplasmic reticulum, and the cell membranes, is involved in lipid synthesis. The role of the microsomal fraction is also to assemble the constituent parts such as amino acids, glucose, and fatty acids into the final products of protein, carbohydrate, and fat for secretion.

Intermediary metabolism of the mammary gland

The pathways identified for milk synthesis and secretion in the mammary alveolus as described by Neville, Allen, and Walters[27] include:

I. Exocytosis of milk protein and lactose in Golgi-derived secretory vesicles
II. Milk fat secretion via the milk fat globule
III. Secretion of ions and water across the apical membrane
IV. Pinocytosis-exocytosis of immunoglobulins
V. Paracellular pathway for plasma components and leukocytes

Glucose

Glucose metabolism is a key function in milk production. Glucose serves as the main source of energy for other reactions as well as a critical source of carbon. Glucose is critical to the volume of milk produced. Glucose is also used in the production of lactose. The

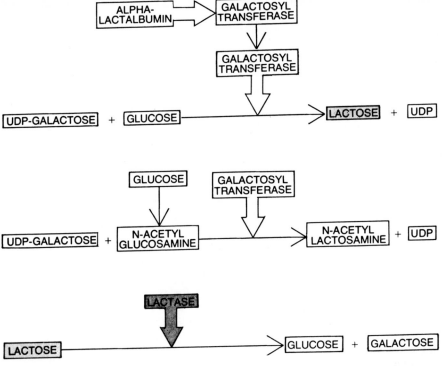

Fig. 3-12.   Synthesis of lactose in mammary gland begins late in pregnancy when specific hormones and protein α-lactalbumin are present. Latter modifies enzyme galactosyl transferase, "specifying" it so that it catalyzes synthesis of lactose from glucose and galactose *(top)*. In nonlactating gland, glucose and galactose *(bottom)*. (From Kretchmer N: Lactose and lactase, Sci Am 227:71, Copyright © 1972 by Scientific American, Inc. All rights reserved.)

synthesis of lactose combines glucose and galactose, the latter originating from glucose-6-phosphate.[13]

Lactose synthesis is carried out by the following equation:

$$\text{UDP-galactose} + N\text{-acetylglucosamine} \rightarrow N\text{-acetyllactosamine} + \text{UDP} \qquad \textbf{(1)}$$

$$\text{UDP-galactose} + \text{Glucose} \rightarrow \text{Lactose} + \text{UDP} \qquad \textbf{(2)}$$

UDP is uridine diphosphogalactose. The catalyst in equation 1 is a galactosyl transferase, *N*-acetyllactosamine synthetase.

Most of the intracellular glucose is derived from blood sugar. A specific whey protein, α-lactalbumin, catalyzes the lactose synthesis (Fig. 3-12). It is a rate-limiting enzyme, which is inhibited by progesterone during pregnancy. In the absence of α-lactalbumin, little lactose is present. With the drop in progesterone and estrogen levels after the removal of the placenta at delivery, there is an increase in prolactin. The synthesis of α-lactalbumin becomes greater, and large amounts of lactose are produced from glucose. Progesterone regulates the onset of lactose synthesis, causing the initiation of production just as the infant is in need of nutrition.

Various aspects of lactose synthesis continue to be vigorously investigated.[13] The molecular mechanism of lactose synthesis is activated by metal ions, manganese (Mn), and calcium (Ca). Lactose synthesis takes place within the Golgi apparatus. The onset of copious milk secretion is dependent upon rapid increase of lactose synthesis. Lactose synthetase performs the rate-limiting step in lactose synthesis. Lactose synthesis is one of the few anabolic reactions involving glucose itself, rather than a phosphorylated derivative. Although progesterone, thyroxine, and lactogenic hormones are important in controlling synthesis, it is not known how they act in this system. The areas available for investigation about lactose synthesis remain vast.

Fat

Fat synthesis takes place in the endoplasmic reticulum. The alveolar cells are able to synthesize short-chain fatty acids, which are derived predominantly from acetate. Long-chain fatty acids, derived chiefly from blood plasma, are used in milk fat. Triglycerides are utilized from the plasma, as well as synthesized from intracellular glucose oxidized via the pentose pathway. Synthesis of fat from carbohydrate plays a predominant role in fat production in human milk.

Two enzymes, lipoprotein lipase and palmitoyl-CoA L-glycerol-3-phosphate palmitoyl transferase, increase markedly after delivery. The lipase acts at the walls of the capillaries to catalyze the lipolysis and uptake of glycerol into the epithelial cells. The transerase catalyzes the process of synthesizing glycerides to triglycerides. It is believed that the marked increase of the lipase and transferase is stimulated by prolactin. Hormonal control of the glycerol precursors and the enzymatic release of fatty acids, leading to the formation of triglycerides, have been associated not only with prolactin but also with insulin, which stimulates the uptake of glucose into the mammary cells.

Esterification of fatty acids takes place in the endoplasmic reticulum. The triglycerides subsequently accumulate into fat droplets in several cisternae. The small droplets sit on the base of the cell and coalesce to large droplets that move toward the apex of the cell. The fat droplets are engulfed in the apical membrane and project into the alveolar lumen. The discharge of fat droplets involves the bulging of the cell apex to envelop the fat globules, protein, and a small amount of cytoplasm; with the pinching off, the globule becomes detached into the lumen. The membrane of the fat globule contains all the normal plasma enzymes. The fat droplets contain predominantly polar lipid and phosphatidyl choline.

Fatty acid synthesis involves a source of substrates and associated enzymes for their conversion to acetyl-CoA and NADPH in the cytoplasm of the cell and the conversion of acetyl-CoA to malonyl-CoA. The newly synthesized fatty acid is then released from the fatty acid synthetase complex.

Protein

Most proteins in milk are formed from free amino acids in the secretory cells of the mammary gland. The definitive data confirming the origin of milk proteins were accumulated in the past two decades. The vast majority of proteins present in normal milk are specific to mammary secretions and are not identified in any quantity elsewhere in nature.[16]

The formation of milk protein and mammary enzymes is induced by prolactin and further stimulated by insulin and cortisol. De novo synthesis of protein uses both essential and nonessential plasma amino acids. Nuclear RNAs, induced by prolactin, stimulate synthesis of messenger and transfer RNA. The *m*RNA conveys the genetic information to

Table 3-2. Alveolar epithelial membrane permeability

Cell ↔ alveolar lumen	Cell → alveolar lumen
Glucose	Lactose
Water	Sucrose
Sodium	Citrate
Potassium	Proteins
Calcium	Fat
Chloride	
Iodine	
Phosphate	
Sulfate	

the protein-synthesizing centers of the cells. The transfer RNA interprets the message to assemble the amino acids in the appropriate sequence of polypeptide chains of the specific milk proteins. The newly synthesized proteins are secreted into the milk during lactation. Casein, α-lactalbumin, and β-lactoglobulin from plasma amino acids are synthesized on the ribosomes of the endoplasmic reticulum, where they are condensed and appear as visible secretory granules moving toward the cellular apex. Proteins are discharged predominantly by apocrine secretion. There is, however, some merocrine secretion, in which proteins and other cellular constituents are secreted, leaving the cell membrane intact. Protein caps or signets, protruding into alveolar lumen, have been described on the outside of the apical membrane. Protein and lactose secreted into the lumen cannot be reabsorbed (Table 3-2).

The synthesis of proteins in the mammary gland follows the general pathway of all proteins under genetic control. Induction of synthesis is under hormonal control. This process involves synthesis from amino acids via the detailed system controlled by RNA and under genetic control of DNA. There is an absolute requirement of glucocorticoid for the expression of the casein gene in the presence of prolactin. In fact, cortisol is the limiting factor for casein gene expression.[10]

Ions and water

Sodium, potassium, chloride, magnesium, calcium, phosphate, sulfate, and citrate pass the membrane of the alveolar cell in both directions. Water also passes in both directions, predominantly from the alveolar cells but also from the interstitial fluid. Plasma water passage depends on the amount of intracellular glucose available for lactose. The aqueous phase of milk is isosmotic to plasma. The major osmole of the aqueous phase of milk is lactose. The concentrations of sodium and chloride are less than those in plasma.

Human milk differs from that of many other species in that the monovalent ions are in low concentration and lactose is in high concentration.[18] The osmolarity is the same, that is, isosmotic with plasma; thus the higher the lactose, the lower the ions. It is presumed that the intracellular concentration of potassium is held high and that of sodium low by a pump on the basal membrane. The sodium and potassium ions are distributed according to the electrical potential gradient. Milk is electrically positive compared to intracellular fluid. The ratio of sodium to potassium is 1:3 in both milk and intracellular fluid. It is thought by Vorherr[41,42] that lactose secretion is responsible for the potential difference across the apical membrane, thus keeping sodium and potassium ion concentration low.

The variation among species in the concentration of lactose and ions is due to the rate of lactose synthesis, the permeability of the membrane, and the number of fixed negative charges on the membrane. The potential difference is higher in the human mammary gland than in any other species evaluated to date.

The relationship between intrastructure and function in the mammary gland changes from pregnancy to lactation. The junction between alveolar cells has attracted much interest. Cell junctions do not merely hold cells together but enable epithelia to function as permeable barriers, allowing communication between cells and coordination of actvities. The three functions of cell junctions are adhesion, occlusion, and communication, which are carried out by desmosomes, tight junctions, and gap junctions, respectively. Changes in tight junctions may provide the basis for a reduction in permeability between cells. For instance, at the initiation of lactation, a tight junction changing from "leaky" to very tight blocks the paracellular movement of lactose and ions. This requires instead transport across cells of these materials and the maintenance of control of high intracellular potassium and low intracellular sodium concentrations.[7]

Citrate is the main buffer system of milk. It is formed within the secretory cell, but how it is secreted into the milk is not clear. It is suggested that citrate and lactose are secreted by a similar route. Following the dilution of milk in the gland with isosmotic lactose, the equilibrium is restored across the apical membrane in experimental models by the entrance of sodium, potassium, and chloride into the milk. No citrate, calcium, or protein enters in excess of the normal secretion rate. Inorganic phosphate is the other major buffer system, but how it is secreted is also unknown.

Calcium, much of which is bound to casein, enters the Golgi apparatus, where it is essentially trapped, and then enters the alveolar milk by unidirectional flow.

Milk enzymes

Some milk enzymes enter the alveolar milk from the mammary blood capillaries via the intercellular fluid. Others come from the breakdown of the mammary secretory cells. The milk enzymes, xanthine oxidase, aldolase, and alkaline phosphatase, are contained in the fat globule, membrane, and milk serum. The most significant enzyme, lipase, splits triglycerides. Amylase, catalase, peroxidase, and alkaline and acid phosphatase are not known to contribute to the infant's digestion of human milk.

Cellular components

Human milk has been called a live fluid by many and "white blood" in many ancient rites. Breast milk contains about 4000 cells/ml, which have been identified with leukocytes and enter the milk via the paracellular pathway, pathway V.[40] The cell number is particularly high in colostrum. The cells in greatest number are the macrophages, which secrete lysozyme and lactoferrin. Lymphocytes, neutrophils, and epithelial cells are also present. Lymphocytes produce IgA and interferon.

REFERENCES

1. Aono T, Shioji T, Shoda T et al: The initiation of human lactation and prolactin response to suckling, J Clin Endocrinol Metab 44:1101, 1977.
2. Baltin DA, Marrs RP, Fleiss PM et al: Effect of suckling on serum prolactin, luteinizing hormone, follicle-stimulating hormone, and estradiol during prolonged lactation, Obstet Gynecol 65:785, 1985.
3. Caldeyro-Barcia R: Milk ejection in women. In Reynolds M and Folley SJ, editors: Lactogenesis, the initiation of milk secretion at parturition, Philadelphia, 1969, University of Pennsylvania Press.

4. Cholst IN, Wardlaw SL, Newman CB et al: Prolactin response to breast stimulation in lactating women is not mediated by endogenous opioids, Am J Obstet Gynecol 150:558, 1984.

5. Cowie AT, Forsyth IA, and Hart IC: Hormonal control of lactation. Monographs in endocrinology, vol 15, New York, 1980, Springer-Verlag.

6. Dawood MY, Khan-Dawood FS, Wahi RS et al: Oxytocin release and plasma anterior pituitary and gonadal hormones in women during lactation, J Clin Endocrinol Metab 52:678, 1981.

7. Falconer IR and Rowe JM: Effect of prolactin on sodium and potassium concentration in the mammary alveolar tissue, Endocrinology 101:181, 1977.

8. Fournier PRJ, Desjardins PD, and Friesen HG: Current understanding of human prolactin physiology and its diagnostic and therapeutic applications: a review, Am J Obstet Gynecol 118:337, 1974.

9. Frantz AG: Prolactin, Physiol Med 298:201, 1978.

10. Ganguly R et al: Absolute requirement of glucocorticoids for expression of the casein gene in the presence of prolactin, Proc Nat Acad Sci USA 77:6003, 1980.

11. Hansen S and Gumme BM: Participation of the lateral midbrain tegmentum in the neuro endocrine control of sexual behavior and lactation in the rat, Brain Res 251:319, 1982.

12. Hartmann PE: Changes in the composition and yield of the mammary secretion of cows during the initiation of lactation, J Endocrinol 59:231, 1973.

13. Healy DL et al: Prolactin in human milk: correlation with lactose, total protein, and of lactalbumin levels, Am J Physiol 238 (Endocrinol Metab 1):E83, 1980.

14. Howie PW, McNeilly AS, McArdle T et al: The relationship between suckling-induced prolactin response and lactogenesis, J Clin Endocrinol Metab 50:670, 1980.

15. Jones DH: The mitochondria of the mammary parenchymal cell in relation to the pregnancy-lactation cycle. In Larson BL, editor: Lactation, vol 4, The mammary gland/human lactation/milk synthesis, New York, 1978, Academic Press, Inc.

16. Larson BL, editor: Lactation, vol 4, The mammary gland/human lactation/milk synthesis, New York, 1978, Academic Press, Inc.

17. Larson BL and Smith VR, editors: Lactation, vol 2, Biosynthesis and secretion of milk/diseases, New York, 1974, Academic Press, Inc.

18. Larson BL and Smith VR, editors: Lactation, vol 3, Nutrition and biochemistry of milk/maintenance, New York, 1974, Academic Press, Inc.

19. Leake RD, Waters CB, Rubin RT et al: Oxytocin and prolactin responses in long term breast-feeding, Obstet Gynecol 62:565, 1983.

20. Lincoln DW and Paisley AC: Neuroendocrine control of milk ejection, J Reprod Fert 65:571, 1982.

21. Lincoln DW and Renfree MB: Mammary gland growth and milk ejection in the agile wallaby, *Macropus agilis,* displaying concurrent asynchronous lactation, J Reprod Fert 63:193, 1981.

22. Lucas A, Drewett RB, and Mitchell MD: Breast-feeding plasma oxytocin concentrations, Br Med J 281:834, 1980.

23. Martin RH, Glass MR, Chapman C et al: Human and lactalbumin and hormonal factors in pregnancy and lactation, Clin Endocrinol 13:223, 1980.

24. McNeilly AS, Robinson ICA, Houston MJ et al: Release of oxytocin and prolactin in response to suckling, Br Med J 281:834, 1980.

25. Meites J: Neuroendocrinology of lactation, J Invest Dermatol 63:119, 1974.

26. Neville MC: Regulation of mammary development and lactation. In Neville MC and Neifert MR, editors: Lactation: physiology, nutrition, and breast-feeding, New York, 1983, Plenum Press.

27. Neville MC, Allen JC, and Walters C: The mechanisms of milk secretion. In Neville MC and Neifett MR, editors: Lactation: physiology, nutrition, and breast-feeding, New York, 1983, Plenum Press.

28. Perry HM and Jacobs LS: Rabbit mammary prolactin receptors, J Biol Chem 253:1560, 1978.

29. Prilusky J and Deis RP: Inhibition of milk ejection by a visual stimulus in lactating rats: implications of the pineal gland, Brain Res 251:313, 1982.

30. Rimoin DL et al: Lactation in the absence of human growth hormone, J Clin Endocrinol Metab 28:1183, 1968.

31. Robinson JE and Short RV: Changes in breast sensitivity at puberty, during the menstrual cycle, and at parturition, Br Med J I:1188, 1977.

32. Robyn C and Meuris S: Pituitary prolactin, lactational performance and puerperal infertility, Semin Perinatol 6:254, 1982.

33. Sherwood LM: Human prolactin, N Engl J Med 284:774, 1971.

34. Smith VR: Lactation, vol 1, The mammary gland/development and maintenance, New York, 1974, Academic Press, Inc.

35. Takeda S, Kuinabara Y, and Mizuno M: Concentrations and origin of oxytocin in breast milk, Endocrinol Japan 33:821, 1986.

36. Tanada T et al: A new sensitive and specific bioassay for lactogenic hormones: measurement of prolactin and growth hormone in human serum, J Clin Endocrinol Metab 51:1058, 1980.

37. Toppozada MK, El-Rahman HA, and Soliman AY: Prostaglandins as milk ejectors: the nose as a new route of administration. In Samuelson B, Paoletti R, and Rawell P, editors: Advances in prostaglandin, thromboxane, and leukotrience research, vol 12, New York, 1983, Raven Press.

38. Tyson JE: Mechanisms of puerperal lactation, Med Clin North Am 61:153, 1977.

39. Vigneri R et al: Spontaneous fluctuations of human placental lactogen during normal pregnancy, J Clin Endocrinol Metab 40:506, 1975.

40. Vorherr H: The breast, morphology, physiology and lactation, New York, 1974, Academic Press, Inc.

41. Vorherr H: Human lactation and breastfeeding. In Larson BL, editor: Lactation IV. The mammary gland/human lactation/milk synthesis, New York, 1978, Academic Press, Inc.

42. Vorherr H: Hormonal and biochemical changes of pituitary and breast during pregnancy. In Vorherr H, editor: Human lactation, Semin Perinatol 3:193, 1979.

43. Weitzman RE, Leake RD, Rubin RT et al: The effect of nursing on neurohypophyseal hormone and prolactin secretion in human subjects, J Clin Endocrinol Metab 51:836, 1980.

44. Widstrom AM, Winberg J, Werner S et al: Suckling in lactating women stimulates the secretion of insulin and prolactin without concomitant effects on gastrin, growth hormone, calcitonin, vasopressin, or catecholamines, Early Hum Develop 10:115, 1984.

Biochemistry of human milk

4

The biochemistry of human milk encompasses a mammoth supply of scientific data and information, most of which has been generated since 1970. Each report or study adds a tiny piece to the complex puzzle of the nutrients that make up human milk. The answers to some questions still elude us. A question as simple as the volume of milk consumed at a feeding remains a scientific challenge. The methodology must be accurate, reproducible, noninvasive, and suitable for home use night or day and must not interrupt breastfeeding. The perfect method has not been found. On the other hand, the precision analysis available for measuring the concentration of the most miniscule of elements is remarkably accurate and reproducible in the laboratory. The discussion in this chapter will be limited to information perceived as immediately useful to the clinician. Considerable detail and species variability will be eliminated to help focus attention on details directly influencing management. A number of extensive and exhaustive reviews will be referenced to provide the reader with easy access to greater detail and validation of the general conclusions reported here.

Human milk is not a uniform body fluid but a secretion of the mammary gland of changing composition. Foremilk differs from hindmilk. Colostrum differs from transitional and mature milks. Milk changes over time of day and as time goes by. As concentrations of protein, fat, carbohydrates, minerals, and cells differ, physical properties such as osmolarity and pH change. The impact of changing composition on the physiology of the infant gut is beginning to be appreciated.

The constituents of milk include a tremendous array of molecules whose descriptions continue to be refined as qualitative and quantitative laboratory techniques are perfected. Resolution of lipid chemicals has advanced dramatically in recent years, but new carbohydrates and proteins have been identified as well. Some of the compounds identified may well be intermediary products in the process that occurs within the mammary cells and may be only incidental in the final product.[128]

Human and bovine milk are known in the greatest detail.[50] There is, however, much information about the milk of five other species: the water buffalo, goat, sheep, horse, and pig. There are miscellaneous data on the milk of 150 more species and no data at all on another 4000 species. Jenness and Sloan[68] have compiled a summary of 140 species from which a sampling has been extracted (Table 4-1). Jenness and Sloan have further pointed out that the constituents of milk can be divided into the following groups, according to their specificity:

1. Constituents specific to both organ and species (example: most proteins and lipids)
2. Constituents specific to organ but not to species (example: lactose)
3. Constituents specific to species but not to organ (example: albumin and some immunoglobulins)

Table 4-1. Constituents of milk of specific mammals

Mammalian species in taxonomic position	Total solids (g/100 g)	Fat (g/100 g)	Casein (g/100 g)	Whey protein (g/100 g)	Total protein (g/100 g)	Lactose (g/100 g)	Ash (g/100 g)
Man	12.4	3.8	0.4	0.6		7.0	0.2
Baboon	14.4	5.0			1.6	7.3	0.3
Orangutan	11.5	3.5	1.1	0.4		6.0	0.2
Black bear	44.5	24.5	8.8	5.7		0.4	1.8
California sea lion	52.7	36.5			13.8	0.0	0.6
Black rhinoceros	8.1	0.0	1.1	0.3		6.1	0.3
Spotted dolphin	31.0	18.0			9.4	0.6	—
Domestic dog	23.5	12.9	5.8	2.1		3.1	1.2
Norway rat	21.0	10.3	6.4	2.0		2.6	1.3
Whitetail jack-rabbit	40.8	13.9	19.7	4.0		1.7	1.5

Modified from Jenness R and Sloan RE: Composition of milk. In Larson BL and Smith VR, editors: Lactation, vol 3, Nutrition and biochemistry of milk/maintenance, New York, 1974, Academic Press, Inc.

NORMAL VARIATIONS IN HUMAN MILK

In defining the constituents of human milk, it is important to recognize that the composition varies with the stage of lactation, the time of day, the sampling time during a given feeding, maternal nutrition, and individual variation. Many early interpretations of the content of human milk were based on spot samples or even pooled samples from multiple donors at different times and stages of lactation. Samples obtained by pumping may vary from those obtained by the suckling infant, since there is some variation in content between the various methods of pumping.

Daytime consumption of milk in a given infant has been shown by Brown et al[11] to be 46% to 58% of the total 24-hour consumption, so that reliance on less than a 24-hour sampling may be misleading. Data from samples taken every 3 hours showed a variation in milk concentration of nitrogen, lactose, and fat, as well as in the volume of milk, by time of day (Fig. 4-1). Furthermore, there were statistically significant diurnal changes in the concentration of lactose and the volume within individual subjects, but the times of those changes were not consistent for each individual. Some individuals varied as much as twofold in volume production from day to day. These investigators also found a significant difference in the concentrations of fat and lactose and in the volume of milk produced by each breast. At the extreme, the less productive breast yielded only 65% of the volume of the other breast.

The variation in the fat content has received some attention. Fat content changes during a given feeding, increasing at the end of the feeding. Fat content rises from early morning to midday; the volume increased from two to five times as reported in early studies when feedings were controlled. Multiple studies in different countries and different decades are summarized by Jackson et al[64] to reveal that some of the variation is related to other factors. Demand feeding (Thai mothers in 1988) has a different circadian variation than scheduled feeding (U.S. mothers in 1932). (See Fig. 4-2.) In the later part of the first year

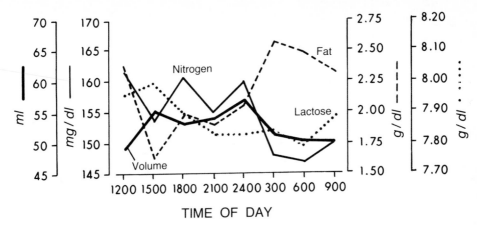

Fig. 4-1. Mean concentrations of nitrogen, lactose, and fat in human milk by time of day. (Modified from Brown KH et al: Am J Clin Nutr 35:745, 1982.)

of lactation, the fat content diminishes. Work done by Atkinson et al[6] and confirmed by other investigators has shown that the nitrogen content of the milk of mothers who deliver prematurely is higher than that of those whose pregnancies reach full term. For a given volume of milk, the premature infant would receive 20% more nitrogen than the full-term infant if each were fed its own mother's milk. Other constituents of milk produced by mothers who deliver prematurely have also been studied and are discussed in Chapter 14.

An additional consideration in reviewing information available on the levels of various constituents of milk is the technique used to derive the data. In 1977, Hambraeus[49] reported that there was less protein in human milk than originally calculated. The present techniques of immunoassay measure the absolute amounts, whereas earlier figures were derived from calculations based on measurements of the nitrogen content. About 25% of the nitrogen in human milk is nonprotein nitrogen. Cow's milk has only 5% nonprotein nitrogen.

A major concern about variation in content of human milk is related to the mother's diet. Maternal diet is of particular concern when the mother is malnourished or eats an unusually restrictive diet. Malnourished mothers have approximately the same proportions of protein, fat, and carbohydrate as well-nourished mothers, but they produce less milk. Water-soluble vitamins, ascorbic acid, thiamin, and B_{12} levels are quickly affected by deficient diets.

COLOSTRUM

The consistently identifiable stages of human milk are colostrum, transitional milk, and mature milk, and their relative contents are significant for the newborn infant and its physiological adaption to extrauterine life.

The first postpartum week's mammary secretion consists of a yellowish, thick fluid, colostrum. The residual mixture of materials present in the mammary glands and ducts at delivery and immediately after is progressively mixed with newly secreted milk, forming colostrum. Human colostrum is known to differ from mature milk in composition, both in the nature of its components and in the relative proportions of these components.

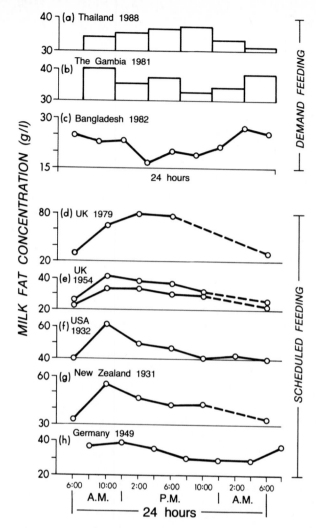

Fig. 4-2. Circadian variation in fat concentration of breast milk from published studies. **A,** Thailand (present study)—Pre-/postfeed expressed samples, 19 mothers studied for 24 h each, infants aged 1 to 9 months. **B,** The Gambia (Prentice et al)—Demand feeding, pre-/post expressed samples, 16 mothers studied for 24 h each, infants aged 1 to 18 months. **C,** Bangladesh (Brown et al)—Samples collected at scheduled intervals by total breast extraction (breast pump), seven mothers studied for 24 h each, infants aged 1 to 9 months. **D,** UK (Hall)—Pre-/post-feed expressed samples, one mother studied for 72 h. **E,** UK (Hytten)—Samples collected by total breast extraction (breast pump). *1,* 29 mothers studied for 24 h each, infants aged 3 to 8 days. *2,* 20 mothers studied for 24 h each, infants aged 21 days to 4 months. **F,** USA (Nims et al)—Samples collected by total breast extraction (manual), three mothers studied, but values only given for one mother, studied for 24 h on six occasions and 72 h on one occasion, infant aged 6 to 60 weeks. **G,** New Zealand (Deem)—Samples collected by total breast extraction (manual), 28 mothers studied for 24 h each, infants aged 1 to 8 months. **H,** Germany (Gunther and Stainier)—Collection of samples by total breast extraction (manual), two mothers studied for 24 h each, six mothers studied for 52 h each, infants aged 8 to 11 days. (Modified from Jackson DA, Imong SM, Sildrasert A et al: Br J Nutr 59:349, 1988.)

Colostrum's specific gravity is 1.040 to 1.060. The mean energy value is 67 kcal/100 ml compared with the 75 kcal/100 ml of mature milk. The volume varies between 2 and 20 dl per feeding in the first 3 days. The volume also varies with the parity of the mother. Women who have had other pregnancies, particularly those who have nursed infants previously, have colostrum more readily available at delivery, and the volume increases more rapidly. The yellow color is due to β-carotene. The ash content is high, and the concentrations of sodium, potassium, and chloride are greater than in mature milk. Protein, fat-soluble vitamins, and minerals are present in greater percentages than in transitional or mature milk.

The higher protein, lower fat, and lactose solution is rich in immunoglobulins, especially sIgA. The number of immunologically competent mononuclear cells is at its highest level. Fat, contained mainly in the core of the fat globules, increases from 2% in colostrum to 2.9% in transitional and to 3.6% in mature milk. Concentration of fat in the prepartum secretion was only 1 g/dl, and the distribution among classes of lipids differed. Prepartum milk was 93% triglycerides, increasing to 97% in colostrum with diglycerides, monoglycerides, and free fatty acids all increasing from pre- to postpartum secretions. Phospholipid levels declined during the same period. Prepartum secretions contain higher amounts of membrane components such as phospholipids, cholesterol, and cholesteryl esters, which decline from colostrum to mature milk.

Cholesterol appears to be synthesized in the mammary gland. The role of cholesterol in human milk beyond its use in brain tissue development remains elusive except the belief that the composition of human milk is best for human infants. Long-range controlled prospective studies may bring the answer closer.

Colostrum facilitates the establishment of bifidus flora in the digestive tract. Colostrum also facilitates the passage of meconium. Meconium contains an essential growth factor for *Lactobacillus bifidus* and is the first culture medium in the sterile intestinal lumen of the newborn infant. Human colostrum is rich in antibodies, which may provide protection against the bacteria and viruses that are present in the birth canal and associated with other human contact.

The progressive changes in mammary secretion in both breastfeeding and nonbreast-feeding women between 28 and 110 days before delivery and up to 5 months after delivery were followed by Kulski and Hartman[79] to study the initiation of lactation. During late pregnancy the secretion contained higher concentrations of proteins and lower concentrations of lactose, glucose, and urea than those contained in milk secreted when lactation was well established. The concentrations of sodium, chloride, and magnesium were higher and those of potassium and calcium were lower in colostrum than in milk. The osmolarity was relatively constant throughout the study. The authors described a two-phase development of lactation with an initial phase of limited secretion in late pregnancy and a true induction of lactation in the second phase, 32 to 40 hours postpartum. Comparison with the nonlactating women revealed similar secretion during the first 3 days postpartum. This, however, was abruptly reversed during the next 6 days as mammary involution progressed. Obtaining samples in these women, however, may have served to prolong the period of production. The authors point out that although breastfeeding was not necessary for the initiation of lactation in this study, it was essential for the continuation of lactation.

The yield of milk has been calculated from absolute values to demonstrate the increase in output of milk constituents during lactogenesis (Fig. 4-3). There were dramatic increases in the production of all the milk constituents. The components synthesized by the mammary epithelium (lactose, lactalbumin, and lactoferrin) increased at a rate greater than those for

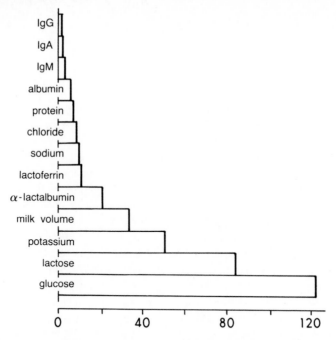

Fig. 4-3. Relative increase in yield of milk components from day 1 to day 7 postpartum. Values presented are for day 7 expressed as percentage increase over day 1. (Modified from Kulski JK and Hartman PE: Aust J Exp Biol Med Sci 59:101, 1981.)

IgA or proteins derived from the serum IgG and IgM. The greatest difference in yield between day 1 and day 7 postpartum was for glucose.

A survey of the fatty acid components by Read and Sarriff[106] showed the lauric acid and myristic acid contents to be low in concentration the first few days. When the lauric and myristic acids increased, C_{18} acids decreased. Palmitoleic acid increased at the same rate as the myristic acid. From this it was concluded that the early fatty acids are derived from extramammary sources, but the breast quickly begins to synthesize fatty acids for the production of transitional and mature milk (Table 4-2). The total fat content may have a predictive value, since it was shown by Hytten[61] that 90% of the women whose milk contained 20 g or more of fat per feeding on the seventh day were successfully breastfeeding 3 months later. Women who only had 5 to 10 g of fat on the seventh day had an 80% dropout rate by 3 months.

Colostrum's high protein and low fat are in keeping with the needs and reserves of the newborn at birth. Although the content of total nitrogen or any amino acid in breast milk in 24 hours is grossly related to the volume produced, the concentration in milligrams per 100 ml is not so related. The relative distribution of the individual amino acids in each 100 ml of milk differs in each mother. The colostrum may actually reflect a transitional maternal blood picture, which is associated with nitrogen metabolism of the postpartum period. The postpartum period is one of involution of body tissue and catabolism of protein in the mother.

The mineral and vitamin reserves of the newborn infant are related to the maternal diet. A fetal supply of vitamin C, iron, and amino acids is adequate, since infant blood

Table 4-2. Fat distribution in milk

	Prepartum		Postpartum		
	Early	Late	Colostrum	Transitional	Mature
Fat (%)			2	2.9	3.6
Fat (g)			2.9	3.6	3.8
Lipid g/dl	1.15	1.28	3.16	3.49	4.14
Phospholipid (mg/dl)	37	40	35	31	27
Percent of total lipid	3.2	3.1	1.1	0.9	0.6
Cholesterol (mg/dl)			29	20	13.5

levels exceed those of the mother. Colostrum is rich in fat-soluble vitamin A, carotenoids, and vitamin E. The average vitamin A level on the third day can be three times that of mature milk. Similarly, carotenoids in colostrum may be ten times the level in mature milk, and vitamin E may be two to three times greater than in mature milk.

TRANSITIONAL MILK

The milk produced between the colostrum and mature milk stages is transitional milk; its content gradually changes. The transitional phase is approximately from 7 to 10 days postpartum to 2 weeks postpartum. The concentration of immunoglobulins and total protein decreases, while the lactose, fat, and total caloric content increase. The water-soluble vitamins increase, and the fat-soluble vitamins decrease to the levels of mature milk.

In a study of transitional milks, breast milk samples were obtained from healthy mothers of term infants on the first, third, fifth, eighth, fifteenth, twenty-second, twenty-ninth, and thirty-sixth days of lactation by Hibberd et al,[59] who defined the first day of lactation to be the third day postpartum. Twenty-four-hour samples were pooled for analysis and the remainder fed to the baby. The authors found a high degree of variability, not only between mothers but also within samples from the same mother. The maximum value in almost every case was more than twice the minimum. They were able to show, however, that the changes in composition were rapid before day 8, and then progressively less change took place until the composition was relatively stable before day 36.

MATURE MILK
Water

In almost all mammalian milks, water is the constituent in the largest quantity, with the exception of the milk of some arctic and aquatic species, who produce milks with high fat content (e.g., the northern fur seal produces milk with 54% fat and 65% total solids) (Table 4-1). All other constituents are dissolved, dispersed, or suspended in water. Water contributes to the temperature-regulating mechanism of the newborn because 25% of his heat loss is from evaporation of water from the lungs and skin. The lactating woman has a greatly increased obligatory water intake. If water intake is restricted during lactation, other water losses through urine and insensible loss are decreased before water for lactation is diminished. Because lactose is the regulating factor in the amount of milk produced, the secretion of water into milk is partially regulated by lactose synthesis. Investigations by Almroth[2] show that the water requirement of infants in a hot humid climate can be provided entirely by the water in human milk.

Lipids

By percentage of concentration, the second greatest constituent in milk is the lipid fraction. Milk lipids also provide the major fraction of kilocalories in human milk and are the most variable constituent.[69,70] Fats are also the most variable constituents in human milk, varying in concentration over a feeding, over a day's time, and over time itself. This information is significant when testing milk samples for energy intake, fat-soluble constituents, and physiologic variation, and for clinically managing lactation problems. Much of the early work was based on lactation in women who "nursed by the clock" rather than tuned into infant needs. When circadian variation in fat content was studied in a rural Thai population who had practiced demand feeding for centuries, Jackson found fat concentrations in feeds in the afternoon and evening (1,600 to 2,000 hours) were higher than those during the night (400 to 800 hours).[64] Fat concentrations at start and finish of feed varied over 24 hours. The most important predictor of fat content was length of time since last feed; the longer the interval, the lower the fat concentration. Fat content at the end of a previous feed and milk intake at previous feed also influenced levels. It is speculated that the altered posture at night, horizontal and relatively inactive, may redistribute fat. The larger the milk consumption at a feed, the greater the increase in fat from the beginning to the end of the feed. There was less fat change during "sleep" feeds than in the daytime.

During the course of a feeding, the fluid phase within the gland was mixed with fat droplets in increasing concentration. The fat droplets are released when the smooth muscle contracts in response to the let-down reflex. The lipid fraction is extractable by suitable solvents and may require more than one technique to extract all the lipids[82] (Table 4-3). Complete extraction in human milk is difficult because of the lipids bound to protein. From 30% to 55% of the kilocalories are derived from fats; this represents a concentration of 3.5 to 4.5 g/100 ml. Milk fat is dispersed in the form of droplets or globules maintained in solution by an absorbed layer or membrane. The protective membrane of the fat globules is made up of phospholipid complexes. The rest of the phospholipids found in human milk are dispersed in the skim milk fraction. Triglycerides, diglycerides, monoglycerides, free fatty acids, phospholipids, glycolipids, sterols, and sterol esters are found in human milk. Vitamin A esters, vitamin D, vitamin K, alkylglyceryl ethers, and glyceryl ether diesters are also in the lipid fraction but do not fall into the classes listed.

Renewed interest in defining the constituents of human milk lipid has developed in recent years as investigators look for the causes of obesity, atherosclerosis, and other degenerative diseases and their relationship to infant nutrition (Table 4-4). A number of reports of historical value are plagued with the technical problems of sampling. Because the fat content of a feeding varies with time, spot samples give spurious results. Jensen and associates[69] have reviewed the literature exhaustively and describe the fractionated lipid constituents in detail.

The average fat content of pooled 24-hour samples has been reported from various sources to vary in mature milk from 2.10% to 3.33%. Maternal diet affects the constituents

Table 4-3. Effects of dietary cholesterol, phytosterol, and polyunsaturate (P)/saturate (S) ratio on human milk sterols

Milk component	Maternal ad lib diet (P/S 0.53) (mg/100 g fat)	Low cholesterol/high phytosterol diet (P/S 1.8) (mg/100 g fat)	High cholesterol/ low phytosterol diet (P/S 0.12) (mg/100 g fat)
Cholesterol	240 ± 40	250 ± 10	250 ± 20
Phytosterol	17 ± 3	220 ± 30	70 ± 10
Dietary cholesterol	450 ± 30	130 ± 5	460 ± 90
Dietary phytosterol	23 ± 8	790 ± 17	80 ± 1
Total fat (%)	3.58 ± 0.56	2.69 ± 0.17	2.66 ± 0.16

From Lammi-Keefe CJ and Jensen RG: J Pediatr Gastroenterol Nutr 3:172, 1984.

Table 4-4. Composition of milks obtained from different mammals and the growth rate of their offspring

Species	Days required to double birth weight	Content of milk (%)			
		Fat	Protein	Lactose	Ash
Man	180	3.8	0.9	7.0	0.2
Horse	60	1.9	2.5	6.2	0.5
Cow	47	3.7	3.4	4.8	0.7
Reindeer	30	16.9	11.5	2.8	—
Goat	19	4.5	2.9	4.1	0.8
Sheep	10	7.4	5.5	4.8	1.0
Rat	6	15.0	12.0	3.0	2.0

From Hambraeus L: Pediatr Clin North Am 24:17, 1977.

of the lipids but not the total amount of fat. A minimal increase in total lipid content was observed when an extra 1000 kcal of corn oil was fed to lactating mothers. A diet rich in polyunsaturated fats will cause an increased percentage of polyunsaturated fats in the milk without altering the total fat content. When the mother is calorie deficient, depot fats are mobilized and milk resembles depot fat. When excessive nonfat kilocalories are fed, levels of saturated fatty acids increase as lipids are synthesized from tissue stores.[62]

The USDA has reported that the average American diet now includes 156 g of fat, up from 141 g in 1947. The significant change is from animal to vegetable fat, which is now 39% of total dietary fats, especially resulting from the switch from butter and lard. The original studies on human milk lipids were done from 1940 to 1950.[62] A change in fatty acid content to more long-chain fatty acids and a twofold to threefold increase in linoleic acid has occurred. Except for 18:2 content in mature milk, the fatty acid composition is remarkably uniform unless the maternal diet is unusually bizarre.[82]

P/S is the ratio of polyunsaturated to saturated fats; polyunsaturated fats include $C_{18:2}$ and $C_{18:3}$, or linoleic and linolenic acid. The bovine P/S ratio is 4. The P/S ratio has shifted as a result of recent dietary changes to 1.3 from 1.35 in human milk. The P/S is significant in facilitating calcium and fat absorption. Calcium absorption is depressed by

Table 4-5. Percent fat in breast milk and percent fatty acids in milk fat

	Vegetarians (N = 79)†		Non-vegetarians (N = 77)	Total sample* (N = 172)
Milk fat	3.21 ± 1.78		3.23 ± 2.13	3.25 ± 1.94
Fatty acids:				
C8:0	0.15 ± 0.10		0.17 ± 0.12	0.16 ± 0.11
C10:0	1.15 ± 0.31	B‡	1.01 ± 0.28	1.10 ± 0.30
C12:0	5.98 ± 1.81	B	5.08 ± 1.49	5.56 ± 1.68
C14:0	8.23 ± 2.39		7.67 ± 2.60	8.01 ± 2.46
De novo§	14.85 ± 3.68		14.60 ± 3.64	14.73 ± 3.71
C16:0	22.50 ± 3.63	B	23.96 ± 2.92	23.28 ± 3.35
C16:1ω9	2.81 ± 0.67	A‖	3.23 ± 0.79	3.02 ± 0.77
C18:0	7.44 ± 1.53	A	8.70 ± 1.31	8.06 ± 1.58
C18:1ω9	30.74 ± 4.13	A	32.98 ± 3.51	31.72 ± 3.81
C18:2ω6	18.38 ± 4.67	A	14.65 ± 4.24	16.49 ± 4.80
C18:3	1.59 ± 0.45		1.51 ± 0.41	1.56 ± 0.43
C20:2ω6	0.41 ± 0.15	A	0.35 ± 0.11	0.38 ± 0.15
C20:3ω6	0.31 ± 0.10	A	0.25 ± 0.08	0.28 ± 0.09
C20:4ω6	0.30 ± 0.10		0.28 ± 0.07	0.29 ± 0.08
C22:6ω3	0.05 ± 0.004		0.06 ± 0.004	0.06 ± 0.004

From Finley DA, Lönnerdal B, Dewey KG, et al: Am J Clin Nutr 41:787, 1985.
*Means for semivegetarians were usually between those of vegetarians and nonvegetarians and were not significantly different from either.
†N = number of samples. Data shown are mean ± SD. Mean ± SD is adjusted for month of lactation.
‡Significant at p ≤ 0.05 when N used to calculate statistic is equal to number of samples. This statistical procedure does not account for the effects of repeated samples from the same woman; differences identified by this test are considered trends.
§Sum of fatty acids synthesized de novo in mammary gland (C8:0, C10:0, C12:0, and C14:0).
‖Significant at p ≤ 0.05 when N used to calculate statistic is equal to the number of women providing samples (vegetarians = 27; nonvegetarians = 23). This statistical procedure accounted for effects of obtaining multiple reports from the same woman.

a 4:5 P/S ratio. The breast can dehydrogenate saturated and monounsaturated fatty acids in milk synthesis.

At least 167 fatty acids have been identified in human milk; possibly others are there in trace amounts. Bovine milk has been identified to have 437 fatty acids. Marked change in fatty acid composition would be the result of major dietary changes.

Essential fatty acid requirements for humans have been studied by many investigators. Diets free from added fats or linoleic acid induce deficiency symptoms in infants. These symptoms include skin lesions, insufficient weight gain, and poor wound healing. Low-fat diets in newborn rats have affected cerebral function. The American Academy of Pediatrics has recommended that infant formulas contain a minimum of 3.3 g of fat/kcal (30% of total kilocalories) and 300 mg of linoleic acid (18.2)/100 kcal (about 1.7% of total kilocalories).[21,22] It did not set a limit on linoleic content of diet, since some human milks have 8% to 10% of the fat as linoleic acid.

Milk from vegetarians (lacto-ovo) contained a lower proportion of fatty acids derived from animal fat and a higher proportion of polyunsaturated fatty acids derived from dietary vegetable fat. Women who consumed 35 g or more of animal fat per day had higher C10:0, C12:0, and C18:3 but lower levels of C16:0 and C18:0. The authors[34] suggest that there is a maximum amount of C16:0 and C18:0 that can be taken up from the blood and subsequently secreted into milk (see Table 4-5).

The milk of strict vegetarians has extremely high levels of linoleic acid, four times that of cow's milk.[114] Some researchers include other long-chain fatty acids such as $C_{20:2}$, $C_{20:3}$, $C_{24:4}$, and $C_{22:3}$ as essential nutrients because they are structural lipids in the brain and nervous tissue. The effects of diet are discussed in Chapter 9.

One important outcome of linoleic and linolenic acids is the conversion of these compounds into longer-chain polyunsaturates. These metabolites have been shown to be important for fluidity of membrane lipids and prostaglandin synthesis. They are present in the brain and visual cells. Long-chain polyunsaturates are needed for development of infant brain and nervous system.[34] When Gibson et al[41] studied fatty acid composition of colostrum and mature milk at 3 to 5 days and later at 6 weeks postpartum, they reported that mature milk had a higher percentage of saturated fatty acids, including medium-chain acids, lower monounsaturates, and higher linoleic and linolenic acids and their long-chain polyunsaturated derivatives. The derivatives of these acids, often ignored by many investigators, have high biologic activity; thus, the reporting of only linoleic acid underestimates the essential fatty acid levels in human milk.[82]

To address the issue of nutrition during brain development it is important to consider the different periods of brain development that have been described biochemically by Sinclair and Crawford.[119] First there is cell division, with the formation of neurons and glial cells, and second, myelination. Sinclair and Crawford showed in the rat brain that 50% of polyenoic acids of the gray matter lipids were laid down by the fifteenth day of life. The fatty acids characteristic of myelin lipids appeared later. Gray matter is largely composed of unmyelinated neurons, whereas white matter contains a very high proportion of myelinated conducting nerve fibers. Normal brain function depends on both.

The fatty acids characteristic of gray matter ($C_{20:4}$ and $C_{22:6}$) accumulate before the appearance of fatty acids characteristic of myelin ($C_{20:1}$ and $C_{24:1}$) in the developing brain. Arachidonic ($C_{20:4}$) and docosahexaenoic ($C_{22:6}$) acids are synthesized from linoleic and linolenic acids, respectively, but the latter two must be obtained in the diet.

The essential fatty acids, linoleic and linolenic acids, may have greater significance in the quality of the myelin laid down. Dick[29] has made a very interesting observation in the geographic distribution of multiple sclerosis worldwide. He notes that the disease is rare in countries where breastfeeding is common. He postulates that the development of myelin in infancy is critical to preventing degradation later. Dick investigated the difference between human milk and cow's milk in relation to myelin production in multiple sclerosis.[29]

Experimental allergic encephalitis is a demyelinating condition, which can be produced by shocking animals that have been sensitized to central nervous system (CNS) antigens. Newborn rats deficient in essential fatty acids are more susceptible to experimental allergic encephalitis, which has been described as resembling multiple sclerosis pathologically.

Widdowson[130] analyzed the body fats of children from Britain and Holland. At birth, body fat was 1.3% linoleic acid for both groups of children. British infants received cow's milk formulas that contained 1.8% linoleic acid. The Dutch infants received corn-oil formulas that were 58.2% linoleic acid. The Dutch infants had body fat that was 25% linoleic acid at 1 month of age and 32% to 37% at 4 months of age. The British infants, receiving cow's milk formulas, had 3% or less linoleic acid in their body fat. The Dutch infants had lower serum cholesterol levels. The children at approximately 10 years of age appeared to be entirely normal.

Cholesterol

The cholesterol content of milk is remarkably stable at 240 mg/100 g of fat when calculated by volume of fat. The range, depending on sampling techniques, is 9 mg to 41 mg/100 ml. The amount of cholesterol changed slightly over time, decreasing 1.7-fold over the first 36 days as reported by Harzer et al,[52] stabilizing at about the fifteenth day postpartum at 20 mg/100 ml. This resulted in a change in the cholesterol/triglyceride ratio. The authors found no uniform pattern of circadian variations between mothers.

Cholesterol has been a factor of great concern because of the apparent association with risk factors for atherosclerosis and coronary heart disease. At present, commercial formulas have high P/S ratios and low cholesterol levels compared with human milk. Dietary manipulation does not change the cholesterol level in the breast milk.[104] When the dietary cholesterol level is controlled, a fall in the infant's plasma cholesterol level is, however, associated with an increase in the amount of linoleic acid in the milk.[103]

No long-range effect of serum cholesterol level has been identified, although Osborn[101] described the pathologic changes in 1500 young people (newborns to age 20). He observed the spectrum of pathologic changes from mucopolysaccharide accumulations to fully developed atherosclerotic plaques. Lesions were more frequent and severe in children who had been bottle fed. Lesions were uncommon or mild in the breastfed children. Investigations done on rats indicated that animals given high levels of cholesterol early in life were better able to cope with cholesterol in later life and maintained a lower cholesterol level.

Proteins

All milks have been evaluated for their protein contents, which vary from species to species. Proteins constitute 0.9% of the contents in human milk and range up to 20% in some rabbit species. Proteins of milk include casein, serum albumin, and α-lactalbumin, β-lactoglobulins, immunoglobulins, and other glycoproteins. Eight of twenty amino acids present in milk are essential and are derived from plasma. The mammary alveolar epithelium synthesizes some nonessential amino acids (Table 4-6). Human milk amino acids occur in proteins and peptides, as well as a small percentage in the form of free amino acids and glucosamine.[1]

Postprandial changes in plasma amino acids in breastfed infants were reported by Tikanoja[126] to be proportional to dietary intake and were highest for the branched-chain amino acids. This was also found to be true for most semiessential and nonessential amino acids.[126] The blood urea levels also reflect dietary intake, with values in breastfed infants being substantially lower than levels in bottle-fed infants. The sum of plasma free amino acids rose and the glycine/valine ratio fell after a feed. When breastfed and formula-fed infants were compared by Järvenpää,[67] concentrations of citrulline, threonine, phenylalanine, and tyrosine were higher in formula-fed than in breastfed infants. Concentrations of taurine were lower in the formula-fed infants. The peak time was different for formula-fed and breastfed infants, which points out the need to standardize sampling times.

Casein

It is well known that milk consists of casein, or curds, and whey proteins, or lactalbumins. The term *casein* includes a group of milk-specific proteins characterized by ester-bound phosphate, high-proline content, and low solubility at pH of 4.0 to 5.0. Caseins form complex particles or micelles, which are usually complexes of calcium caseinate and

Table 4-6. Human milk-free amino acid concentrations

	Colostral milk (μmol/dl)	Transitional milk (μmol/dl)	Mature milk (μmol/dl)
Glutamic acid	36-68	88-127	101-180
Glutamine	2-9	9-20	13-58
Taurine	41-45	34-50	27-67
Alanine	9-11	13-20	17-26
Threonine	5-12	7-8	6-13
Serine	12	6-11	6-14
Glycine	5-8	5-10	3-13
Aspartic acid	5-6	3-4	3-5
Leucine	3-5	2-6	2-4
Cystine	1-3	2-5	3-6
Valine	3-4	3-6	4-6
Lysine	5	1-11	2-5
Histidine	2	2-3	0.4-3
Phenylalanine	1-2	1	0.6-2
Tyrosine	2	1-2	1-2
Arginine	3-7	1-5	1-2
Isoleucine	2	1-2	1
Ornithine	1-4	1	0.5-0.9
Methionine	0.8	0.3-3	0.3-0.8
Phosphoserine	8	5	4
Phosphethanolamine	4	8	10
α-Aminobutyrate	1	0.4-1.4	0.4-1
Tryptophan	5	1	1
Proline	—	6	2-3

From Carlson SE: Adv Pediatr 32:43, 1985.

calcium phosphate. When milk clots or curdles as a result of heat, pH changes, or enzymes, the casein is transformed into an insoluble calcium caseinate-calcium phosphate complex. There are physiochemical differences between human and cow caseins.

When Lönnerdal and Forsum[87] measured the casein content of human milk by three different methods—isoelectric precipitation, sedimentation by ultra centrifuge and indirect analysis—they consistently had three separate results. They report the correct ratio of casein nitrogen: whey nitrogen is 20:80. Casein has a species-specific amino acid composition.

Methionine/cysteine ratio. The cysteine content is high in human milk, whereas it is very low in cow's milk. Instead, the methionine content is high in bovine milk, thus the methionine/cysteine ratio is two to three times greater in cow's milk than in the milk of most mammals and seven times that in human milk. Human milk is the only animal protein in which the methionine/cysteine ratio is close to 1. Otherwise, this ratio is seen only in plant proteins. Two significant characteristics of amino acid composition of human milk are the ratio between the sulfur-containing amino acids, methionine and cysteine, and the low content of the aromatic amino acids, phenylalanine and tyrosine. The newborn and especially the premature infant are ill prepared to handle phenylalanine and tyrosine because of low levels of the specific enzymes required to metabolize them.

Taurine. Taurine is a third sulfur-containing amino acid that has been found in high concentrations in human milk and is virtually absent in cow's milk. It is now being added to some prepared formulas. Free taurine and glutamic acid have been measured in breast milk in high concentration. Taurine has been associated in the body at all ages with bile acid conjugation; in the newborn, bile acids are almost exclusively conjugated with taurine. It has been suggested by the work of Sturman and associates[123] that taurine may also be a neurotransmitter or neuromodulator in the brain and retina. Taurine in the nutrition of the human infant was reviewed by Gaull,[40] who reports that evidence is accumulating that taurine has a more general biologic role in development and membrane stability. Taurine is found in very high concentrations in the milk of cats.[105] Kittens deprived of taurine by feeding with purified taurine-free casein diets after weaning develop retinal degeneration and blindness. The process can be reversed by feeding taurine, but not by feeding methionine, cysteine, or inorganic sulfate.[93] The structural integrity of the retina of the cat has been shown to be taurine dependent. The taurine levels were more severely depleted in the brain tissue, but its significance has not been identified yet.[123] Both humans and cats are unable to synthesize taurine to any degree and are therefore wholly dependent on a dietary supply. The process requires cystathionase and cysteinesulfinic acid decarboxylase, which are enzymes that convert methionine, cysteine, or cystine to taurine.

In studies of amino acid levels, only the concentrations of taurine in plasma and urine of breastfed term infants were higher than those of preterm infants fed formula. Levels in term infants were higher than those of preterm infants fed pooled human milk at a fixed volume. The effects of feeding taurine-deficient formula to the human infant, which was happening prior to the addition of taurine to infant formula, are not as severe as seen in the kitten. The presence of taurine in human milk and predominance of taurine conjugates in the gut at birth suggest that bile acid conjugate status may be a control factor. When bile acid metabolism was measured in infants fed human milk, they consistently had higher intraluminal bile acid concentrations at all ages (1 week to 5 weeks) than did formula-fed infants with and without additional taurine. Human milk also facilitated intestinal lipid absorption.[129]

The human infant conjugates bile acids predominantly with taurine at birth but quickly develops the capacity to conjugate with glycine. Those infants fed human milk continue to conjugate with taurine, whereas those fed formulas soon conjugate with glycine predominantly. The cat, in contrast, uses only taurine throughout life.[123] In the human the various pools of taurine in the body cannot be predicted by measurement of plasma taurine alone. Because of the growing evidence for the role of taurine during development, the requirement for taurine for the neonate remains under investigation[123] although taurine has been added to some formulas.

Whey proteins

When clotted milk stands, the clot contracts, leaving a clear fluid called *whey,* which contains water, electrolytes, and proteins. The ratio of whey proteins to casein is 1.5 for breast milk and 0.25 for cow's milk, that is, 40% of human milk protein is casein and 60% lactalbumin, and cow's milk is 80% casein and 20% lactalbumin.[87]

Human milk forms a flocculent suspension with 0 curd tension. The curds are easily digested. The total amount of protein has been recently measured to be 0.9%, which is lower than the previously reported figure of 1.2%. The discrepancy is due to recalculation

Table 4-7. Composition of protein nitrogen and nonprotein nitrogen in human milk and cow's milk*

	Human milk		Cow's milk	
Protein nitrogen		1.43 (8.9)		5.3 (31.4)
Casein nitrogen	0.40	(2.5)	4.37	(27.3)
Whey protein nitrogen	1.03	(6.4)	0.93	(5.8)
α-Lactalbumin	0.42	(2.6)	0.17	(1.1)
Lactoferrin	0.27	(1.7)	Traces	
β-Lactoglobulin	—		0.57	(3.6)
Lysozyme	0.08	(0.5)	Traces	
Serum albumin	0.08	(0.5)	0.07	(0.4)
IgA	0.16	(1.0)	0.005	(0.03)
IgG	0.005	(0.03)	0.096	(0.06)
IgM	0.003	(0.02)	0.005	(0.03)
Nonprotein nitrogen		0.50		0.28
Urea nitrogen	0.25		0.13	
Creatine nitrogen	0.037		0.009	
Creatinine nitrogen	0.035		0.003	
Uric acid nitrogen	0.005		0.008	
Glucosamine	0.047		?	
α-Amino nitrogen	0.13		0.048	
Ammonia nitrogen	0.002		0.006	
Nitrogen from other components	?		0.074	
Total nitrogen		1.93		5.31

Courtesy Forsum E and Lönnerdal B: Protein evaluation of breast milk and breast milk substitutes with special reference to the nonprotein nitrogen, unpublished data.
*Values refer to grams of nitrogen per liter; values within parentheses, to grams of protein per liter.

of the data in which the total amount of protein was determined by measuring the nitrogen content and multiplying by 6.25. Of the nitrogen content 25% is nonprotein nitrogen, whereas in bovine milk 5% of the nitrogen is from nonprotein nitrogen. Hambraeus[49] has reported the composition of the nonprotein fraction to be urea, creatine, creatinine, uric acid, small peptides, and free amino acids (Table 4-7).

Closer examination of the whey proteins shows α-lactalbumin and lactoferrin to be the chief fractions, with no measurable β-lactoglobulin. β-Lactoglobulin is the chief constituent of cow's milk. The term *lactalbumin* includes a mixture of whey proteins found in bovine milk and should not be confused with α-*lactalbumin*, which is a specific protein that is part of the enzyme lactose synthetase. The α-lactalbumin content parallels lactose levels in different species. Human milk is high in both lactose and α-lactalbumin.

Lactoferrin. Lactoferrin is an iron-binding protein that is part of the whey fraction of proteins in human milk. It is in very low amounts in bovine milk. Lactoferrin has been observed to inhibit the growth of certain iron-dependent bacteria in the gastrointestinal tract. It has been suggested that lactoferrin protects against certain gastrointestinal infections in breastfed infants. Giving iron to newborn infants appears to inactivate the lactoferrin by saturating it with iron.

Immunoglobulins

The immunoglobulins in breast milk are distinct from those of the serum. The main immunoglobulin in serum is IgG, which is present in the amount of 1210 mg/100 ml. IgA is found in the serum at 250 mg/100 ml, a fifth the level of IgG. The reverse is true of human colostrum and milk. Colostrum has 1740 mg of IgA/100 ml, and milk has 100 mg/100 ml. Colostrum has 43 mg of IgG/100 ml, and milk has 4 mg of IgG/100 ml. The IgA and IgG in human milk are derived from serum and from synthesis in the mammary gland. The IgA is secretory IgA (sIgA), the principal immunoglobulin in colostrum and milk. Secretory IgA contains an antigenic determinant associated with a secretory component. It is synthesized in the gland from two molecules of serum IgA linked by disulfide bonds. The sIgA levels are very high in colostrum the first few days and then decline rapidly, disappearing almost completely by the fourteenth day. Secretory IgA is very stable at low pH and resistant to proteolytic enzymes. It is present in the intestine of breastfed infants and provides a protective defense against infection by keeping viruses and bacteria from invading the mucosa. The protective qualities are further described in Chapter 5.

Lysozyme

Lysozyme is a specific protein found in high concentration in egg whites and human milk but in low concentration in bovine milk. It has been identified as a nonspecific antimicrobial factor. This enzyme is bacteriolytic against *Enterobacteriaceae* and gram-positive bacteria. It has been found in concentrations up to 0.2 mg/ml. Lysozyme is stable at 100° C and at an acid pH. Lysozyme contributes to the development and maintenance of specific intestinal flora of the breastfed infant. It will be further described under enzymes and in Chapter 5.

Nonprotein nitrogen

Nonprotein nitrogen (NPN) accounts for 18% to 30% of the total nitrogen in human milk.[15] Although these are large interindividual variations, the range is from 350 to 530 mg/L. The total nitrogen ranges from 1700 to 3700 mg/L depending upon length of gestation, duration of lactation, and maternal diet. Some of the nitrogen contributes to the pool available for synthesis of nonessential amino acids in the neonate. Those compounds having more specialized roles are peptide hormone/growth factors, epidermal growth factor, amino sugars of oligosaccharides, free amino acids, amino alcohols of phospholipids, nucleic acids, nucleotides, and carnitine. Their importance is not based on percent concentration, as they may serve roles as catalysts. Many protein factors in human milk serve roles other than growth, such as the host resistance factors (lactoferrin, sIgA, and lysozyme).

The significance of these compounds and their relative concentrations are presented in Table 4-8. The wide variety of nitrogenous compounds within the fraction of human milk is only beginning to be investigated and understood. This information clearly widens the chemical gap between human milk and proprietary formulas. Increasing evidence suggests that the prematurely born reaps even more benefit than the term infant from mother's milk, based on the investigations of nonprotein nitrogen alone.[15]

Nucleotides

Nucleotides are compounds derived from nucleic acid by hydrolysis and consist of phosphoric acid combined with a sugar and a purine or pyrimidine derivative. The level and components of acid-soluble nucleotides of several species, including humans, have

Table 4-8. Levels and significance of nonprotein nitrogen constituents of human milk

NPN	Concentration in milk		Significance
	Under 30 days	**Over 30 days**	
Amino sugars			
N-Acetylglucosamine	230 mg N/L	150 mg N/L	Low oral osmotic load; control gut colonization; constituents of gangliocides for brain development
N-Acetylneuraminic acid	63 mg N/L	3-27 mg N/L	Substrate for gut epithelium
Peptides	—	60 mg N/L	
Epidermal growth factor	88 ng/ml	—	Regulates intestinal mucosal development (see text)
Somatomedin-C/insulin-like growth factor	18 ng/ml	6-8 ng/ml	Stimulates DNA synthesis and cell division in the gut
Delta sleep-inducing peptide	30 ng/ml	5 ng/ml	Diurnal pattern highest at 2 PM and 8 PM. ? influence sleep/awake patterns
Insulin	21 ng/ml	2 ng/ml	? regulates development of gut
Free amino acids			
Taurine	41-45 μmol/dl	27-67 μmol/dl	See text
Glutamic acid/glutamine	2-9 μmol/dl	13-58 μmol/dl	Improves zinc absorption; precursor to brain glutamate
Carnitine	1.0 mg N/L	0.7 mg N/L	Brain lipid synthesis (see text)
Choline and ethanolamine	7-20 mg N/L	10-20 mg N/L	Possible growth requirement
Nucleic acid	—	19 mg N/L	Pool of DNA and RNA
Nucleotides	3 mg N/L	3 mg N/L	Growth advantage (see text)
Polyamines	0.1 mg N/L	0.2 mg N/L	Increase rate of transcription, translation, and amino acid activation

been studied, since recent work has shown a characteristic nucleotide composition in the milk that differed from that of the mammary gland. Johke[72] reviewed the existing knowledge on nucleotides in milk. The large numbers of purine and pyrimidine nucleotides present in various tissues have a number of functions in the cell. They are part of nucleic acid synthesis and metabolism and are also part of milk synthesis. It is well known that adenosine triphosphate (ATP) supplies usable energy for biosynthetic reactions.

Human milk has been recorded to have 6.1 to 9.0 μmol of free nucleotides/100 ml, according to Johke.[72] The levels in colostrum and mature milk are similar. The conspicuous difference in quality and quantity of nucleotides between the mammary gland and its secretion would indicate that nucleotides are secreted from the epithelial cells of the gland into the milk. There are distinct species differences in composition and content of nucleotides as well. Cytidine monophosphate (CMP) and uracil are the nucleotides in the highest concentration in human milk, which also contains uridine diphosphate-N-acetyllactosamine and other oligosaccharides. Human milk contains only a trace of orotic acid and no gua-nosine diphosphate-fucose. Orotic acid is the chief nucleotide of bovine milk. Nucleotide levels fall rapidly in bovine milk to minimal levels in mature bovine milk.

When the nitrogen fraction of human milk was further identified over time by Janas and Picciano,[65] a variance was noted in the pattern of nucleotides. Levels of cytidine-5'-monophosphate and adenosine-5'-monophosphate declined from 594 to 321 μg/100 ml and from 244 to 143 μg/100 ml, respectively, whereas levels of inosine-5'-monophosphate increased from 158 to 290 μg/100 ml. The total nucleotide nitrogen remained constant, accounting for 0.10% to 0.15% of the total nonprotein nitrogen. The average intake per day of a normal breastfed infant would be 1.4 to 2.1 mg of nucleotide nitrogen. Measurement of adenosine monophosphate (AMP) and cyclic guanosine monophosphate (GMP) by Skala et al[120] showed variation in concentration within 15 minutes, which fluctuated over 24 hours. Milk concentration differed widely from maternal plasma levels collected at the same time. Whether inosine-5'-monophosphate contributes to the superior iron absorption is still unanswered (see discussion on p. 96).

Nucleotides are important in the process of protein synthesis, which is enhanced in the newborn infant by a dietary supply of nucleotides. A statistically significant increase in weight was observed by György[45] and his colleagues when weanling rats who had been fed a low-protein diet (10% casein) were given added nucleotides as compared with controls without supplements of nucleotides. A high-protein diet (20%) did not produce significant growth increase when nucleotides were added.

Carnitine

Carnitine is Y-trimethylamino-B-hydroxybutrate and is essential for the catabolism of long-chain fatty acids. Only two conditions in life have been described where carnitine is indispensable: total parenteral nutrition lasting over 3 weeks and early postnatal life. In older individuals it is synthesized in liver and kidney from essential amino acids lysine and methionine. Carnitine serves as an essential carrier of acyl groups across the mito-chondrial membrane to sites of oxidation and therefore has a central role in the mitochondrial oxidation of fatty acids in the human.[100] The newborn undergoes major metabolic changes during transition from fetal to extrauterine life, including the rapid development of the capacity to oxidize fatty acids and ketone bodies as fuel alternatives to glucose. The fatty acids derived from high-fat milk and endogenous fat stores become the preferred fuel of the heart, brain, and tissues with high-energy demands. There is, in addition, a dramatic increase in serum fatty acids in the first hours of life. After the interruption of the feto-placental circulation and in the absence of an exogenous supply of carnitine, neonatal plasma levels of free carnitines and acylcarnitines decrease very rapidly. Carnitine admin-istration seems to act by increasing ketogenesis and lipolysis.[98] When serum carnitine and ketone body concentrations were measured in breastfed and formula-fed newborn infants, lower carnitine levels were found in infants fed formulas than in those fed breast milk.[115]

The levels of carnitine range from 70 to 95 nmol/ml in breast milk (up to 115 nmoles/ml in colostrum) and from 40 to 80 nmol/ml in commercial formula (Enfamil). The bioavailability of carnitine in human milk may be a significant factor in the higher carnitine and ketone body concentrations in breastfed babies. In omnivorous mothers, L-carnitine levels do not vary considerably over time. Levels in the milk of lacto-ovo-vegetarian mothers were always consistently lower than omnivores. The lower serum level of lysine in these women is a possible cause of lower carnitine.

The carnitine levels in human milk were followed for 50 days postpartum by Sandor et al,[115] who found the mean level to be 62.9 nmol/ml (56.0-69.8 nmol/ml range) during the first 21 days and 35.2 ± 1.26 nmol/ml until the fortieth to fiftieth day. Levels were not related to volume of milk secreted.

Carbohydrates

The predominant carbohydrate of milk is lactose, or milk sugar. It is present in high concentration (6.8 g/100 ml in human milk and 4.9 g/100 ml in bovine milk). Lactose is a disaccharide compound of two monosaccharides, galactose and glucose. Lactose is synthesized by the mammary gland. A number of other carbohydrates are present in milk. They are classified as monosaccharides, neutral and acid oligosaccharides, and peptide- and protein-bound carbohydrates. There are small amounts of glucose (14 mg/100 ml) and galactose (12 mg/100 ml) present in breast milk also. There are other complex carbohydrates present in free form or bound to amino acids or protein, such as *N*-acetylglucosamine. The concentration of oligosaccharides is about 10 times greater than in cow's milk. This difference arises, no doubt, from biosynthetic control mechanisms yet to be described. These carbohydrates and glycoproteins possess bifidus factor activity. There is also fucose, which is not present in bovine milk and may be important to the early establishment of *L. bifidus* as gut flora. The nitrogen-containing carbohydrates are 0.7% of milk solids.

Lactose is hydrolyzed selectively by a brush border enzyme called lactase located predominantly in the tip of the intestinal villi. Digestion of lactose is the rate-limiting step in its absorption. Although lactase activity develops later in fetal life than that of other disaccharidases, it is present by 24 weeks of fetal life. Lactase concentration is greatest in the proximal jejunum. Levels continue to increase throughout the last trimester, reaching concentrations at term two to four times those levels at 2 to 11 months of age. Prematures rapidly increase their lactase levels given a lactose challenge. A well-fed breast-fed infant ingesting 150 ml of milk/kg/day receives 10 g of lactose/kg/day, which ensures the normal unstressed infant at least 4 mg/kg/min of glucose, which is considered optimal rate.[84]

Lactose does appear to be specific, however, for newborn growth. It has been shown to enhance calcium absorption and has been suggested as being critical to the prevention of rickets, in view of the relatively low calcium levels in human milk. Lactose is a readily available source of galactose, which is essential to the production of the galactolipids, including cerebroside. These galactolipids are essential to CNS development.

Interesting correlations have been made between the amount of lactose in the milk of a species and the relative size of the brain[78] (Fig. 4-4). The fact that lactose is found only in milk and not in other animal and plant sources enhances the significance of its high level in human milk. Lactose levels are quite constant throughout the day in a given mother's milk. Even in poorly nourished mothers, the levels of lactose do not vary. Because lactose is influential in controlling volume, the total output for the day may be diminished, but the concentration of lactose in human milk will be 6.2 to 7.2 g/100 ml.[17]

Minerals

The total ash content of milk is species specific and parallels the growth rate and body structure of the offspring. There are a number of metallic elements and organic and inorganic acids in milk. They may be present as ions, un-ionized salts, and weakly ionized

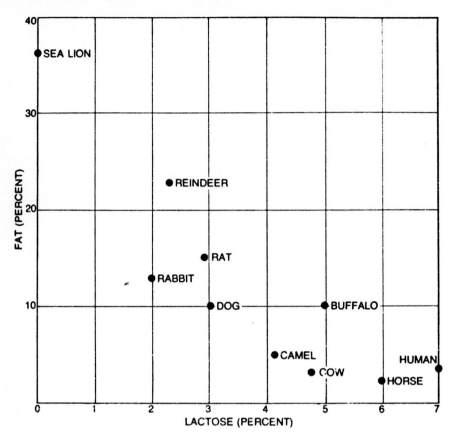

Fig. 4-4. Concentration of lactose varies with source of milk. In general, less lactose, more fat, which can also be used by newborn animal as energy source. (From Kretchmer N: Lactose and lactase, Sci Am 227:73, Copyright © 1972 by Scientific American, Inc. All rights reserved.)

salts. Some are bound to other constituents. Sodium, potassium, calcium, and magnesium are the major cations. Phosphate, chloride, and citrate are the major anions. High-lactose milks, in general, contain less total ash than low-lactose milks, which have high total salt content.

Daily intakes of calcium, phosphorus, zinc, potassium, sodium, iron, and copper were found to decrease significantly over the first 4 months of life, with only magnesium increasing. Despite seemingly low mineral intakes, growth was found satisfactory by Butte et al.[13] This maintains osmolality close to that of serum. The high mineral content is associated with a rapid growth rate of the specific species as well.

Potassium and sodium

Potassium levels are much higher than those of sodium, which are similar to the proportions in intracellular fluids (Table 4-9). Although sodium, potassium, and chloride are present as free ions, the other constituents appear as complexes and compounds. Ions can pass through the secretory cell membrane in both directions and in and out of the lumen. Intracellular sodium, chloride, and potassium are in equilibrium with the ions of

Table 4-9. Minerals in human milk and cow's milk (per 100 ml)

Minerals	Colostrum	Transitional	Mature	Cow's milk
Calcium (mg)	39.0	46.0	35.0	130.0
Chlorine (mg)	85.0	46.0	40.0	108.0
Copper (μg)	40.0	50.0	40.0	14.0
Iron (μg)	70.0	70.0	100.0	70.0
Magnesium (mg)	4.0	4.0	4.0	12.0
Phosphorus (mg)	14.0	20.0	15.0	120.0
Potassium (mg)	74.0	64.0	57.0	145.0
Sodium (mg)	48.0	29.0	15.0	58.0
Sulfur (mg)	22.0	20.0	14.0	30.0
Total ash (mg)	—	—	200.0	700.0

From Food and Nutrition Board, National Research Council, National Academy of Sciences: Recommended dietary allowances, ed 9, Washington DC, 1980, US Government Printing Office.

Table 4-10. Recommended dietary intake of electrolytes for infants

Age (yr)	Sodium (mg)	Potassium (mg)	Chloride (mg)
0-0.5	115-350	350-925	275-700
0.5-1.0	250-750	425-1275	400-1200

From Food and Nutrition Board, National Research Council, National Academy of Sciences: Recommended dietary allowances, ed 9, Washington DC, 1980, US Government Printing Office.

the plasma and alveolar milk. An apical pumping mechanism has been calculated for chloride release, whereas sodium, potassium, and intracellular chloride pass into milk because of their electrochemical gradients. The cellular pumping mechanism maintains the ionic concentrations in the extracellular fluid and alveolar milk.

The Committee on Nutrition of the Academy of Pediatrics[23] has stated that the daily requirement of sodium for growth is 0.5 mEq/kg/day between birth and 3 months of age, decreasing to 0.1 mEq/kg/day after 6 months of age (Table 4-10). To cover dermal losses, an additional 0.4 to 0.7 mEq/kg/day is needed, with little for urine and stool losses. Infants fed human milk receive enough sodium to meet their needs for growth, dermal losses, and urinary losses. Studies by Keenan et al[75] have demonstrated an apparent regulation of milk sodium and potassium concentrations by adrenal corticosteroids as well as a circadian rhythm in the levels.

Sodium levels in cow's milk are 3.6 times those in human milk (human, 7 mEq/L or 16 mg/dl; bovine, 22 mEq/L or 50 mg/100 ml). Hypernatremic dehydration has been associated with cow's milk feedings. Experiments with newborn rats on high salt intakes have shown that hypertension can develop.

The diurnal variation in milk electrolytes was found to vary between 22% and 80%,[75] and these changes varied as the lactation period progressed but were independent of mother's diet. Sodium restriction did not influence milk levels. In a longitudinal study Hazebroek and Hofman[54] found sodium levels fell from 20 mEq/L to 15 mEq/L in the first week. On day 8, levels were 8 mEq/L, and by the fifth week they were stabilized at 6 mEq/L.

At a constant sodium intake, decreasing the Na/K ratio in the diet by increasing potassium lowers blood pressure. The dietary Na/K ratio has an important role in determining the severity, if not the development, of salt-induced hypertension. The mechanism of potassium's antihypertensive effect is unclear, but the higher potassium and lower sodium levels of breast milk appear to be physiologically beneficial.

Chloride

Little attention has been paid to the adequacy of chloride in the diet, and it has always been assumed to be sufficient until recent events focused attention on this cation.

Chloride deficiency in infants has become associated with a syndrome of failure to thrive with hypochloremia and hypokalemic metabolic alkalosis. This was first described in infants fed formula that was deficient in chloride but has also been described in a breastfed infant whose mother's milk contained less than 2 mEq/L chloride (normal >8 mEq/L).[5] This is a rare phenomenon caused by unexplained maternal production. This mother had previously successfully nourished five other infants.

Total ash

Cow's milk has three times the total salt content of human milk (Table 4-11). All the minerals that appear in cow's milk also appear in human milk. The phosphorus level is six times greater in cow's milk; the calcium level is four times higher (Table 4-12).

The renal solute load of cow's milk is considerably higher than that of breast milk. This is magnified by the metabolic breakdown products of the high protein content, which are in increased amounts, also. This is shown in the high urea levels in formula-fed infants (Table 4-26). Although the mean urea levels in breast milk are 37 mg/100 ml and only 15 mg/100 ml in cow's milk, the blood urea levels in breastfed infants are about 22 mg, whereas infants fed formula are 47 mg and those fed formula plus solids are 52 mg/100 ml (Table 4-13). The plasma osmolarity of infants fed breast milk is lower and approximates the physiological level of plasma.

Calcium/phosphorus ratio

The ratio of calcium to phosphorus is considerably lower in cow's milk (1.4) than in human milk (2.2). Many investigators have studied calcium and phosphorus values in human milk and found some variation from mother to mother and from study to study. The Ca/P ratio varied from 1.8 to 2.4, with the absolute values for calcium varying from 20 to 34 mg/100 ml and those for phosphorus varying from 14 to 18 mg/100 ml. Data compiled by Forfar[36] demonstrate the variation. Fetal and newborn plasma concentrations for calcium decline sharply from 10.4 mg/100 ml at birth to 8.5 mg/100 ml by day 4. Unlike calcium, phosphorus concentrations rise in the postnatal period. The drop in serum calcium levels in the bottle-fed infants was more marked than in the breastfed infants. Infant serum phosphorus concentrations rise during the postnatal period. When gestation is prolonged or the mother has preeclampsia, the concentrations are even higher at birth.

Longitudinal studies by Greer et al,[42] measuring calcium and phosphorus in human milk and maternal and infant sera, have shown progressive increases in infant serum calcium in association with decreasing phosphorus content of breast milk and infant serum. Maternal serum calcium also increased, although the mother's dietary intake was below recommended levels for lactating women.

Although the Ca/P ratio has been stressed in the past, recent investigations have not found a statistical correlation between the calcium and phosphorus contents of plasma and

Table 4-11. Principal salt constituents in bovine and human milks

Constituent	Bovine (mg/100 ml)	Human (mg/100 ml)
Calcium	125	33
Magnesium	12	4
Sodium	58	15
Potassium	138	55
Chloride	103	43
Phosphorus	96	15
Citric acid	175	20-80
Sulfur	30	14
CO_2	20	—

From Jenness R and Sloan RE: Composition of milk. In Larson BL and Smith VR, editors: Lactation, vol 3, Nutrition and biochemistry of milk/maintenance, New York, 1974, Academic Press, Inc.

Table 4-12. Recommended dietary intake of minerals for infants*

Age (yr)	Calcium (mg)	Phosphorus (mg)	Magnesium (mg)	Iron (mg)	Zinc (mg)	Iodine (μg)
0-0.5	360	240	50	10	3	40
0.5-1	540	360	70	15	5	50

From Food and Nutrition Board, National Research Council, National Academy of Sciences: Recommended dietary allowances, ed 9, Washington DC, 1980, US Government Printing Office.
*Because there is little information on which to base allowances, these amounts are provided in the form of ranges of recommended intakes.

Table 4-13. Statistical analysis by Student's "t" test of blood urea levels in 61 healthy infants aged 1 to 3 months

Infant group	Number	Blood urea, mean ± SE (mg/100 ml)	Individual values >40 mg/100 ml Number	Total observations (%)
A: breastfed	12	22.7 ± 1.6*	0	0‡
B: artificial milk alone	16	47.4 ± 2.0†	12	75§
C: artificial milk + solid foods	33	51.9 ± 1.8	29	88

From Davies DP and Saunders R: Arch Dis Child 48:563, 1973.
*When compared with group B and group C: $p < 0.001$ ($t = 9.7$) and $p < 0.001$ ($t = 11.5$), respectively.
†When compared with group C: $p > 0.05$ ($t = 1.6$).
‡When compared with group B and group C: $p < 0.001$ ($t = 6.9$) and $p < 0.001$ ($t = 15.5$), respectively.
§When compared with group C: $p > 0.05$ ($t = 1.1$).

corresponding breast milk Ca/P. This suggested that Ca/P ratio is not critical in the low mineral loads present in breast milk. When human milk was fractionated and analyzed for distribution of calcium, whole milk contained 241.2 ± 61.9 μg/ml, with most of the calcium in the skim fraction. Significant amounts were also found in the fat; less than 4% was found in the casein. A low-molecular-weight fraction contained 34% calcium, which may explain calcium's bioavailability. The total calcium requirements for maximum growth have been questioned by those who believe the total amount of calcium is too low in breast milk. The fact that rickets has not been seen in infants totally breastfed by well-nourished mothers is supportive circumstantial evidence.

Magnesium and other salts

Magnesium is present as a free ion and in complexes with casein and phosphate in caseinate micelles or citrate complexes. Cow's milk has three times as much magnesium as human milk (12 mg/100 ml compared with 4 mg/100 ml) (Table 4-11). Magnesium was measured in human milk by Fransson and Lönnerdal,[39] who found 41.4 ± 15.4 μg/ml in whole milk samples, with most of the magnesium in the skim milk fraction but significant amounts in the fat fraction and less than 4% in the casein. The bound fraction was associated with low-molecular-weight proteins, thus enhancing bioavailability. Mineral intakes were shown to increase between 1 and 3 months postpartum (1.15 to 1.36 mmol/L).[102]

Longitudinal magnesium concentrations were measured by Greer et al[42] in milk and maternal sera and in the infants over a 6-month period. Progressive increases in serum magnesium level were seen in the breastfed infants in association with decreasing phosphorus content of the milk. Milk magnesium levels did not change significantly between 3 and 26 weeks. The authors suggested that the rising magnesium levels in infant serum may in part be due to a decrease in dietary phosphorus in breastfed infants.

Citrate is found in the milks of many species and is three to four times higher in cow's milk than in human milk (Table 4-11). The distribution of ions and salts differs among various milks and depends on the relative concentrations of casein and citrate.

Most of the sulfur in milk is in the sulfur-containing amino acids, with only about 10% present as sulfate ion. There are some organic acids present, and they appear as anions in milk.

Trace elements

The recommended daily intake of trace elements for infants is given in Tables 4-12 and 4-14.

Iron. Because of the great emphasis on iron in the modern diet, and especially in the diet of the infant in the first year of life, the iron in human milk has been closely scrutinized.[21] It has been determined that normal infants need 1500 mg of exogenous elemental iron in the first year of life, which can be translated into 8 to 10 mg/day (Table 4-12). Prepared infant formulas currently supply 10 to 12 mg/day. Human milk has 100 μg/100 ml, which does not meet the requirements just given. Historically, however, breastfed infants have not been anemic (Table 4-9).

In 350 samples of breast milk there was a variation between <0.1 and 1.6 μg of iron/ml. Age, parity, and lactation history influenced the levels in some studies. The distribution of iron in various fractions of human milk of Swedish women was determined using multiple methods by Fransson and Lönnerdal,[38] who also found low levels, 0.26 and 0.73 ng/ml. The lipid fraction bound 15% to 46% of the iron; 18% to 56% of the iron

Table 4-14. Recommended dietary intake of trace elements for infants*

Age (yr)	Copper (mg)	Manganese (mg)	Fluoride (mg)	Chromium (mg)	Selenium (mg)	Molybdenum (mg)
0-0.5	0.5-0.7	0.5-0.7	0.1-0.5	0.01-0.04	0.01-0.04	0.03-0.06
0.5-1.0	0.7-1.0	0.7-1.0	0.2-1.0	0.02-0.06	0.02-0.06	0.04-0.08

From Food and Nutrition Board, Nutritional Research Council, National Academy of Sciences: Recommended dietary allowances, ed 9, Washington DC, 1980, US Government Printing Office.
*Because the toxic levels for many trace elements may be only several times usual intakes, the upper levels for the trace elements given in this table should not be habitually exceeded.

was in the low-molecular-weight protein fraction, with only a small amount bound to lactoferrin. Feeley et al[32] studied 102 American women by stage of lactation; 96% of the women took prenatal iron supplements. A diurnal variation was observed, and a significant decrease occurred from 4 to 45 days postpartum. The authors estimated that fully breastfed infants would receive 0.10 mg/kg/day of iron.

The effects of maternal iron nutrition in rats during lactation was studied by Anaokar and Garry,[4] who fed three groups of dams control amounts of 250 ppm iron, high-iron diets of 2500 ppm, and no-iron diets. Milk iron concentration decreased in all diet groups during lactation. The rate of decrease was diet dependent. Furthermore, iron levels in the dams were influenced by diet and correlated with levels in their pups.

Iron absorption from human milk is more efficient and has been noted to be 49% of iron available, whereas only 10% of cow's milk iron and 4% of iron in iron-fortified formulas is absorbed. Hematologic values of bottle-fed infants were abnormal, whereas those of breastfed infants were not. The breastfed infants had high ferritin levels, indicating a long-term adequacy of iron assimilation.

The infant who is exclusively breastfed for the first 6 months of life is not at risk for iron deficiency anemia or the depletion of iron stores during that time according to iron depletion studies of Duncan et al.[30] These findings were confirmed in iron balance studies on exclusively breastfed infants by Schulz-Lell,[117] who also cautioned against supraphysiological iron supplementation (10 to 12 mg/L), which they found leads to a 12- to 40-fold increase in iron retention compared to well-nourished exclusively breastfed infants. Studies in adults given tagged iron in human milk and in cow's milk show better absorption from the human milk solution. Other factors that influence iron absorption include higher amounts of vitamin C. Lactose, which promotes iron absorption, is in higher concentration in breast milk, especially as compared with prepared formulas, which may not contain lactose. Phosphorus may interfere with iron absorption, as may high protein levels. There is still considerable doubt as to whether it is physiologically sound to increase the hemoglobin of an infant with exogenous iron. All species of mammals have low iron content in their milks. All mammals investigated so far have a drop in their hemoglobin levels after birth and a gradual rise to adult levels for the species. The relationship between plasma concentration of ferritin and body iron stores has not been clearly established; the explanation of iron absorption and use in breastfed infants is still under study.

Zinc. Zinc has been identified as essential to the human. Its chief roles described to date are as part of the enzyme structure and as an enzyme activator. Zinc deficiency has been described as well, most recently in newborns and premature infants on hyperalimentation regimens. The chief clinical symptoms are failure to thrive and typical skin lesions. Milk has been identified as a food with bioavailable zinc.[73]

Zinc absorption from human milk, cow's milk, and infant formula was tested in healthy adults with labeled zinc chloride, Zn 65. The absorption was 41% from human milk, 28% from cow's milk, 31% from standard infant formula, and 14% from soy formula. The dietary zinc intake of both lactating and nonlactating postpartum women was found by Moser and Reynolds[96] to be 42% of recommended allowances. There was no correlation of maternal dietary zinc and maternal plasma and erythrocyte zinc with the concentrations of zinc in breast milk.

Changes in hair zinc concentrations of breastfed and bottle-fed infants during the first 6 months of life were measured by MacDonald et al.[92] Only the bottle-fed males had a significant decline in hair zinc concentration. There was no decline of zinc in any breastfed infant, which supports the concept of the superior bioavailability of zinc in breast milk.

Picciano and Guthrie[102] studied milk from 50 mothers in 350 samples. They found zinc levels to average 3.95 µg/ml and to be consistent regardless of time of day, duration of lactation, or other variables. They estimated that breastfed infants receive 0.35 mg of zinc/kg/day. They found zinc levels to decline slightly from the first to the third month postpartum (33.8 to 29.5 µmol/L). Longitudinal changes in dietary zinc requirements for infants acquiring new lean body mass through growth were studied by Krebs et al.[77] As growth velocity declines, zinc requirements decline in the male infant from a high of 780 µg/day at 1 month to 480 µg/day in the fifth through twelfth months. Meanwhile, the percentage of absorption increased over time.

Human milk was fractionated and analyzed by Frannsson and Lönnerdal[39] for the distribution of zinc. Most of the zinc was found in the skim milk fraction, but significant amounts were found in the fat associated with the fat globule membrane; less than 4% was found in the casein.

Cow's milk zinc is associated with high-molecular-weight fractions, and zinc in human milk is associated with low-molecular-weight fractions. The association of zinc with low-molecular-weight components of milk is related in part to protein content and composition and to the relative zinc concentration. When adult females were given oral doses of zinc with human milk, cow's milk, casein hydrolysate formula, and soy-based formula, the plasma response with human milk was significantly (three times) greater than with any of the others.[19]

The low-molecular-weight ligand has been proved to be readily absorbed. Breast milk has been therapeutic in the treatment of acrodermatitis enteropathica, an inherited zinc-metabolism disorder, whereas cow's milk formulas are ineffective.

Copper, selenium, aluminum, titanium, chromium, manganese, molybdenum, and nickel

Picciano and Guthrie[102] studied copper levels in human milk and noted that the content varied considerably among women and within each woman. The range was 0.09 to 0.63 µg/ml. Copper levels were higher in the morning. Dietary supplements did not alter results. Age, parity, and lactation history showed that older mothers and multiparas had higher levels. The fully breastfed infant would receive 0.05 mg of copper/kg/day (Table 4-14).

Fractionated analysis by Frannsson and Lönnerdal[39] revealed whole milk concentration of copper to be 0.27 ± 0.13 µg/ml with most of the copper in the skim milk fraction, significant amounts in the fat, and little in the casein. The predominant binding was with low-molecular-weight proteins, which would enhance bioavailability. Changes in hair copper concentrations were also studied among breastfed and bottle-fed infants.[92] Hair copper levels rose in the first 3 months in all infants and then declined, regardless of feeding or sex of infant. The authors associated this with the redistribution of copper in early infancy (Table 4-9).

The bioavailability of selenium depends on the sources and chemical form, and the quantitative significance is under investigation. Except for Keshan's disease, a potentially fatal cardiomyopathy seen in infants in China, there has not been a convincingly associated clinical deficiency syndrome. Dietary recommendations have been based on those for adults. Dietary intakes less than the lower limits, however, should not be considered deficient, especially in breastfed infants.[131]

Selenium concentrations in human milk are consistent in samples collected from many parts of the world, according to work by Hadjimarkos and Shearer.[46] The mean value was 0.020 ppm, which was similar to the value from many parts of the United States, where the range was 0.007 to 0.033 ppm.

Selenium is considered an essential nutrient in humans. It is an integral component of glutathione peroxidase, an enzyme known to metabolize lipid peroxides, and deficiency states have been described. Questions have been raised about the detrimental effects of high selenium intake on dentition. Selenium status was assessed in infants exclusively fed human milk or infant formula for 3 months by Smith et al.[121] Foremilk samples had a mean concentration of 15.7 ng/ml, hindmilk mean concentration was 16.3 ng/ml, and mean formula concentration was 8.6 ng/ml. The breastfed infants had greater intakes and higher serum levels of selenium than the formula-fed infants in the first 3 months (Table 4-14).

The concentration of chromium is highest in the organs of the newborn and declines rapidly during the first years of life. A longitudinal study of chromium in human milk was undertaken by Kumpulainen and Vuori.[80] Mothers collected samples at 8 to 18 days, 47 to 54 days, and 128 to 159 days postpartum, representing every feed during a 24-hour period with equal portions of fore- and hindmilk. The mean concentration was 0.39 (SD = 0.15) ng/ml and the intake 0.27 (SD = 0.11) µg/day. The values did not change over time. These values are the same as those in human serum and urine. The mothers' dietary intake averaged about 30 µg/day, which is lower than the 50 to 200 µg recommended daily allowance.

A high-density lipoprotein-cholesterol level can be increased with chromium supplementation. Chromium also is reported to have a favorable effect on serum lipid profiles. Deficiency of chromium in infancy may be an issue with low-birth-weight infants or those with inadequate fetal stores.[80]

Due largely to a lack of information, there is little understanding regarding manganese in infant nutrition.[88] In human milk, the major fraction of manganese is 71% found in the whey, 11% in the casein, and 18% in the lipid. Levels in human milk in the first month of lactation decreased from a mean of 5.4 ± 1.6 ng/ml on day 1 to 2.7 ± 1.6 ng/ml from day 5 through day 28. The average intake of the infant in the first month was 2.0 g/day.

The main biochemical role of molybdenum in mammalian systems is as a cofactor for several enzymes. Deficiencies are rare, usually in those on total parenteral nutrition. Molybdenum levels in human milk were measured from day 1 through day 38. Levels began at 15.0 ± 6.1 ng/ml and leveled off at 1 to 2 ng/ml at 1 month.

Nickel is generally accepted as an essential trace element for animals, but its role in humans is undefined. Levels in human milk are stable over time at 1.2 ng/ml. The average daily intake of nickel at 1 month was 0.8 µg.

Fluorine. Fluorine has been widely accepted as a significant dietary factor in decreasing dental caries (Table 4-14). The effect has been associated with the conversion of the enamel hydroxyapatite to fluorapatite with a reduction in acid solubility. It has been suggested that the presence of fluorine during the formation of hydroxyapatite creates less soluble, more resistant crystals.

Conflicting reports of the fluorine levels in human milk had led to the belief that breastfed infants needed supplementation.[86] More accurate studies in communities where fluoride has been in the public drinking water supply show 7 μg of fluorine per liter (range 4 to 14 μg/L).[31] The Academy of Pediatrics no longer recommends supplementing breastfed infants with fluorine (see Chapter 9).

The significant development of deciduous and permanent teeth is after birth and depends on fetal stores as well as on fluorine available in the diet. Studies comparing breastfed and bottle-fed infants show a distinct difference, with fewer dental caries and better dental health in breastfed infants. The role of fluorine and other factors, such as selenium, that predispose the breastfed infant to healthier teeth have yet to be defined completely. Nursing-bottle caries add to the total dental caries of the bottle-fed infant.

Iodide

Iodide levels have rarely been studied, although it was recognized that levels in the milk could be raised above those in the serum (in which radioactive iodine compounds have been examined). Mean breast milk iodide levels were 178 μg/L (range 29 to 490 μg/L), which is about four times the recommended daily allowance for infants.[44] Levels in milk were unrelated to the age of the infant but directly related to maternal intake calculated in the diet.

pH and osmolarity

The pH range in human milk is 6.7 to 7.4, with a mean of 7.1. The mean pH of cow's milk is 6.8. The caloric content of both human and cow's milk is 65 kcal/100 ml or 20 kcal/oz. The specific gravities are 1.031 and 1.032, respectively.

The osmolarity of human milk approximates that of human serum, or 286 mosmol/kg of water, whereas that for cow's milk is higher, 350 mosmol.[25] The renal solute load of human milk is considerably lower than that of cow's milk. Renal solute load is roughly calculated by totaling the solutes that must be excreted by the kidney. It consists primarily of nonmetabolizable dietary components, especially electrolytes, ingested in excess of body needs, and metabolic end products, mainly from the metabolism of protein. It can be estimated by adding the dietary intake of nitrogen and three minerals, sodium, potassium, and chloride. Each gram of protein is considered to yield 4 mosmol (as urea), and each milliequivalent of sodium, potassium, and chloride is 1 mosmol, according to Fomon.[35] The renal solute load of cow's milk is 221 mosmol, compared with 79 mosmol for human milk.

Osmoregulation in human lactation was investigated by Dearlove[27] in an effort to determine whether fluid loading was a valid clinical maneuver. It is known that an oral hypotonic fluid load results in suppression of prolactin in adults. After an intravenous hypotonic saline infusion, there was a significant correlation between serum osmolarity and prolactin. No changes in serum prolactin, milk yield, serum, or breast milk osmolarity were noted when normal lactating women were given a hypotonic fluid load in a controlled study.

Table 4-15. Vitamins and other constituents of human milk and cow's milk (per 100 ml)

Milk elements	Colostrum	Transitional	Mature	Cow's milk
Vitamins				
Vitamin A (µg)	151.0	88.0	75.0	41.0
Vitamin B₁ (µg)	1.9	5.9	14.0	43.0
Vitamin B₂ (µg)	30.0	37.0	40.0	145.0
Nicotinic acid (µg)	75.0	175.0	160.0	82.0
Vitamin B₆ (µg)			12.0-15.0	64.0
Pantothenic acid (µg)	183.0	288.0	246.0	340.0
Biotin (µg)	0.06	0.35	0.6	2.8
Folic acid (µg)	0.05	0.02	0.14	0.13
Vitamin B₁₂ (µg)	0.05	0.04	0.1	0.6
Vitamin C (mg)	5.9	7.1	5.0	1.1
Vitamin D (µg)	—	—	0.04	0.02
Vitamin E (mg)	1.5	0.9	0.25	0.07
Vitamin K (µg)	—	—	1.5	6.0
Ash (g)	0.3	0.3	0.2	0.7
Calories (kcal)	57.0	63.0	65.0	65.0
Specific gravity	1050.0	1035.0	1031.0	1032.0
Milk (pH)	—	—	7.0	6.8

Table 4-16. Recommended daily dietary allowances for fat-soluble vitamins for infants*

Age (yr)	Weight		Height		Protein (g)	Vitamin A (µg R.E.)†	Vitamin D (µg)‡	Vitamin E (mg αT.E.)§
	(kg)	(lb)	(cm)	(in)				
0.0-0.5	6	13	60	24	kg × 2.2	420	10	3
0.5-1.0	9	20	71	28	kg × 2.0	400	10	4

From Food and Nutrition Board, National Research Council, National Academy of Sciences: Recommended dietary allowances, ed 9, Washington DC, 1980, US Government Printing Office.

*The allowances are intended to provide for individual variations among most normal persons as they live in the United States under usual environmental stresses. Diets should be based on a variety of common foods in order to provide other nutrients for which human requirements have been less well defined.

†Retinol equivalents. 1 retinol equivalent = 1 µg retinol or 6 µg carotene.

‡As cholecalciferol, 10 µg cholecalciferol = 400 IU vitamin D.

§α-Tocopherol equivalents 1 mg d-α-tocopherol = 1 αT.E.

Vitamins
Vitamin A

Vitamin A content is 75 µg/100 ml or 280 international units (IU) in mature human milk and 41 µg/100 ml or 180 IU in cow's milk (Table 4-15). Thus the supply of vitamin A and its precursors, carotenoids, is considered adequate to meet the estimated daily requirement, which varies from 500 IU to 1500 IU/day if the infant consumes at least 200 ml of breast milk per day (Table 4-16). There is twice as much vitamin A in colostrum as in mature milk.

Vitamin D

Vitamin D has always been included in the fat-soluble vitamin group because that is the form in which it had been identified in nature. The levels in human milk were 0.05 μg/100 ml, previously reported in the fat fraction. Human milk was shown by Lakdawala and Widdowson[81] in 1977 to have vitamin D in both the fat and the aqueous fractions. The water-soluble sulfate conjugate of vitamin D was measured. Other investigators have attempted to repeat this work, but, more important, they have evaluated the biologic activity of any water-soluble metabolites. When activity is measured by an assay that measures stimulation of intestinal calcium transport, human milk is found to contain 40 to 50 IU/L of vitamin D activity. The metabolite 25-hydroxyvitamin D_3 accounts for 75% of the activity; vitamin D_2 and vitamin D_3 account for 15% activity. Vitamin D sulfate, or any other as yet unidentified water-soluble metabolite of vitamin D, has not been proven to have significant biologic activity.

The impact of the maternal diet content of vitamin D was measured in a double-blind study of white mothers in a temperate climate in the winter.[110] A direct relationship was seen between maternal and infant levels of 25-hydroxyvitamin D_3 and maternal diet. An additional group of infants, whose mothers' diets were unsupplemented, received 400 IU vitamin D/day and had even higher serum concentrations of 25-hydroxyvitamin D_3. When mothers have been given large doses of vitamin D, the content of vitamin D and D_3 in their milk increases as it does with exposure to sunshine. The level of 25-OH vitamin D does not change. The majority of the activity in human milk is in the form of 25-OH vitamin D. This may be an advantage for the breastfed infant who utilizes this form most readily. Clearly the levels vary and may be inadequate in human milk in some situations, especially in cold climates in the winter when there is little sunshine, especially for dark-skinned individuals. The level of 40 IU/100 ml or 1.00 μg/100 ml may provide adequate amounts in the fully breastfed infant to meet the requirements of 400 IU or 10 mg/day. See Table 4-16 for recommended daily allowances. Levels of vitamin D are also higher in colostrum than in mature milk.

Vitamin E

Vitamin E has been a subject of much interest. Levels in colostrum are 1.5 mg/100 ml, whereas transitional milk has 0.9 mg/100 ml and mature milk has 0.25 mg/100 ml. The difference at different stages has been found to be due to α-tocopherol, because the contents of β- and γ-tocopherol are similar. Total tocopherol in mature milk correlates with total lipid and linoleic acid contents. Significantly higher tocopherol/linoleic acid ratios are found in both colostrum and transitional milk than in mature milk.[66]

Cow's milk has 0.07 mg/100 ml of vitamin E (Table 4-15). Correspondingly, serum levels in breastfed infants rise quickly at birth and maintain a normal level, whereas cow's milk–fed infants have depressed levels. Vitamin E includes a group of fat-soluble compounds, α-, β-, γ-, and δ-tocopherol, and their unsaturated derivatives, α-, β-, γ-, and δ-tocotrienol. An international unit of vitamin E is equal to 1 mg of synthetic α-tocopherol or 0.74 mg of natural α-tocopherol acetate. Vitamin E is required for muscle integrity, resistance of erythrocytes to hemolysis, as well as for other biochemical and physiologic functions. The requirement for vitamin E is related to the polyunsaturated fatty acid (PUFA) content of the cellular structures and of the diet (see Table 4-16). Satisfactory plasma levels are 1 mg/100 ml, and these can be maintained by feedings with a vitamin E/PUFA ratio of 0.4 mg/g.

Table 4-17.   Recommended daily dietary allowances for vitamins for infants*

Age (yr)	Vitamin K (μg)	Biotin (μg)	Pantothenic acid (mg)
0-0.5	12	35	2
0.5-1.0	10-20	50	3

From Food and Nutrition Board, National Research Council, National Academy of Sciences: Recommended dietary allowances, ed 9, Washington DC, 1980, US Government Printing Office.
*The allowances are intended to provide for individual variations among most normal persons as they live in the United States under usual environmental stresses. Diets should be based on a variety of common foods in order to provide other nutrients for which human requirements have been less well defined.

An estimate of the tocopherol/linoleic acid ratio in mature milk is 0.79 mg α-tocopherol equivalents/g, which is comparable to a daily requirement of 0.5 mg for term infants but may be low for prematures, especially those on iron supplementation.[82] Ordinarily, this would be supplied by 4 IU of vitamin E/day. Since human milk contains 1.8 mg/L or 40 μg of vitamin E/g of lipid, it supplies more than adequate levels of vitamin E.

Vitamin K

Vitamin K is essential for the synthesis of blood clotting factors, which are normal in the serum at birth. The old levels of vitamin K reported in human milk (15 μg/100 ml) have been replaced with those done by more accurate techniques and are lower, i.e., 2.1 μg/L for mature milk and 2.3 μg/L for colostrum,[82] which is less than the recommended daily intake of 12 μg/day. The measurement of the homologues of vitamin K have been equivocal. When mothers are given a single dose of 20 mg phylloquinone (K_1), the milk level increases from 1 μg/L to 140 μg/L in 12 hours, dropping to 5 μg/L in 48 hours.[43] When infants are given 1 mg vitamin K_1 at birth as is the practice in many countries, the concentration of K_1 in both breastfed and formula-fed infants in the first week of life remains elevated. When no neonatal prophylaxis is given, Büller et al[12] reported no difference in coagulating factors among a sample of 113 breastfed, formula-fed, or combination-fed infants. They reported a case of low vitamin K levels in the milk of a mother whose infant died at 6 weeks of an intracranial bleed without neonatal prophylaxis. See Table 4-17 for recommended daily dietary allowances. Vitamin K is produced by the intestinal flora but takes several days in the previously sterile gut to be effective. Vitamin K–dependent clotting factors in normal breastfed infants were studied by Jimenez et al,[71] who reported that no infant studied had clinical evidence of bleeding. The prothrombin time and partial thromboplastin time were similar in breastfed and bottle fed infants. The normotest and thrombotest were significantly prolonged in the breastfed group. The authors concluded that 5% of breastfed children have possible vitamin K deficiency. There are several case reports[89,99] of infants exclusively breastfed with no vitamin K given at birth who developed late-onset hemorrhagic disease that responded to vitamin K administration. The report by O'Connor et al[99] points out the association of vitamin K deficiency with home birth and suggests that the physician give vitamin K as recommended by the Academy of Pediatrics if it has been omitted (Table 4-17). It is recommended that all infants receive vitamin K at birth, regardless of feeding plans, to prevent hemorrhagic disease of the newborn caused by vitamin K deficiency in the first few days of life.[20]

Table 4-18. Recommended daily dietary allowances for water soluble vitamins for infants*

Age (yr)	Vitamin C (mg)	Thiamin (mg)	Riboflavin (mg)	Niacin (mg N.E.)†	Vitamin B₆ (mg)	Folacin‡ (μg)	Vitamin B₁₂ (μg)
0-0.5	35	0.3	0.4	6	0.3	30	0.58
0.5-1.0	35	0.5	0.6	8	0.6	45	1.5

From Food and Nutrition Board, National Research Council, National Academy of Sciences: Recommended dietary allowances, ed 9, Washington DC, 1980, US Government Printing Office.
*The allowances are intended to provide for individual variations among most normal persons as they live in the United States under usual environmental stresses. Diets should be based on a variety of common foods to provide other nutrients for which human requirements have been less well defined.
†INF. (niacin equivalent) is equal to 1 mg of niacin or 60 mg of dietary tryptophan.
‡The folacin allowances refer to dietary sources as determined by *Lactobacillus casei* assay after treatment with enzymes ("conjugases") to make polyglutamyl forms of the vitamin.

Vitamin C

Vitamin C is part of several enzyme and hormone systems as well as of intracellular chemical reactions. It is essential to collagen synthesis (Table 4-18).

Human milk is an outstanding source of water-soluble vitamins and reflects maternal dietary intake (Table 4-15). Increased vitamin C has been measured in the milk within 30 minutes of a bolus of vitamin C being given to the mother. Human milk contains 43 mg/ 100 ml (fresh cow's milk contains up to 21 mg). Levels obtained in normal lactating women 6 months postpartum were 35 mg/L in those on normal diets and 38 mg/L in those supplemented with multivitamins containing 90 mg vitamin C.[125] Levels obtained in 16 low-socioeconomic level lactating women were 53 mg/L for unsupplemented and 65 mg/L for supplemented mothers at 1 week postpartum and 61 mg/L and 72 mg/L, respectively, at 6 weeks postpartum. Several subjects in the unsupplemented low socio-economic group had levels too low to provide 35 mg vitamin C/day to their infants.

When lactating women were given 250, 500, or 1000 mg/day vitamin C for 2 days, milk levels remained within the range of 44 to 158 mg/L and did not differ significantly between dosages even at ten times the RDA.[14] Total intake of the infant via the milk ranged from 49 to 86 mg/day. These findings suggest a regulatory mechanism for vitamin C levels in milk. When women received high doses of vitamin C, levels of the vitamin excreted in the urine also increased proportionately.

Vitamin B complex
Vitamin B₁

Vitamin B₁, or thiamin, levels increase with the duration of lactation but are lower in human milk (160 μg/100 ml) than in cow's milk (440 μg/100 ml). In a study by Nail et al,[97] levels obtained by normal lactating women showed significant increases between 1 and 6 weeks postpartum, but there was no difference in levels between supplemented (1.7 mg daily) and unsupplemented women.

Since urinary excretion of thiamin is significantly higher in supplemented than in unsupplemented women, there appears to be a limit on the amount of vitamin transferred into milk. Malnourished women show significant increases in their milk when supplemented.[86] Thiamin is essential for the use of carbohydrates in the pyruvate metabolism (cofactor in pyruvic acid decarboxylation) and for fat synthesis. Insufficient thiamin produces insufficient carbohydrate oxidation with accumulation of intermediary metabolites such as lactic acid. See Table 4-18 for recommended daily allowances.

Vitamin B_2

Vitamin B_2, or riboflavin, is significant for the newborn in whom intestinal tract bacterial synthesis is minimal (see Table 4-18 for recommended daily allowances). Riboflavin is involved in oxidative intracellular systems and is essential for protoplasmic growth. There are 36 μg/100 ml in human milk and 175 μg/100 ml in cow's milk (Table 4-15).

Levels obtained in normal lactating women showed significantly lower levels of riboflavin in the milk of the unsupplemented women (36.7 μg/100 ml) at 1 week as compared with the milk of the supplemented women, who received 2 mg/day in a multivitamin (80.0 μg/100 ml). There was no significant difference between 1 and 6 weeks in either group.[97]

Niacin

Niacin (nicotinamide) is an essential part of the pyridine nucleotide coenzymes and is part of the intracellular respiratory mechanisms. There is 147 μg/100 ml in human milk and 94 μg/100 ml in cow's milk (Table 4-15). Levels respond to dietary supplementation.

Vitamin B_6

Vitamin B_6 (pyridoxine) forms the enzyme group of certain decarboxylases and transaminases involved in metabolism of nerve tissue. The supply of vitamin B_6 is vital to DNA synthesis, which is needed to form the cerebrosides in the myelination of the central nervous system (see Table 4-18 for recommended daily allowances). There is 12 to 15 μg/100 ml of vitamin B_6 in human milk and 64 μg/100 ml in cow's milk. The principal form of B_6 in human milk is pyridoxal (PL), whereas pyridoxine (PN) is the principal form of vitamin B_6 fortification in infant formulas.[127] Levels of vitamin B_6 in the milk of mothers consuming more than 2.5 mg of the vitamin daily (RDA for lactating women is 2.5 mg/day) were significantly higher in the first week than were levels in the unsupplemented mothers' milk. Average maternal diets in several studies were consistently below the recommended levels of vitamin B_6.[108] The recommended daily intake for infants under 6 months of age is 0.30 mg.

Long-term use of oral contraceptives has been shown to result in low levels of vitamin B_6 in maternal serum in pregnancy and at delivery and low levels in the milk of these mothers.[109] The relationship of B_6 supplements to suppression of prolactin and the treatment of galactorrhea is discussed under lactation failure (see Chapter 15). The doses used to suppress lactation (600 mg/day) far exceed the levels in multiple vitamins (1 to 10 mg).

Pantothenic acid

Pantothenic acid is part of coenzyme A, a catalyst of acetylation reactions. The reaction of coenzyme A with acetic acid to form acetyl-CoA is prime to intermediary metabolism. The levels of pantothenic acid in human milk were restudied by Johnston et al[74] because of the range of values in the literature. They found the mean to be 670 μg/100 ml in fore- and hindmilk samples. No change occurred in concentrations from 1 to 6 months postpartum. They did find a positive correlation with dietary intake. Recommended daily allowances appear in Table 4-17.

Folacin

Folacin (folic acid) is part of the conversion of glycine to serine. It is also involved in the methylation of nicotinamide and homocystine to methionine. It is essential for erythropoiesis. There is 4.0 to 7.0 μg of folic acid/100 ml of breast milk. Colostrum is relatively low in folacin, but levels increase as lactation proceeds. Supplementation with folic acid in deficient mothers caused prompt increase in levels in the milk. When mothers and their infants were evaluated, folate levels were two to three times higher in the breastfed infants than in their mothers, and there was a correlation between levels in the milk and in the infants' plasma. Folic acid has also been identified as a critical element in deficiency states during pregnancy, being associated with abruptio placentae, toxemia, and intrauterine growth failure as well as megaloblastic anemia.

Vitamin B_{12}

Early studies reported that vitamin B_{12} is found in human milk in low concentration, 0.3 μg/100 ml, whereas cow's milk has 4.0 μg/ml. Well-nourished mothers on balanced diets appear to have adequate amounts for their infants. Microbiologic assay has demonstrated that very high concentrations of vitamin B_{12} appear in early colostrum but level off in a few days to those of serum. Colostric samples reported by Samson and McClelland[112] have a mean binding capacity of 72 ng/ml; in mature milk the capacity is one third of this value. Vitamin B_{12} levels were compared by Sandberg et al[113] in supplemented and unsupplemented mothers and were not significantly different. Levels were 33 to 320 ng/100 ml, with a mean of 97 ng/100 ml. When nutritionally deficient low-socioeconomic-group lactating women were studied by Sneed et al,[122] supplementation with a multivitamin did indeed result in elevated vitamin B_{12} levels. This was true for folate as well.

Although cow's milk has five to ten times more vitamin B_{12} than mature human milk, cow's milk has little vitamin B_{12}–binding capacity, which is substantial in human milk. Vitamin B_{12} functions in transmethylations such as synthesis of choline from methionine, serine from glycine, and methionine from homocysteine. It is involved in pyrimidine and purine metabolism. Vitamin B_{12} also affects the metabolism of folic acid. Megaloblastic anemia is a common symptom of vitamin B_{12} deficiency. Vitamin B_{12} occurs exclusively in animal tissue, is bound to protein, and is minimal or absent in vegetable protein. The minimum daily requirement for infants is 0.58 μg/day in the first year of life, when growth is rapid. (See Table 4-17.)

Enzymes

Until recently little effort has been applied to studying the activities of enzymes in humans, although considerable data have been collected on the enzymatic activities of many milks. Jenness and Sloan[68] report 44 enzymes detected so far in bovine, human, and some other milks. Xanthine oxidase, lactoperoxidase, uridine diphosphogalactose, glucose, galactosyl transferase, ribonuclease, lipase, alkaline phosphatase, acid phosphatase, and lysozyme have been isolated, in crystalline form.

The role and significance of enzymes in human milk were reviewed by Hamosh,[51] who confirmed that there are over 20 active human-milk enzymes (Table 4-19). They can be categorized into three general groups by their activity: mammary gland function, which reflects physiologic changes occurring in the mammary gland itself during lactation; compensatory digestive enzymes in human milk, which have digestive functions in the neonate; and milk enzymes, important in neonatal development.[51] Some enzyme levels are signif-

Table 4-19. Functions of enzymes in human milk

Enzyme	Function
Antiproteases	Prevent proteolytic activity in mammary gland. Protect bioactive proteins (enzymes, immunoglobulins) from hydrolysis in milk and in the intestine of the newborn.
α-Amylase	Facilitates digestion of polysaccharides (in milk, formula and beikost) by the infant.
Lipase, bile salt stimulated	Hydrolysis of fat in the intestine of the newborn. Bactericidal activity.
Lipase, serum stimulated	Regulates long-chain triglyceride, phospholipid, and cholesterol concentration in milk.
Sulfhydryl Oxidase	Catalyzes oxidation of SH groups: possible role in maintaining structure and function of proteins containing disulfide bonds.
Lysozyme	Bactericidal.
Peroxidase	Bactericidal, present in milk leukocytes.

From Hamosh M: Enzymes in human milk. In Howell RR, Morriss FH, and Pickering LK, editors: Human milk in infant nutrition and health, Springfield Ill, 1986, Charles C Thomas, Publisher.

icantly higher in colostrum than in mature milk. Most are whey proteins and contribute minimally to milk proteins. Some enzymes, like other proteins in milk, are probably produced elsewhere and are transported to the breast via the bloodstream.[63] The evidence to support the concept of local synthesis includes the demonstration of secretory tissue in the mammary gland. Amylase levels are twice as high in milk as in serum.[56,85] Casein proteins have been synthesized in vitro in cell-free mammary-derived mRNA-enriched systems. Mammary explants from mice, monkeys, and humans have accumulated lactose synthetase B. The enzymes of possible importance in infant digestion are those with pancreatic analogues: amylase, lipases, protease(s), and ribonuclease.[118]

Amylase

Amylase, the chief polysaccharide-digesting enzyme, is not developed at birth even in full-term infants who have only 0.2% to 0.5% of adult values. Mammary amylase is present, however, throughout lactation, with levels higher in colostrum than in mature milk. Human milk levels are 0.5 to 1.0 g/dl oligosaccharides of varying chain length. The levels in milk of preterm mothers were comparable to term milk levels.

Milk levels are twice those of serum in the first 90 days and remain higher than serum over 6 months. When exposed to a pH of 5.3, this salivary-type amylase remains active; at a pH of 3.5, one half the original activity is present at 2 hours and one third at 6 hours. Much milk amylase activity remains in the duodenum after a meal of human milk. This is significant for the digestion of starch because pancreatic amylase is still low in infants. It has been suggested that mammary amylase may be an alternate pathway of digestion of glucose polymers as well as of starch.

Lipases

Milk fat is almost completely digestible. The emulsion of fat in breast milk is greater than in cow's milk, resulting in smaller globules. Milk lipases play an active role in creating the emulsion, which yields a finer curd and facilitates the digestion of triacylglycerols.

The newborn easily digests and completely uses the well-emulsified small fat globules of human milk. Free fatty acids are important sources of energy for the infant.

Lipase in human milk was first described in 1901. At least two different lipases (glycerol ester hydrolases) were described then. The lipases in human milk make the free fatty acids available in a large proportion even before the digestive phase of the intestine. The lipolytic milk-enzyme activity is similar to the activity of pancreatic lipase, breaking down triglycerides to free fatty acids and glycerol. One enzyme is present in the fat fraction and is inhibited by bile salts.

It appears that the function of this enzyme is to facilitate the uptake by the mammary gland of fatty acids from circulating triglycerides for incorporation with milk lipids because it is dependent in vivo on added serum for activity. Its presence in milk probably represents "leakage" from the mammary gland, and it is unlikely to play a major physiologic role in the lipolysis of milk triglycerides.[57]

There are additional lipases in the skim milk fraction, and these are stimulated by bile salts. The lipase stimulated by bile salts has greater activity and splits all three ester bonds of the triglyceride. This lipase is also stable in the duodenum and contributes to the hydrolysis of the triacylglycerols in the presence of the bile salts.[57]

Investigators have continued to study the action of these lipases in the presence of bile salts.[47,48,57,58] The lipase remains active during passage through the stomach because it is stable above pH 3.5 and only slowly inactivated by pepsin. The optimal bile-salt concentration for activity is about 2 mmol/L, which is within the physiologic range in the newborn. Bile salts protect the enzyme from tryptic activity.[57,58] It is reported that glycine rather than taurine conjugates are essential for activity. The lipid concentration and lipolytic activity increase significantly over the course of the feed, the latter remaining constant in samples collected early and late in the postpartum period.[52] The main lipolytic products are fatty acids with little specificity for different fatty acids of triglyceride. In vitro studies of bile salt–stimulated lipase demonstrate that activity is closely controlled by components found in the milk. It is suggested by Hall and Muller[48] that human milk lipase in the small intestine complements rather than duplicates pancreatic lipase activity.

Diastase

Diastase catalyzes the hydrolysis of starch to maltose and may indeed be α-amylase or a mixture of α- and β-amylase. There is a high level of diastase in colostrum, with an initial rapid fall and a constant level for the next 6 months. Since most infants are deficient in diastase initially, this may account for the lack of apparent digestive disturbances when starch gruels are introduced early in breastfed infants.[118]

Glucose-6-phosphate dehydrogenase

Glucose-6-phosphate dehydrogenase (G-6-PD) is rich in the milk of mothers with normal red cell dehydrogenase and absent in mothers with G-6-PD deficiency. Its levels are dependent on the increased rate of carbohydrate metabolism in the mammary gland.[118]

Lactic and malic acid dehydrogenases

Lactic and malic acid dehydrogenase levels are high in colostrum, are lower in mature milk, and increase at the end of a feeding. The levels are higher in species with small body size; thus, mice and humans have more than cows. Since there is no correlation with serum levels, it is believed to be synthesized in the mammary gland. There is a change in these enzymes during lactation.

Lactose synthetase

Lactose synthetase catalyzes the synthesis of lactose from UDP-galactose and glucose. This enzyme has two components: A-protein, a glycoprotein, and B-protein, which is an α-lactalbumin. The control mechanism for lactose biosynthesis by the A-protein and α-lactalbumin ensures that lactose is synthesized in the mammary gland only in response to specific hormones.

Lysozyme

Lysozyme is a thermostabile nonspecific antimicrobial factor that catalyzes the hydrolysis of β-linkage between *N*-acetyl glucosamine and *N*-acetyl muramic acid in the bacterial cell wall. It is bacteriolytic toward *Enterobacteriaceae* and gram-positive bacteria and is considered to play a role in the antibacterial activity of milk as well as a significant role in the development of intestinal flora. It also hydrolyzes mucopolysaccharides. Human lysozyme is antigenically and serologically different from the bovine enzyme. The content in human milk is 3000 times that in bovine milk and the activity 100 times that of bovine milk. It is considered to be a spillover product from breast epithelial cells.

Phosphatases

Acid phosphatase is similar in human and bovine milk, but alkaline phosphatase is much less active in human milk by a factor of 40. Its level increases with the increase in fat concentration and increases as the feeding progresses. In 199 samples from 20 donors, there was no relationship to age, nationality, or other characteristics of the donor, except for a tendency to increase over time. Alkaline phosphatase concentrations appeared to be related to the fat concentration in human milk. Levels increased as lactation progressed.[1]

Protease

Protease catalyzes the hydrolysis of proteins. There are high levels of protease in human milk, which suggests that enzymes may provide the breastfed infant with significant digestive assistance immediately after birth.

Xanthine oxidase

Xanthine oxidase catalyzes the oxidation of purines, pyrimidines, and aldehydes. Although bovine milk contains high levels, it was only after much effort that investigators were able to identify it in human milk.[132] The activity in human milk peaks on the third day after birth and decreases with the progression of lactation. It differs from that in bovine milk in that it is not of bacterial origin and its activity is correlated with protein concentration.

Hormones

Protein hormones, especially prolactin, and steroid hormones such as gestagens, estrogens, corticords, androgens, and opiate-like peptides can be detected in milk.[116]

Hormones are present in human milk and in the milk of other mammals. Animal studies have shown that at least some of these hormones retain physiological activity when ingested but not when pasteurized. Although their presence was recognized in the 1930s, advances in hormone assay techniques have brought more information to light.[76] Hormones with simple structures, such as steroids and thyroxine (T$_4$), can pass easily by diffusion into the milk from circulating blood. Peptide hormones such as hypothalamic-releasing hormones, because of their small size, would be expected to appear in milk. Of the larger-molecular-weight pituitary hormones, only prolactin has been found so far. The hormones identified in human milk include gonadotropin-releasing hormone, thyroid-releasing hormone (TRH), thyroid-stimulating hormone (thyrotropin, TSH), prolactin, gonadotropins, ovarian hormones, corticosteroids, erythropoietin, cyclic adenosine monophosphate (cAMP), and cyclic guanosine monophosphate (cGMP).

The concentration of hormones changes during lactation, with prolactin decreasing over time and triiodothyronine (T_3) and T_4 increasing. There is information demonstrating that the gastrointestinal tract of suckling mammals possesses the ability to absorb various proteins with substantial preservation of their immunologic properties. The absorption of large-molecular-weight hormones has been demonstrated in suckling rats and mice with measurable amounts appearing in serum and other tissues.

The thyroid hormones have received considerable attention because of the apparent protection of hypothyroid infants who are breastfed. TSH content was investigated by both direct ^{125}I-TSH radioimmunoassay and radioimmunoassay.[124] TSH was present in human milk in low concentrations comparable to those normally found in the serum of euthyroid adults. Experimentally, thyroidectomy of the lactating rat led to the disappearance of measurable T_4 and an increase in the level of TSH in the milk. In contrast, administration of T_3 decreased the TSH in the rat model.

Prolactin has been identified as a normal constituent of human milk. Levels are high in the first few days postpartum but subsequently decline rapidly. There is "prolactin-like" biological activity measurable in human colostrum with the highest levels on day 1. Concentrations in the milk tend to parallel concentrations in the blood plasma among different species.

The exact mechanism by which prolactin enters the milk is unclear. Prolactin-binding sites have been identified within the alveolar cells.[55] The functional significance of prolactin also remains unclear. In rodents, milk prolactin influences fluid and ion absorption from the jejunum. It may influence gonadal and adrenal function as demonstrated in other species.

Endocrine responses in the neonate differ between breastfed and formula-fed infants.[90] In a study of 34 6-day-old healthy, full-term infants who were formula fed, there were significant changes in the plasma concentrations of insulin, motilin, enteroglucagon, neurotensin, and pancreatic polypeptide following a feeding. Similar levels were measured in 43 normal breastfed infants, and little or no change was noted. Further, the basal levels of gastric inhibitory polypeptide, motilin, neurotensin, and vasoactive intestinal peptide were also higher in the bottle-fed than in the breastfed infants. Whether pancreatic and gut hormone-release changes affect postnatal development is yet to be determined.

Prostaglandins

In the investigation of the factors in human milk that may modify or supplement physiological functions in the neonate, the role of prostaglandins comes under review. Prostaglandins include any of a class of physiologically active substances present in many tissues and originally described in genital fluid and accessory glands. Among the many effects are those of vasodepression, stimulation of intestinal smooth muscle, uterine stimulation, aggregation of blood platelets, and antagonism to hormones influencing lipid metabolism. Prostaglandins are a group of prostanoic acids often abbreviated PGE, PGF, PGA, and PGB with numeric subscripts according to structure.

The synthesis of prostaglandins occurs when dietary linoleic acid is converted in the body by a series of steps involving chain lengthening and dehydration to arachidonic acid, the principal (but not the only) precursor of prostaglandins. Although the prostaglandins are similar in structure, the biologic effects of various prostaglandins produced from a single unsaturated fatty acid can be profoundly different and, in some cases, antagonistic.

Because of the possible beneficial effects of prostaglandins on the gastrointestinal tract of infants, several investigators[3,91,107] have measured levels in human milk. The measurements were made in colostrum, transitional milk, and mature milk with collections of both fore- and hindmilk. PGE and PGF have been shown to be present in breast milk in over 100 times the concentration in adult plasma (Fig. 4-5). The ratio of the principal metabolite of PGFM to PGF itself suggests a relatively long half-life (Fig. 4-6). Although prostaglandins occur in cow's milk, none was measurable in cow's milk–based formulas. Two inactive metabolites were found in milk in levels similar to those in the control adult plasma.

It is thought that prostaglandins play a role in gastrointestinal motility, possibly assisting peristalsis physiologically. Infantile diarrhea may occasionally be due to excessive prostaglandin secretion into the mother's milk during menstruation, when maternal plasma levels of PGF may be raised. The difference in stool patterns between breast and formula feeds may be partially attributable to the presence of prostaglandins in human milk and not in formulas. The role of prostaglandins in the pathogenesis of food intolerance is also under study, since prostaglandins have a cytoprotective effect on the upper bowel and reportedly are increased in patients with abnormal peristalsis and irritable bowel syndrome.[83]

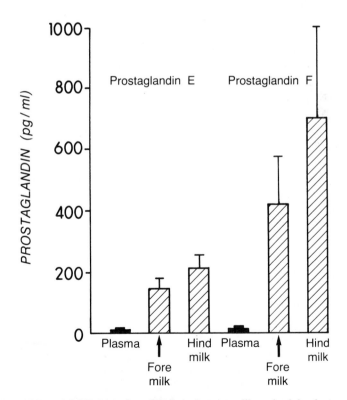

Fig. 4-5. PGE and PGF (pg/ml ± SEM) in human milk and adult plasma. (From Lucas A and Mitchell MD: Arch Dis Child 55:950, 1980.)

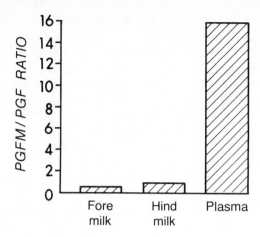

Fig. 4-6. PGFM/PGF ratio in human milk and adult plasma. (From Lucas A and Mitchell MD: Arch Dis Child 55:950, 1980.)

It appears that in addition the human infant may require PGE_2 for maintenance of its gastric mucosal integrity, as do adults, and therefore it is not surprising that the use of prostaglandin synthesis inhibitors as indomethacin for closure of a patent ductus is associated with necrotizing enterocolitis. PGE_2 in human milk may also promote the accumulation of phospholipids in the neonatal stomach, enhancing the gastric mucosal barrier.

Bile salts

Another limiting factor in digestion in the newborn is the decreased bile-salt pool and the low concentration of bile salts in the duodenum. The presence of some biologically active substances in human milk contributes to digestion in the newborn. For this reason the role of bile salts was investigated, and cholate and chenodeoxycholate were found in all samples of milk obtained from 28 lactating women in the first postpartum week.[37] In both colostrum and milk there was a predominance of cholate. Samples were randomly collected, and the range of concentration was wide. The ratio of maternal serum to milk was 1:1 for cholate and 4:1 for chenodeoxycholate. The significance of these findings is under study.

Epidermal growth factor

Epidermal growth factor (EGF) is a small polypeptide mitogen that has been identified in many species and isolated and characterized in human milk. Of the growth factors that have been purified to date, EGF is one of the most biologically potent and best characterized as to its physical, chemical, and biologic properties. It is well established that EGF stimulates the proliferation of epidermal and epithelial tissues and has significant biologic effects in the intact mammal, particularly in the fetus and the newborn.[16] Effects verified in humans also include increased growth and maturation of the fetal pulmonary epithelium, stimulation of ornithine decarboxylase activity and DNA synthesis in the digestive tract, and acceleration of the healing of wounds of the corneal epithelium. Quite unrelated is the observation that EGF inhibits histamine- or pentagastrin-induced secretion of gastric acid. It has a maturational effect on duodenal mucosal cells and increased lactase activity and net calcium transport in suckling rats. EGF has been identified in plasma, saliva, urine, amniotic fluid, and milk. Human milk is known to be mitogenic for cultured cells. EGF is active when administered orally, stable in acid, and resistant to trypsin digestion.

Newborn puppies, fed their mother's milk, were found to have hyperplasia of the enteric mucosa as compared with formula-fed littermates. Furthermore, the intestinal weight, length, and DNA and RNA content were greater in the puppies fed their mother's milk.

Studies of EGF in human milk first reported the fact that human milk stimulates DNA synthesis in cell cultures in which growth had been arrested.[94] The mitogenic activity of the milk was neutralized by the addition of antibody to human EGF. These findings support the concept that EGF is a major growth-promoting agent in breast milk. Actual measurements of EGF in the milk of 11 mothers who delivered at term and 20 who delivered prematurely were also done. EGF concentrations were 68 ± 19 ng/ml (mean $\pm$ SEM) in those who delivered at term and 70 ± 5 ng/ml (mean $\pm$ SEM) in the milk of those who delivered prematurely. There was no significant change over 7 weeks and no diurnal variation. The total EGF content was closely correlated with the volume of milk expressed, suggesting to the authors that EGF has a passive transport from the circulation as a function of plasma concentration.[16,94] Little change occurred with refrigeration or freezing. The role of EGF in promoting normal growth and functional maturation of the intestinal tract continues under study.

REFERENCES

1. Adcock EW, Brewer ED, Caprioli RM et al: Macronutrients, electrolytes and minerals in human milk: differences over time and between population groups. In Howell RR, Morriss FH, and Pickering LK, editors: Human milk in infant nutrition and health, Springfield Ill, 1986, Charles C Thomas, Publisher.
2. Almroth SG: Water requirements of breastfed infants in a hot climate, Am J Clin Nutr 31:1154, 1978.
3. Alzina V, Puig M, de Echániz L et al: Prostaglandins in human milk, Biol Neonate 50:200, 1986.
4. Anaokar SG and Garry PJ: Effects of maternal iron nutrition during lactation on milk iron and rat neonatal iron status, Am J Clin Nutr 34:1505, 1981.
5. Asnes RS et al: The dietary chloride deficiency syndrome occurring in a breastfed infant, J Pediatr 100:923, 1982.
6. Atkinson SA, Bryan MH, and Anderson GH: Human milk: differences in nitrogen concentration in milk from mothers of term and premature infants, J Pediatr 93:67, 1978.
7. Auricchio S, Rubino A, and Mürset E: Intestinal glycosidase activities in the human embryo, fetus, and newborn, Pediatrics 35:944, 1965.
8. Barth CA, Roos N, Nottbohn B et al: L-Carnitine concentrations in milk from mothers on different diets. In Schaub J, editor: Composition and physiological properties of human milk, Amsterdam, 1985, Elsevier.
9. Bitman J, Wood DL, Mehta NR et al: Comparison of the phospholipid composition of breast milk from mothers of term and preterm infants during lactation, Am J Clin Nutr 40:1103-19, 1984.
10. Bitman J, Wood DL, Neville MC et al: Lipid composition of prepartum, preterm and term milk. In Hamosh M and Goldman AS, editors: Human lactation, vol 2, Maternal and environmental factors, New York, 1986, Plenum Press.
11. Brown KH et al: Clinical and field studies of human lactation: methodological considerations, Am J Clin Nutr 35:745, 1982.
12. Büller H, Peters M, Burger B et al: Vitamin K status beyond the neonatal period, Eur J Pediatr 145:496, 1986.
13. Butte NF, Garza C, and Smith EO: Macro- and trace mineral intakes of exclusively breastfed infants, Am J Clin Nutr 45:42, 1987.
14. Byerley LO and Kirksey A: Effects of different levels of vitamin C intake on the vitamin C concentration in human milk and the vitamin C intakes of breastfed infants, Am J Clin Nutr 41:665, 1985.
15. Carlson SE: Human milk nonprotein nitrogen: occurrence and possible function, Adv Pediatr 32:43-70, 1985.
16. Carpenter G: Epidermal growth factor is a major growth-promoting agent in human milk, Science 210:198, 1980.
17. Casey CE and Hambidge KM: Nutritional aspects of human lactation. In Neville MC and

Neifert MR, editors: Lactation, physiology, nutrition, and breastfeeding, New York, 1983, Plenum Press.

18. Casey CE and Neville MC: Studies in human lactation. III. Molybdenum and nickel in human milk during the first month of lactation, Am J Clin Nutr 45:921, 1987.
19. Casey CE, Walravens PA, and Hambidge KM: Availability of zinc: loading tests with human milk, cow's milk, and infant formulas, Pediatrics 68:394, 1981.
20. Committee on Nutrition, American Academy of Pediatrics: Vitamin K supplementation for infants, Pediatrics 48:483, 1971.
21. Committee on Nutrition, American Academy of Pediatrics: Commentary on breast-feeding and infant formulas, including proposed standards for formulas, Pediatrics 57:278, 1976.
22. Committee on Nutrition, American Academy of Pediatrics: Nutrition and lactation, Pediatrics 68:435, 1981.
23. Committee on Nutrition, American Academy of Pediatrics: Sodium intake of infants in the United States, Pediatrics 68:445, 1981.
24. Forbes GB, editor: Pediatric nutrition handbook, ed 2, Elk Grove Village Ill, 1985, American Academy of Pediatrics.
25. Dale G et al: Plasma osmolality, sodium, and urea in healthy breastfed and bottle-fed infants in Newcastle-upon-Tyne, Arch Dis Child 50:731, 1975.
26. Davies DP and Saunders R: Blood urea: normal values in early infancy related to feeding practices, Arch Dis Child 48:563, 1973.
27. Dearlove JC: Prolactin, fluid balance, and lactation, Br J Obstet Gynaecol 88:652, 1981.
28. Dial EJ and Lichtenberger LM: Gastric protective properties of human milk. In Howell RR, Morriss FH, and Pickering LK, editors: Human milk in infant nutrition and health, Springfield Ill, 1986, Charles C Thomas, Publisher.
29. Dick G: The etiology of multiple sclerosis, Proc R Soc Med 69:611, 1976.
30. Duncan B, Schifman RB, Corrigan JJ et al: Iron and the exclusively breastfed infant from birth to six months, J Pediatr Gastroenterol 4:421, 1985.
31. Ekstrand J, Spak CJ, Falch J et al: Distribution of fluoride to human breast milk following intake of high doses of fluoride, Caries Res 18:93, 1984.
32. Feeley RM et al: Copper, iron, and zinc contents of human milk at early stages of lactation, Am J Clin Nutr 37:443, 1983.
33. Ferris AM and Jensen RG: Lipids in human milk: a review. I. Sampling, determination and content, J Pediatr-Gastroenterol Nutr 3:108, 1984.
34. Finley DA, Lönnerdal B, Dewey KG et al: Breast

milk composition: fat content and fatty acid composition in vegetarians and non-vegetarians, Am J Clin Nutr 41:787, 1985.
35. Fomon SJ: Infant nutrition, ed 2, Philadelphia, 1974, WB Saunders Co.
36. Forfar JO: Calcium, phosphorus, magnesium metabolism. In Forfar JO, editor: Aspects of neonatal metabolism, Clin Endocrinol Metab 5(1):123, 1976.
37. Forsyth JS, Ross PE, and Bouchier IAD: Bile salts in breast milk, Eur J Pediatr 140:126, 1983.
38. Fransson GB and Lönnerdal B: Iron in human milk, J Pediatr 96:380, 1980.
39. Fransson GB and Lönnerdal B: Zinc, copper, calcium and magnesium in human milk, J Pediatr 101:504, 1982.
40. Gaull GE: Taurine in the nutrition of the human infant, Acta Paediatr Scand (Suppl) 269:38, 1982.
41. Gibson RA and Kneebore GM: Fatty acid composition of human colostrum and mature breast milk, Am J Clin Nutr 34:252, 1981.
42. Greer FR et al: Increasing serum calcium and magnesium concentrations in breastfed infants: longitudinal studies of minerals in human milk and in sera of nursing mothers and their infants, J Pediatr 100:59, 1982.
43. Greer FR, Mummah-Schendel LL, Marshall S et al: Vitamin K (phylloquinone) and vitamin K (menaquinone) status in newborns during the first week of life, Pediatrics 81:137, 1988.
44. Gushurst CA, Mueller JA, Green JA et al: Breast milk iodide: reassessment in the 1980's, Pediatrics 73:354, 1984.
45. György P: Biochemical aspects. In Jelliffe DB and Jelliffe EFP, editors: The uniqueness of human milk, Am J Clin Nutr 24:970, 1971.
46. Hadjimarkos DM and Shearer TR: Selenium in mature human milk, Am J Clin Nutr 26:583, 1973.
47. Hall B: Changing composition of human milk and early development of appetite control, Lancet 1:779, 1975.
48. Hall B and Muller DPR: Studies on bile-salt-stimulated lipolytic activity in human milk. II. Demonstration of two groups of milk with different activities. Pediatr Res 17:716, 1983.
49. Hambraeus L: Proprietary milk versus human milk in infant feeding: a critical approach from a nutritional point of view, Pediatr Clin North Am 24:17, 1977.
50. Hambraeus L, Forsum E, and Lönnerdal B: Nutritional aspects of breast milk and cow's milk formulas. In Hambraeus L, Hanson L, and MacFarlane H, editors: Symposium on food and immunology, Stockholm, 1975, Almqvist and Wiksell.

51. Hamosh M: Enzymes in human milk. In Howell RR, Morriss FH, and Pickering LK, editors: Human milk in infant nutrition and health, Springfield Ill, 1986, Charles C Thomas, Publisher.

52. Harzer G et al: Changing patterns of human milk lipids in the course of the lactation and during the day, Am J Clin Nutr 37:612, 1983.

53. Harzer G and Kauer H: Binding of zinc to casein, Am J Clin Nutr 35:981, 1982.

54. Hazebroek A and Hofman A: Sodium content of breast milk in the first six months after delivery, Acta Paediatr Scand 72:459, 1983.

55. Healy DL et al: Prolactin in human milk: correlation with lactose, total protein, and α-lactalbumin levels, Am J Physiol 238 (Endocrinol Metab 1): E83, 1980.

56. Heitlinger LA et al: Mammary amylase: a possible alternate pathway of carbohydrate digestion in infancy, Pediatr Res 17:15, 1983.

57. Hernell O and Bläckberg L: Digestion of human milk lipids: physiologic significance of sn-2 monoacyl glyceral hydrolysis by bile-salt-stimulated lipase, Pediatr Res 16:882, 1982.

58. Hernell O and Olivecrona T: Human milk lipases. II. Bile-salt-stimulated lipase, Biochim Biophys Acta 369:234, 1974.

59. Hibberd CM et al: Variation in the composition of breast milk during the first five weeks of lactation: implications for the feeding of preterm infants, Arch Dis Child 57:658, 1982.

60. Howell RR, Palma PA, West MS et al: Trace elements in human milk: differences over time and between population groups. In Howell RR, Morriss FH, and Pickering LK, editors: Human milk in infant nutrition and health, Springfield Ill, 1986, Charles C Thomas, Publisher.

61. Hytten FE: Clinical and chemical studies in human lactation. VII. The effect of differences in yield and composition of milk on the infant's weight gain and duration of breastfeeding, Br Med J 1:1410, 1954.

62. Insull W and Ahrens EH: The fatty acids of human milk from mothers on diets taken ad libitum, Biochem J 72:27, 1959.

63. Isaacs CE et al: Sulfhydryl oxidase (SHO) in human milk and induction in kidney and skin at weaning (Abstract), Pediatr Res 15:112A, 1981.

64. Jackson DA, Imong SM, Silprasert A et al: Circadian variation in fat concentration of breast milk in a rural northern Thai population, Br J Nutr 59:349, 1988.

65. Janas LM and Picciano MF: The nucleotide profile of human milk, Pediatr Res 16:659, 1982.

66. Jansson L, Akesson B, and Holmberg L: Vitamin E and fatty acid composition of human milk, Am J Clin Nutr 34:8, 1981.

67. Järvenpää AL et al: Milk protein quantity and quality in the term infant. II. Effects on acidic and neutral amino acids, Pediatrics 70:221, 1982.

68. Jenness R and Sloan RE: Composition of milk. In Larson BL and Smith VR, editors: Lactation, vol 3, Nutrition and biochemistry of milk/maintenance, New York, 1974, Academic Press, Inc.

69. Jensen RG, Clark RM, and Ferris AM: Composition of the lipids in human milk: a review, Lipids 15:345, 1980.

70. Jensen RG, Hagerty MM, and McMahon KE: Lipids of human milk and infant formulas: a review, Am J Clin Nutr 31:990, 1978.

71. Jimenez R et al: Vitamin K–dependent clotting factors in normal breastfed infants, J Pediatr 100:424, 1982.

72. Johke T: Nucleotides of mammary secretions. In Larson BL, editor: Lactation, vol 4, Mammary gland/human lactation/milk synthesis, New York, 1978, Academic Press, Inc.

73. Johnson PE and Evans GW: Relative zinc availability in human breast milk, infant formulas, and cow's milk, Am J Clin Nutr 31:416, 1978.

74. Johnston L, Vaughn L, and Fox HM: Pantothenic acid content of human milk, Am J Clin Nutr 34:2205, 1981.

75. Keenan BS, Buzek SW, and Garza C: Cortisol and its possible role in regulation of sodium and potassium in human milk, Am J Physiol 244: (Endocrinol Metab 7): E253, 1983.

76. Koldovsky O: Hormones in milk, Life Sci 26:1833, 1980.

77. Krebs NF and Hambidge KM: Zinc requirements and zinc intakes in breastfed infants, Am J Clin Nutr 43:288, 1986.

78. Kretchmer N: Lactose and lactase, Sci Am 227:73, 1972.

79. Kulski JK and Hartmann PE: Changes in human milk composition during the initiation of lactation, Aust J Exp Biol Med Sci 59:101, 1981.

80. Kumpulainen J and Vuori E: Longitudinal study of chromium in human milk, Am J Clin Nutr 33:2299, 1980.

81. Lakdawala DR and Widdowson EM: Vitamin D in human milk, Lancet 1:167, 1977.

82. Lammi-Keefe CJ and Jensen RG: Lipids in human milk, a review. II. Composition and fat-soluble vitamins, J Pediatr-Gastroenterol Nutr 3:172, 1984.

83. Lessof MH, Anderson JA, and Youlten LJF: Prostaglandins in the pathogenesis of food intolerance, Ann Allergy 51:249, 1983.

84. Lifschitz CH: Carbohydrate needs in preterm and term newborn infants. In Tsang RC and Nichols BL, editors: Nutrition during infancy, St. Louis, 1988, The CV Mosby Co.

85. Lindberg T and Skude G: Amylase in human milk, Pediatrics 70:235, 1981.

86. Lönnerdal B: Effects of maternal dietary intake on human milk composition, J Nutr 116:499, 1986.

87. Lönnerdal B and Forsum E: Casein content of human milk, Am J Clin Nutr 41:113, 1985.

88. Lönnerdal B, Keen CL, and Hurley LS: Manganese binding proteins in human and cow's milk, Am J Clin Nutr 4:550, 1985.

89. Lorber J, Lilleyman JS, and Peile EB: Acute infantile thrombocytosis and vitamin K deficiency associated with intracranial haemorrhage, Arch Dis Child 54:47, 1979.

90. Lucas A et al: Breast vs bottle: endocrine responses are different with formula feeding, Lancet 1:1267, 1980.

91. Lucas A and Mitchell MD: Prostaglandins in human milk, Arch Dis Child 55:950, 1980.

92. MacDonald LD, Gibson RS, and Miles JE: Changes in hair zinc and copper concentrations of breastfed and bottle fed infants during the first six months, Acta Paediatr Scand 71:785, 1982.

93. Malloy MH et al: Development of taurine metabolism in beagle pups: effects of taurine-free total parenteral nutrition, Biol Neonate 40:1, 1981.

94. Moran JR, Courtney ME, and Orth DN: Epidermal growth factor in human milk: daily production and diurnal variation during early lactation in mothers delivering at term and at premature gestation, J Pediatr 103:402, 1983.

95. Morriss FH: Physical-chemical changes in human milk during the course of lactation. In Howell RR, Morriss FH, and Pickering LK, editors: Human milk in infant nutrition and health, Springfield Ill, 1986, Charles C Thomas, Publisher.

96. Moser PB and Reynolds RD: Dietary zinc intake and zinc concentrations of plasma, erythrocytes, and breast milk in antepartum and postpartum lactating and nonlactating women: a longitudinal study, Am J Clin Nutr 38:101, 1983.

97. Nail PA, Thomas MR, and Eakin R: The effect of thiamin and riboflavin supplementation on the level of those vitamins in human milk and urine, Am J Clin Nutr 33:198, 1980.

98. Novak M et al: Carnitine in the perinatal metabolism of lipids. I. Relationship between maternal and fetal plasma levels of carnitine and acylcarnitines, Pediatrics 67:95, 1981.

99. O'Connor ME et al: Vitamin K deficiency and breastfeeding, Am J Dis Child 137:601, 1983.

100. Orzali A et al: Effect of carnitine on lipid metabolism in the newborn, Biol Neonate 43:186, 1983.

101. Osborn GR: Relationship of hypotension and infant feeding to aetiology of coronary disease, Coll Int Cont Natl Res Sci 169:193, 1968.

102. Picciano MF et al: Milk and mineral intakes of breastfed infants, Acta Paediatr Scand 70:189, 1981.

103. Picciano MF, Guthrie HA, and Sheehe DM: The cholesterol content of human milk, Clin Pediatr 17:359, 1978.

104. Potter JM and Nestel PJ: The effect of dietary fatty acids and cholesterol on the milk lipids of lactating women and the plasma cholesterol of breastfed infants, Am J Clin Nutr 29:54, 1976.

105. Rassin DK, Sturman JA, and Gaull GE: Taurine in milk: species variation, Pediatr Res 11:449, 1977.

106. Read WWC and Sarriff A: Human milk lipids. I. Changes in fatty acid composition of early colostrum, Am J Clin Nutr 17:177, 1965.

107. Reid B, Smith H, and Friedman Z: Prostaglandins in human milk, Pediatrics 66:870, 1980.

108. Roepke JLB and Kirksey A: Vitamin B_6 nutriture during pregnancy and lactation. I. Vitamin B_6 intake, levels of the vitamin in biological fluids, and condition of the infant at birth, Am J Clin Nutr 32:2249, 1979.

109. Roepke JLB and Kirksey A: Vitamin B_6 nutriture during pregnancy and lactation. II. The effect of long-term use of oral contraceptives, Am J Clin Nutr 32:2257, 1979.

110. Rothberg AD et al: Maternal-infant vitamin D relationships during breastfeeding, J Pediatr 101:500, 1982.

111. Salmenperä L, Perheetupa J, and Siimes MA: Folate nutrition is optimal in exclusively breastfed infants but inadequate in some of their mothers and in formula-fed infants, J Pediatr-Gastroenterol Nutr 5:283, 1986.

112. Samson RR and McClelland DBL: Vitamin B_{12} in human colostrum and milk, Acta Paediatr Scand 69:93, 1980.

113. Sandberg DP, Begley JA, and Hall CA: The content, binding, and forms of vitamin B_{12} in milk, Am J Clin Nutr 34:1717, 1981.

114. Sanders TAB et al: Studies of vegans: the fatty acid composition of plasma choline phosphoglycerides, erythrocytes, adipose tissue, and breast milk, and some indicators of susceptibility to ischemic heart disease in vegans and omnivore controls, Am J Clin Nutr 31:805, 1978.

115. Sandor A et al: On carnitine content of human breast milk, Pediatr Res 16:89, 1982.

116. Schams D and Karg H: Hormones in milk, Ann NY Acad Sci 464:75, 1986.

117. Schulz-Lell G, Buss R, Oldigs HD et al: Iron balances in infant nutrition, Acta Paediatr Scand 76:585, 1987.

118. Shahani KM, Kwan AJ, and Friend BA: Role and significance of enzymes in human milk, Am J Clin Nutr 33:1861, 1980.

119. Sinclair AJ and Crawford MA: The accumulation of arachidonate and docosahexaenoate in the developing rat brain, J Neurochem 19:1753, 1972.

120. Skala JP, Koldovsky O, and Hahn P: Cyclic nucleotides in breast milk, Am J Clin Nutr 34:343, 1981.

121. Smith AM, Picciano MF, and Milner JA: Selenium intakes and status of human milk and formula-fed infants, Am J Clin Nutr 35:521, 1982.

122. Sneed SM, Cane C, and Thomas MR: The effects of ascorbic acid, vitamin B_6, vitamin B_{12} and folic acid supplementation on the breast milk and maternal nutritional status of low socioeconomic lactating women, Am J Clin Nutr 34:1338, 1981.

123. Sturman JA, Rassin DK, and Gaull GE: Taurine in the developing kitten: nutritional importance, Pediatr Res 11:450, 1977.

124. Tenore A et al: Thyrotropin in human breast milk, Hormone Res 14:193, 1981.

125. Thomas MR et al: The effects of vitamin C, vitamin B_6, and vitamin B_{12}, folic acid, riboflavin, and thiamin on the breast milk and maternal status of well-nourished women at 6 months postpartum, Am J Clin Nutr 33:2151, 1980.

126. Tikanoja T et al: Plasma amino acids in term neonates after a feed of human milk or formula. II. Characteristic changes in individual amino acids, Acta Paediatr Scand 71:391, 1982.

127. Vanderslice JT et al: Form of vitamin B_6 in human milk, Am J Clin Nutr 37:867, 1983.

128. Vorherr H: The breast: morphology, physiology, and lactation, New York, 1974, Academic Press, Inc.

129. Watkins JB: Bile acid metabolism in the human infant: role of taurine supplementation and human milk. In Filer LJ and Fomon SJ, editors: The breastfed infant: a model for performance, Columbus Ohio, 1986, Ross Laboratory.

130. Widdowson EM et al: Body fat of British and Dutch infants, Br Med J 1:653, 1975.

131. Young VR, Nahapetian A, and Janghorbani M: Selenium bioavailability with reference to human nutrition, Am J Clin Nutr 35:1076, 1982.

132. Zikakis JP, Dougherty TM, and Biasotto HO: The presence and some properties of xanthine oxidase in human milk and colostrum, J Food Sci 41:1408, 1976.

Host-resistance factors and immunologic significance of human milk

5

As early as 1892, medical literature carried the data that proved that milk from various species, including humans, was protective for the offspring, containing antibodies against a vast number of antigens.[32] Veterinarians have known the urgency of the offspring's receiving the early milk of the mother. Death among newborns not suckled at the breast in the Third World is at least five times higher than among those who receive colostrum and mother's milk. Evidence that lack of breastfeeding and poor environmental sanitation have a pernicious synergistic effect on infant mortality has been presented by Habicht et al[31] after studying 1,262 women in Malaysia. Lower incidence of diarrheal disease in breastfed infants is well established worldwide, even in North America where the American Indian and Alaskan have high risk for infection. The lowest incidence of breastfeeding in the United States is among the indigent and disadvantaged urban and rural, yet no data on infection rate in these groups are available. Day-care children are a new population at extremely high risk for infection, and it is speculated these children benefit from at least partial breastfeeding. Protection against respiratory tract infections and otitis media are less well established for the United States despite a number of investigatory efforts all well reviewed by Cunningham.[13]

Using a self-administered questionnaire completed by parents when their infant was 18 months old in Shanghai, Republic of China, Chen et al[12] studied the protective effect of breastfeeding against one or more episodes of hospitalization for infection. The definition of breastfeeding was "ever breastfeed," which would bias the data against breastfeeding, and yet those infants "never breastfed" were twice as likely to be hospitalized for respiratory infections and approximately one third more likely to be hospitalized for gastroenteritis or other infections in the first 18 months of life. The design of the study clearly biased against breastfeeding, Kramer[44] points out, and still the results are clear: Breastfeeding is protective.

Breastfeeding is effective in minimizing infection in infants by decreasing the exposure to enteropathogens that may contaminate other foods or formula, providing nutrition, and providing special unique protective factors, which can be loosely grouped as antibody and nonantibody.[60] The protection provided varies by the pathogen and by the chronological age and maturity of the infant.

As the newborn infant prepares for existence outside the uterus, various organ systems adjust and adapt. It had been suggested that protection against infection was provided by the mother transplacentally, since it has been established that the neonate is immunologically immature at birth.

The neonate does not have sufficient innate defenses to protect himself against the highly contaminated environment he enters from the usually sterile environment of the uterus. The incidence of infection in the newborn infant is significant. It has been estimated that up to 10% of newborns are infected during delivery or in the first few months of life. It is generally believed that the newborn cannot muster the same level of defense against infection that an adult is capable of developing. The diminished phagocytic function of newborn cells is an example. This maturational defect is attributed to both cellular and extracellular factors.

Maternal antibody is transmitted to the fetus by different pathways in different species. An association has been recognized between the number of placental membranes and the relative importance of the placenta and the colostrum as sources of antibodies. By this analysis it is noted that the horse, with six placental membranes, passes little or no antibodies transplacentally and relies on colostrum for protection of the foal. Humans and monkeys, having three placental membranes, receive more of the antibodies via the placenta and less from the colostrum. The transfer of IgG in the human is accomplished by active transport mechanism of the immunoglobulin across the placenta. Secretory IgA immunoglobulins are found in human milk and provide local protection on the mucous membranes of the gastrointestinal tract. It has been established by other investigations that the mammary glands and their secretion of milk are important in protecting the infant not only through the colostrum but also through mature milk from birth through the early months of life. Some information has been available for decades to support the acknowledgment of the protective role of human milk.[37] Many recent discoveries, however, have further broadened this knowledge.[22]

Although the predominance of IgA in human colostrum and milk had been described, the importance of this phenomenon was not fully appreciated until the discovery that IgA is a predominant immunoglobulin present in mucosal secretions of other glands in addition to the breast. Mucosal immunity has become the subject of extensive research.[42] The data produced suggest that there may be considerable traffic of cells between secretory sites. These data support the concept of a general system of mucosa-associated lymphoid tissue (MALT), which includes the gut, lung, mammary gland, salivary and lacrimal glands, and the genital tract. This concept of MALT implies that immunization at one site may be an effective means of producing immunity at distant sites. Antibodies found in the milk have also been found in the saliva, for instance. There is evidence available to suggest that the mammary glands may act as extensions of the gut-associated lymphoid tissue (GALT) and possibly the broncho-associated (immunocompetent) lymphoid tissue (BALT). The ability of epithelial surfaces exposed to the external environment to defend against foragers has been well established for the gastrointestinal, genitourinary, and respiratory tracts. The common defense is secretory IgA. Direct contact with the antigen and the lymphoid cells of the breast is unlikely.[54]

All mysteries of the protective value of human milk, however, have not been unraveled. The protective properties of human milk can be divided into cellular factors and humoral factors for facility of discussion, although they are closely related in vivo. A wide variety of soluble and cellular components and microbial agents have been identified in human milk and colostrum (Table 5-1).

Table 5-1. Immunologically active components in human colostrum and milk

Soluble	Cellular	Microbial agents
Secretory component		
Immunoglobulins sigA, 7S	Monocytic phagocytes	Bacterial agents
IgA, IgG, IgM	macrophage	
Immunoregulatory mediators		
Complement	Neutrophils	Hepatitis B surface antigen
Chemotactic factors	B lymphocytes	Rubella
Lactoferrin	Plasma cells	Cytomegalovirus
Lysozyme	T lymphocytes	Other vaccine viruses
Lactoperoxidase	Transplantation antigens	
Interferon		
Bifidus factor		

From Ogra SS and Ogra PL: Components of immunology reactivity in human colostrum and milk. In Ogra PL and Dayton D, editors: Immunology of breast milk, New York, 1979, Raven Press.

CELLULAR COMPONENTS OF HUMAN COLOSTRUM AND MILK

Cells do constitute an important postpartum component of maternal immunologic endowment. Over 100 years ago, cell bodies were described in the colostrum of animals. As with much lactation research, further study of colostral corpuscles was undertaken by the dairy industry for commercial reasons in the early 1900s. This research afforded an opportunity to make major progress in the understanding of cells in milk. Initially it was believed that these cells represented a reaction to infection in the mammary gland and were even described as "pus cells."

It has become clear that the cells of milk are normal constituents of that solution in all species. Cells include macrophages, lymphocytes, neutrophils, and epithelial cells, and they total 4000/mm.[3] Cell fragments and epithelial cells were examined by electron microscope in fresh samples from 30 women by Brooker.[7] He found that that membrane-bound cytoplasmic fragments in the sedimentation pellet outnumbered intact cells. The fragments were mostly from secretory cells that contained numerous cisternae of rough endoplasmic reticulum, lipid droplets, and Golgi vesicles containing casein micelles. Secretory epithelial cells were found in all samples and, after the second month postpartum, began to outnumber macrophages. Ductal epithelial cells were about 1% of the population of cells for the first week or so and then disappeared. All samples contained squamous epithelial cells originating from galactophores and the skin of the nipple.

Living leukocytes are normally present in human milk. The overall concentration of these leukocytes is of the same order of magnitude as that seen in peripheral blood, although the predominant cell in milk is the macrophage rather than the neutrophil. Macrophages comprise about 90% of the leukocytes, and 2000 to 3000/mm^3 are present. Lymphocytes make up about 10% of the cells (200 to 300/mm^3), which is much lower than in human blood. There are large and small lymphocytes. By indirect immunofluo-rescence with anti-T antibody to identify thymus-derived lymphocytes, it has been shown that 50% of human colostral lymphocytes are T cells. By immunofluorescence procedures to detect surface immunoglobulins characteristic of B-lymphocytes, 34% were identified as B-lymphocytes.

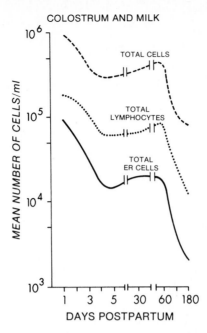

Fig. 5-1. Geometric mean concentration of total cells, lymphocytes, and E rosette-forming cells *(ER)* in the colostrum and milk of 200 lactating women. (Modified from Ogra SS and Ogra PL: J Pediatr 92:546, 1978.)

The number of leukocytes and the degree of mitogenic stimulation of lymphocytes sharply decline during the first 2 or 3 months of lactation to essentially undetectable levels according to Goldman et al[25] (Fig. 5-1). Enumeration of the total cell numbers in milk has been difficult, but when various techniques are compared (Coulter electronic particle counter, visual cell counting with special stains, filter trapping with fluorescent detection, and automated fluorescent cell counting), stains for DNA were superior.

Macrophages

Macrophages are large-complex phagocytes that contain lysosomes, mitochondria, pinosomes, ribosomes, and a Golgi apparatus. The monocytic phagocytes are lipid laden and were previously called the colostral bodies of Donne. They have the same functional and morphologic features as those in other human tissue sources. These features include ameboid movement, phagocytosis of microorganisms (fungi and bacteria), killing of bacteria, and production of complement components C3 and C4, lysosome, and lactoferrin. Other milk macrophage activities include the following[60]:

Phagocytosis of latex, adherence to glass
Secretion of lysozyme, complement components
C3b-mediated erythrocyte adherence
IgG-mediated erythrocyte adherence and phagocytosis
Bacterial killing
Inhibition of lymphocyte mitogenic response
Release of intracellular IgA in tissue culture
Giant cell formation
Interaction with lymphocytes

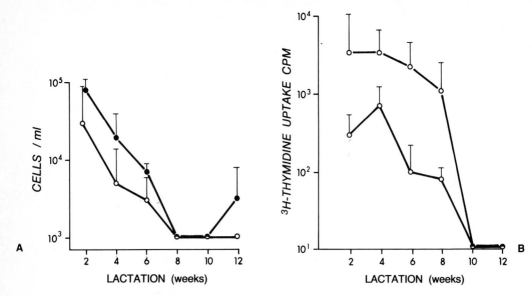

Fig. 5-2. Longitudinal study of cells. Same subjects were examined during the second through the twelfth week of lactation. Data are presented as means ± SD of macrophages-neutrophils (●——●) and lymphocytes (○——○) and of stimulated (●——●) and unstimulated (○——○) lymphocytes. **A,** Longitudinal study of numbers of leukocytes. **B,** Longitudinal study of uptake of ³H-thymidine in lymphocytes. (From Goldman AS, Garza C, Nichols BL et al: J Pediatr 100:563, 1982.)

There are data to suggest these macrophages also amplify T-cell reactivity by direct cellular cooperation or by antigen processing. The colostral macrophage has been suggested as a potential vehicle for the storage and transport of immunoglobin. A significant increase in IgA and IgG immunoglobin synthesis by colostral lymphocytes when incubated with supernatants of cultured macrophages has been reported.[61]

The macrophage may also participate in the biosynthesis and excretion of lactoperoxidase and cellular growth factors that enhance growth of intestinal epithelium and maturation of intestinal brush-border enzymes.

The mobility of macrophages is inhibited by the lymphokine migration inhibitor factor (MIF), which is produced by antigen-stimulated sensitized lymphocytes. The activities of macrophages have been demonstrated in both fresh colostrum and in colostral cell cultures.

Polymorphonuclear leukocytes

Colostrum (1 to 4 days postpartum) contains 10^5 to 5×10^6 leukocytes/ml, and 40% to 60% are polymorphonuclear (PMN). Mature milk (i.e., beyond 4 days) has fewer cells (Fig. 5-2), ranging 10^5/ml with 20% to 30% PMN. Beyond 6 weeks there are few PMN. The functions of the PMN normally include microbial killing, phagocytosis, chemotactic responsiveness, stimulated hexose monophosphate shunt activity, stimulated nitroblue tetrazolium dye reduction, and stimulated oxygen consumption.[9] When milk PMN are compared with those in the serum, their activity is often less than that of serum PMN cells. Whether milk PMNs actually perform a role in protection of the infant has been studied by many investigators using many techniques. Animal studies, in summary, have shown that the mammary gland is susceptible to infection in early lactation, dramatic increase in PMN occurs with mammary inflammation, and, in the presence of peripheral neutopenia during chronic mastitis, severe infection of the gland occurs. This implies, according to Buescher and Pickering,[9] that the primary function of milk PMN is as defense of the mammary tissue per se and not to impart maternal immunocompetence to the newborn. This may explain the presence of large numbers of PMN that are relatively hypofunctional early and then disappear over time.

Lymphocytes

It has been established that both T- and B-lymphocytes are present in human milk and colostrum. They synthesize IgA antibody. Human milk lymphocytes respond to mitogens by proliferation, with increased macrophage-lymphocyte interaction and the release of soluble mediators, including MIF. Cells destined to become lymphopoietic cells are derived from two separate influences, the thymus (T) and the bursa (B) or bursal equivalent tissues. The population of cells called B cells comprises the smaller part of the total. The term *B cell* is derived from its origination in a different anatomic site from the thymus; in birds it has been identified as the bursa of Fabricius. The B cells can be identified by the presence of surface immunoglobulin markers. The B cells in human milk include cells with IgA, IgM, and IgG surface immunoglobulins.

T-cell system

More rapid mitotic activity occurs in the thymus gland than in any other lymphatic organ, yet 70% of the cells die within the cell substance. Thymosin has recently been identified as a hormone produced by thymic epithelial cells to expand the peripheral lymphocyte population. After emergence from the thymus gland, T cells acquire new surface antigen markers. The T cells circulate through the lymphatic and vascular systems as long-lived lymphocytes, which are called the recirculating pool. They then populate restricted regions of lymph nodes, forming thymic-dependent areas.

The significance of the leukocytes in human milk in affording immunologic benefits to the breastfed infant continues to be investigated. It is suggested that the lymphocytes can sensitize, induce immunologic tolerance, or incite graft-versus-host reactions. According to Head and Beer, lymphocytes may be incorporated into the suckling's tissues, achieving short-term adoptive immunization of the neonate.[34]

Studies of the activities of lymphocytes have been carried out by a number of investigators who collected samples of milk from lactating women at various times postpartum, examined the number of cell types present, and then studied the activities of these cells in vitro. Ogra and Ogra[53] collected samples from 200 women and measured the cell content from 1 through 180 days (Fig. 5-1). They then compared the response of T-lymphocytes in colostrum and milk with that of the T cells in the peripheral blood (Fig. 5-1). T-cell subpopulations have also been shown by surface epitopes to be similar to those in the peripheral blood.

The greatest number of cells appeared on the first day, with the counts ranging from 10,000 to 100,000/mm³ for total cells. By the fifth day, the count had dropped to 20% of the first day's count. In addition, the number of E rosette-forming cells was determined by using sheep erythrocyte-rosetting technique. The E rosette formation (ERF) lymphocytes constituted a mean $100/mm^3$ on the first day and a tenth of that by the fifth day.

At 180 days, total cells were $100,000/mm^3$, lymphocytes were $10,000/mm^3$, and ERF lymphocytes were $2000/mm^3$. The investigators compared the values to those in the peripheral blood of each mother where the levels remained essentially constant.

In a similar study, Bhaskaram and Reddy[5] sampled milk over time from 74 women and found comparable cell concentrations. They examined the bactericidal activity of the milk leukocytes and found it to be comparable to that of the circulating leukocytes in the blood, irrespective of the stage of lactation or state of nutrition of the mother.

Ogra and Ogra[52] also studied the lymphocyte proliferation responses of colostrum and milk to antigens. Their data show response to stimulation from the viral antigens of rubella, cytomegalovirus, and mumps. Analysis of cell-mediated immunity to microbial antigens shows milk lymphocytes are limited in their potential for recognizing or responding to certain infectious agents as compared with cells from the peripheral circulation. This is believed to be an intercellular action and not due to lack of external factors. On the other hand, the T cells and B cells have been shown to have unique reactivities not seen in peripheral blood.

The effect of human milk on B-cell function was studied by Juto.[39] Cell-free, defatted, filtered colostrum as well as mature breast milk showed an enhancing effect on B-cell proliferation and generation of antibody secretion. This was not seen with formula. Juto suggested that this could represent an important immunological mechanism.[39] Goldblum et al[23] were able to show a response in human colostrum to *Escherichia coli* given orally, which was not accompanied by a systemic response in the mother. This suggests that milk provides a site for local humoral or cell-mediated immunity induced at a distant site such as the gut with the reactive lymphoid cells migrating to the breast. This concept has been further refined to suggest that IgA and IgM immunoglobulin in colostrum may represent migration of specific antibody-producing cells from the gut lymphoid tissue, specifically Peyer's patches, to the mammary gland. Ogra and Ogra[52,53] suggest that the cells may be selectively accumulated in the breast during pregnancy. The responses of milk cells and their antibodies are not representative of the total immunity of the individual.[57] Head and Beer[34] have provided a scheme to describe this mechanism (Fig. 5-3). The diagram depicts the progeny of specifically sensitized lymphocytes that originated in the lymphoid tissue of the gut as they migrate to the mammary gland. As they infiltrate the mammary gland and its secretion, they supply the breast with immune cells capable of selected immune responses.

Most of these immunocompetent cells recirculate to the external mucosal surface and populate the lamina propria as antibody-producing plasma cells. A substantial number of these antigen-sensitized cells selectively home to the stroma of the mammary glands and initiate local IgA antibody synthesis against the antigens initially encountered in the respiratory or intestinal mucosa.

Colostral lymphocytes are derived from mature rather than immature T-cell subsets. The distribution of T-cell subsets in colostrum includes both T_4 and T_8 positive cells.[64] The distribution in colostrum of T_4 cells is lower than in the serum, and there are fewer than there are T_8 cells. The percentage is higher than in the serum of either postpartum donors or normal controls. There is no correlation with length of gestation and number of cells (in normal blood there are usually twice as many T_4 as T_8 positive lymphocytes).[39]

Parmely et al[56] partially purified and propagated milk lymphocytes in vitro to study their immunologic function. Milk lymphocytes responded in a unique manner to stimuli known to activate T-lymphocytes from the serum. Parmely et al[57] found milk lymphocytes

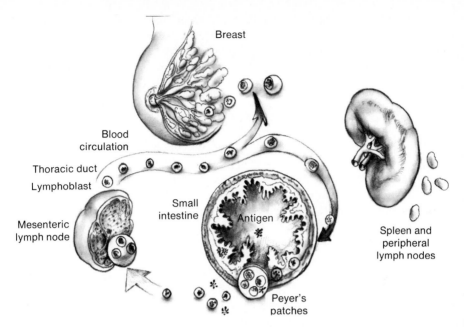

Fig. 5-3. Schema of mechanism by which progeny of specifically sensitized lymphocytes originating from gut-associated lymphoid tissue may migrate to and infiltrate mammary gland and its secretions, supplying breast with immune cells. (Modified from Head JR and Beer AE: The immunologic role of viable leukocytic cells in mammary exosecretions. In Larson BL, editor: Lactation, vol 4, Mammary gland/human lactation/ milk synthesis, New York, 1978, Academic Press, Inc.)

to be hyporesponsive to nonspecific mitogens and histocompatible antigens on allogenic cells in their laboratory. They found them unresponsive to *Candida albicans*. Significant proliferation of lymphocytes occurred in response to K_1 capsular antigen of *E. coli*.[35] Lymphocytes from blood failed to respond. This supports the concept of local mammary tissue immunity at the T-lymphocyte level.

More recent experiments in rodents have provided evidence that T-lymphocytes reactive to transplantation alloantigens can adoptively immunize the suckling newborn. Foster nursing experiments performed in rodents have shown that newborn rats exposed to allogenic milk manifested alterations in their reactivity to skin allografts of the foster mother's strain. In animals, mothers may give their suckling newborn immunoreactive lymphocytes. The influence of maternal milk cells on the development of neonatal immunocompetence has been demonstrated in several different immunologic contexts. Congenitally, athymic nude mice nursed by their phenotypically normal mothers or normal foster mothers had increased survival. The mothers contributed their T cell–helper activity to the suckling newborn.

Colostral lymphocytes proliferate in response to various mitogens, alloantigens, and conventional antigens. Colostral cells survive in the neonatal stomach and in the gut of experimental animals, some remaining viable in the upper gastrointestinal tract for a week. On the other hand there is no evidence that transepithelial migration takes place when neonatal mice are foster-nursed by newly delivered animals whose colostral cells were tagged with ^{3}H-thymidine.[9]

The accumulated research data support the concept that lymphocytes from colostrum and milk provide the human infant with immunologic benefits. Both T- and B-lymphocytes are reactive against organisms invading the intestinal tract. Investigations on allergy, necrotizing entercolitis, tuberculosis, and neonatal meningitis support the concept that milk fulfills a protective function.

SURVIVAL OF MATERNAL MILK CELLS

Although it is clear that cells are provided in the colostrum and milk, the effectiveness and impact of these cells on the neonate depend on their ability to survive in the gastrointestinal tract. It has been demonstrated in several species, including the human, that the pH of the stomach can be as low as 0.5, but the output of HCl is minimal for the first few months, as is the peptic activity. Immediately after a feeding begins, the pH rises to 6.0 and returns to normal in 3 hours. The cells from milk tolerate this. Studies have also shown that intact nucleated lymphoid cells are found in the stomach and intestines.[3] These cells, when removed from rat stomachs, are capable of phagocytosis. Lymphoid cells in milk have been shown to traverse the mucosal wall.

When human milk is stored, however, it has been shown that the cellular components do not tolerate heating to 63° C, cooling to −23° C, or lyophilization. Although a few cells may be identified, they are not viable.[24]

HUMORAL FACTORS
Immunoglobulins

All classes of immunoglobulins are found in human milk. The study of immunoglobulins has been enhanced through electrophoresis, chromatographics, and radioimmunoassays. More than 30 components have been identified; of these, 18 are associated with proteins in the maternal serum, and the others are found exclusively in milk.

The concentrations are highest in the colostrum of all species, and the concentrations change as lactation proceeds.[49]

IgA, principally secretory IgA (sIgA) and lactoferrin, are highest in colostrum, and although their levels fall over the next 4 weeks, substantial levels are maintained throughout the first year, during gradual weaning between 6 and 9 months, and in fact during partial breastfeeding (where infant receives solid foods) in the second year of life (Figs. 5-4 and 5-5). Specific sIgA antibodies to *E. coli* persist through lactation and may even rise. Lysozyme also trends from initial values of 85 to 90 mg/ml down to 25 mg/ml at 2 to 4 weeks and then over 6 months rises to 250 mg/ml.[25]

The main immunoglobulin in human serum is IgG; IgA is only one fifth the level of IgG. In milk, however, the reverse is true. IgA is the most important immunoglobulin in milk, not only in concentration but also in biologic activity. Of the IgA immunoglobulins, secretory IgA is the most significant and is likely synthesized in the mammary alveolar cells.

Quantitative determinations of immunoglobulins in human milk were made from milk collected at birth up to as long as 27 months postpartum by Peitersen et al[59] and by Goldman et al.[25] The IgA content was high immediately after birth, dropping in 2 to 3 weeks, and then remaining constant. Similar observations were made on IgG levels and IgM levels. Milk and serum values were found to be comparable to standard adult levels. Ogra and Ogra[52,53] have compared serum and milk levels at various times postpartum. Samples obtained separately from the left and right breasts showed similar values. The levels

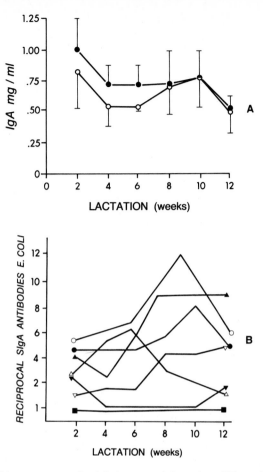

Fig. 5-4. Same subjects were examined during second through twelfth week of lactation. Total (●) and secretory IgA (○) data were presented as mean ± SD. sIgA antibody titers to *E. coli* somatic antigens from each subject are represented by different symbols. **A,** Longitudinal study of total and secretory IgA. **B,** Longitudinal study of reciprocal of sIgA antibody titers to *E. coli* somatic antigens in human milk. (From Goldman AS, Garza C, Nichols BL et al: J Pediatr 100:563, 1982.)

remained constant during a given feeding and for a 24-hour period as a whole. In all quantitative determinations, IgA is the predominant immunoglobulin in breast milk, constituting 90% of all the immunoglobulins in colostrum and milk (Fig. 5-4).

Ogra and Ogra[53,54] studied the serum of postpartum lactating mothers and nonpregnant matched controls and noted that the individual and mean concentrations of all classes of immunoglobulin were lower in the postpartum subjects. The levels were statistically significant in IgG, being 50 to 70 mg higher in the nonpregnant women.

It is important to note, in recording the fact that immunoglobulin levels, particularly IgA and IgM, are very high in colostrum and drop precipitously in the first 4 to 6 days, that the volume of mammary secretion also increases dramatically in this same period; thus, the absolute number is more nearly constant than it would first appear. IgG does not show this decline. Local production and concentration of IgA and probably IgM may take place in the mammary gland at the time of delivery.

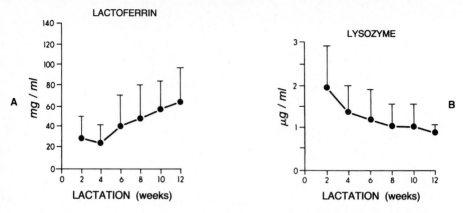

Fig. 5-5. Same subjects were examined during second through twelfth week of lactation. Concentration of lactoferrin progressively decreased through first eight weeks (r = 0.69) (2 vs 8 weeks; $P < 0.02$), but not thereafter. In contrast, lysozyme levels steadily increased from fourth through twelfth week (r = 0.76) (4 vs 12 weeks; $P < 0.01$). **A,** Longitudinal study of lactoferrin. **B,** Longitudinal study of lysozyme in human milk (means ± SD). (From Goldman AS, Garza C, Nichols BL et al: J Pediatr 100:563, 1982.)

IgE and IgD have also been measured in colostrum and milk. Using radioimmunoassay techniques, colostrum was found to contain concentrations of 0.5 to 0.6 IU/ml IgE in 41% of samples and less in the remainder.[1] IgD was found in all samples in concentrations of 2 to 2000 µg/100 ml. Plasma levels were poorly correlated. The findings suggest possible local mammary production rather than positive transfer. Whether IgE or IgD antibodies in breast milk have similar specificities for antigens as the IgA antibodies in milk is unanswered.[48] Keller et al[41] examined the question of local mammary production of IgD and possible participation of IgD in a mucosal immune system by comparing colostrum and plasma levels of total IgD with specific IgD antibodies.

To address the question of total quantities of immunologic components secreted into human milk per day and available to the infant, Butte et al[11] measured the amounts of sIgA, sIgA antibodies to *E. coli,* lactoferrin, and lysozyme ingested per day and per kilogram per day in the first 4 months of life (Figs. 5-6 to 5-10). Lactoferrin, sIgA, and sIgA antibodies gradually declined in amount ingested per day and per kilogram per day. Lysozyme, on the other hand, rose during the same period in total amount available and amount per kilogram per day. The authors[11] suggest that production and secretion of these immunologic factors by the mammary gland may be linked to the catabolism of the components at the mucosal tissues of the infant. When concentrations of 11S, IgA, IgG, IgM, alpha[1] antitrypsin, lactoferrin, lysozyme, and globulins C_3 and C_4 were compared in relationship to parity and age of the mother, there was no consistent trend. When maturity of the pregnancy was considered, however, mean concentrations of all these proteins was higher, except for IgA, when the delivery was premature. Because several proteins in human milk have physiological function in the infant, Davidson and Lönnerdal[14] examined the survival of human milk proteins through the gastrointestinal tract. Crossed immunoelectrophoresis showed that three human milk proteins transversed the entire intestine and were present in the feces: lactoferrin, sIgA, and alpha[1] antitrypsin.

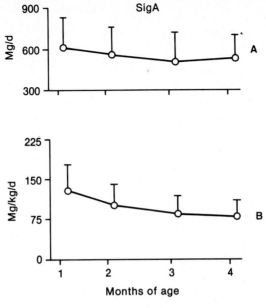

Fig. 5-6. Amounts of sIgA in human milk. Amounts of sIgA and of sIgA antibodies to *E. coli* somatic antigens in human milk ingested per day, **A,** and per kilogram per day, **B.** Data are presented as mean ± SD. (From Butte NF, Goldblum RM, Fehl LM et al: Acta Paediatr Scand 73:296, 1984.)

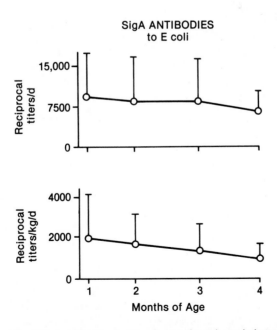

Fig. 5-7. Amount of sIgA antibodies to *E. coli* somatic antigens in human milk. (From Butte NF, Goldblum RM, Fehl LM et al: Acta Paediatr Scand 73:296, 1984.)

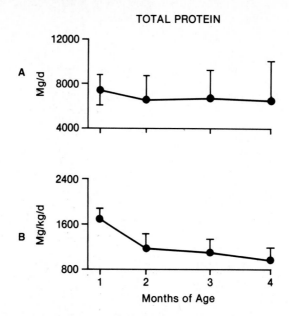

Fig. 5-8. Amount of total protein in human milk ingested per day, **A,** and per kilogram per day, **B.** Data are presented as mean ± SD. (From Butte NF, Goldblum RM, Fehl LM et al: Acta Paediatr Scand 73:296, 1984.)

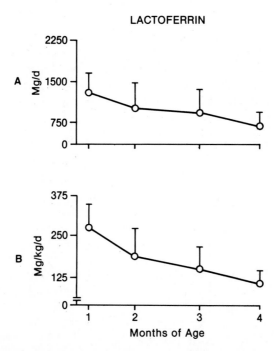

Fig. 5-9. Amount of lactoferrin in human milk ingested per day, **A,** and per kilogram per day, **B.** Data are presented as mean ± SD. (From Butte NF, Goldblum RM, Fehl LM et al: Acta Paediatr Scand 73:296, 1984.)

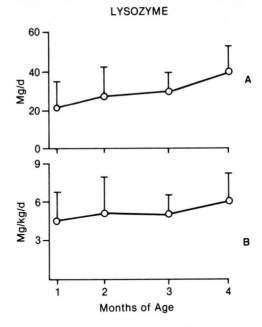

LYSOZYME

Fig. 5-10. Amount of lysozyme in human milk ingested per day, **A,** and per kilogram per day, **B.** Data are presented as mean ± SD. (From Butte NF, Goldblum RM, Fehl LM et al: Acta Paediatr Scand 73:296, 1984.)

The effect of maternal nutritional status on immunological substances in human colostrum and milk was reported by Miranda et al.[50] Maternal malnutrition was characterized as lower weight/height ratio, creatine/height index, total serum proteins, and IgG and IgA. The colostrum contained one third the normal concentration of immunoglobulin G, less than half the normal level of albumin, and lower IgA and complement (C_4). Lysozyme, complement C_3, and IgM levels were normal. Levels improved with development of mature milk and/or improvement in maternal nutrition.

Immunologic components in human milk during the second year of lactation become a significant point as more infants are nursed longer. Subjects were part of a longitudinal study, had fully breastfed their infants for 6 months to a year, and were continuing to partially breastfeed.[26] Samples were collected by fully emptying the breast by electric pump. Concentrations are summarized in Table 5-2. No leukocytes were detected. Concentrations of total and secretory IgA, lactoferrin, and lysozyme were similar to those 7 to 12 months of age and during gradual weaning. sIgA antibodies to *E. coli* were produced in the second year, demonstrating that there is significant benefit immunologically to continued breastfeeding.[26]

Immunoglobulins A, M, and G were measured in nursing women from the beginning of lactation and simultaneously in the feces of their children by Jatsyk et al[36] in the Academy of Medicine in Moscow. They reported IgA to be very high in the milk and rapidly increasing in the feces. IgG and IgM levels, however, were low in both milk and feces. In normal full-term bottle fed infants, they found IgA appeared in the feces at 3 to 4 weeks of age but at much lower levels than in the breastfed infants.

Table 5-2. Concentrations of immunologic components in human milk collected during second year of lactation

Component	Duration of lactation (months)		
	12	13-15	16-24
IgA (mg/ml)			
Total	0.8 ± 0.3	1.1 ± 0.4	1.1 ± 0.3
Secretory	0.8 ± 0.3	1.1 ± 0.3	1.1 ± 0.2
Lactoferrin (mg/ml)	1.0 ± 0.2	1.1 ± 0.1	1.2 ± 0.1
Lysozyme (μg/ml)	196 ± 41	244 ± 34	187 ± 33
SIgA antibodies (reciprocal titers to *E. coli* somatic antigens)	5 ± 6	9 ± 10	6 ± 3

From Goldman AS, Goldblum RM, and Garza C: Acta Paediatr Scand 72:461, 1983. Data are presented as the mean ± SD.

Serum levels of IgG, IgA, and IgM were measured in 198 infants at 2, 4, 6, 9, and 12 months by Savilahti et al.[65] By 9 months the infants exclusively breastfed had IgG and IgM levels significantly lower than those who had been weaned early (before 3.5 months) to formula. Six infants were still exclusively breastfed at 12 months, and their IgA levels had also lowered to levels found at 2 months with bottle feeders. Infection rates were similar. Two months after weaning to formula, the IgG and IgM levels were comparable. Iron and zinc levels were the same in all children.

Stability of immunoglobulins

Preservation of human milk at $-20°C$ alters the levels of IgA, IgM, C-3, C-4, alpha$_1$ antitrypsin, and sIgA antibodies to *E. coli* and lactoperoxidase.[18] Heat treatments include low-temperature, short-time (LTST), 56° C for 15 minutes, Holder pasteurization (HP) 62.5° C for 30 minutes and high-temperature, short-time (HTST) 70° C for 15 seconds. Boiling essentially destroys 100% of immunologic activity. Secretory IgA and lysozyme activities drop by 20% with Holder pasteurization and by 50% at 65° C. Neither LTST nor HTST reduces the sIgA or lysozyme content. IgG and IgM are marked and reduced by Holder pasteurization (Table 5-3).

Secretory IgA differs antigenically from serum IgA. Secretory IgA can be synthesized in the nonlactating as well as in the lactating breast. It is a compact molecule and resistant to proteolytic enzymes of the intestinal tract and the low pH of the stomach. It is manufactured by the mammary gland and by the cellular lymphocytes in milk. Levels in milk are 10 to 100 times higher than in serum. Levels in cow's milk are very low, that is, a tenth the level in mature human milk (0.03 mg/100 ml). Later in life, the intestinal tract's subepithelial plasma cells secrete IgA, but this does not occur in the neonatal period.

Discussion continues as to whether antibodies are absorbed from the intestinal tract. There is, however, a wealth of evidence to demonstrate the activity of the immunoglobulins, especially secretory IgA, at the mucosal levels. These antibodies provide local intestinal protection against viruses such as poliovirus and bacteria such as *E. coli,* which may infect the mucosa or enter the body via the gut.

Table 5-3. Antiviral antibody in human milk

Factor	Shown, in vitro, to be active against:	Assay*	Effect of heat
Secretory IgA	Enteroviruses		
	Poliovirus types 1, 2, 3	ELISA, NA, Precipitan	Stable at 56° C for 30 min;
	Coxsackie virus types	NA	some loss (0-30%)
	A₉, B3, B₅	NA	At 62.5° C for 30 min; de-
	Echovirus types 6 and 9		stroyed by boiling
	Herpes virus		
	Cytomegalovirus	ELISA, IFA, NA	
	Herpes simplex virus	NA	
	Semliki Forest virus	IFA	
	Respiratory syncytial virus	IFA	
	Rubella	IFA, HAI	
	Reovirus type 3	ELISA, NA	
	Rotavirus		
IgM, IgG	Cytomegalovirus		Stable at 56° C for 30 min;
	Respiratory syncytial virus		IgG decreased by a third
	Rubella		at 62.5° C for 30 min

*ELISA, enzyme linked immunosorbent assay; NA, neutralizing assay; IFA, immunofluorescent assay; HAI, hemagglutination inhibition.

Table 5-4. Distribution of the different *Bifidobacterium* species in feces of breastfed or artificially fed infants

Feeding	Artificial	Maternal
No. of feces	39	12
No. of *Bifidobacterium* strains isolated	153	81
B. bifidum	20 = 13%	58 = 72%
B. infantis	28 = 18%	0
B. longum	91 = 60%	23 = 28%
B. adolescentis	2 = 1%	0
B. breve	12 = 8%	0

From Beerens H, Romond C, and Nevi C: Am J Clin Nutr 33:2434, 1980.

Bifidus factor

It has been established since the work of Tissier in 1908 on the intestinal flora of the newborn infant that the predominant bacteria of the breastfed infant are bifid bacteria. Bifid bacteria are gram-positive, nonmotile anaerobic bacilli. Many observers have shown the striking difference between the flora of the guts of breastfed and bottle fed infants. György[30] demonstrated the presence of a specific factor in colostrum and milk that supported the growth of *Lactobacillus bifidus*. Bifidus factor has been characterized as a dialyzable nitrogen-containing carbohydrate that contains no amino acid.

In vitro studies by Beerens et al[4] showed the presence of a specific growth factor for *Bifidobacterium bifidum* in human milk, which they called BB. Other milks, including

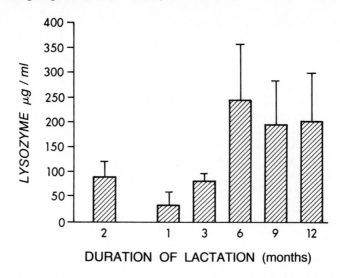

Fig. 5-11. Lysozyme content during period of lactation. In period from 15 to 27 months of lactation, lysozyme was found in only three samples, values varying considerably. (Modified from Peitersen B et al: Acta Paediatr Scand 64:709, 1975.)

cow's milk, sheep's milk, pig's milk, and infant formulas, did not promote the growth of this species but did show some activity supporting *B. infantis* and *B. longum*. This growth factor was found to be stable when the milk was frozen, heated, freeze-dried, and stored for 3 months (Table 5-7). There were growth-promoting factors present for the six strains studied, which varied in their resistance to physical change. Since all these factors were active in vitro, they did not require the presence of intestinal enzymes for activation. It has not been possible to show the presence of this factor in other mammalian milks; thus it is possible that it contributes to the implantation and persistence of *B. bifidum* in the breastfed infant's intestine (Table 5-4).

Resistance factor

The fact that human milk protects the human infant against staphylococcal infection was well known in the preantibiotic era. The protection continued throughout the lactation period. György[30] identified the presence of an "antistaphylococcal factor" in experiments with young mice who had been stressed with staphylococci. This factor has no demonstrable direct antibiotic properties. It was termed a *resistance factor* and described as nondialyzable, thermostable, and part of the free fatty acid part of the phosphide fraction, probably $C_{18:2}$, distinct from linoleic acid.

Lysozyme

Human milk contains a nonspecific antimicrobial factor, lysozyme, which is a thermostable, acid-stable enzyme. It is found in large concentrations in the stools of breastfed infants and not in stools of formula-fed infants; it thus is thought to influence the flora of the intestinal tract. Lysozyme levels show an increase over time during lactation (Fig. 5-11); this finding is more apparent in Indian women than in those of the Western world. Reddy et al[63] studied the levels of lysozyme in well-nourished and poorly nourished women in India and found no difference between them (Table 5-5). As shown in this study, lysozyme

Table 5-5. Antibacterial factors in colostrum and mature milk in nourished and undernourished women

| Group | Hemoglobin (g/100 ml) | Serum albumin (g/100 ml) | Immunoglobulins (mg/100 ml) | | | Lysozyme (mg/100 ml) | Lactoferrin (mg/100 ml) |
			IgA	IgG	IgM		
Colostrum (1 to 5 days)							
Well-nourished women	11.5 ± 0.37	2.49 ± 0.065	335.9 ± 37.39 (17)*	5.9 ± 1.58 (17)	17.1 ± 4.29 (17)	14.2 ± 2.11 (15)	420 ± 49.0 (28)
Undernourished women	11.3 ± 0.60	2.10 ± 0.081	374.3 ± 42.13 (10)	5.3 ± 2.30 (10)	15.3 ± 2.50 (10)	16.4 ± 2.39 (21)	520 ± 69.0 (19)
Mature milk (1 to 6 months)							
Well-nourished women	12.8 ± 0.43	3.39 ± 0.120	119.6 ± 7.85 (12)	2.9 ± 0.92 (12)	2.9 ± 0.92 (12)	24.8 ± 3.41 (10)	250 ± 65.0 (17)
Undernourished women	12.6 ± 0.56	3.47 ± 0.130	118.1 ± 16.2 (10)	5.8 ± 3.41 (10)	5.8 ± 3.41 (10)	23.3 ± 3.53 (23)	270 ± 92.0 (13)

From Reddy V et al: Acta Paediatr Scand 66:229, 1977.
*Figures in parentheses indicate number of samples analyzed.

Table 5-6.   Effect of iron therapy on lactoferrin in milk*

	Total lactoferrin (mg/100 ml)	Saturated lactoferrin (% of total)
Before iron therapy	240 ± 29.0	9.0 ± 7.15
After iron therapy	260 ± 80.0	8.6 ± 3.32

From Reddy V et al: Acta Paediatr Scand 66:229, 1977.
*Values are mean ± SE of 11 subjects.

levels increase during lactation. Levels in human milk are 300 times the level in cow's milk. Lysozyme is bacteriostatic against *Enterobacteriaceae* and gram-positive bacteria.[60]

In a study of immunologic components in human milk in the second year of lactation, Goldman et al[26] reported that concentrations of lysozyme, lactoferrin, and total and secretory IgA were similar to those in uninterrupted lactation and in gradual weaning at 6 to 9 months. sIgA antibodies to *E. coli* were also produced during the second year. The authors state that "this supports the idea that the enteromammary lymphocyte traffic pathway which leads to the development of lymphoid cells in the mammary gland that produce IgA antibodies to enteric organisms, operates throughout lactation."[26]

Lactoferrin

Lactoferrin is an iron-binding protein that has a strong bacteriostatic effect on staphylococci and *E. coli,* apparently by depriving the organism of iron. Lactoferrin is normally unsaturated with iron. It has been suggested that oral iron therapy can interfere with the bacteriostatic function of lactoferrin, which depends on its unsaturated state. Reddy et al[63] showed that giving iron to the mother, however, did not interfere with the saturation of lactoferrin in the milk or therefore its potential microbicidal effect (Table 5-6). Lactoferrin is less than 50% saturated with iron in human milk.

The concentration of lactoferrin is high in colostrum, 600 mg/100 ml, and then progressively declines over the next 5 months of lactation, leveling off at about 180 mg/100 ml (Table 5-5). It also contains small amounts of transferrin (10 to 15 µg/ml).

Unsaturated lactoferrin has been demonstrated by Kirkpatrick et al[43] to inhibit the growth of *C. albicans*. A combination of lactoferrin and specific antibody had a powerful bacteriostatic effect on *E. coli*. Inhibited *E. coli* appears to be markedly iron deficient. A significant factor that has been clearly demonstrated in preserving the bacteriostatic properties of human milk is that milk proteins, including lysozyme and lactoferrin, reach the duodenum without any digestion. They are stable in the acid pH of the stomach. Trypsin inhibitor, which has been identified in human milk, temporarily delays the hydrolysis of protein. Brock et al[6] attempted to demonstrate a relationship between lactoferrin-mediated inhibition of *E. coli* and the presence of antibodies against the serologically important *E. coli* antigens, O, K, and H. They further investigated the role of enterobactin (enterochelin) in the ability to overcome the inhibitory effect wherein *E. coli* removes iron from lactoferrin and transferrin. The role of lactoferrin in human milk is to sequester exogenous iron reaching the gut rather than to bind or transport the endogenous iron of milk, since the iron in human milk is bound to fat and casein and not to lactoferrin.

Interferon

Colostrum cells in culture have been shown[60] to be stimulated to secrete an interferon-like substance with strong antiviral activity up to 150 NIH units/ml. This property is not found in the supernatant of colostrum or milk. Interferon is a potent stimulator of leukocytes' cytotoxicity in the absence of antibody.

Complement

The C3 and C4 components of complement, known for their ability to fuse bacteria bound to a specific antibody, are present in colostrum in low concentrations as compared with the levels in serum. IgG and IgM activate complement. C3 proactivator has been described, and IgA and IgE have been identified as stimulating the system. Activated C3 has opsonic, anaphylactic, and chemotactic properties and is important for the lysis of bacteria bound to a specific antibody.

B$_{12}$-binding protein

Unsaturated B$_{12}$-binding protein of high molecular weight has been found in very high levels in human milk and in the meconium and stools of breastfed infants as compared with infant formulas and the infants who are formula fed. The protein binding renders the B$_{12}$ unavailable for bacterial growth of *E. coli* and bacteroides.[29]

Gangliosides

Gangliosides are glycolipids found particularly in the plasma membrane of cells of the grey matter. They have sialic acids, hexoses, and hexos amines in the carbohydrate part and ceramide as the lipid. Ganglioside-like components, which were extracted from human fat and skim milk in trace amounts, inhibit *E. coli* and cholera toxin in vitro and in vivo.[56] Human milk gangliosides may be important in protecting infants against endo-toxin-induced diarrhea.

FLORA OF THE INTESTINAL TRACT

As has been pointed out, the normal flora of the intestinal tract of the breastfed infant is *L. bifidus*. The Gram-negative population in the gut is kept small.

In a prospective study of breastfed Mayan Indian infants from birth to 3 years of age, bifid bacteria predominated and constituted 95% to 99% of the flora. Other culturable microorganisms were streptococci, bacteroides, clostridia, micrococci, enterococci, and *E. coli*. A change occurred when large amounts of solid foods were added at about 1 year of life. The solids were notably protein poor. *E. coli* progressively increased in numbers. *L. bifidus* metabolizes milk saccharides, producing large amounts of acetic acid, lactic acid, and some formic and succinic acids, which create the low pH of the stool of breastfed infants. The intestinal flora of bottle fed infants is gram-negative bacteria, especially coliform organisms and bacteroides.

The flora of bifid bacteria is inhibitory to certain pathogenic bacteria. Substantial clinical evidence is available to demonstrate that there is a resistance mechanism against intestinal infections from *Staphylococcus aureus*, *Shigella*, and *Protozoa*.

Newer techniques have shown that intestinal flora is *Bifido-bacterium* or *Eubacterium,* which are obligatory anaerobes and not *E. coli* as previously believed. More recently, work by Yoshioka et al[69] in 1983, using prereduced anaerobically sterilized media, demonstrated the development of stool bacterial flora in both breastfed and bottle fed infants. In both groups, the initial colonization was the enterobacteria in concentrations of $10^9/g$ in specimens collected from the rectum using a sterile glass tube. Both groups of infants were also given 5% glucose water ad libitum. By day 6, bifidobacteria were the predominant organisms in the breastfed infants in a ratio of 1000 to 1 with enterobacteria. In formula-fed infants, the predominant organisms were enterobacteria by a ratio of 10 to 1. By 1 month of age, however, bifidobacteria were most prevalent in both groups, but the number in breastfed infants was ten times that in the bottle fed infants. In the bottle fed infants, the numbers of enterobacteria, bacteroides, and staphylococci were isolated in a constant number in both groups.

Two actions are apparent. The first encourages the growth of *L. bifidus* and thus crowds out the growth of other bacteria. In the second, the number of pathogens is further kept low by the direct action of lysozyme and lactoferrin. When the number of pathogenic bacteria is kept low, the immune antibodies can keep the growth under control and prevent the absorption of bacteria through the gut wall into the bloodstream.

EVIDENCE OF EFFECTIVENESS OF HUMAN MILK IN CONTROLLING INFECTION

The properties of human milk do appear to control infection. Specific disease entities have shown a clear differential in the incidence between infants fed cow's milk and those fed human milk.[47,52]

Bacterial infection

Breast milk IgA has antitoxin activity against enterotoxins of *E. coli* and *Vibrio cholerae* that may be significant in preventing infantile diarrhea. Antibodies against O antigen of some of the most common serotypes of *E. coli* were found in high titer in breast milk samples collected from healthy mothers in Sweden. The infants who had consumed reasonable amounts of breast milk with high titers of *E. coli* antibodies had antibodies in their stool.[32]

Protection against cholera in breastfed children by antibodies in breast milk was studied by Glass et al.[22] A prospective study in Bangladesh showed cholera antibody levels to vary in the colostrum and milk. The correlation among colonization, disease, and milk antibodies led the authors to conclude that breast milk antibodies against cholera do not protect children from colonization with *V. cholera,* but they do protect against disease.

Salmonella infection was similarly studied by France et al[19] to evaluate the immunologic mechanisms in host colostrum and milk specific for salmonellae. Vigorous responses of colostral and milk cells against these organisms and nonspecific opsonizing capacity of the aqueous phase of colostrum and milk were demonstrated.

In studies by Gothefors et al,[28] it was shown that *E. coli* isolated from stools of breastfed infants differed from strains found in formula-fed infants in two respects: They were more sensitive to the bactericidal effect of human serum. More often, spontaneously agglutinated bacteria from other sites, such as the prepuce or periurethral area, were less sensitive in breastfed infants. These findings support the theory that breast milk favors proliferation of mutant strains, which have decreased virulence. This mutation of bacterial strains is another way breastfeeding may protect against infection.

It has been suggested that milk immunization is a dynamic process because a mother's milk has been found to contain antibody to virtually all her infant's strains of intestinal bacteria. The mother exposed to the infant's microorganisms either via the breast or the gut responds immunologically to those microorganisms and thus automatically protects her immunologically immature infant.

The orderly review of data on the presence of antibodies in human milk has produced a substantial list of affected organisms. In addition to *E. coli*, there have been identified antibodies to *Bacteroides fragilis, Clostridium tetani, Haemophilus pertussis, Diplococcus pneumoniae, Corynebacterium diphtheriae, Salmonella, Shigella, Chlamydia trachomatis, V. cholerae, S. aureus*, and several strains of *Streptococcus* (Table 5-7).

A study in Oslo by Hanson[32] of an outbreak of severe diarrhea due to *E. coli* strain 0111 showed that six severely ill children were formula fed. Two infants who were breastfed had *E. coli* strain 0111 in their stools but showed few symptoms. Their mothers had no detectable antibodies for strain 0111 in their milk, which would suggest that other factors in human milk protect the infant from serious illness when there are no antibodies in the milk. Hanson[32] also showed in another study that after colonization with a specific strain of *E. coli*, mothers had large numbers of lymphoid cells in their milk with antibodies to that *E. coli*. Their serum produced no such response. This supports the concept that antigen-triggered lymphoid cells from Peyer's patches seek out lymphoid-rich tissue, producing IgA in the mammary gland. The mother is immunized in the gut at the same time her milk is. It has also been shown that *E. coli* enteritis can be cured by feeding human milk.

A study of possible cell-mediated immunity in breastfed infants was undertaken by Schlesinger and Covelli.[66] They showed that tuberculin-positive nursing mothers had reactive T cells in their colostrum and early milk. Furthermore, eight of thirteen infants nursed by tuberculin-positive mothers had tuberculin-reactive peripheral blood T cells after 4 weeks. Cord blood had no such activity.

Viral infection

Protection against viruses has been the subject of similar studies. Breast milk contains antibodies against poliovirus, coxsackievirus, echovirus, influenza virus, reovirus, and rhinovirus. It has been confirmed that human milk inhibits the growth of these viruses in tissue culture. Nonspecific substances in human milk are active against arbo-virus and murine leukemia virus, according to work by Fieldsteel.[16]

A high degree of antiviral activity against Japanese B encephalitis virus as well as the two leukemia viruses has been found in human milk. The factor was found in the fat fraction and was not destroyed by extended heating, which distinguishes it from antibodies. The nonimmunoglobulin macromolecule antiviral activity in human milk is thought by May[47] to be due to specific fatty acids and monoglycerides (Table 5-8).

Specimens of human colostrum have been found to contain neutralizing activity against respiratory syncytial virus (RSV). RSV has become a major threat in infancy and is the most common reason for hospitalization in infancy in some developed countries. It has a high mortality. Epidemics have occurred in special-care nurseries. Statistically significant data collected by Downham[15] showed that few breastfed babies (8 of 115) were among the infants hospitalized for RSV infection, compared with uninfected controls who were breastfed (46 of 167).

Table 5-7. Nonantibody, antibacterial protective factors in human milk

Factors (references)	Proposed mechanisms of action	Organisms affected	Effect of heat
Bifidus factor	Inhibits replication of certain bacteria in the gastrointestinal tract by causing a proliferation of lactoba-cilli	Enterobacteriaceae including shigella, salmonella, and some *Escherichia coli*	Stable to boiling
Complement components	Opsonic, chemotatic and bacterioly-tic activity	*E. coli*	Destroyed by heating at 56° C for 30 min
Lysozyme	With IgA, peroxide or ascorbate, causes lysis of bacteria	*E. coli* Salmonella	Same loss (0-23%) at 62.5° C for 30 min; essentially destroyed by boiling for 15 min
Lactoferrin (nutrient binders)	Binds ferric iron	*E. coli* *Candida albicans*	Two thirds destroyed at 62.5° C for 30 min
Lactoperoxidase	Oxidation of bacteria	*E. coli* *Salmonella typhimurium*	Presumably destroyed by boiling
Nonantibody proteins: receptor-like glycolipid or glycopro-tein	Inhibit bacterial adherence	*V. cholerae*	Stable to boiling for 15 min
Gangliosides (GM 1 like)	Interfere with attachment of entero-toxin to GM₁ cell membrane gan-glioside receptors	*E. coli* and *V. cholerae* en-terotoxins	Stable to boiling
Nonlactose carbohydrate factors	Prevent action of stable toxin	*E. coli* ST	Stable at 85° C for 30 min
Milk cells (macrophages, poly-morphonuclear leucocytes, B & T lymphocytes)	By phagocytosis and killing, *E. coli*, *S. aureus*, *S. enteritidis* By sensitized lymphocytes: *E. coli* By phagocytosis: *C. albicans* lymphocyte stimulation by *E. coli* K antigen		Destroyed by 62.5° C for 30 min

Modified from May JT: Aust Paediatr J 20:265, 1984; Pickering LK and Kohl S: Human milk humoral immunity and infant defense mechanisms. In Howell RR, Morriss RH Jr, and Pickering LK, editors: Human milk and infant nutrition and health, Springfield Ill, 1986, Charles C Thomas, Publisher.

Table 5-8. Nonantibody, antiviral and antiprotozoan factors in human milk

Factors (references)	Proposed mechanisms of action	Viruses that factors are effective against	Effect of heat
Lipid (unsaturated fatty acids and monoglycerides)	Inactivate lipid-enveloped virus	Herpes simplex Simliki Forest Influenza Ross River	Stable to boiling for 30 min
Macromolecules	Inhibit attachment and penetration	Herpes simplex Coxsackie B4 CMV Rotavirus	Most stable at 56° C for 30 min destroyed by boiling for 30 min
Alpha-2, macroglobulin protein	Inhibits hemagglutinin activity	Influenza Parainfluenzae	Stable to boiling for 15 min
Alpha-1 antitrypsin	Trypsin-dependent inhibition	Rotavirus	Stable to boiling for 10 min
Bile salt stimulated lipase	May generate fatty acids and monoglycerides that inactivate organisms	Giardia lamblia Entamoeba histolytica	
Nonlipase macromolecule	Unknown	G. lamblia	
Milk cells	Induced interferon by virus or PHA, induced lymphokine (LDCF) by phytohaemagglutinin (PHA), induced cytokine by herpes simplex virus, lymphocyte stimulation by rubella, cytomegalovirus, herpes, measles, mumps		Destroyed at 62.5° C for 30 min

Modified from May JT: Aust Paediatr J 20:265, 1984; Pickering LK and Kohl S: Human milk humoral immunity and infant defense mechanisms. In Howell RR, Morriss RH Jr, and Pickering LK, editors: Human milk and infant nutrition and health, Springfield III, 1986, Charles C Thomas, Publisher.

The immune response to RSV was studied prospectively in 26 nursing mothers over several months by Fishaut et al.[17] Antiviral IgM and IgG were rarely found in colostrum or milk. RSV specific IgA was identified, however, in 40% to 75% of specimens. Two mothers with the disease had specific IgG, IgM, and IgA antibody in serum and naso-pharyngeal secretions, but only IgA was found in their milk. This confirms that IgA antibody to specific respiratory tract pathogens is present in the products of lactation. Since RSV appears to replicate only in the respiratory tract, the authors suggest that viral-specific antibody activity in the mammary gland may be derived from the BALT.

Necrotizing enterocolitis has been a serious threat to premature infants in acute-care newborn nurseries in recent years. Animal studies have demonstrated a protective quality to breast milk. Efforts to confirm a similar relationship in human infants have been encouraging but not conclusive. Leukocytes in milk fulfill a protective function in premature infants, possibly as a consequence of their natural transplantation, according to Beer and Billingham.[3]

In a controlled prospective study of high-risk, low-birth-weight infants in India using donor human milk, there were significantly fewer infections and no major infections in the group receiving human milk, although the controls experienced diarrhea, pneumonia, septicemia, and meningitis.

The relationship of sudden infant death to formula feeding is supported by circumstantial evidence and retrospective studies. The fact remains that in all series reported, sudden infant death is rare in breastfed infants. Whether this is related to protection against infection is not clear.

The apparent predisposition of bottle fed infants to purulent otitis media as compared with breastfed infants may be due to IgA-conferred immunity in human milk. It may also be due to the mechanics of bottle feeding. Of a group of infants with otitis media, 85% had had their bottles propped up, whereas only 8% of a matched bottle feeding control group who did not have otitis media had had their bottles propped. When an infant swallows fluid lying flat on the back, it is possible to regurgitate it into the eustachian tube.[2]

Antiprotozoan factors in human milk

In human milk, bile salt–stimulated lipase has been found to be the major factor inactivating protozoans[47] (Table 5-9). The mechanism by which lipase acts is not known, although it may generate fatty acids and monoglycerides, which inactivate the enveloped bacteria, viruses, or protozoan. A nonimmunoglobulin nonlipase, heat-stable factor has been identified in human milk that can inactivate *Giardia lamblia*.

Transmission of disease via the milk

Transmission of disease via the milk in the animal kingdom is a significant source of persistent viral infections, especially retroviruses.[33] In addition to tumors of the mammary gland in mice, which were the first viruses noted to be transmitted via the milk, type B retrovirus and murine leukemia viruses have also been noted to be transmitted via the milk in animals. Infection of lambs with visna virus and of kids with caprine arthritis-encephalitis virus can be prevented according to Haywood by withholding colostrum from the offspring. It has been suggested that infected monocytes are the vehicle of transmission. Human experience with transmission of cytomegalovirus via the milk has been well documented.[47] Now AIDS is reported to be similarly transmitted. Viruses know to produce persistent infections in humans and to appear in milk such as CMV, herpes, hepatitis, and

Table 5-9. Antiprotozoan factors in breast milk

Factor	Shown, in vitro, to be active against	Effect of heat
Bile salt–stimulated lipase	G. lamblia E. histolytica T. vaginalis	Destroyed at 62.5° C for 1 min
Nonimmunoglobulin, nonlipase macromolecule	G. lamblia	Stable to boiling for 20 min

From May JT: Aust Paediatr J 20:265, 1984.

Table 5-10. Microbial contaminant in human milk*

Contaminant	Number of infections	Effect of heat
Cytomegalovirus	69% of infants consuming cytomegalovirus milk excrete virus	Inactivated at 62.5° C for 30 min
Rubella	25% of infants seroconvert after consuming rubella milk	Inactivated at 62.5° C for 30 min
Herpes simplex type 1	Rare	Inactivated at 62.5° C for 30 min
Hepatitis B	?	
Coxiella burnetti	?	
Group B streptococci†	Rare	
Staphylococci†	Rare	62.5° C for 30 min decreases bacteria 85-100%

From May JT: Aust Paediatr J 20:265, 1984.
*Excluding human milk collected for milk banks.
†Breast also infected.

AIDS will require careful monitoring in relation to breastfeeding on a case-by-case basis (Table 5-10). Milk contains a variety of cell types that could harbor other viruses.[58]

Anti-inflammatory properties of human milk

Human milk protects against many intestinal and respiratory pathogens without evidence of inflammation. Goldman and colleagues[27] hypothesize that human milk is poor in initiators and mediators of inflammation but rich in anti-inflammatory agents.

The major biochemical pathways of inflammation, they point out, include the coagulation system, the fibrinolytic system and complement, all of which are poorly represented in human milk. The anti-inflammatory properties of various constituents are outlined in the boxed material on p. 144. The interaction of factors in the milk with one another or with host defenses cannot be entirely predicted by examining each factor separately. When the decreased response of human milk leukocytes to chemoattractant peptides was demonstrated by Thorpe et al,[68] the failure of the response of human milk leukocytes was not due to alterations in maternal peripheral blood leukocytes. It suggested that inhibitors are in the milk and that the human milk leukocytes may be modified in the mammary gland to protect by noninflammatory mechanisms.[68]

Anti-inflammatory features of human milk

A. Paucity of initiators and mediators
   1. Foreign antigens
   2. IgG antibodies
   3. Complement system
   4. Fibrinolytic system
   5. Coagulation system
   6. Kallikrein system

B. Anti-inflammatory agents

1. Lactoferrin	Inhibits complement
2. Secretory IgA	Prevents bacterial adherence
	Inhibits neutrophil chemotaxis
	Limits antigen penetration
3. Lysozyme	Inhibits neutrophil chemotaxis generation of toxic 0 radicals
4. Catalase	Destroys hydrogen peroxide
5. Alpha tocopherol Cysteine Ascorbic acid	Scavangers of oxygen radicals
6. Histaminase	Degrades histamine
7. Arylsulfatase	Degrades leukotrienes
8. Alpha 1-antichymotrypsin Alpha 1-antitrypsin	Neutralize enzymes which act in inflammation
9. Prostaglandins (E2, F2a)	Cytoprotective. Inhibit neutrophil degranulation, lymphocyte activation
10. Pregnancy associated alpha 2-glycoprotein	Inhibits lymphocyte blastogenesis
11. Oligosaccharides	Inhibits microbial attachment
12. Epithelial growth factors	Strengthens mucosal barriers

C. Special features of leukocytes
   1. No basophils, mast cells, eosinophils, or platelets
   2. T lymphocytes respond poorly to allogeneic cells
   3. Low natural killer cells or antibody dependent cytotoxicity
   4. Poor response of neutrophils and macrophages to chemoattractants

From Goldman AS et al: Acta Paediatr Scand 75:689, 1986.

The antioxidant properties of human colostrum were demonstrated by Buescher and McIlheran[8] using aqueous human colostrum on human PMNs. The colostrum significantly interfered with PMN oxygen metabolic and enzymatic activities that are important in the mediation of acute inflammation.

Human milk appears to protect the recipient infant and also the mammary gland by providing anti-infective agents and also by minimizing inflammation.

ALLERGIC PROTECTIVE PROPERTIES

In discussing the antiallergic properties of human milk, it is more difficult to identify specific protective properties. During the neonatal period, the small intestine has increased permeability to macromolecules. Infants have more serum and secretory antibodies against dietary proteins than do children or adults. Production of secretory IgA in the intestinal tract is delayed until 6 weeks to 3 months of age. Secretory IgA in colostrum and breast milk prevents the absorption of foreign macromolecules when the infant's immune system is immature. Protein of breast milk is species specific and therefore nonallergic for the human infant. No antibody response has been demonstrated to occur with human milk in human infants. It has also been shown that macromolecules in breast milk are not absorbed.

Indirect evidence can be inferred from a demonstration of the response to cow's milk protein. Within 18 days of taking cow's milk, the infant will begin to develop antibodies. Since the advent of prepared formulas, in which the protein has been denatured by heating and drying, the incidence of cow's milk allergy has been considered to be 1%. The most reliable means of diagnosing it is by challenging with isolated cow's milk protein. Although circulating antibodies and coproantibodies have been identified, these are not reliable techniques for the clinician involved in patient care.

The allergic syndromes that have been associated with cow's milk allergy include gastroenteropathy, atopic dermatitis, rhinitis, chronic pulmonary disease, eosinophilia, failure to thrive, and sudden death, or cot death, which has been attributed to anaphylaxis to cow's milk.[38,45] The gastrointestinal symptoms have received the greatest attention and include spitting, colic, diarrhea, blood in the stools, frank vomiting, weight loss, malabsorption, colitis, and failure to thrive. Cow's milk has been associated in the gastrointestinal protein and blood loss. The diagnosis is best made by elimination from diet and, when appropriate, challenge tests. Cutaneous testing is of little help.

The association of nasal-secretion eosinophilia with infants freely fed feeding cow's milk or solid foods as compared with eosinophilia in strictly breastfed infants was shown by Murray.[51] Of free-fed infants, 32% had high eosinophilic secretions, and only 11% of breastfed infants had eosinophils in nasal secretions.

It is not surprising that many different antigenic specificities are recognized when the colostrum or milk of one species is fed to or injected into another species. Cow's milk is high on the list of food allergens, particularly in children; sensitivity to cow's milk is responsible for at least 20% of all pediatric allergic conditions, according to Gerrard.[20] Evidence exists that IgA antibodies play an important role in confining food antigens to the gut. Food antigens given to a bottle fed infant before he can make his own IgA, and when he is deprived of that in human milk and the plasma cells, may be expected to be more readily absorbed.

The association of the drop in breastfeeding and the rise in allergy was first made by Glaser.[21] He pioneered the theory of prophylactic management of allergy. The prophylactic management of the potentially allergic infant will be discussed in Chapter 16. The management of specific syndromes such as colic and colitis is discussed in Chapters 8 and 14.

REFERENCES

1. Bahna SI, Keller MA, and Heiner DC: IgE and IgD in human colostrum and plasma, Pediatr Res 16:604, 1982.
2. Beauregard WG: Positional otitis media, J Pediatr 79:294, 1971.
3. Beer AE and Billingham RE: Immunologic benefits and hazards of milk in maternal-paternal relationships, Ann Intern Med 83:865, 1975.
4. Beerens H, Romond C, and Nevi C: Influence of breast-feeding on bifid flora of the newborn intestine, Am J Clin Nutr 33:2434, 1980.
5. Bhaskaram P and Reddy V: Bactericidal activity of human milk leukocytes, Acta Paediatr Scand 70:87, 1981.
6. Brock JH et al: Role of antibody and enterobactin in controlling growth of Escherichia coli in human milk and acquisition of lactoferrin- and transferrin-bound iron by Escherichia coli, Infect Immun 40:453, 1983.
7. Brooker BE: The epithelial cells and cell fragments in human milk, Cell Tissue Res 210:321, 1980.

8. Buescher ES and McIlheran SM: Antioxidant properties of human colostrum, Pediatr Res 24:14, 1988.

9. Buescher ES and Pickering LK: Polymorphonuclear leukocytes in human colostrum and milk. In Howell RR, Morriss RH, and Pickering LK, editors: Human milk in infant nutrition and health, Springfield Il, 1986, Charles C Thomas, Publisher.

10. Bullen JJ: Iron-binding proteins and other factors in milk responsible for resistance to *E. coli*. In Ciba Foundation Symposium, no 42, New York, 1976, Elsevier North Holland, Inc.

11. Butte NF, Boldblum RM, Fehl LM et al: Daily ingestion of immunologic components in human milk during the first four months of life, Acta Paediatr Scand 74:655, 1984.

12. Chen Y, Yu S, and Li W: Artificial feeding and hospitalization in the first 18 months of life, Pediatrics 81:58, 1988.

13. Cunningham AS: Morbidity in breast fed and artificially fed infants. II, J Pediatr 95:685, 1979.

14. Davidson LA and Lönnerdal B: Persistence of human milk proteins in the breast-fed infant, Acta Paediatr Scand 76:733, 1987.

15. Downham MAPS et al: Breast feeding protects against respiratory syncytial virus infections, Br Med J 2:274, 1976.

16. Fieldsteel AH: Nonspecific antiviral substance in human milk active against arbovirus and murine leukemia virus, Cancer Res 34:712, 1974.

17. Fishaut M et al: Bronchopulmonary axis in the immune response to respiratory syncytial virus, J Pediatr 99:186, 1981.

18. Ford JE et al: Influences of the heat treatment of human milk on some of its protective constituents, J Pediatr 90:29, 1977.

19. France GL, Marmer DJ, and Steele RW: Breast feeding and *Salmonella* infection, Am J Dis Child 134:147, 1980.

20. Gerrard JW: Allergy in infancy, Allerg Pediatr Ann 3:9, October 1974.

21. Glaser J: The dietary prophylaxis of allergic disease in infancy, J Asthma Res 3:199, 1966.

22. Glass RI et al: Protection against cholera in breast-fed children by antibodies in breast milk, N Engl J Med 308:1389, 1983.

23. Goldblum RM et al: Antibody-forming cells in human colostrum after oral immunization, Nature 257:797, 1975.

24. Goldman AS: Immunologic system in human milk (editorial), J Pediatr Gastr Nutr 5:343, 1986.

25. Goldman AS, Garza C, Nichols BL et al: Immunologic factors in human milk during the first year of lactation, J Pediatr 100:563, 1982.

26. Goldman AS, Goldblum RM, and Garza C: Immunologic components in human milk during the

second year of lactation, Acta Paediatr Scand 72:461, 1983.

27. Goldman AS, Thorpe LW, Goldblum RM, and Hanson LA: Anti-inflammatory properties of human milk, Acta Paediatr Scand 75:689, 1986.

28. Gothefors L, Olling S, and Winberg J: Breast feeding and biological properties of faecal *E. coli* strains, Acta Paediatr Scand 64:807, 1975.

29. Gullberg R: Possible influence of vitamin B_{12} binding protein in milk on the intestinal flora in breast-fed infants. II. Contents of unsaturated B_{12} binding protein in meconium and faeces from breast-fed and bottle-fed infants, Scand J Gastroenterol 9:287, 1974.

30. György P: A hitherto unrecognized biochemical difference between human milk and cow's milk, Pediatrics 11:98, 1953.

31. Habicht J-P, DaVanzo J, and Butz WP: Mother's milk and sewage: their interactive effects on infant mortality, Pediatrics 81:456, 1988.

32. Hanson LA: The mammary gland as an immunological organ, Immunol Today 3:168, 1982.

33. Haywood AM: Patterns of persistent viral infections, N Eng J Med 315:939, 1986.

34. Head JR, and Beer AE: The immunologic role of viable leukocytic cells in mammary exosecretions. In Larson BL, editor: Lactation, vol IV, Mammary gland/human lactation/milk synthesis, New York, 1978, Academic Press, Inc.

35. Ho PC and Lawton JWM: Human colostral cells: phagocytosis and killing of *E. coli* and *C. albicans*, J Pediatr 93:910, 1978.

36. Jatsyk GV, Kuvaeva IB, and Gribakin SG: Immunological protection of the neonatal gastrointestinal tract: the importance of breast feeding, Acta Paediatr Scand 74:246, 1985.

37. Jelliffe DB and Jelliffe EFP: Human milk in the modern world, Oxford, 1978, Oxford University Press.

38. Johnstone DE and Dutton AM: Dietary prophylaxis of allergic disease in children, N Engl J Med 274:715, 1966.

39. Juto P: Human milk stimulates B cell function, Arch Dis Child 60:610, 1985.

40. Keller MA, Faust J, Rolewic LJ et al: T-cell subsets in human colostrum, J Pediatr Gastr Nutr 5:439, 1986.

41. Keller MA, Heiner DC, Myers AS et al: IgD in human colostrum, Pediatr Res 19:122, 1985.

42. Kirkpatrick CH et al: Inhibition of growth of *Candida albicans* by iron-unsaturated lactoferrin: relation to host-defense mechanisms in chronic mucocutaneous candidiasis, J Infect Dis 124:539, 1971.

43. Kleinman RE and Walker WA: The enteromammary immune system: an important concept in

breast milk host defense, Digest Dis Sci 24:876, 1979.

44. Kramer MS: Infant feeding, infection, and public health, Pediatrics 81:164, 1988.

45. Lebethal E: Symposium on gastrointestinal and liver disease, cow's milk protein allergy, Pediatr Clin North Am 22:827, 1975.

46. Lewis-Jones DI et al: The influence of parity, age, and maturity of pregnancy on antimicrobial proteins in human milk, Acta Paediatr Scand 74:655, 1985.

47. May JT: Antimicrobial properties and microbial contaminants of breast milk—an update, Aust Paediatr 20:265, 1984.

48. McClelland DBL: Antibodies in milk, J Reprod Fert 65:537, 1982.

49. Michael JG, Ringenback R, and Hottenstein S: The antimicrobial activity of human colostral antibody in the newborn, J Infect Dis 124:445, 1971.

50. Miranda R, Saravia NG, Ackerman R et al: Effect of maternal nutritional status on immunological substances in human colostrum and milk, Acta Paediatr Scand 72:461, 1983.

51. Murray AB: Infant feeding and respiratory allergy, Lancet 1:497, 1971.

52. Narayanan I, Prakash K, and Gujral VV: The value of human milk in the prevention of infection in the high-risk low-birth weight infants, J Pediatr 99:496, 1981.

53. Ogra SS and Ogra PL: Immunologic aspects of human colostrum and milk. I. Distribution characteristics and concentrations of immunoglobulins at different times after the onset of lactation, J Pediatr 92:546, 1978.

54. Ogra SS and Ogra PL: Immunologic aspects of human colostrum and milk. II. Characteristics of lymphocyte reactivity and distribution of E-rosette forming cells at different times after the onset of lactation, J Pediatr 92:550, 1978.

55. Ogra SS and Ogra PL: Components of immunology reactivity in human colostrum and milk. In Ogra PL and Dayton DH, editors: Immunology of breast milk, New York, 1979, Raven Press.

56. Otnaess AK, Laegreid A, and Ertresvag K: Inhibition of enterotoxin from Escherichia coli and Vibrio cholerae by gangliosides from human milk, Infect Immunol 40:563, 1983.

57. Parmely MJ, Beer AE, and Billingham RE: In vitro studies of the T-lymphocyte population of human milk, J Exp Med 144:358, 1976.

58. Pass RF: Transmission of viruses through human milk. In Howell RR, Morriss RH Jr, and Pickering LK, editors: Human milk in infant nutrition and health, Springfield Ill, 1986, Charles C Thomas, Publisher.

59. Peitersen B, Bohn L, and Andersen H: Quantitative determination of immunoglobulins, lysozyme, and certain electrolytes in breast milk during the entire period of lactation, during a 24-hour period, and in milk from the individual mammary gland, Acta Paediatr Scand 64:709, 1975.

60. Pickering LK and Kohl S: Human milk humoral immunity and infant defense mechanisms. In Howell RR, Morriss RH Jr, and Pickering LK, editors: Human milk in infant nutrition and health, Springfield Ill, 1986, Charles C Thomas, Publisher.

61. Pitt J: The milk mononuclear phagocyte, Pediatrics Suppl 64:745, 1979.

62. Pittard WB III: Breast milk immunology: a frontier in infant nutrition, Am J Dis Child 133:83, 1979.

63. Reddy V et al: Antimicrobial factors in human milk, Acta Paediatr Scand 66:229, 1977.

64. Richie ER: Lymphocyte subsets in colostrum. In Howell RR, Morriss RH, and Pickering LK, editors: Human milk in infant nutrition and health, Springfield Ill, 1986, Charles C Thomas, Publisher.

65. Savilahei E, Salmenpera L, Tainio VM et al: Prolonged exclusive breastfeeding results in low serum concentrations of immunoglobin G, A, and M, Acta Paediatr Scand 76:1, 1987.

66. Schlesinger JJ, and Covelli HD: Evidence for transmission of lymphocyte responses to tuberculin by breast-feeding, Lancet 2:529, 1977.

67. Stoliar OA et al: Secretory IgA against enterotoxins in breast milk, Lancet 1:1258, 1976.

68. Thorpe LW, Rudloff HE, Powell LC et al: Decreased response of human milk leukocytes to chemoattractant peptides, Pediatr Res 20:373, 1986.

69. Yoshioka H, Isekl KI, and Fujita K: Development and differences of intestinal flora in the neonatal period in breast-fed and bottle-fed infants, Pediatrics 72:317, 1983.

Psychologic bonding 6

Although the previous chapters provide more than adequate information to support the urgency of breastfeeding in almost every case, the critical impact in the return to breastfeeding in modern cultures rests with the issue of the mother's role and her perception of breastfeeding as a biologic act. The maternal influences include psychophysiologic reactions during nursing, long-term psychophysiologic effects, maternal behavior, sexual behavior, and attitudes toward men. All professionals providing support care in the perinatal period need to have a clear view not only of the biologic benefits but also of their own psychologic attitudes about the breast itself. The breast has been regarded as a sex object in the Western world for almost a century, and its biologic benefits have been downplayed. This is clearly demonstrated by the conflicting mores that permit pornographic pictures in newspapers, movies, and nude theaters but arrest a mother, discreetly nursing her baby in public, for indecent exposure.

It has been generally accepted by proponents of breastfeeding, even before the upsurge of interest and research in bonding, that the major reason to breastfeed is to provide that special relationship and closeness that accompany nursing. Conversely, the major contraindication to breastfeeding was lack of desire to do so. This was evidenced by the fact that it was considered more appropriate to present breastfeeding as a matter of personal choice with no compelling reasons to urge a mother to consider nursing. The concern over creating guilt in the mother who chose not to nurse has been significant and often resulted in a passive attitude on the part of the clinician so that the mother received no prenatal counseling at all about infant feeding.[29]

MOTHER-INFANT INTERACTION

The studies performed to understand bonding have largely been done without reference to breastfeeding. It has been pointed out that a comprehensive book, *Attachment and Loss* by Bowlby,[8] which reviews early mother-infant interactions extensively, never mentions breastfeeding. In addition, sucking is given extensive treatment without making a distinction between bottle and breast or implying that there is an alternative to the bottle. The emphasis in the 1940s was on the effects of disrupting already formed attachments. Separation in the neonatal period was ignored, and infant socialization was studied from 6 months of age on.

Work by Spitz[46] and others has identified the devastating effects on the infant deprived of long-term material contact. These investigators demonstrated major deficits in both mental and motor development, as well as general failure to thrive. What had yet to be described was the impact on the mother. Klaus and Kennell[25] have provided those data in their many writings on mother-infant interaction, which are summarized in their book, *Parent-Infant Bonding*. There is reason to believe that the maternal-infant bond is the strongest human bond, when two major facts are considered: The infant's early growth is within the mother's body, and survival after birth depends on her care. Although the process had not been meticulously described yet, it had been noted by Budin[10] in 1907 that when a mother was separated from her infant and was unable to provide the early care of her sick child, she lost interest and even abandoned the infant.

The immediate emotional reactions of mothers to their newborns were studied by Robson and Kumar[41] in 193 women (two groups of primiparas, $n = 112$ and $n = 41$, and one group of multiparas, $n = 40$). About 40% of the primiparas and 25% of the multiparas recalled that their predominant emotional reaction when holding their babies for the very first time had been indifference. Maternal affection was more likely to be lacking if the mother had had an amniotomy or painful labor or had received more than one dose of pethidine unrelated to cesarean section or forceps delivery. There was no difference between breastfeeding and bottle feeding mothers. The feelings of indifference persisted for a week or longer. This study points out that normal women may be indifferent toward their babies intitially, while others experience great elation. The development of positive feelings in primiparous women toward their normal newborns occurred before delivery in a third of women, immediately at birth or in the first day for 42%, and by the second or third day for 19% in a study by Pascoe and French.[36] Breastfeeding mothers were more likely to express positive feelings. Labors of less than nine hours were associated with positive feelings, but there was no association with social class, infant gender, type of delivery, or duration of initial mother-infant contact.

Klaus and Kennell[25] suggested that there may be a critical period in which ideal bonding takes place in the human. This critical period has been described for many animal species in which the mother rejects or even destroys her offspring if they are taken from her at a critical early postpartum time. For the goat, this time is the first 5 minutes. For the human, Kennell et al.[24] described this critical period as within the first 12 hours. Further, they noted that mothers in the United States showed different attachment behavior when permitted early contact with their premature infants compared with mothers who had first contact at 3 weeks of age. Mothers of full-term infants who were allowed contact within the first 2 hours and subsequent extra contact behaved differently at 1 month and 1 year with their babies, compared with controls. Actually, Jackson et al.[23] made similar observations in the Yale Rooming-In Unit from 1945 to 1955, but had failed to provide control observations.

As a result of the thought-provoking work of Klaus and Kennell in the 1970s, remarkable changes have taken place in labor, delivery, and postpartum services in hospitals in the United States and around the world. Mothers have been "allowed" to have their infants to hold and cuddle as soon as possible after delivery, and fathers have been "allowed" to participate in the birth experience. The "take charge" attitude of health care professionals has relaxed, and gradually hospital perinatal care has been humanized. In the meantime a number of investigators have challenged the power of "bonding" and failed to identify an early critical time when bonding takes place in the human mother-infant couple. In a critical review of early and extended maternal-infant contact research, Siegel[43] suggests that although many longitudinal experiences affect parenting behavior in complex ways, reasonable judgment supports early and extended contact whenever possible. He further states, however, that "over-reliance on a simple solution for prevention of parenting inadequacy carries the serious risk of disillusionment." Lozoff et al.[31] suggest: "In view of the widespread disturbances in this society's families, it seems unwise to await the demonstration of long-term irreversible consequences of separation before early and extended contact are offered to all families. It should become hospital routine for families to be together and for separation to occur only upon specific request. There is no medical reason why healthy mothers and babies should not be together from the time of birth to the time of discharge from the hospital."

The impact of early mother-infant interaction and breastfeeding on the duration of breastfeeding has been reported; no data appear to be available as to whether mothering is different between breastfeeding and bottle feeding mothers. Sosa et al.[45] reported the effect of early mother-infant contact on breastfeeding, infection, and growth. Breastfeeding mothers who were permitted early contact but not early breastfeeding were compared with mothers without early contact who also breastfed. The mothers with early contact were observed to nurse 50% longer than the controls. The early-contact infants were heavier and had fewer infections. Sosa et al[45] conducted a similar study in Brazil, in which each mother nursed immediately on delivery and the infant was kept beside the mother's bed until they went home. At home they had a special nurse make continual contacts to help in the breastfeeding. The control had traditional therapy, that is, contact at feeding times after an early glimpse. Infants were housed in a separate nursery. At 2 months, 77% of the early-contact mothers and only 27% of the controls were successfully nursing. It is quite possible that the early and continued contact was accompanied by increased support and assistance from the nursery staff. This added support could facilitate breastfeeding and thus be the cause of the improved outcome.

An additional study by DeChateau[16] in Sweden investigated a group of 21 mothers with early contact and 19 control mothers, all of whom were breastfeeding in the hospital. The only difference in management was the first 30 minutes of early contact, since 24-hour rooming-in was provided for all mothers after 2 hours postpartum. The length of breastfeeding differed: for the early-contact group, 175 days, and for the controls, 105 days. Follow-up observations at 3 months showed different mothering behavior. The study group showed more attachment behavior, fondling, caressing, and kissing than the controls.

Unless heavy medication or difficult delivery intervenes, an infant experiences a period when his eyes are wide open and he can see, has visual preferences, turns to the spoken word, and responds to his environment. A similar period in the state of consciousness of the infant may last only a few seconds or minutes at a time over the next one to two days.

When Klaus and Kennell[25] diagrammed the reciprocal interaction in the first few hours of life, they chose a nursing mother-infant couple. They included in their scheme the factors limited to breastfeeding, such as the transfer of lymphocytes and macrophages from mother to infant and the stimulation of oxytocin and prolactin by suckling of the infant as part of the reciprocal interaction (Fig. 6-1).

Many mothers who did not have the privilege of early contact because of hospital policy, cesarean section, or adoption of the baby have been led to feel they have missed the single opportunity to establish model parenting. Lamb[28] and others[2,3,13] have been critical of the earlier work on the value of early contact, pointing out the weakness in the study design. Lamb[28] has, however, been supportive of the trend toward humanizing childbirth to provide a rich emotional experience for parents.

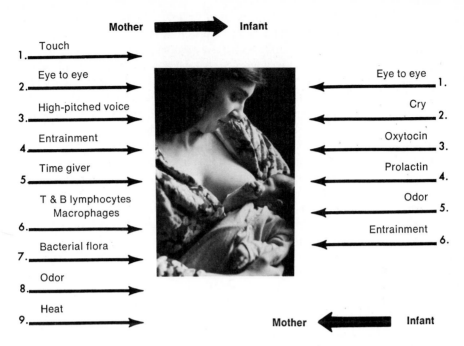

Mother ➡ **Infant**

1. Touch ➡
2. Eye to eye ➡
3. High-pitched voice ➡
4. Entrainment ➡
5. Time giver ➡
6. T & B lymphocytes Macrophages ➡
7. Bacterial flora ➡
8. Odor ➡
9. Heat ➡

Eye to eye ⬅ 1.
Cry ⬅ 2.
Oxytocin ⬅ 3.
Prolactin ⬅ 4.
Odor ⬅ 5.
Entrainment ⬅ 6.

Mother ⬅ **Infant**

Fig. 6-1. Mother-to-infant and infant-to-mother interactions that can occur simultaneously in first days of life. (From Klaus MH and Kennell JH: Parent-infant bonding, St. Louis, 1982, The CV Mosby Co.)

Human relationships are complex. A newborn brings joy, fear, anxiety, frustration, and triumph, reminds Richards.[40] Adaptability and compensation in the developmental processes are part of human existence. The concept of bonding has drawn attention to this period of life and begun the process of understanding the mother-infant relationship.[26]

BODY CONTACT AND CULTURAL TRADITION

If we look at other mammals, lactation behavior—including the duration and frequency of feedings—is species specific and predictable because it is a genetically controlled behavioral characteristic of the species. Only those animals kept in zoos or laboratories reject their young. Among higher primates, learning plays a significant role; monkeys reared without role models have to be taught how to groom and feed their young. In the human, breastfeeding behavior is highly variable from one culture to the next. Different cultures of the world have different sets of "rules" about lactation as they do about many other aspects of life and even death. Cultural tradition dictates the initiation, frequency, and termination of breastfeeding. Learning plays a key role in the lactation process, but the learning is focused on the beliefs, attitudes, and values of the culture.

The degree of body contact permitted by the culture is a fundamental difference among these cultures. Simpson-Herbert[44] describes the degree of mother-infant body contact as the physical and social distance that mothers keep from their babies. The physical distance is viewed as a reflection of the social distance sanctioned by the culture.

Cultures prescribe how often an infant will be held or carried and how he will be carried (e.g., in the arms, a pouch, or a sling, or on a cradleboard). How the infant is clothed, where he is placed when not held, and where he spends the night are all culturally determined and also affect breastfeeding. The cultural constraints that control maternal behavior include those on the kinds and amounts of maternal clothing, acceptability of breast exposure, and beliefs on frequency and length of feedings.

The effect of increased carrying of infants was studied by Hunziker and Barr[21] in a group of primiparous breastfeeding women in Montreal. The crying pattern of normal infants in industrialized societies has been reported to increase until 6 weeks of age, followed by a decline to 4 months with most crying occurring in the evening. The investigators had the study families increase carrying the infants either in the arms or in a carrier to a minimum of 3 hours a day, whereas control infants were placed in a crib or a seat with a mobile in view. At 6 weeks there was significantly less (43%) crying in the "carried" infants, especially in the evening. Similar but smaller differences were noted at 4, 8, and 12 weeks. When Cunningham and colleagues[15] randomly provided either soft baby carriers (Snugglis) or plastic infant seats to a group of low-income women in a clinic in New York City, they found the infants carried in a soft carrier were more securely attached than those placed in a seat when tested with the Ainsworth strange-situation study. The study and control infant groups had an equal number of breastfeeders. The authors found no effect of breastfeeding on study results and concluded that in low-income groups, mother-infant relationships benefited from early use of soft carriers and "contact comfort."

Anthropologic studies of 60 societies by Whiting[51] considered mother-infant body contact. He classified these cultures as high or low in contact as follows:

Culture classification	Minimum distance between mother and child
High contact: ↓ Symbiotic identification ↓ Long breastfeeding	1. Infant almost continuously carried by mother in the early months. 2. Little or no clothing separates the mother and infant so that they are in skin-to-skin contact. 3. Infant sleeps with mother.
Low contact: ↓ Ambivalent dependency ↓ Early weaning	1. Infant is separated from mother at birth. 2. Infant is often swaddled or elaborately clothed. 3. Infant is kept in a crib or cradleboard. 4. Infant does not sleep with mother at night.

Other factors influence the development of cultural mores, including climate and means of food gathering. Simpson-Herbert[44] points out that when infants are heavily clothed and swaddled, as in cold climates, they are neat packages that can be put down easily. The Eskimo is an exception, however, keeping the infant inside her parka for warmth and frequent feeding. Breastfeeding is almost continuous in warm climates where clothing is loose or absent, there is frequent holding and carrying, and the breast is readily accessible.

The diet of the hunter-gatherer society is not conducive to early weaning because meat, roots, nuts, and berries are difficult for infants to chew and digest, whereas the softer foods of the agricultural societies can be prepared for early infant feeding.

Study of specific world societies reveal that North American and European women are concerned with the beliefs that it is indecent to expose the breast, it is possible to spoil an infant with too much handling, and early weaning is a sign of infant development. Western mothers keep their distance from their babies. Mothers in high–body contact societies spend at least 75% of the time in contact with their babies, while low-contact societies spend less than 25%.

PSYCHOLOGIC DIFFERENCE BETWEEN BREASTFEEDING AND BOTTLE FEEDING

Professionals have spent decades reassuring mothers that they can capture the same emotional and behavioral experience by feeding an infant a bottle as they can feeding at the breast and that the same warmth and love are there. Technically speaking, the same warmth is not there, because the lactating breast has been shown to be warmer than the nonlactating breast. This can be demonstrated by infrared pictures.

Newton and Newton[34] suggest that special caution should be used in evaluating statistical associative studies that purport to study the hypothesis that breastfeeding and bottle feeding are psychologic equivalents. "Because breastfeeding involves a large measure of personal choice and because it is related to attitudinal and personality factors, no groups of breastfeeders and bottle feeders are likely to be equal in other respects. Therefore the relation of breastfeeding to any particular psychosocial measure may not be cause and effect, but simply the differences due to other uncontrolled covariables."[34] A human mother's care of her infant is derived from a complex mixture of her genetic endowment, the response of the infant, a long history of interpersonal relationships with others, her family constellation, this and previous pregnancies, and the community and culture.

The method chosen to feed a baby is but one item in a whole style of maternal-child interaction. It is unlikely that this style is determined by the method of feeding, according to Richards.[39] Breastfeeding is a very different activity when it is carried out by a small minority compared to breastfeeding when it is commonplace in the community.

Before reviewing specific psychologic attributes relating to breastfeeding, the distinction between styles of nursing in Western societies should be considered. Newton[34] has described two distinct groups: unrestricted breastfeeding and token breastfeeding.

Unrestricted breastfeeding

Unrestricted breastfeeding means the infant is put to the breast whenever he cries or fusses. Feeding is ad lib and not by the clock, usually leading to 10 or more feedings a day. The infant receives no bottles, and solids are not introduced until the second half of the first year. Breast milk continues to be a major source of nourishment beyond the first year of life. It is interesting to note that this was routine practice in the United States in the beginning of this century, as attested by writings on the subject of child rearing.

Token breastfeeding

Token breastfeeding means feeding characterized by rules and regulations. Both frequency and duration of feeding are determined by the clock. It is deemed unnecessary to permit unlimited suckling. Weaning usually occurs by the third month, if not before. Supplementary bottles and solids are not uncommon. As a result, the let-down reflex is never well established. Engorgement is not uncommon. The infant is frequently too frantic from crying or too sleepy to feed well at the appointed times.

A University of Rochester study[29] of urban physicians revealed that many of the pediatricians prescribed solids by 3 months or earlier and suggested supplementary bottles. Most of the physicians in the family medicine program in the same community, however, provided no supplements and no solids until 6 months. Over 50% of mothers in that community who planned to breastfeed had made contact with some childbirth or breast-feeding program and chose their physician according to practice style.

Let-down reflex

The unrestricted breastfed infant cries, and his mother has the urge to suckle him because the cry has triggered her let-down reflex. The breast is turgescent and ready for the infant. Unrestricted crying is rarely seen in these infants. With token breastfeeding such a response does not occur on schedule, and from feeding to feeding the milk supply may be little, or conversely, gushing. The infant is unable to cope with the unpredictability.

PERSONALITY DIFFERENCES BETWEEN BREASTFEEDING AND BOTTLE FEEDING MOTHERS

There are clear differences between mothers who practice unrestricted breastfeeding and those who bottle feed. There are even some distinctions between token breastfeeders and bottle feeders. It has been said that maternal personality is more important than either breastfeeding or bottle feeding per se to the development of the infant's personality. Experimenters looking at these questions have provided a wealth of somewhat conflicting information. Chamberlain[12] undertook to decipher the differences between mothers who bottle fed and those who practiced unrestricted breastfeeding with their second child. The groups were similar in age, education, parity, intelligence, and socioeconomic status. The breastfeeding mothers were less defensive about their method of feeding, were more oriented toward home life, and had higher radicalism scores. The bottle feeding mothers confirmed the hypothesis that they had problems in trying to breastfeed their first child due to inadequate lactation, possibly a psychosomatic reaction. They also had a greater incidence of sexual anomalies, as indicated from a higher surgency score. The breastfeeding mothers wanted their children to do things typical of children; the bottle feeding mothers preferred their children to be conservative and other-person oriented, and urged them to be more adult.

Call[11] had studied the emotional factors favoring successful breastfeeding and noted that of 104 consecutive mothers delivering at an Air Force hospital, 42.6% of the multiparas and 50% of the primiparas chose bottle feeding. Of the breastfeeding mothers, 48% of those multiparas and 40% of the primiparas were successful beyond 3 weeks. Failure was associated with engorgement, lack of let-down reflex, and psychologic conflict. The two conflicts seen in those who did not nurse and those who failed were as follows:

1. They had a conflict in accepting the biologic maternal role in relation to the infant versus other roles society holds for women. The maternal role is considered a general class attitude in middle-class American society.
2. They had a conflict regarding the functioning of the breast itself, that is, as an organ for nourishment of the young versus a sexual organ, affording the breast the same psychologic value as the penis in the male. Nursing thus became a "castration" threat.

POSTPARTUM DEPRESSION

Much has been written in the lay press about "baby blues," and many mothers will admit to a few hours or a day of incredible emotional seesawing some time in the first week after delivery. Episodes in which a mother dissolves in tears when she has "so much to be thankful for" is the usual description. This is a transient state that has been attributed to the tremendous change in hormonal levels after the delivery of the placenta. It is usually successfully treated with reassurance and rest. True postpartum depression does occur, however, and, contrary to popular fantasy, it occurs in women who are breastfeeding. The incidence of psychiatric disorders, especially depression, is known to increase postpartum.[2]

The relationship between breastfeeding and depression was studied by Kumar and Robson[27] among mothers who totally breastfed and those who totally bottle fed. No relationship was found between depression and feeding method. A prospective study following 103 women postpartum recorded a 13% incidence of marked postnatal depressive illness and an additional 16% of minor depressive illness of at least 4 weeks' duration. No correlation was made with method of feeding until the mothers were asked about their feeding methods and oral contraceptive use in an attempt to determine the influence of hormones on depression. The authors speculated that the prolactin, estrogen, and progesterone levels would vary with the amount of breastfeeding, amount of other foods consumed by the baby, and amount of hormones taken in the form of contraceptives. In this study the bottle feeders received estrogen and progesterone, but breastfeeders received only progesterone as contraceptives. Total breastfeeders who were not taking contraceptives were somewhat more likely to report depressive symptoms. Feelings of fatigue may have influenced this. The mothers least likely to be depressed were those who were likely to have normal hormonal levels, that is non-pill taking partial breastfeeders. Clearly, breastfeeding women are not immune to postpartum depression.[14]

PSYCHOPHYSIOLOGIC REACTIONS DURING NURSING

Newton and Newton[34] have equated psychophysiologic reactions during nursing to the degree of successful lactation. During unrestricted suckling the gentle stroking of the nipple occurs 3,000 to 4,000 times. This should result in an increase in temperature of the mammary skin and rhythmic contraction of the uterus. Failure to experience these signs is related to failure to produce adequate milk.

The role of various hormones in inducing maternal behaviors in animals has been extensively studied. Rosenblatt[42] showed that both male and female rats, including virgin females, manifest maternal behavior after 5 to 7 days contact with foster pups. Manipulation of estrogen, progesterone, and prolactin has demonstrated that estrogen is the most potent inducer of maternal behavior, progesterone usually is inhibitory, and prolactin strangely ineffective. The induction of maternal behavior after administration of oxytocin experimentally in rats by Pedersen and Prange[37] demonstrated that estrogen priming is necessary for the effect, but oxytocin may be the triggering hormone for maternal behaviors. A strong relationship between the peptide hormones native to the central nervous system and the reproductive hormones results not only in endocrine effects but also in behavior.

The long-term psychophysiologic reaction of unrestricted nursing is a more even mood cycle compared with the mood swings associated with ovulation and menstruation.

Unrestricted nursing is associated with secondary amenorrhea for as long as 16 months.

From studies in animals, Thoman et al.[49] have stated, "The present experiments do indicate that there is a unique buffering system which appears to protect the lactating female from large variations in responsiveness during the process of lactating. Inasmuch as there exists considerable information that indicates that maternal factors have profound and long-lasting effects on the psychophysiologic function of offspring in adulthood, the existence of such buffering systems in the lactating females would appear to be of importance in the mother-young interaction."

In relating the rate of success in breastfeeding to experiences at birth, Jackson et al.[23] reported that the more difficult the labor, the less successful the breastfeeding. A direct correlation has also been made with the amount of medication and anesthetic given during labor and delivery and subsequently the sleepiness of the infant and, ultimately, the inadequacy of the suckling. Newton observed that mothers who talked to their babies on the second day nursed their babies longer, that is, beyond the second month.[34]

Modahl and Newton[32] measured mood state differences between breast and bottle feeding mothers when feeding and not feeding. They used the Curran and Cattep questionnaire, which measures transient mood states rather than personality traits. Bottle feeders showed significantly more anxiety, stress, depression, regression, fatigue, and guilt than women did while breastfeeding. Mothers measured while bottle feeding had more anxiety, stress, depression, regression, fatigue, guilt, and extroversion than the control group of bottle feeders tested in a nonfeeding situation. Another control group who were lactating but also gave bottles were measured while not feeding and showed less anxiety, stress, depression, regression, fatigue, and guilt than the average population. Measurements were taken at home with no examiner present.

The psychophysiological responses of breast and bottle feeding mothers to their infants' signals were measured by Wiesenfelt et al.[52] using physiologic monitoring, while mothers observed previously prepared videotapes of their own infants while they smiled, were quiescent and cried. Strikingly different response patterns characterized breast and bottle feeding mothers across all response measures. Breastfeeding mothers were physiologically more relaxed but were more apt to want to interact with their child and expressed greater satisfaction with the feeding experience. The authors interpreted these patterns as suggesting differential physiology rather than personality factors operating on choice of feeding mode.

IMPACT OF SOCIETY, MEDICAL PROFESSION, AND FAMILY
Society

Newton[33] has pointed out that a woman's joy in and acceptance of the female biologic role in life may be an important factor in her psychosexual behavior, which includes lactation. She found that women who wished to bottle feed also often believed that the male role was the more satisfying role. Nulliparous women who planned to breastfeed their children more often stated their satisfaction with the female role, according to Adams.[1] Breastfeeding behavior has been related to a woman's role in life as influenced by her cultural locale, education, social class, and work. Breastfeeding rates and weaning times vary in the United States by geographic area. The smaller the community, the longer the duration of breastfeeding. Cross-cultural studies in large cities show variation in rates of nursing. These rates are influenced by education and, in this generation, the higher the education, the higher the incidence of breastfeeding.

The attitudes of the husband, close family, and friends have an influence on the mother's attitude toward breastfeeding. More important, these attitudes influence the rate of success and the age at weaning more negatively than positively. One study showed that a grandmother's interest did not influence the mother's decision to nurse as frequently as did a friend's (peer's) decision to bottle feed.

Medical profession

The enthusiastic physician can influence the number of breastfeeding mothers in his practice; this has been demonstrated. If the physician provides knowledgeable medical and psychologic support, the success rate of the patients who intended to breastfeed will increase. Some patients who had not formed an opinion or given it any thought in their preparation for motherhood will be persuaded to try. In addition, this physician will attract patients to the practice who are already successfully breastfeeding but find their own physician unable or unwilling to support their efforts.

A study was done at the University of Rochester in a small city where over 50 pediatricians practiced. The pediatricians described their own practices according to the number of breastfeeding mothers (high, 75%; moderate, 50%; low, 25%). They were also asked when they started solid foods, general practice "regulations," and, finally, how their own children were fed. The physicians with a high incidence of breastfeeding in their practices started solids after 4 months, had few rules and regulations about the office, and usually their own children had been breastfed. The physicians with a high number of bottle feeders started solids by 6 weeks, had many rules and regulations about the practice, and their own children had been bottle fed. When asked about using lay groups to help their patients breastfeed, the female physicians were more apt than the male physicians to discredit what these mothers could do to help other mothers.

A national survey conducted among a representative sample of obstetricians, pediatricians, and family physicians by mailed questionnaire reinforced the observation that the physician's attitude and personal beliefs about breastfeeding influence the advice given.[27] It further confirmed that not all physicians were informed about current knowledge on human lactation, not all physicians discussed lactation with their pregnant patients, and not all felt it was worth counseling time when problems arose.

The family
Impact on the infant

For the infant, there are differences between breastfeeding and bottle feeding in the alleviation of hunger, the mother-infant interaction, oral gratification, activity, development, personality, and adaptation to the environment. Often mother and baby are alone together during breastfeeding, and the mother gives her full attention to the baby with stroking and fondling. Social interaction with the baby is less frequent when he is bottle fed, and the mother is often in a distracting social situation. The breastfed infant has control of what is happening, or at least shares control, whereas the mother controls the bottle and the bouts of sucking.

Development. Early assessment of newborns in the first and second weeks of life shows more body activity with breastfed than bottle fed infants. They are more alert and have stronger arousal reaction. Statistics reported by Douglas[17] on age of learning to walk in Great Britain showed a distinct difference, with breastfed infants starting 2 months earlier than bottle fed. The longer the infant was nursed, the more striking the differences. Thus, prolonged breastfeeding does not impede development, as has been implied by advocates of early weaning. A study in Illinois[19] in 1929 compared children exclusively breastfed for 4 months, 9 months, and over a year to bottle fed infants. The children who were exclusively breastfed for 4 and 9 months scored significantly higher on achievement tests, but the difference was reversed beyond a year. Exclusively breastfeeding beyond a year increased morbidity as well, which is in keeping with the concept that solids should be added in the second half of the first year.

Animal work has also shown a relationship of weaning time to learning skills. Since it has become evident that there are species-specific proteins and amino acids, it is possible that the brain develops more physiologically with the precise basic nutrients. Comparisons with animal species show that the more intelligent and skillful groups within a species are nursed longer.

Personality. The personality and adjustment of infants as related to their early feeding experiences have been the subject of much discussion. It must be acknowledged that the personality of the mother and the temperament of the child need to be considerd. Some conflicting information is reported in studies analyzing retrospectively the effects of breastfeeding on outcome in terms of security and behavior. The emphasis has been on the duration of the breastfeeding rather than the quality of the relationship. When abrupt weaning takes place, it may be psychologically very traumatic for the infant and the mother. In animals, when the mother is stressed while lactating, the nursling's plasma cortisone levels are elevated. The psychologically depressed mother may not experience postpartum depression until the infant is weaned from the breast. It has been accepted that early experience, including feeding experience, does influence later behavior in the long run. The performance in young women on an anxiety scale questionnaire (IPAT) and a personality inventory (EPI) showed that those women who had been bottle fed had higher anxiety scores and greater neuroticism than the women who had been breastfed, irrespective of duration of breastfeeding.[20] But much more study must be done before the impact of nursing at the breast is truly understood in the complexity of life's events.

Impact on the father

Since the birthing process moved into the hospital setting, fathers have been moved further from the nucleus of the new family. In recent years this trend has been reversed. Research on interaction with the infant had focused on the mother until Parke and associates[35] observed all three together. In the triadic situation, the father tends to hold the baby twice as much, touches the baby slightly more, but smiles significantly less than the mother. The father plays the more active role when both are present. The study was conducted with middle-class participants who had been to childbirth classes, but the same results were obtained among low-income families without preparation or the presence of the father in the labor and delivery room. The infant had to be relatively active and responsive to capture the father's attention. The investigators felt fathers were far more involved in and responsive toward their infants than our culture had acknowledged. Other studies have shown that when fathers were asked to undress their babies and establish eye contact with them in the first few days of life, they showed more caregiving behavior 3 months later than did controls.

Newton[34] describes the early attachments of the new family as follows:

Father	interacts with baby	engrossment
Mother	interacts with baby	bonding
Baby	interacts with mother	attachment

The father has been brought back into the childbirth scene as a coach. The coach role has been described as the father's role in shared childbirth. The idea of coaching has negative connotations, since a coach is one who develops the players to work and try harder but always to win. Ideally, the father should be a partner and supporter in labor, delivery, and breastfeeding. Raphael[38] has suggested that the father may well play the role of the doula. The doula is one who provides psychologic encouragement and physical assistance to the newly delivered mother. Raphael further indicates that it is the lack of a doula to support the mother that predisposes her to failure with breastfeeding.

The stress placed on sharing responsibilities of parenthood implies an across-the-board division of labor. This implies that parenting is equal for women and men. There are complementary activities for fathers and mothers. Parents are not equally able to do all things. There is more to nurturing the infant than feeding. The father therefore should play a very significant role with the infant. For instance, when the infant is fussy and does not need to be fed, comforting is often best done by the father.

The father's most common negative reaction to breastfeeding according to Waletsky[50] is jealousy of the physical and emotional closeness of the nursing mother and child. The degree of jealousy may reflect how much and how happily the mother breastfeeds. Actually, fathers may express distress because they have no similar way to bring food and contentment to their baby. Male envy of female sex characteristics and reproductive capacity has been identified by Lerner[30] as "a widespread and conspicuously ignored dynamic." Improving the birth experience for husbands is a significant means of helping them feel closer to their baby and better about themselves as fathers, according to Waletsky.[50]

Fathers who object to their wives' breastfeeding may do so because they do not want to share this part of their lover with an infant. Some fathers express concern that the breast will leak and destroy any sexual mystique. On the other hand, many men take great pride in the knowledge that their infants will be breastfed and support their wives in this effort. The decision to breastfeed should be made with the full involvement of the father.

Impact on siblings

Although there is some information about siblings and breastfeeding with regard to behavior patterns, there are no known studies comparing siblings of bottle fed and breastfed infants. Just as siblings frequently wish to try the infant's bottle, they may wish to nurse at the breast. The child will reflect the mother's attitude toward the breast and nursing. If the mother nurses secretly or in private and isolates herself from the family, it may cause concern in the sibling and produce feelings of shame or guilt toward the breasts.

WHY WOMEN DO NOT BREASTFEED

Before the trend toward bottle feeding can be reversed, one has to understand why some women do not breastfeed. It cannot be blamed on society or the medical profession when a woman cannot accept this as part of the biologic role of a mother. A physician who does not understand the complexities of rejecting breastfeeding cannot hope to assist a mother to succeed in breastfeeding.

Our society has assumed that there is no valid intellectual stimulation to be had in the company of young children. Mothers are made to feel intellectually stagnant and uncreative while breastfeeding. Indeed, they are also made to feel asexual at the peak of their sexual cycle. In response, new mothers panic to maintain their social and professional ties. They feel they must produce tangible works to be productive. Bloom[7] points out poignantly that one of the greatest intellectual voyages of our time was undertaken when Jean Piaget sat at his son's crib and observed the child's successive attempts to grasp a rattle. A nursing mother learns about her child through many internal, subjective, and kinesthetic modes that were not open to Piaget. When a mother wrote of her observations in this setting, her writing was ignored as unscientific and trivial.

Bentovim[6] has taken a systems approach, pointing out that a range of physical, psychologic, and sociologic factors are involved. "Breastfeeding is a systemic product of many interacting factors rather than a product of individual behavior only,"[6] according to Bentovim. A good experience with breastfeeding can ensure an intense interaction and synchronous response of giving and taking. According to Brazelton,[9] this is the essence of the infant's beginning to create a secure world for himself.

It is clear that beliefs and attitudes toward breastfeeding influence the choice and the success of breastfeeding. Bentovim points out that it may be possible to restore breastfeeding as the natural choice. This would depend on society's finding a system in which the breast can be accepted not only as good for the infant and his development, but also as the object of less ambivalent and secret pleasure. Bentovim suggests, "The role of the health professionals in this area is important in that only through the right relationship with the mother will a new source of mothering be found that can act as a form of extended family for the woman to identify with and to counteract personal, family, and cultural influences."[6] Hendricks[18] confirms this view and states that the biggest block in the minds of women relates to feelings of shame associated with breastfeeding. More than half the women in the Newcastle[4] survey were prevented from breastfeeding because of a sense of shame. The shame is a result of relating the breast to concepts of sexuality.

Failure at breastfeeding

When a mother who had planned to breastfeed is unable to because of illness in herself or her baby, or when a mother begins to breastfeed and must stop, there is a grief reaction. The mother experiences a great loss. Prolonged mourning and depression are not uncommon. Some women report feeling more distant from this child than from her others if the others had been successfully breastfed. The stronger the commitment had been to breastfeed, the stronger the grief reaction. Few mothers found help, according to Richards[39] in this study, from either professionals or lay support groups. Professionals failed to understand the feeling of failure or loss. The support groups tended to magnify the guilt and sense of failure. The emotions are complex surrounding this intimate activity. Physicians who must recommend discontinuing breastfeeding for medical reasons should be aware of the impact and provide for appropriate support for the mother.

REFERENCES

1. Adams AB: Choice of infant feeding technique as a function of maternal personalty, J Consult Clin Psychol 23:143, 1959.
2. Alder EM and Cox JL: Breast feeding and postnatal depression, J Psychosom Res 27:139, 1983.
3. Anisfeld E and Lipper E: Early contact, social support; and mother-infant bonding, Pediatrics 72:79, 1983.
4. Bacon CJ and Wylie JM: Mothers' attitudes to infant feeding at Newcastle General Hospital in summer 1975, Br Med J 1:308, 1976.
5. Barr RG and Elias MF: Nursing interval and maternal responsivity: effect of early infant crying, Pediatrics 81:529, 1988.
6. Bentovim A: Shame and other anxieties associated with breast feeding: a systems theory and psychodynamic approach. In Ciba Foundation Symposium, no. 45, Breast feeding and the mother. Amsterdam, 1976, Elsevier Scientific Publ. Co.
7. Bloom M: The romance and power of breast feeding, Birth Fam J 8:259, 1981.
8. Bowlby J: Attachment and loss, London, 1969, The Hogarth Press Ltd.
9. Brazelton TB: The early mother-infant adjustment, Pediatrics 32:931, 1963.
10. Budin P: The nursling, London, 1907, The Caxton Publishing Co.
11. Call JD: Emotional factors favoring successful breast feeding of infants, J Pediatr 55:485, 1959.
12. Chamberlain RE: Some personality differences between breast and bottle feeding mothers, Birth Fam J 3:31, 1976.
13. Chess S and Alexander T: Infant bonding: mystique and reality, Am J Orthopsychiatr 52:213, 1982.
14. Cox JL, Connor Y, and Kendall RE: Prospective study of the psychiatric disorders of childbirth, Br J Psychiatr 140:111, 1982.
15. Cunningham N, Anisfeld E, Casper V et al: Infant carrying, breastfeeding and mother-infant relations (letter), Lancet 1:379, 1987.
16. deChâteau P et al: A study of factors promoting and inhibiting lactation, Dev Med Child Neurol 19:575, 1977.
17. Douglas JWB: Extent of breast feeding in Great Britain in 1946 with special reference to health and survival of children, J Obstet Gynaecol Br Empire 57:335, 1950.
18. Hendrickse RG: Discussion from Ciba Foundation Symposium, no. 45, Breast feeding and the mother, Amsterdam, 1976, Elsevier Scientific Publ. Co.
19. Hoeffer C and Hardy MC: Later development of breast fed and artificially fed infants, JAMA 92:615, 1929.
20. Hughes RN and Hawkins AB: EPI and IPAT anxiety scale performance in young women as related to breastfeeding during infancy, J Clin Psychol 31:663, 1975.
21. Hunziker VA and Barr RG: Increased carrying reduces infant crying: a randomized controlled trial, Pediatrics 77:64, 1986.
22. Hwang CP: Aspects of the mother-infant relationship during nursing, 1 and 6 weeks after extended post-partum contact, Early Hum Dev 5:279, 1981.
23. Jackson EB, Wilkin LC, and Auerbach H: Statistical report on incidence and duration of breast feeding in relation to personal, social, and hospital maternity factors, Pediatrics 17:700, 1956.
24. Kennell JH, Trause MA, and Klaus MH: Evidence for a sensitive period in the human mother. In Ciba Symposium, no. 33, Parent-infant interaction, Princeton, NJ, 1975, Excerpta Medica, Associated Scientific Publishers.
25. Klaus M and Kennell J: Parent-infant bonding, St Louis, 1982, The CV Mosby Co.
26. Klaus M and Kennell J: Parent to infant bonding: setting the record straight, J Pediatr 102:575, 1983.
27. Kumar R and Robson K: Neurotic disorders during pregnancy and the puerperium: preliminary report of a prospective study of 119 primigravidae. In Sandler MJ, editor: Mental illness in pregnancy and the puerperium, London, 1978, Oxford University Press.
28. Lamb M: Early contact and material-infant bonding: one decade later, Pediatrics 70:763, 1982.
29. Lawrence RA: Practices and attitudes toward breast feeding among medical professionals, Pediatrics 70:912, 1982.
30. Lerner H: Early origins of envy and devaluation of women: implications for sex role stereotypes, Bull Meninger Clin 38:538, 1974.
31. Lozoff B, Brittenham GM, Trause MA et al: The mother-newborn relationship: limits of adaptability, J Pediatr 91:1, 1977.
32. Modahl C and Newton N: Mood state differences between breast and bottle feeding mothers. In Carenza L and Zinchella L, editors: Emotion and Reproduction, Proceedings of the Serano Symposia: 20B-819, 1979.
33. Newton N: Psychologic differences between breast and bottle feeding. In Jelliffe DB and Jelliffe EFR, editors: Symposium, the uniqueness of human milk, Am J Clin Nutr 24:993, 1971.

34. Newton N and Newton M: Psychologic aspects of lactation, N Engl J Med 277:1179, 1967.

35. Parke RD, O'Leary S, and West S: Mother-father-newborn interaction: effects of maternal medication, labor and sex of infant, J Perspect Soc Psychol 23:243, 1972.

36. Pascoe JM and French J: The development of positive feelings in primiparous mothers toward their normal newborns: a descriptive study, AJDC 142:382 (abst), 1988.

37. Pedersen CA and Prange AJ: Induction of maternal behavior in virgin rats after intracerebroventricular administration of oxytocin, Proc Nat Acad Sci USA 76:6661, 1979 (Neurobiology).

38. Raphael D: The tender gift, breastfeeding, New York, 1976, Schocken Books, Inc.

39. Richards MPM: Breast feeding and the mother-infant relationship, Acta Paediatr Scand Suppl 299:33, 1982.

40. Richards MPM: Bonding babies, Arch Dis Child 60:293, 1985.

41. Robson KM and Kumar R: Delayed onset of maternal affection after childbirth, Br J Psychiatr 136:347, 1980.

42. Rosenblatt JS: Nonhormonal basis of maternal behavior in the rat, Science 156:1512, 1967.

43. Siegel E: Early and extended maternal-infant contact, Am J Dis Child 136:251, 1982.

44. Simpson-Herbert M: Breast feeding and body contact, Populi 7:17, 1980.

45. Sosa R et al: The effect of early mother-infant contact on breast feeding, infection and growth. In Ciba Foundation Symposium, no. 45, Breast feeding and the mother, Amsterdam, 1976, Elsevier Scientific Publ. Co.

46. Spitz RA: An inquiry into the psychiatric conditions in early childhood, Psychoanal Study Child 1:53, 1945.

47. Taylor PM, Maloni JA, Taylor FH et al: II. Extra early mother-infant contact and duration of breast-feeding, Acta Paediatr Scand (suppl) 316:15, 1985.

48. Taylor PM, Taylor FH, Maloni JA et al: I. Effect of extra early mother-infant contact, Acta Paediatr Scand (suppl) 316:3, 1985.

49. Thoman EB, Wetzel A, and Levine S: Lactation prevents disruption of temperature regulation and suppresses adrenocortical activity in rats, part A, Commun Behav Biol 2:165, 1968.

50. Waletsky LR: Husbands' problems with breast feeding, Am J Orthopsychiatr 49:349, 1979.

51. Whiting JWM: Causes and consequences of the amount of body contact between mother and infant. In Munroe RL, Munroe RD, and Whiting BB, editors: Handbook of cross-culture human development, New York, 1980, Garland Publishing Co.

52. Wiesenfeld AR, Malatesta CZ, Whitman PB et al: Psychophysiological response of breast and bottle-feeding mothers to their infant's signals, Psychophysiology 22:79, 1985.

Contraindications to and disadvantages of breastfeeding

7

In reviewing the contraindications to breastfeeding, it is important to look at the entities that put the mother or infant at significant risk and are not remedial. Contraindications are medical; the disadvantages of breastfeeding are a second group of factors to be considered. The disadvantages tend to be social. The physician needs to have a clear understanding of the benefits of breastfeeding and the risks in a particular mother-infant dyad. The risk-benefit ratio can only be determined by the clinician in a position to weigh all the data, usually the pediatrician for the infant or the obstetrician for the mother.

CONTRAINDICATIONS
Breast cancer

A mother with a diagnosis of breast cancer should not nurse her infant in the interest of having definitive treatment immediately, since prolactin levels remain very high during lactation, and the role of prolactin in the advancement of mammary cancer is still in dispute. Although endogenous prolactin by itself may not be a risk factor, it could, along with sex steroids, contribute to the acceleration of malignant growth.[33] All lumps in the lactating breast are not cancer and are not even benign tumors. The lactating breast is lumpy, and the "lumps" shift day by day. If a mass is located and the physician thinks it should be biopsied, this can be done under local anesthesia without weaning the infant. Rochester surgeons have performed many such procedures following referrals in the past 30 years without postoperative complications. The diagnosis of benign masses was made in almost all cases. The performance of immediate surgery relieved tremendous anxiety without unnecessarily sacrificing breastfeeding. With noninvasive mammary imaging techniques such as ultrasound, computerized axial tomography (CAT) scanning, and magnetic resonance imaging, careful diagnosis can be carried out without interfering with lactation and without delaying diagnosis.

Is cancer more or less common in women who breastfeed? The answer is not easy to find, but in countries where breastfeeding is common, breast cancer is uncommon. In the United States, the incidence of breast cancer has steadily risen while the frequency of breastfeeding has declined. At one time it had been suggested that nursing protected a women against breast cancer, but this concept was investigated in an international study and shown to be invalid.[28] Breastfeeding, however, does not predispose a woman to cancer.[18]

A case-controlled study of 453 white females with breast cancer and 1,365 white females without breast cancer from upstate New York showed a negative association between length of breastfeeding and breast cancer in premenopausal women that has not been seen in postmenopausal women. The authors[7] found this apparent protective effect persisted throughout statistical control for age, parity, age at first pregnancy, age of menarche, and education. The women with cancer had a higher incidence of lactation failure due to "insufficient milk." The authors[7] suggest that the significance of this study may be that women who are unsuccessful at lactation are at increased risk for cancer rather than that breastfeeding is protective. Kalache et al.[24] studied 707 married women ages 16 to 50 years presenting with breast cancer in eight teaching hospitals in Oxford and London. Data were collected on duration of breastfeeding of each child and on detailed medical information on study patients and 707 controls. They found no correlation between breastfeeding and cancer. The combination of low parity and late age at first birth was associated with a sevenfold increase in risk of breast cancer at ages 66 to 80 in a study by Luben et al.[27] of over 1,400 women in Canada. At all ages the authors found an increased cancer risk associated with relative infertility, benign breast disease, and not breastfeeding.

Marriage has been established as a negative risk factor for breast cancer. Mortality rates for most causes of death are higher among single women than among ever-married women. Evidence for a crossover in breast cancer risk factors was reported by Janerich and Hoff,[23] who studied women under and over age 40 and who suggest this point has significance for understanding the etiology of mammary cancer. They did not report breastfeeding rates, however, in their detailed study of the factor of pregnancy.

The statistics associating pregnancy and breast cancer influence the picture. In an epidemiologic study, the risk of breast cancer had a linear relationship to the time interval between puberty and childbirth.[20] The risk was reduced by one third for women who bear their first child before 18 years of age compared with those women who have their first baby when they are older. The risk of breast cancer for women who become pregnant before age 20 was about half that of those who first become pregnant after 25 years of age. Births after the first full-term pregnancy did not influence the statistics. Women whose first pregnancy appeared after 30 to 35 years of age had a risk of breast cancer four times that of nulliparous women in the same age group.[46]

The critical question remains—does breastfeeding increase any child's risk of breast cancer, especially in female offspring? This haunting question, first posed by an experimental scientist, created tremendous publicity and genuine concern among physicians asked this question by patients. One needs to explore the available data.

Virus in breast milk

There is no documented evidence in women with breast cancer that there is RNA of tumor virus in human milk. No correlation between RNA-directed DNA polymerase activity has been found in women with a family history of breast cancer. RNA-directed DNA polymerase activity, a reserve transcriptase, is a normal feature of the lactating breast.[11,15,36]

Epidemiologic study

Epidemiologic data conflict with the suggestion that the tumor agent is transmitted via the breast milk. The incidence of breast cancer is low among groups that had nursed their infants, including lower economic groups, foreign-born groups, and those in sparsely populated areas.[28] The frequency of breast cancer in mothers and sisters of a women with breast cancer is two to three times that expected by chance. This could be genetic or environmental. Cancer actually is equally common on both sides of the family of an affected woman. If breast milk were the cause, it should be transmitted from mother to daughter. When mother-daughter incidence of cancer was studied, there was no relationship found to breastfeeding.

Sarkar et al.[38] reported that human milk, when incubated with mouse mammary tumor virus, caused degradation of the particle morphology and decreased infectivity and reverse transcriptase activity of the virions. They suggest that the significance of this destructive effect of human milk on mouse mammary tumor virus may account for the difficulty in isolating the putative human mammary tumor agent. Sanner[37] has provided data to show that the inhibitory enzymes in milk can be removed by special sedimentation technique. He ascribes the discrepancies in isolating virus particles in human milk to these factors, which inhibit RNA-directed DNA polymerase.

Current position

It has been concluded that breast cancer is not related to breastfeeding; further, the fear of cancer in the breastfed female offspring does not justify avoiding breastfeeding. Breastfed women have the same breast cancer experience as nonbreast fed women. There is no increase in benign tumors, either. Daughters of breast cancer patients have an increased risk of developing benign and malignant tumors by merit of their heredity, not their breastfeeding history.[31,32]

Unilateral breastfeeding (limited to the right breast) is a custom of Tanka women of the fishing villages of Hong Kong. Ing et al.[22] investigated the question, Does the unsuckled breast have an altered risk of cancer? They studied breast cancer data from 1958 to 1975. Breast cancer occurred equally on the left and the right breast. Comparison of patients who had nursed unilaterally with nulliparous patients and with patients who had borne children but not breastfed indicated a highly significantly increased risk of cancer in the unsuckled breast. The authors conclude that in postmenopausal women who have breastfed unilaterally, the risk of cancer is significantly higher in the unsuckled breast. They believed that breastfeeding may help protect the suckled breast against cancer.

Other authors[30] have suggested that Tanka women are ethnically a separate people and that it is possible that left-sided breast cancer is related to their genetic pool and not to their breastfeeding habits. No mention has been made of other possible influences, for instance, the impact of their role as "fishermen" or any inherent trauma to the left breast.[34]

Papaioannou,[34] in a collective review of the etiologic factors in cancer of the breast in humans, concludes, "Genetic factors, viruses, hormones, psychogenic stress, diet and other possible factors, probably in that order of importance, contribute to some extent to the development of cancer of the breast."

Wing[48] concludes in her update on human milk and health that "in view of the complete absence of any studies showing a relationship between breastfeeding and increased risk of breast cancer, the presence of virus-like particles in breast milk should not be a contraindication to breastfeeding."

Henderson et al.[20] make a similar statement, and Vorherr[46] concludes that the roles of pregnancy and lactation in the development and prognosis of breast cancer are not determined.

Radiation therapy to the breast

Ionizing radiation is carcinogenic to the female mammary tissue. Women in Hiroshima and Nagasaki and those subjected to therapeutic radiation for mastitis were followed for many years.[41] The risk of cancer is 3.2 times greater in irradiated breasts, increasing over time since the irradiation treatment. There is also a linear relationship to radiation dose.

Radiation usually causes destruction to lobules, condensation of the cytoplasm in cells lining the ducts and fibrosis. Successful lactation following radiation for carcinoma has been reported[14] in a 36-year-old woman with one previous pregnancy and lactation experience 6 years previously.

Hepatitis B virus

The transmission of hepatitis B from mothers whose blood contains hepatitis B antigen to their infants has been described in several parts of the world.[26] Such transmission of an infectious agent from mother to infant is termed *vertical transmission*. The mode of transmission is transplacentally in utero, at delivery, or shortly after delivery. Horizontal transmission occurs between two individuals in close contact. Taiwan and Japan report a high incidence of transmission from carrier mothers to their infants, in contrast to reports from the rest of the world.[44] Follow-up from 4 to 12 months of age indicated the infants of carrier mothers in most studies remained serum negative. In the United States, the rate of transmission to infants from carrier mothers is very low.

Transmission from mothers with acute hepatitis B in pregnancy is very different. It was shown that in mothers with active disease just before, during, or after pregnancy, the infants had up to a 50% chance of being hepatitis B antigen positive. Hepatitis was acquired transplacentally or at birth, but not by breast milk because the infants were not breastfed. There is a 50% risk of hepatitis if a mother has the disease at the end of pregnancy.[13]

In addition to transplacental infection there is the risk of fecal-oral transmission at delivery and transcolostrally. Hepatitis B antigen has been found in saliva, stool, urine, prostatic fluid, and seminal fluid. Some infants do pick up the virus at birth. Hepatitis B antigen is found in breast milk.[43] Transmission by this route has not been well documented. The mothers of some infants who did become infected did not have the virus in the colostrum.[3]

Beasley et al.[4] write that although breast milk transmission is possible, their work showed no difference in frequency of antigenemia among breastfed and nonbreastfed babies in a long-term follow-up study of 147 mothers who were carriers of hepatitis B antigen. The time of transfer of the antigen from mother to infant may be during labor and delivery, when microscopic blood leaks may occur across the placenta, rather than via the breast milk.

All infants born to mothers who have active disease or are carriers now receive both hepatitis B immune globulin (HBIG 0.5 ml/M) immediately in the delivery room, plus the first dose of human hepatitis B vaccine followed by a second dose at 1 week of age or later. The HBIG should not be postponed and should occur within an hour of birth.[12] This decreases the risk of acquiring the infection to almost zero, and breastfeeding is permitted in all protected infants in all countries. The newborn should receive a total of three doses of 10 µg (0.5 ml or half the adult dose) of HB vaccine 1 month and 6 months after the dose at birth.

The *Redbook of the Committee on Infection of the Academy of Pediatrics* has stated in the 1988 edition[12]: "Studies in Taiwan and England do not demonstrate that breastfeeding by mothers who are HBsAg positive increases the risk of HBV infection in their newborn infants."

Mothers who are at high risk for hepatitis should be screened prenatally so that proper precautions to protect health care workers is provided and the neonate receives HBIG promptly. Mothers at high risk are women of Asian descent, IV drug abusers, women born in Haiti or sub-Saharan Africa, women with liver disease, and those exposed on the job to blood products.

Cytomegalovirus infection

Cytomegalovirus (CMV) has been identified in human milk of women with CMV-CF (complement fixation) antibody. Hayes and associates[19] showed 10.8% incidence at 1 to 6 days and 50% incidence at 1 to 13 weeks. There is no correlation between the presence of viruria and the finding of CMV in the milk. Breast milk ranks with cervical secretions as a potential source of CMV infection in infants according to these researchers.[19] The risk of CMV infection and/or serious consequences to the infant of a lactating woman with CMV in her milk is negligible because the milk also contains appropriate antibodies that protect the infant. The risk of milk containing CMV is for a donor recipient such as a premature or other high-risk infant who receives some virus but not a daily dose of antibodies (see Chapter 19, Milk Banking).

β-Streptococcal disease

A case of recurrent β-streptococcal disease in an infant who was breastfed has been reported.[39] The infant was infected at birth and treated with antibiotics. Six weeks later the mother developed bilateral mastitis, and the infant became moribund 2 days later. The infant and the milk grew out β-streptococcus. In the same journal, two other cases of β-streptococcal infection in breastfed infants are reported. The same type of β-streptococcus was found in mother and infant. It is highly likely that the mother was infected by the infant. It is rare to see bilateral mastitis in humans, but in all three cases of streptococcal mastitis, it was bilateral. Any time there is streptococcal disease in the newborn, there is potential for recurrence. Bilateral mastitis should be considered a suspicious sign.

Acquired immune deficiency syndrome (AIDS)

Embryopathy associated with human T-cell lymphotropic virus type III has been described to include growth failure, microcephaly, hypertelorism, prominent forehead, flat nasal bridge, obliquity of the eyes, long palpebral fissures, blue sclerae, and patulous lips. The greater the dysmorphism, the sooner clinical manifestations of the disease seem to appear. About 50% of mothers of infants with congenital manifestations are still asymptomatic at birth but almost always positive for HIV antibodies. For women who are seropositive at delivery, 30% to 60% of their infants will develop acquired immune deficiency syndrome (AIDS) or AIDS-related complex (ARC). The virus can be acquired in utero, from infected blood during delivery, or postnatally. Cesarean section does not appear to change the rate in high-risk pregnancies. Of children under the age of 13 years with a parent with AIDS or a mother in the high-risk group, 80% will develop the disease. The incubation period for perinatally acquired AIDS is 6 to 8 months, compared to 28 months in adolescents and adults.

HIV has been isolated from blood, semen, vaginal secretions, saliva, tears, cerebrospinal fluid, amniotic fluid, urine, and breast milk. Only blood, semen, vaginal secretions, and possibly breast milk, have been implicated in person-to-person transmission. Careful study has not revealed nonsexual spread in households.

The first case of breastfeeding-associated disease was reported by Ziegler et al.[49] in 1985, and attention became sharply focused on the potential of spread to infants through mother's milk. A healthy mother was delivered by emergency cesarean section because of placenta previa and fetal distress with a blood loss of 1500 cc. Fifteen minutes after the delivery a two-unit transfusion was begun. The next day she received two more units. The donor of one unit was identified 13 months later as having antibody to AIDS-related virus. The infant was healthy and was successfully breastfed for 6 weeks. At 3 months the infant developed atopy and failure to thrive. When tested at 13 months, mother and infant had antibody to AIDS virus. Mother and infant have generalized adenopathy. The father and siblings tested negative. Two additional cases of AIDS in breastfeeding infants whose mothers were not at risk but received contaminated blood at delivery were reported.[25]

Eighty-three children enrolled in the European collaborative study of infants born to HIV-positive mothers were studied by Senturia et al.[40] for a history of breastfeeding. Eleven infants were breastfed for 1 week to 7 months, of which six "lost antibody," i.e., are now sero-negative and clinically well. Three infants are well but remain sero-positive. Two had AIDS or ARC, one with first symptoms at 2 weeks, the second at 8 weeks (died at 7 months). The AIDS virus has been isolated from cell-free breast milk of three healthy virus carriers.

Thoughtful consideration regarding perinatal transmission of AIDS has led the Centers for Disease Control (CDC) and the Public Health Service to recommend that women who test positive for HIV antibody in the United States should be counseled to avoid breastfeeding to avoid postnatal transmission to a child who may not be infected.[1,8,9] In countries where the risk of death in the first year is 50% from diarrhea and other disease (exclusive of AIDS), breastfeeding is still the feeding of choice because the risk of dying from AIDS when born to an infected mother is only 18%. Breastfeeding should be encouraged in developing countries even when the mother has hepatitis or AIDS.[8,9,10] Barrett,[2] in his excellent review of pediatric AIDS, offers an algorithm for the clinical evaluation and management of high-risk mothers and infants (see Fig. 7-1). As in any other clinical situation, the pediatrician in conjunction with the obstetrician should review all the available data in the case and facilitate the mother's (parents') making an informed decision in the light of current clinical information and medical options.

Life-threatening illnesses

Life-threatening or debilitating illness in the mother may necessitate avoiding lactation.[5] This is a clinical judgment that should be made with the mother and father, with all the facts presented. Although some woman with the same diagnosis may be able to overcome all obstacles and prove she can nurse her baby, it does not necessarily mean that this patient's situation is identical.[6] If the mother wishes some lay reading on the subject, the clinician should be familiar with the text of the material so that any apparent inconsistencies of opinion can be discussed.

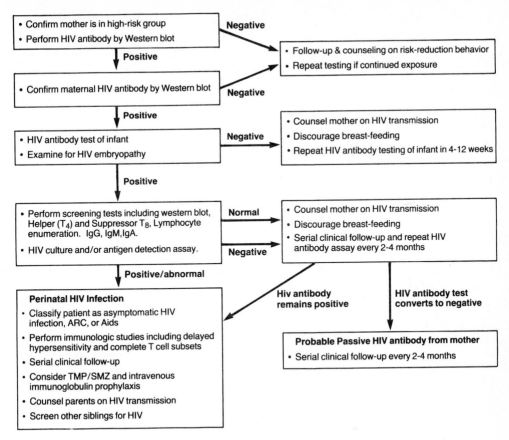

Fig. 7-1. Algorithm for the clinical evaluation and management of high-risk mothers and infants. (Modified from Barrett DJ: Contemp Pediatr 5:24, 1988.)

DISADVANTAGES

Disadvantages to breastfeeding are those factors perceived by the mother as an inconvenience to her, since there are no known disadvantages for the normal infant. (In the rare circumstance of galactosemia in the neonate, which involves an inability to tolerate lactose, breastfeeding is contraindicated [see Chapter 14]). In cultures in which nursing in public is commonplace, nursing is not considered inconvenient, since the infant and the feeding are always available.

The fact that the mother is committed to the infant for six to twelve feedings a day for months is overwhelming to a women who has been free and independent. Motherhood, itself, changes one's life-style.

Guilt from failure, shame, and other anxieties are of considerable concern. Surveys evaluating the decline of breastfeeding have revealed that feelings of shame, modesty, embarrassment, and distaste have been described. These feelings are more common in lower social groups. Research on wider sociologic and psychologic factors regarding the feelings and attitudes toward breastfeeding can have a considerable influence on the choice to breastfeed and will be helpful in dealing with these issues.

As the incidence and duration of breastfeeding increase and professionals and lay people alike are caught up in the rush to convert all parents and change all hospital routines and recommendations, a sense of balance must be maintained. It is necessary to appreciate that there are normal women who cannot or will not nurse their babies. Their babies will survive and grow normally. The sharp letter by Fisher[17] brings this to focus when she describes the frustrations and disappointments of others and dispels what she calls the myths about breastfeeding.

The popular press[28] has drawn attention to parenting trends that divide responsibility for the infant equally between mother and father after the birth. This, of course, necessitates bottle feeding. The justification is division of labor and equal opportunity for both parents to do good things for the baby. This is probably another way of expressing breast envy and jealousy. Some husbands are jealous because they have no similar way to bring food and contentment to their infant, according to Waletzky.[47] "A certain manliness was required to foster breastfeeding in one's family when society as a whole was hostile to it," according to Pittenger and Pittenger.[35] They point out that the perinatal period is a breeding ground for marital and parental maladjustment. Many writers, on the other hand, have described participation in childbirth as a potentially beneficial experience for men. The father's feelings are useful during labor and delivery. These experiences contribute to heightened self-concepts and better adjustments to roles as husband and father. The quality of the birth experience has been cited as the major determinant of paternal attachment. Paternal attachment has led to a greater pride in breastfeeding and a more secure, self-confident support person for the mother who is breastfeeding their infant. Perinatal counseling of prospective new parents may anticipate these reactions, and in turn the professional will have an opportunity to facilitate the best experience possible.

REFERENCES

1. Ammann AJ: The immunology of pediatric AIDS. In Report of the Surgeon General's workshop on children with HIV infection and their families, DHHS pub no HRS-D-MC 87-1:13, 1987.
2. Barrett DJ: The clinician's guide to pediatric AIDS, Contemp Pediatr 5:24, 1988.
3. Beasley RP: Transmission of hepatitis by breast feeding (letter to the editor), N Engl J Med 292:1354, 1975.
4. Beasley RP et al: Evidence against breast feeding as a mechanism for vertical transmission of hepatitis B, Lancet 2:740, 1975.
5. Berger LR: When should one discourage breastfeeding, Pediatrics 67:300, 1981.
6. Brewster DP: You can breast feed your baby . . . even in special situations, Emmaus Pa, 1979, Rodale Press.
7. Byers T, Graham S, Rzepka T et al: Lactation and breast cancer, Am J Epidemiol 121:664, 1985.
8. Centers for Disease Control: Recommendation for assisting in the prevention of perinatal transmission of human T-lymphotropic virus type III/lymphadenopathy-associated virus and acquired immunodeficiency syndrome, MMWR 34:721, 1985.
9. Centers for Disease Control: Public Health Service guidelines for counseling and antibody testing to prevent HIV infection and AIDS, MMWR 36:509, 1987.
10. Centers for Disease Control: Recommendations for prevention of HIV transmission in health-care settings, MMWR 36(suppl no 25):35, 1987.
11. Chopra H et al: Electron microscopic detection of Simian-type virus particles in human milk, Nature N Biol 243:159, 1973.
12. Committee on Infectious Disease: Report of the Committee on Infectious Disease, American Academy of Pediatrics Redbook, ed 21, Evanston Ill, 1988, American Academy of Pediatrics.
13. Crumpacker CS: Hepatitis. In Remington JS and Klein JO, editors: Infectious diseases of the fetus and newborn infant, Philadelphia, 1971, WB Saunders Co.

14. David FC: Lactation following primary radiation therapy for carcinoma of the breast, Int J Radiat Oncol Biol Phys 11:1425, 1985.

15. Fieldsteel AH: Nonspecific antiviral substances in human milk active against arbovirus and murine leukemia virus, Cancer Res 34:712, 1974.

16. Fischl MA, Dickinson GM, Scott GB et al: Evaluation of heterosexual partners, children and household contacts of adults with AIDS, JAMA 257:640, 1987.

17. Fisher PJ: Breast or bottle: a personal choice, (letter to the editor), Pediatrics 72:435, 1983.

18. Fraumeni JF and Miller RW: Breast cancer from breast feeding, Lancet 2:1196, 1971.

19. Hayes K et al: Cytomegalovirus in human milk, N Engl J Med 287:177, 1972.

20. Henderson BE et al: An epidemiologic study of breast cancer, J Nat Cancer Inst 53:609, 1974.

21. Hornstein E, Skornick Y, and Rozin R: The management of breast carcinoma in pregnancy and lactation, J Surg Oncol 21:179, 1982.

22. Ing R, Ho JHC, and Petrakis NL: Unilateral breast feeding and breast cancer, Lancet 2:124, 1977.

23. Janerich DT and Hoff MB: Evidence for a crossover in breast cancer risk factors, Am J Epidemiol 116:737, 1982.

24. Kalache A, Vessey MP, and McPherson K: Lactation and breast cancer, Br Med J 1:223, 1980.

25. Lepage P, Van de Perre P, Carael M et al: Postnatal transmission of HIV from mother to child, Lancet 2:400, 1987.

26. Linnemann CC and Goldberg S: HBAg in breast milk, Lancet 2:155, 1974.

27. Lubin JH, Burns PE, Blot NJ et al: Risk factors for breast cancer in women in northern Alberta, Canada, as related to age at diagnosis, J Nat Cancer Inst 68:211, 1982.

28. MacMahon B et al: Lactation and cancer of the breast: a summary of an international study, Bull WHO 42:185, 1970.

29. Marion RW, Wiznia AA, Hutcheon RG et al: Human T-cell lymphotropic virus type III (HTLV-III) embryopathy, AJDC 140:638, 1986.

30. McManus IC: Predominance of left-sided breast tumours, Lancet 2:297, 1977.

31. Miller RW and Fraumeni JF: Does breast feeding increase the child's risk of breast cancer? Pediatrics 49:645, 1972.

32. Morgan RW, Vakil DV, and Chipman ML: Breast feeding, family history, and breast disease, Am J Epidemiol 99:117, 1974.

33. Ory H et al: Oral contraceptives and reduced risk of benign breast disease, N Engl J Med 294:419, 1976.

34. Papaioannou AN: Etiologic factors in cancer of the breast in humans: collective review, Surg Gynecol Obstet 138:257, 1974.

35. Pittenger JE and Pittenger JG: The perinatal period: breeding ground for marital and parental maladjustment, Keeping Abreast J 2:18, 1977.

36. Roy-Burman P et al: Attempts to detect RNA tumour virus in human milk, Nature N Biol 244:146, 1973.

37. Sanner T: Removal of inhibitors against RNA-directed DNA polymerase activity in human milk, Cancer Res 36:405, 1976.

38. Sarkar NH et al: Effect of human milk on mouse mammary tumor virus, Cancer Res 33:626, 1973.

39. Schreiner RL, Coates T, and Shackelford PG: Possible breast milk transmission of group B streptococcal infection (letter to the editor), J Pediatr 91:159, 1977.

40. Senturia YD, Ades AE, Peckham CS et al: Breast-feeding and HIV infection, Lancet 2:400, 19187.

41. Shore RE, Hildreth N, Dvoretsky P et al: Breast cancer among women given x-ray therapy for acute postpartum mastitis, J Nat Cancer Inst 77:689, 1986.

42. Smith JL and Hindman SH: Transmission of hepatitis by breast-feeding (letter to the editor), N Engl J Med 292:1354, 1975.

43. Stevens CE et al: Vertical transmission of hepatitis B antigen in Taiwan, N Engl J Med 292:771, 1975.

44. Stone E: A feminist fad? Ms 11(8):68, 1983.

45. Thiry L, Sprecher-Goldberger S, Jonckheer T et al: Isolation of AIDS virus from cell-free milk of three healthy virus carriers, Lancet 2:891, 1985.

46. Vorherr H: Pregnancy and lactation in relation to breast cancer risk, Semin Perinatol 3:299, 1979.

47. Waletzky LR: Husbands' problems with breast-feeding, Am J Orthopsychiatr 49:349, 1979.

48. Wing JP: Human versus cow's milk in infant nutrition and health: update 1977, Curr Prob Pediatr 8(1):entire issue, November 1977.

49. Ziegler JB, Cooper DA, Johnson RO et al: Postnatal transmission of AIDS-associated retrovirus from mother to infant, Lancet 1:896, 1985.

Management of the mother-infant nursing couple

8

Successful nursing depends on the successful association of mother and infant with appropriate support from the father and available medical resources. Since both mothers and infants vary, a simple set of rules cannot be outlined to guarantee success for everyone. In fact, one of the difficulties has been that a rigid system was established in hospitals for initiating lactation that did not fit all mother-infant couples. Furthermore, physicians do not receive formal education on breastfeeding; thus they resort to gaining information from nonmedical sources and assume that this is the only way to approach the situation.

Nowhere in medicine do one's personal interests or prejudices become more evident than in the area of counseling about childbirth and breastfeeding. Having a child does not make one an expert on the subject. Conversely, not having a child does not preclude the development of unexcelled skills. Some of the world's most revered experts in human lactation have not had a child or nursed an infant, but they have brought the eye of a skilled observer and experience of a broadly trained clinician to the situation unencumbered by emotional bias and personal prejudices.

The key to the management of the nursing couple is establishing a sense of confidence in the mother and supporting her with simple answers to questions when they arise. Good counseling also depends on understanding the science of lactation. Then in the situation where a problem arises, there is already in place a mechanism for the mother to receive help from her physician's office before the problem creates a serious medical complication.

THE SCIENCE OF SUCKLING

The ability to lactate is characteristic of all mammals from the most primitive to the most advanced. The divergence of suckling patterns, however, makes it urgent that the human be studied specifically to understand human patterns.[14] Some aquatic mammals such as whales nurse under water; others such as the seal and sea lion nurse on land. A variety of erect or recumbent postures are assumed by different terrestrial mammals.[29] Nursing may be continuous, as in the joey attached to a marsupial teat, or at widely different intervals characteristic of the species. The interval may be a half hour in the dolphin, an hour in the pig, a day in the rabbit, 2 days in the tree-shrew, or a week in the northern fur seal. There are many anatomic distinctions as well. The principal mechanism of milk removal common to all mammals is the contractile response of the mammary myoepithelium under the hormonal influence of oxytocin released from the neurohypophysis.

The functional implications in all species is the effective control of milk delivery to the young in the right amount and at the appropriate intervals, which requires a storage system, exit channels, a prehensile appendage, an expulsion mechanism, and a retention mechanism. The primary, secondary, and tertiary ducts form an uninterrupted channel for the passage of milk from the alveoli to the mammary sinuses. A process of erection of the areolar region facilitates prehension by the young during suckling. The principal object of the suction produced by the facial musculature of the young is to draw the nipple into the mouth and retain it there. Positive pressure is used to expel milk from the gland by the contractile changes in the mammary gland provided by the myoepithelial cells (see Fig. 2-10). The sympathetic nervous stimuli can oppose milk ejection by increasing vasoconstrictor tone, thereby reducing access of circulating oxytocin to the mammary myoepithelium. Sympathetic activity also can occur during conditions of apprehension or muscular exertion. The milk-ejection reflex can be blocked by emotional disturbance or reflex excitation of the neurohypophysis. The central nervous system control of milk ejection indeed suggests that restraining mechanisms exist to ensure that milk ejection can only occur under circumstances wholly conducive to the effective removal of milk by the suckling young.

In all species that have been studied, a rise in intramammary pressure and flow of milk occur as a reflex event in suckling. The excitation of the neurohypophysis results in the release of oxytocin, which is conveyed in the bloodstream to mammary capillaries, where it evokes contraction of the myoepithelium.[27] The successive ejection pressure peaks demonstrated in lactating women can be duplicated more accurately by a series of separate oxytocin injections than by the same total dose as a single injection or by a continuous infusion of the hormone. This strongly suggests that oxytocin is released from the neurohypophysis in spurts. The study of suckling patterns in all species shows a high degree of ritualization, which in turn suggests a close neural connection between cognitive or behavioral and hormonal responses.

Attention has focused on the mechanisms that control suckling behavior, on its incidence, on the events that precipitate and terminate it, on the effects of stress, and on how development modifies it. Suckling is characteristic of each species and vital for survival. Although suckling has been studied in other species with the young and the mother, much of human data has been collected using a rubber nipple and bottle. Other mammals sucked only in the nutritive mode, whether receiving milk from the nipple or not. Human infants were noted to have two distinct patterns with rubber nipples: a nutritive mode and a nonnutritive mode.[109,110] When this work was repeated using the breastfeeding model, there was no difference between nutritive and nonnutritive suckling rates but rather a continuous variation of suckling rate in response to milk-flow rate.[15] Suckling rates in other species correlate with milk composition and species-specific feeding schedules (one suck per second in great apes and four to five sucks per second in sheep and goats). In further experiments, there was a linear relationship between milk flow and suckling rate. Thus, the higher the milk flow, the lower the suckling rate. In human infants younger than 12 weeks of age, suckling will terminate with sleep and be reinstated on awakening, a pattern that is well described in other species.[14] In infants older than 12 weeks, suckling is not terminated by sleep. At 12 to 24 weeks, infants will play with the nipple and explore the mother and not always elicit nipple attachment. During a given feeding from one breast during continuous measurement of milk intake, a progressive reduction in intake volume per suck and an increase in the proportion of time spent pausing between bursts of sucking was seen. Using the miniature Doppler ultrasound flow transducer, Woolridge et al.[113] have studied 32 normal mother-baby pairs from 5 to 9 days postpartum. Intakes during trials averaged 34.2 g (± 3.7 g) on the first breast and 26.2 g (± 3.5 g) on the second breast. At the start of feeds the average suck volume was about 0.14 ml/suck, which decreases to about 0.01 ml/suck or less. The mean latency for release of milk was 2.2 minutes after the infant began to suckle. The researchers also noted that on the first breast the flow increased and stabilized after 2 minutes, with concomitant slowing and stabilizing of sucking pattern over the remainder of the feed. On the second breast, the suck volume fell off dramatically toward the end of the feed (50% reduction from peak to end of feed). (See Fig. 8-15.) These observations support the theory that infants become satiated at the breast and milk remains unconsumed in the breast.[113] Over the first month of life, infants consume a given amount of fluid with decreasing investment of time. The amount of fluid per suck increases over time. The control of intake appears to come under intrinsic control during the first month of life.[84]

When sucking was studied using a multisensor nipple for recording oral variables such as lip and tongue movements and fluid flow, it was observed that fluid flow begins as the intranipple pressure decreases and tapers off as the intranipple pressure increases.[18] One flow pattern is seen in each sucking movement.

The development of the sucking response in the normal newborn with a rubber nipple transducer in a nonnutritive mode has been reported immediately after birth.[6] Pressure exerted immediately was 5 torr at birth, peaking to 103 at 90 minutes. There are no data on optimal pressures or on pressures developed with immediate breastfeeding.

The movement of the lips and tongue have been more difficult to study. A cineradiographic study of breastfeeding was done by Ardran and colleagues in 1957 and compared with a similar study of bottle feeding.[9,10] The nipples and areolas of 41 breastfeeding mothers were coated with a paste of barium sulfate in lanolin, and cineradiographic films were taken with the infant at breast. These were then reviewed meticulously. The authors concluded in their original description as shown in the box, top of p. 175.

In a similar study of bottle feeding by Ardran et al.[9] cineradiographic films were taken of infants, lambs, and kid goats, taking a mixture of milk and barium from a bottle. In the 1950s when Ardran et al.[9] made their landmark studies of bottle feeding, the rubber nipples used were different in size, shape, and consistency, so some of their observations may not pertain to present equipment. They had concluded that gravity was key to the operation and that infants are not able to suck and swallow while taking a breath.

With the development of real-time ultrasound with improved definition of image, several studies have been published using this noninvasive technique to observe the action of the infant's tongue and buccal mucosa and the maternal nipple areola. Using a video-recorder that allowed frame-by-frame analysis and recording simultaneous respiration, the pattern of suck, swallow, and breathing was documented over a period of active suckling at the breast. A suck was defined by Weber et al.[106] as the beginning of one indentation of the nipple by the tongue to the beginning of the next. Weber et al.[106] had examined six breastfed and six bottle fed infants between 1 and 6 days of life. Not all sucks were associated with a swallow. The process is summarized in the boxed material in the middle of p. 175.

The process has been described as a pulsating process similar to peristalsis along the

---

Radiographic interpretation of suckling at the breast

1. The nipple is sucked to the back of the baby's mouth and a teat is formed from the mother's breast.
2. When the jaw is raised this teat is compressed between the upper gum and the tip of the tongue resting on the lower gum. The tongue is applied to the lower surface of the teat from before backwards, pressing it against the hard palate: the teat is reduced to approximately half its former width. As the tongue moves towards the posterior edge of the hard palate the teat shortens and becomes thicker.
3. When the jaw is lowered the teat is again sucked to the back of the mouth and restored to its previous size.
4. Each cycle of jaw and tongue movement takes place in approximately 1.5 seconds. The pharyngeal cavity becomes airless and the larynx closed every time the upward movement of the tongue against the teat and hard palate is completed.
5. The teat is formed from the nipple and the adjacent areola and underlying tissues.

From Ardran GM, Kemp FH, and Lind J: Br J Radiol 31:156, 1958.

Ultrasound interpretation of suckling at the breast

1. The lateral margins of the tongue cup around the nipple, creating a central trough.
2. The suck is initiated by the tip of the tongue against the nipple followed by pressure from the lower gum.
3. There is peristaltic action of the tongue toward the back of the mouth.
4. The tongue elevation continues to move the bolus of milk into the pharynx.

Adapted from Weber F, Woolridge MW, and Baum JD: Dev Med Child Neurol 28:19, 1986.

---

rest of the gastrointestinal tract. This undulating motion as described by cineradiography does not involve stroking or friction, as is clearly pointed out by Woolridge.[112] The nipple should not move in and out of the infant's mouth if the breast is positioned correctly. The tip of the tongue does not move along the nipple. The positive pressure of the tongue against the teat (areola and nipple), coupled with ejection of the milk from increased intraductal pressure, evacuates the milk, not suction. The negative pressure created in the mouth holds the nipple and breast in place and reduces the "work" to refill the ampullae and ducts. Visual observations and videotapes made in our laboratory to study suckling show the undulating motion of the external buccal surfaces even in the newly born. Ultrasound confirms the molding of buccal mucosa and tongue around the teat, leaving no space.

In breastfeeding, the tongue action is a "rolling," or peristaltic, action. In the bottle feeder the tongue action is more piston-like or squeezing. When resting between sucks, the human nipple is indented by the tongue, and the latex teat is expanded in the bottle fed. (See Figs. 8-1 and 8-9.) The change in nipple dimensions during suckling is detailed by Smith et al.,[94,95] who also used ultrasound and examined 16 term infants aged 60 to 120 days and their mothers. They demonstrated that the human nipple is highly elastic and elongates during active feeding including about 2 cm of areola to form a teat approximately twice its resting length. They also showed that the cheeks (bucchal membranes) with their thick layer of fatty tissue, known as sucking fat pads, act to make a passive seal to create a vacuum (as opposed to the concept that the cheeks are sucked in by the negative pressure).

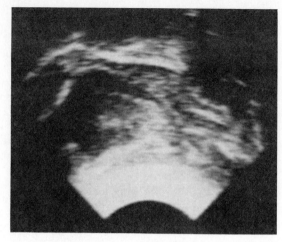

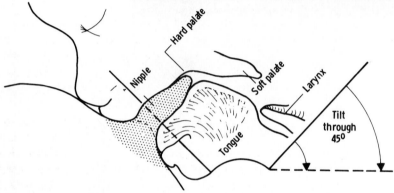

Fig. 8-1. Ultrasound of infant at breast. Still picture of ultrasound scan frame from videorecording. Scanhead is at bottom with a sector view of 90°. Below is artist's impression of image showing key features. Image is seen best when tilted through 45°, so that infant's head is vertical. Picture corresponds to point in sucking cycle when maximum point of compression of nipple by tongue has almost reached tip of nipple. Once nipple has become fully expanded, fresh cycle of compression will be initiated at base of nipple and will then move back. (From Weber F, Woolridge MW, and Baum JD: Dev Med Child Neurol 28:19, 1986.)

Milk ejection was noted to occur after maximal compression of the nipple. Although the firm texture of the latex teat was harder for the infant to compress, Weber et al.[106] did not observe any practical differences in sucking between breast and bottle. Softer latex nipples do not readily reexpand and so do not solve the suckling problem. Ultrasound as a study tool will continue to clarify sucking patterns in neonates and can also be useful as a diagnostic tool in presumed sucking disorders before "suck training or retraining" is considered.

Coordination of suck and swallow

The ability to swallow is developed in utero during the second trimester and has been well demonstrated by fetal ultrasound. Fetal swallowing of amniotic fluid is an important part of the complex regulation of amniotic fluid. The suck is actually part of the oral phase of the swallow. Little was done to examine the role of swallowing on the suckling rate until Burke[20] studied the role of swallowing in the organization of suckling behavior, albeit with a bottle and solutions of 5% and 10% sucrose solution. The author reports two major observations: "First, the frequency of swallowing in newborns increased significantly as a function of increasing concentration and amount of sucrose solution given per criterion suck. Second, there was a significant difference in the duration of the sucking interresponse times which immediately followed the onset of swallowing and the duration of interresponse times not associated with swallowing." Those observations explain those of previous investigators regarding nutritive and nonnutritive sucking.

The coordination of sucking and swallowing was observed by ultrasound by Weber et al.[106] as a movement of the larynx. By 4 days of age, both breast and bottle fed infants were swallowing with every suck. Later in the feeding the ratio of sucks to swallows changed to 2:1 or more until sucking stopped. Swallowing occurred in the end expiratory pause between expiration and inspiration (see Fig. 8-1). The change in suck-swallow ratio seemed to be a function of the availability of milk.

Factors influencing sucking

As one manages infants with difficulty feeding, a number of rituals are often initiated to enhance infant behavior. Only a few of these have been evaluated for their effect. The effect of position of the infant—that is, flat, supine, and supported upright to 90° angle—was found to have no influence on the sucking pattern or pressure.[36] An effect of temperature was found, however. Sucking pressure decreased as environmental temperature increased from 80° F to 90° F, which may have application in encouraging an infant to nurse. This effect was shown to increase from the third to the fifth day of life. Higher sucking pressures have been recorded in the morning than in the afternoon.

When the size of latex nipples was studied, it was observed that the large nipple elicits fewer sucks and a slower sucking rate than smaller nipples, although the volume of milk delivered is the same with all nipple sizes.[26] Although it is not possible to alter human nipple size, this knowledge may help in assessing the response of a newborn in specific situations.

The volume of each swallow was calculated during breastfeeding in 1905 by Süsswein,[96] who counted swallows and made test weighings. His observations have now been confirmed with elaborate electronic equipment.[115] The average swallow of a new newborn is 0.6 ml, which is also the exact amount drawn from a bottle equipped with an electromagnetic flowmeter transducer and a valve that responded to negative pressure at each suck in modern studies, even though the sucking mechanism between breast and bottle is different.[91] When a conventional bottle without a valve is used, the volume is reduced to one third and to 0.19 ml/suck. The valve removed the need for the infant to suck against the negative pressure created in the bottle. This supports the fact that a bottle fed infant with a poor suck does better with a boat-shaped bottle, in which the distal end is kept open, or with a collapsible bag as a source of milk. The size of the hole in the nipple influenced the volume of the suck only in the valved bottle. When breastfed infants were compared with a group fed by cup from birth and a group fed by bottle, the breastfed infants had a stronger suck than either of the other two groups, who did not differ from each other in sucking skill.[29,30]

Patterns of milk intake were studied by electronic weighings in interrupted feeds by Lucas et al.[67] They reported that 50% of a feed from each breast was consumed in 2 minutes, 80% to 90% by 4 minutes, and the last 5 minutes of a feed was minimal from each breast. Bottle fed infants, evaluated with the same technique of test weighings, took 84% of the feeding in the first 4 minutes. Bottle feeding patterns were linear, whereas the breastfed infant had a biphasic pattern when nursed on both breasts. The total intake of the two types of feeds was similar in volume in the same 25 minutes of total time.

Fat content and infant sucking

The high concentration of fat in breast milk toward the end of a feed was hypothesized as a satiety signal to terminate the feeding.[47] When this was studied using high- and low-fat formulas, it was found that high-fat milk did not act to cue babies to slow or stop feeding.[35,81,82] In fact, babies appeared to feed more actively on high-fat milk, sucking in longer bursts with less resting. When human milk of low and high fat content was fed from bottles, switching the baby from low-fat breast milk to high-fat breast milk, the babies did not alter either milk intake rate or sucking patterns. To fully test the hypothesis, a study carefully observed infants switching from the first to the second breast and back to the first breast.[81,82] Infants were 2 months old and well established at exclusive breastfeeding. There was no significant difference in the time taken to attach to the new breast and the time taken to reattach to the previously sucked breast. Mean milk intake from the first breast was 91.7 g (range 58 to 208 g), higher than that from the second breast (mean 52.5 g, range 8 to 75 g). The mean fat contents before and after nursing on the first breast were 23 g/L and 52 g/L, whereas on the second breast they were 24 g/L and 48 g/L. This shows that infants will nurse when fat content is higher, contrary to the theory that increasing fat causes satiation[81] (Fig. 8-15).

Studies of 3-day-old bottle fed infants fed sucrose and glucose solutions show that they manifest tongue movements of greater amplitude when fed stronger concentrations of carbohydrate.[62,109] Sensory apparatus responsible for assessing sweetness is apparently competent in the newborn.

Breathing and sucking during feeding

Breathing and sucking during feeding were addressed by Johnson and Salisbury,[62] who studied normal full-term infants from 1 to 10 days of age, measuring breathing, sucking, and flow of fluid from a feeding bottle with a flowmeter. No infant aspirated water, but 8 of 18 infants inhaled saline. Even from a bottle, breast milk was associated with more regular breathing than was formula feeding. It has been demonstrated in other species that the newborn will become apneic when fed milk from species other than his own. The coordination of breathing and swallowing improves with increase in milk availability and with the maturity of the infant according to Weber.[106]

Sucking patterns as indicators of pathologic conditions

Newborn infants whose mothers received a single dose of 200 mg secobarbital as obstetric sedation during labor sucked at significantly lower rates and pressures and consumed less nutrient than did infants whose mothers received no medication.[62] The effect persisted for 4 days. Similar effects have been seen in Brazelton's examination.[16] It is important for the clinician to be aware of the perinatal history of medication during labor so that early identification of any effect on suckling can be made. The mother of an infant with a poor suck may need some additional stimulus by electric pump to facilitate milk production. The infant may require extra assistance in latching on and in obtaining sufficient nourishment the first few days. Work of Aono and others[8,22,75] suggests that prolactin levels in early lactation are a function of the effectiveness of the sucking stimulus.

The sucking rhythms of infants with a normal perinatal course were compared to those of infants with perinatal distress. The analysis showed that rhythms of nonnutritive sucking were significantly different from rhythms of normal controls even when there were no gross neurologic signs.[65,110]

Perioral stimulation facilitated nutritive sucking abilities in high-risk newborns when analyzed with 29- to 30-week gestation sick newborns with each subject serving as his own control.[68] The stimulation was applied manually with quick touch-pressure stimulus for 1 second over the buccal fat pad. Similar stimulation has been used in children with central nervous system dysfunction in an effort to facilitate better sucking and swallowing. Such studies have not been reported during breastfeeding.[39]

Sucking stimulus and prolactin

When lactating postpartum women nurse their infants, the prolactin level increases from a high baseline level to levels several times mean baseline. When nursing women played with but did not feed their infants, prolactin did not rise despite the initiation of a let-down. Substitution of a breast pump at regular intervals caused prolactin elevations similar in timing and magnitude to those induced by sucking. When normal, menstruating, nonlactating adult women were stimulated with the breast pump for 30 minutes, there were significant prolactin increases in 7 of the 18 women. No response was obtained in normal men (see Fig. 8-14).

When the prolactin response was used as a measure of "success" in establishing lactation in the first week postpartum, there was no difference in prolactin levels between women who had been considered good producers and those who were considered poor feeders.[56] Mothers whose infants were in the special care unit and who were using a breast pump to establish lactation had minimal prolactin response to pumping but produced a mean of 86 g of milk per pumping. A similar study had been carried out previously, in which different responses to suckling were found in prolactin levels in good, fair, and poor producers.[55] When prolactin levels were measured following use of the breast pump at uniform settings, all three groups were similar.[8] This suggests that infant suckling plays a significant role in adequate milk production.

Conclusions

Knowledge about infant suckling has been accumulating rapidly, but little of it involves study of suckling at the breast. It has been established that the patterns are different mechanically. At the breast, nutritive and nonnutritive suckling vary only in rate, not in pattern. Infants can suck immediately at birth and tolerate mother's milk (colostrum) best as the pattern of respirations remains physiologic. Inadequate suckling can influence maternal production, but inadequate suckling can be improved.

Management of breastfeeding is best discussed in terms of the three stages: (1) the prenatal period, (2) the immediate postpartum, or hospital, management, and (3) the postnatal, or post hospital, period.

PRENATAL PERIOD

It is most effective to prepare for breastfeeding well in advance of delivery. Prospective parents should consider feeding plans for the infant during the prenatal period, after the pregnancy is well established. Once quickening has occurred, the infant becomes more of a reality for the mother and she can relate to planning. Except in sophisticated cultures, the parents will not initiate this decision-making discussion, and it is appropriately introduced by the obstetrician in the second trimester. Particularly with first children, it is appropriate to suggest to the parents that they select a pediatrician early. They should request a prenatal conference with the pediatrician to discuss not only feeding but also points of management and child rearing about which they might have questions. If the mother is receiving prenatal care from a family practice physician, this step is automatic.

Many studies of infant feeding choices have been reported in the literature reviewing the reasons women breastfeed. Universally, mothers do it because it is best for the infant. Many decided long before the pregnancy, but those who chose bottle feeding admit they could have been persuaded if only someone had cared enough to tell them how important breastfeeding is to the infant. All women know mother's milk is best. Clearly, health care providers have made breastfeeding too complicated and burdened mothers with so many rules and regulations that they cannot cope and default to bottle feeding. When health care workers try to persuade a woman to breastfeed, they perpetuate the image of an impossible feat by saying, "Why not give it a try? It's not that bad," or "You'll be surprised. It isn't that hard," instead of conveying opportunity and good experience with, "It is a marvelous opportunity for you and your baby," or "It will be a special joy." Employment rarely cuts breastfeeding opportunities short, as it is usually unemployed women who are at home bottle feeding. (See Chapter 13.) Any time spent breastfeeding is worthwhile for the working mother.

The medical profession has been hesitant to take anything but a neutral position in such discussions for fear of pressuring the mother. The evidence is stronger than ever that there are distinct advantages to the infant and mother in breastfeeding. Parents have the right to hear the data. They can make their own choice. Fear of instilling guilt is a poor reason to deprive a mother of an informed choice.

The prenatal discussion should also include any questions the parents may have about the lactation process and mother's ability to provide adequately for the infant. An examination of the breasts is part of good prenatal care and an excellent opportunity to discuss breastfeeding. If there are any anatomic abnormalities, they should be discussed. The breast tissue should be checked for lumps and cysts that might need treatment. The size of the mass of mammary tissue is not correlated with the ability to produce milk. The more generous gland is usually due to a more geneous fat pad. During pregnancy the fat is replaced by proliferating acini. A woman with small breasts should not be discouraged from nursing; she may be the mother who most needs to prove herself.

Breast texture should be assessed by palpation. The inelastic breast gives the impression it is firmly knit together and the overlying skin is taut and firm so it cannot be picked up. The elastic breast is looser and the overlying skin free, and the tissue is more easily picked up. Inelastic breasts are more prone to engorgement and seem improved by prepartum massaging and close attention to prevention of engorgement (Fig. 8-2).

Examination of the areola and nipple is equally important to identify any anatomic problems that may need some preparation before delivery. Gross malformations and inversion of the nipple will be easily detected, but lesser problems may go unnoticed. One must test for freedom of protusion. When the areola is squeezed and it retracts, it indicates a "tied nipple" or inverted nipple caused by the persistence of the original invagination of the mammary dimple (Fig. 8-3).

The physician may provide literature on breastfeeding or suggest reading sources for the patient. One should avoid dismissing the parents' questions by merely suggesting appropriate readings, since their decision making will be enhanced by open discussion

A   B

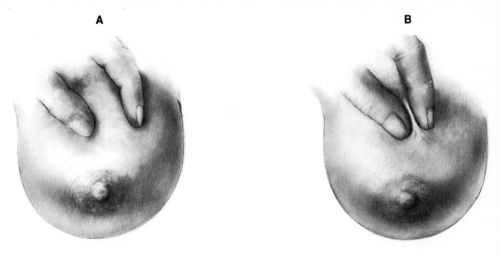

Fig. 8-2. Texture of breast tissue can be assessed by picking up skin of breast. **A,** Inelastic breast tissue; **B,** elastic breast tissue.

A   B

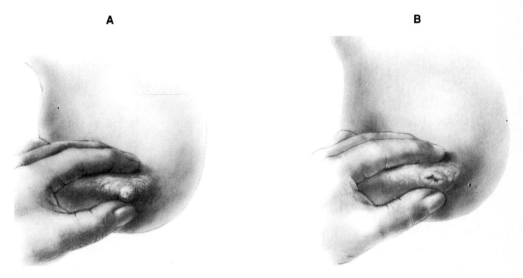

Fig. 8-3. A, Normal nipple everts with gentle pressure. **B,** Inverted or tied nipple inverts with gentle pressure.

with a knowledgeable professional. Although parents may have access to childbirth preparation programs in the community, the parents should not be put off to seek all their information from such sources. When parents have no opportunity to discuss with their care provider such issues as early infant contact, nursing the infant in the delivery room, and family-centered maternity care, they often experience tremendous disappointment and misunderstanding. Although the most vocal groups on the subject of childbirth and the family in our society today lump all these options, including breastfeeding, together as a package, many mothers want to breastfeed but do not wish to have rooming-in, for instance.

Therefore, all patients should be provided with adequate information to make a choice in each matter separately.

The concerns most frequently expressed by mothers considering breastfeeding are related to the mother, not the infant. Mothers who are more concerned about their own well-being have more trouble adjusting to motherhood and should be provided with more support in adapting to the role. They may be helped by selecting a doula to support them, since our modern culture tends to isolate the young couple. Raphael[87] describes a doula as one of "those individuals who surround, interact with, and aid the mother at any time within the perinatal period, which includes pregnancy, birth and lactation."

Concerns most frequently expressed prenatally include the following:

1. What is the effect on the figure? Data indicate that the breast is affected by heredity, age, and pregnancy in that order and only minimally by lactation. Women who have never borne children may "lose their figures" long before a grand multipara who nurses her infants. Pregnancy enlarges breasts temporarily, as does early lactation, but the effect is temporary. Poor diet and lack of exercise will destroy a figure in both male and female long before any other influence.

2. What is the effect on the mother's freedom? Obviously, only a mother can breast-feed the infant; however, ample data support the fact that it is possible to maintain a career, keep a job, or just get away from the house and still nurse one's infant in today's world. Actually, mothers in primitive cultures have returned to the fields or some form of productivity outside the home out of sheer necessity for generations. Mothers concerned about this often are best reassured by their peers, that is, mothers who are nursing. In communities with nursing mother groups, it is a simple referral. Employment statistics have revealed that women do successfully return to the work force and continue breastfeeding. Employment is rarely a reason for not breastfeeding. In most communities the blue-collar mother is unemployed and bottle feeding.

3. Many women are concerned with exposing the breasts. Despite the constant barrage of publicity about the breast in the modern press, many women are embarrassed to consider baring their breasts. As pointed out in Chapter 5, shame is an important consideration when helping a mother accept breastfeeding. Bentovim[13] suggests that shame and anxieties arise from the influence of one's life history and current events; thus, intervention is necessary at many levels. Clothes that make discreet breastfeeding possible are readily available and fashionable. Considerable body exposure is not necessary for breastfeeding. In a public survey performed in the Midwest in 1985, few people, male or female, in any age group considered breastfeeding embarrassing, and 82% would want their child breastfed.

Preparation of the breasts

The prenatal period is a time for the couple to prepare for their new role as parents and to learn as much as possible about breastfeeding. Most mothers do no special preparation and are very successful. Carefully controlled studies do not support the contention that fair-skinned women, especially redheads, are more prone to developing cracked, sore nipples than are others. Mothers who have had trouble with tender, cracked nipples when nursing a previous infant will need extra assistance in putting the infant to breast properly in the first few days, but elaborate rituals prenatally rarely make a difference. Nipple preparation has a negative effect on some women who are not ready to handle their breasts so aggressively as required for "nipple exercises."

Bathing should be as usual, with minimal or no soap directly on the nipples and thorough rinsing. Patting the nipple dry with a soft towel is recommended by some, but this should not be done except following a shower or bath. Persistent removal of natural oils of the nipple and areola actually predisposes the skin to irritation. Montgomery glands in the areola secrete a sebaceous material for the cleansing and lubrication of the areola and nipple. This should not be removed by soaps or chemicals. Tincture of benzoin, alcohol, and other drying agents are contraindicated because they predispose the nipples to cracking during early lactation. Wearing protective brassieres, modern women do not get the friction to the nipples that looser clothing provides, which may be why cracked nipples are a common problem. In Scandinavia, it is suggested that the pregnant women get as much air and sunshine as possible directly on the breasts before delivery. In countries where this is not possible, a cautiously used sunlamp or hair dryer can provide the same effect. Wearing a nursing brassiere with the flaps down to expose the nipples under loose clothing will serve the same purpose. In any case, aggressive and abrasive treatment of the nipples does not prevent nipple pain postpartum and may actually enhance it. Gentle love making involving the breasts is usually safe and is the most effective preparation.[52]

The use of hydrous lanolin, which is miscible with water and thus allows normal evaporation from the skin, does no apparent harm but in controlled studies also made no difference. Women allergic to wool will also be allergic to lanolin. Lanolin has been confirmed to contain insecticide residuals such as DDT and dioxins because sheep are routinely dipped in insecticides before shearing. Lanolin should not be routinely used, according to the FDA. Use of A and D ointment prophylactically made no difference, having an effect only in the treatment of fissures later. Mothers disliked the odor of this ointment as well. Petrolatum and other ointments made the skin more macerated and susceptible to irritation. Ointment should not be applied over the end of the nipple and the ducts.[90]

Soap, alcohol, and tincture of benzoin have been shown to cause damage to tissue of areola and nipple.[75]

Gentle traction to the point of discomfort, but not pain, has been shown by some to improve perception of pain in the first week of lactation.[19] A study carefully controlled to eliminate subjective discrepancies of interpretation revealed no significant difference in nipple sensitivity or trauma in those who practiced prenatal nipple rolling, application of breast cream, or expression of colostrum, as compared with those who had untreated breasts.[52] There was no increased pain or trauma among the fair-skinned participants in this study, treated or untreated. Since many women are not inclined to manipulate their breasts before delivery and might be discouraged from breastfeeding if it is implied that this must be done, physicians should prescribe treatment only when there is an indication for it.[111] The physician should specifically inform the patient about protecting the nipple from soaps, ointments, tinctures, and excessive manipulation, since there has never been evidence to suggest it is safe, much less beneficial.

Preparation of the nipples

Flat nipples or inverted nipples do not preclude breastfeeding, but it is important to prescribe some form of treatment before delivery rather than wait until the infant is frustrated and the breast engorged. Flat nipples respond to the same passive treatment with a breast shell that works for inverted nipples. The shells can be worn during the last trimester.

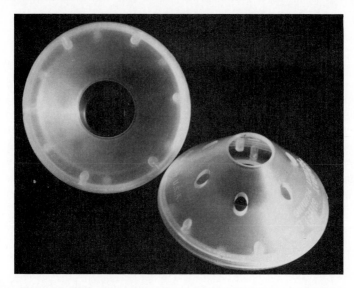

Fig. 8-4. Breast shells: vented domes worn over ring that allows nipple to evert. Shell is slipped into cup of well-fitting brassiere. Available in several styles and designs.

Inverted nipples (Fig. 8-3) can be diagnosed by pressing the areola between the thumb and the forefinger. A flat or normal nipple will protrude; a truly inverted nipple will retract. True inverted nipples are actually rare. Inverted nipples can be treated with a nipple shell (Fig. 8-4 and 8-5) available at pharmacies or breastfeeding supply stores in several shapes and designs. The inner ring fits over the areola, and the nipple can protrude through the hole in the center. A dome is placed over the ring and worn within a well-fitting brassiere, taking up additional space. Constant, gentle pressure around the nipple causes it to evert. The shells are usually worn during the last trimester, and nipples are usually well everted by delivery. Small air vents in the plastic dome admit air to the skin and avoid maceration. They can be used between feedings postpartum also.

Exercises for the nipple

Exercises to evert the nipples are rarely successful and may be dangerous. The obstetrical literature abounds with articles about the use of nipple stimulation in place of the traditional oxytocin challenge test; only a few are quoted here.[7,9,16,19,25,73] Using the breast pump or manual expression to produce colostrum is reported in the literature to induce labor or increase the strength of contractions in desultory labor. A case of severe abruptio placentae following nipple stimulation is reported by Taylor and Green.[98] A series of patients induced labor with self-manipulation of the breasts with a 45% success rate. All patients in the series showed some ripening of the cervix with dilation and effacement over a 3-day period of breast stimulation. A relatively high incidence (45.5%) of exaggerated uterine activity in response to a breast-stimulation stress test, usually within 7 minutes of initiation of stimulation, was reported by Lipitz et al.[66] and others.[19,37,98] Although all the cases and series cannot be reported here, it is clear that nipple stimulation in the third trimester can initiate uterine contractions and, in some, labor. Under the direction of an obstetrician, breast stimulation can be used effectively therapeutically, but it should not be recommended without obstetrical evaluation when safer, more effective methods (breast

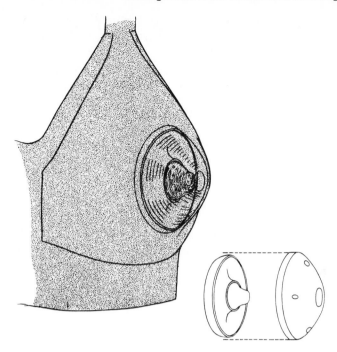

Fig. 8-5.   Nipple shield in place inside brassiere to evert nipple.

shells) are available. Suggesting stretching (Hoffman) exercises is unwise, especially in women with a tendency to early labor. No study since Hoffman's initial report of two cases has shown the process to be effective. Stretching the areola forcefully can damage the delicate Montgomery glands. Prepartum mastitis has also occurred with prenatal expression of colostrum. Whether manipulating the breast prenatally provides the mother with greater comfort in breastfeeding has not been demonstrated. Mothers who choose to bottle feed have told us that having to "exercise" their breasts is one of the "rules" that kept them from breastfeeding.

The Hoffman exercises[54] involve placing the thumbs or forefingers opposite each other close to the base of the nipple and slowly pushing away from the areola. Done in a vertical line and then a horizontal line in the form of an imaginary cross, this is intended to stretch and break the fibers that "tie" the inverted nipple. Nipple rolling is another technique of nipple stimulus or "preparation" that involves grasping nipple with thumb and forefinger while supporting the breast with the other three fingers. The nipple is drawn out to the point of discomfort and released. The exercise is repeated 10 to 20 times several times a day.[75]

Surgical correction of permanently inverted nipples

Inverted nipples have been known to medicine for centuries, and treatment has long been described to include various exercises or the use of older vigorous infants to suckle and the use of adults who hired out for this purpose in difficult cases. The first surgical procedure was described in 1873. Other techniques have since been advanced.[48,88,93] A primary indication of the inverted nipple has been the chronic occurrence of central pockets of inflammation of the nipple, leading to spread of infection and suppurative mastitis. A simple method for correction without division of the lactiferous ducts involves using a purse-string suture and traction of holding sutures. The procedure can be done in the office under local anesthesia, accoding to Hauben.[48] A truly inverted nipple may have fewer ducts. The microscopic pathology of severely inverted nipples indicates the ducts are abnormal.[48,88,93]

Hand expression

Some breastfeeding instructions suggest hand expressing the breast to produce a few drops of colostrum every day for the last few weeks of pregnancy. Fortunately, the instructions usually suggest the patient consult her physician first. Manual or any kind of pumping of the breasts may, indeed, stimulate the uterus to contract. It has no particular benefit and means that the early sequestered cells are expressed away in the drops of colostrum before delivery and are lost to the infant. Occasionally, prepartum mastitis has developed from this treatment. The risks far outweigh any seeming benefit.

Summary

Following is a summary of prenatal preparation:
1. During the first trimester, make the initial breast examination. Suggest considering how the infant is to be fed. If anatomic variations may interfere with lactation, mention them and discuss possible remedies.
2. At each prenatal visit offer information about breastfeeding, which is part of preparations for birthing center, rooming-in, and discharge plans.
3. Investigate mother's knowledge of breastfeeding and document her information base to fill in the gaps and correct misinformation. Also inquire about any treatments or routines she has initiated on her own so that the total management is appropriate.
4. Once quickening has been experienced, the parents are ready to plan more concretely about the baby. Suggest a visit with the pediatrician.
5. As delivery approaches, initiate discussion about feeding immediately after birth, feeding protocols, and the mother's special needs or requests.
6. Be familiar with community resources so that patients can be wisely referred for peer support or assistance unavailable from office staff.

IMMEDIATE POSTPARTUM, OR HOSPITAL, PERIOD

Immediately after the placenta has separated, the establishment of lactation begins. This is a critical period because many mothers who do not receive the proper support in the hospital are driven to failure by inept management.

Nursing in the delivery room

The mother will probably want to nurse her infant immediately after birth, if she has read the current literature. If she does not ask, the obstetrician should suggest it and the delivery room staff facilitate it.

Disease-oriented physicians who have been trained to give trials of water first, hours after delivery, are always concerned that the infant may aspirate. Clinical signs of potential for aspiration include low Apgar score, increased secretions, and polyhydramnios. Actually, all infants born elsewhere in the world go straight to the breast on delivery, which has a physiologic effect on the uterus, causing it to contract. Because sugar water and cow's milk formulas are very irritating if aspirated, delay in feeding has been the rule in the United States, where most infants are bottle fed. Colostrum is not irritating, however, and is readily absorbed by the respiratory tree if aspirated. There are a few contraindications to immediate nursing: (1) a heavily medicated mother, (2) an infant with a 5-minute Apgar score under 6, or (3) a premature infant under 36 weeks of gestation. The concern for the infant with a tracheoesophageal (TE) fistula is important, but a few precautions should suffice. If there is hydramnios or excess secretions at birth, a tube should be passed to the stomach to make sure the esophagus is patent. If all is well, the infant may nurse. If there is the TE fistula, it is a surgical emergency. Choanal atresia is another anomaly that would be of concern, but an infant cannot suck on the breast or anything if he cannot breathe through his nose. Usually an infant with choanal atresia has a low Apgar score or needs some assistance in establishing respirations.

For this first breastfeeding, it may be best to have the mother on a stretcher or a bed wide enough to have the infant lie beside her. Some newer delivery tables are wide enough. The infant should not be dangled in midair over the breast. The mother should be assisted to turn onto her side and the infant presented to the breast, with the ventral surface to the ventral surface of the mother. The infant should not have to turn his head toward the breast. The mother may need assistance in holding her breast so as to present the nipple squarely into the infant's mouth, which is stimulated to open by stroking the lips with the nipple.

Both mother and infant will do better if there is an atmosphere of tranquility in the room. The only other risk to the infant is thermal stress. If the room is air-conditioned, it may be necessary to provide a radiant warmer over the infant, especially if the infant is naked for skin-to-skin contact. Some mothers have shaking chills following the strenuous event of labor and cannot provide adequate warmth for the infant without some external source of heat.

Chilling an infant may set off a chain of events from hypothermia to hypoglycemia to tachypnea to mild acidosis to the extent of requiring a septic workup. Hypothermia therefore is more easily prevented than treated.

If possible, mother, father, and infant should remain together for the next hour or so. The first hour for the infant is usually one of quiet alertness, a state that will usually recur only briefly for the next few days. It is important to delay the instillation of prophylactic eye drops until after this time spent with the mother. If the drops are put into the eyes, blepharospasm will prevent the infant from opening his eyes and mar the eye-to-eye contact. Only if there is a known risk of gonorrhea should the drops be put in immediately. If the mother has delivered in a birthing center, early contact and nursing should be part of the routine.

Two natural hand positions for the mother are used most commonly. With attention to a few details, either position works (one is not right and the other wrong). The scissor grasp is the placement of the thumb and index finger above the areola and the other three fingers below the breast for support, thus allowing some compression of the areola. Care should be taken that the hand is not in the way of the infant's getting sufficient areola into the mouth (see Fig. 8-6). This grip has been used for centuries and was shown in sketches and paintings even before the Christian era. If the hand is large or the breast small, it may not work as well as the palmar grasp. The *palmar grasp* is the placement of all the fingers under the breast and only the thumb above. This gives firm support to the breast. It permits

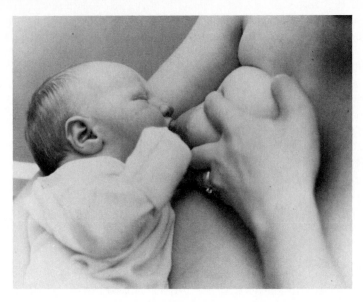

Fig. 8-6. Scissor grasp, presenting breast while supporting infant.

directing the breast squarely into the infant's mouth and avoids the need to press the breast away from the infant's nose. The palmar grasp is similar to the prehensile grasp of the apes when they nurse their young, and it has been found especially helpful when there is nipple pain, soreness, or trauma. It is also useful when mother's hand is too small for a large breast (Fig. 8-7).

Days in the hospital

The physician should see that patients are permitted to have their infants with them as much as they wish, within the guidelines of reasonable medical care. Only the few patients with difficult deliveries, cesarean sections with medication, postpartum complications, or eclampsia need to be excluded, but the physician should make that judgment. An experienced nursing staff is critical to the management of the nursing mother at this point.[77] Advice should be reasonable and consistent, and nurses should be cautioned against interjecting their own personal opinion or experience, as too many individuals are involved in postpartum care and mothers are easily overwhelmed with information.

Key points in management should include the following:
1. Help the mother find a comfortable position. There should be no rules about sitting up or lying down.
2. Help the infant to the breast. The infant should be held so that the ventral surface of the infant faces the mother.
3. Help the mother hold her breast for her baby, choosing the better grasp for the situation.
4. Help the mother reposition the infant on the second breast, since moving may be hard at first.
5. If the infant falls asleep after the first breast, the mother should be shown how to break the suction with her fingers. Nonnutritive suckling while asleep is es-

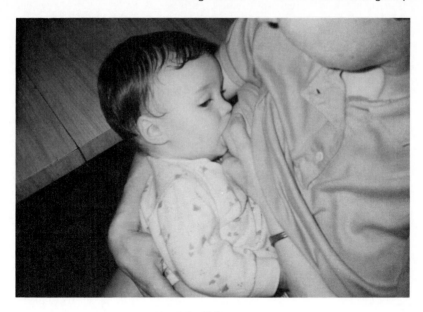

Fig. 8-7. Palmar grasp.

pecially irritating to the nipple in the first few days. Wait a little, wake the baby, and then move him to the second side.

6. When waking an infant, unwrapping the blanket and using gentle stimulus are appropriate. Jackknifing is never appropriate and may cause regurgitation, aspiration, or trauma to vital organs.

7. Allow the infant to nurse about 5 minutes per side at first. This will usually assure that the infant takes both sides and will help the breasts adapt gradually. Timing should be casual and not with stopwatch rigidity. It takes 2 to 3 minutes for the let-down reflex to be effective in early lactation. Frequent small feedings will provide good stimulation to the breast without stressing the mother. The milk supply is best stimulated by suckling. The policy of the nursery should be to have all breastfed infants taken to their mothers when they awaken during the night,[69] if they have not roomed-in.

If the physician believes that until the milk is in, the 2 AM feeding can be replaced by water in the nursery if the infant wakes up so that the mother gets a full night's sleep, there should be a written order. A mother should be given the infant if she requests to have him. On the other hand, modern hospitals are a hubbub of activity, and with liberalized visiting hours there is no time for the mother to rest unless naps are scheduled. In the early days of the Rooming-In Unit at the Yale–New Haven Hospital, Jackson[12] insisted that all postpartum mothers have a nap after lunch. Every day the shades were drawn and traffic decreased on the unit for an hour. This is part of mothering the mother. In primitive cultures, mothers are groomed, fed, and protected after delivery, often for weeks. Furthermore, adequate rest is essential to successful lactation. In 1953 Jackson, with her colleagues Barnes et al.,[12] prepared a classic description of the management of breastfeeding that remains the single most valuable source of information.

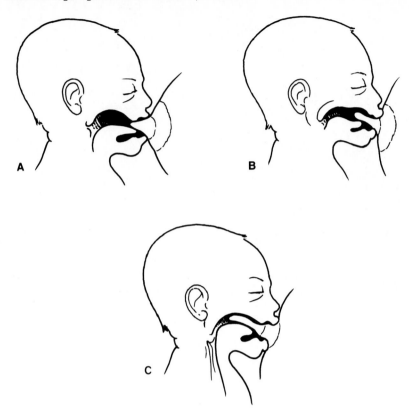

Fig. 8-8. A, As infant grasps breast, tongue moves forward to draw nipple in. **B,** Nipple and areola move toward palate as glottis still permits breathing. **C,** Tongue moves along nipple, pressing it against hard palate and creating pressure. Ductules under areola are milked and flow begins as a result of peristaltic movement of tongue. Glottis closes. Swallow follows.

Diagnosing problems with breastfeeding

To solve the problem of unsuccessful nursing, observe the mother feeding the infant. Often the problem is a simple one such as a mother so uncomfortable and tense that the let-down reflex will not trigger or perhaps an infant with a poor suck. In these cases and others the diagnosis will be made most easily by direct observation.

Understanding the mechanism of suckling in the neonate, however, is essential to recognize ineffective sucking on the part of the infant (Fig. 8-8). As the breast is offered to the infant, the lips gently clamp the areola to hold it in place as the tongue thrusts forward to grasp the nipple and areola. In a rhythmic motion, the tongue moves up against the hard palate, drawing the nipple and areola into the mouth, creating an elongated teat. The cheeks fill the mouth because of the sucking fat pads and provide further negative pressure. The tongue undulates along the teat, compressing the collecting ductules in the areola and "milking" them toward the nipple. Milk flows from the nipple and is swallowed as a response of the swallowing reflex. If the infant has a fluttering tongue that is discoordinate, it may not be as productive in stimulating ejection. If the infant cannot coordinate suck and swallow, choking occurs. Sometimes if ejection is strong, the first rush

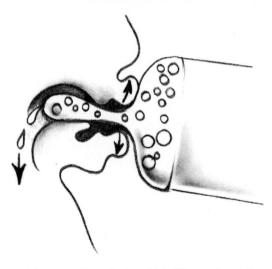

Fig. 8-9. Infant suckling on rubber nipple, which fills mouth and thus prevents tongue action and provides flow without tongue movement. Flow occurs even if lips not tight around rubber hub.

of milk will cause choking. Stopping and starting again should solve the problem. If the mother's milk flows abundantly with first let-down, she may need to manually express (and save) the first few milliliters to avoid choking the infant. Usually the flow moderates quickly. This problem is only temporary or limited to times when the infant has not been nursed for an unusually long interval.

If the infant's jaw is slightly receding, the nipple may not stay in place. Gentle support at the angle of the jaw will help.

An infant who is given a bottle or rubber nipple to suck can become confused because the milking action is different (Fig. 8-9). The relatively inflexible rubber nipple may keep the tongue from its usual rhythmic action. In addition, the flow may be so rapid, even without sucking, that the infant learns to put the tongue against the rubber nipple to slow down the flow. Some infants who have been breastfed gag when the relatively large rubber nipple is put in their mouths. When an infant uses the same tongue action he has needed for a rubber nipple at the breast, he may even push the human nipple out of the mouth. When he cannot grasp an engorged areola properly, he will clamp down on the nipple with his jaws, causing pain in the nipple and disrupting the ejection reflex. Manual expression of a little milk will soften the areola.

When observing an infant being breastfed, take note of the following:
1. Position of mother, her body language and tension.
2. Position of infant—his ventral surface should be to mother's ventral surface, lower arm, if not swaddled, around mother's thorax; infant cannot swallow if head has to turn to breast, and grasp of areola will be poor.
3. Position of mother's hand on breast (not in way of proper grasp by infant).
4. Position of infant's lips on areola about 1 to 1½ inches from base of nipple.
5. Lower lip should not be folded in so infant sucks lip.

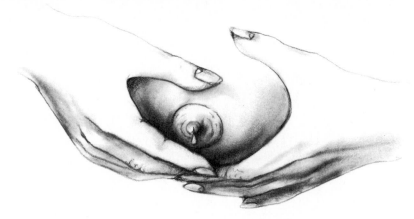

Fig. 8-10. Position for manual expression of breast. Thumbs are brought toward areola, compressing areola between thumb and supporting fingers. With areola grasped, pressure is applied toward chest wall, and then pressure is released. This compression and pressure stimulate milking action (also see Appendix H).

Engorgement

The best management of engorgement is prevention. The degree of engorgement lessens with each infant because the time at which the milk comes in seems to shorten in multiparas. The primipara suffers most from engorgement. Engorgement involves two elements: one, congestion and increased vascularity, is physiologic; the second is accumulation of milk. Engorgement may involve only the areola, only the body of the breast (so-called peripheral engorgement), or both. Some engorgement is normal. No response of breast with "fullness" is abnormal.

Areolar engorgement. When the areola is engorged, it obliterates the nipple and makes properly grasping the areola impossible for the infant. If he sucks only the nipple, it is exquisitely painful, since that is the only area of the breast where there are pain fibers. In addition, the collecting ductules are not "milked" and therefore do not empty, and the infant is frustrated by lack of milk.

The treatment is directed toward reducing the engorgement so that the infant can nurse effectively, which will further reduce the overdistended ducts. Gentle manual expression by the mother herself will usually produce a small amount of flow and soften the areola. The presence of milk on the nipple will further encourage the infant's sucking. Warm soaks just before a feeding may facilitate manual expression. A mother should be taught how to manually express (Fig. 8-10). Placing the thumb and forefinger at the margins of the areola and pressing back in toward the chest and then bringing the fingers together, rhythmically simulating the action of the infant's jaw, will start the flow and soften the tense tissue (see Appendix H). When the infant is put to the breast, the mother should compress the areola between two fingers to make it easier for the infant to grasp. Offering the breast this way makes it easier for any infant to grasp, especially when he needs encouragement to nurse (Fig. 8-11).

Peripheral engorgement. Initially, the breasts increase in vascularity and begin to swell. This usually starts in the second 24-hour period after delivery. Initially, engorgement is vascular; thus pumping mechanically briefly to stimulate the breast when the infant is

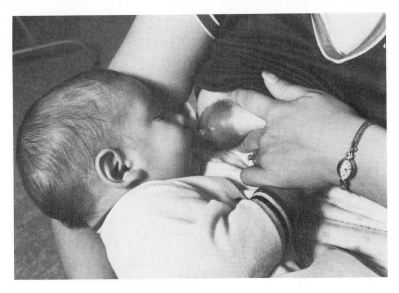

Fig. 8-11. When breast is offered to infant, areola is gently compressed between two fingers and breast supported to assure that infant is able to grasp areola adequately.

not nursing adequately is appropriate. Pumping "to relieve engorgement" will yield little milk and may traumatize the breast that is hypervascular.

The mother should be advised to wear a well-fitting but adjustable nursing brassiere that does not have thin straps or permanent plastic lining. She should wear it 24 hours a day. With moderately severe engorgement, the breasts become full, hard, and tender. The swelling starts at the clavicle and goes to the lower rib cage and from the midaxillary line to the midsternum. The breasts may even become hard, tense, and warm. The mother complains of throbbing and aching pain and can find no comfortable position except to lie flat on her back and very still.

Management is centered on making the mother comfortable so that she can continue to nurse and stimulate milk production as well as nourish the infant. Proper support to elevate the breasts is important. The axilla are particularly painful, probably as a result of the tension on Cooper's ligament. Cold packs may help initially to reduce vascularity. Warm packs may help some patients. Having the mother stand in a warm shower and manually express some milk at the same time may be the best preparation to feed the infant. Some find comfort in alternating hot and cold water. Aspirin may give the mother some relief and should not bother the infant. An aspirin-codeine preparation has been recommended as well. It may be necessary to provide the mother with some sleep medication. Medications should be timed so that the least amount possible reaches mother's milk and the baby. If medication is taken immediately before nursing, the pain will be relieved, but the drug will not reach the milk for more than ½ hour in the case of aspirin, acetaminophen, codeine, or short-acting barbiturates.

It is important to maintain drainage during this period of engorgement to prevent back pressure in the ducts from developing and eventually depressing milk production. Intraductal pressure can lead eventually to atrophy of both the secreting and myoepithelial cells and a diminishing milk supply. The best treatment is frequent breastfeeding around the clock because suckling by the infant is the most effective mechanism for removal of milk. Relief is based on establishment of flow. The infant may have trouble grasping or not be interested in nursing frequently in the first few days, so manual expression may also be necessary. Every mother should be taught this technique by the perinatal nursing staff.[90]

The mother should support the breast with her fingers and place her thumbs distally and massage gently toward the areola, rotating gradually around the breast to include all quadrants. Then, once the peripheral lobules have been softened, areolar expression as previously described should be used to encourage complete emptying of the collecting ducts in the areola. This is a procedure best done by the mother, but it may take a skilled and experienced nurse to teach this technique. Further description of manual expression of milk is illustrated in Appendix H. In cases of engorgement it may be helpful to use an electric pump, which is very effective because of its gentle milking action (see Chapter 19).

Hand pumps can be used but exert only negative pressure on the areola. Unless accompanied by manual expression of the distal segments, they are only temporizing.

Currently maternity patients are going home in 2 to 3 days or sooner, which is certainly before lactation is well established, but it may also be before engorgement is full-blown. At the time when maternity floors were run so rigidly that ad lib breastfeeding was an impossible feat, it was often suggested that a mother go home and get away from the negative hospital atmosphere to a place where she could relax and concentrate on feeding the infant and resting. This is a point at which the doula, so well described by Raphael,[87] could make the difference between success and failure. It may be appropriate for the obstetrician to order the mother to have some assistance at home, whether it is her husband, her mother, or a friend. "The common denominator for success in breastfeeding is the assurance of some degree of help from some specific person for a definite period of time after childbirth," according to Raphael.[87] She studied mothers in the cycle of anxiety while she became the doula for the individuals she studied at about 6 to 10 days postpartum. The calm that can be experienced in the presence of a confident, caring person will relax the mother. The infant senses the calm and confidence and sleeps. When he feeds again, he nurses well. Breaking the cycle of panic that seizes a new mother when she finds herself home alone with a new infant who needs frequent feeding requires an ability to instill confidence.

Although the physician cannot be the doula, he can be sure that the family understands the need and can suggest community resources if no personal ones are available. Successful breastfeeding is not automatic, as is demonstrated by the failure rate. Some problems have been generated by the disturbance of the synchronization of interaction between mother and infant by rigid hospital protocol. This is continued at home when feeding is by the clock rather than by instinct. A program developed in the Rochester community for early discharge called Perinatal Homecare, where nursing, laboratory, and homemaker services are provided under insurance coverage, has proved especially conducive to successful breastfeeding.[4]

Nipples

Painful nipples. Presumably the nipples will adapt to the nursing experience naturally; however, often there are discomforts. It is common for the initial grasp of the nipple and first suckles to cause discomfort in the first few days of lactation. It is not cause for alarm, but it requires reassurance. The sensation is created by the negative pressure on the ductules, which are not yet filled with milk. Later, when lactation is well established and the let-down reflex is experienced, mothers will describe a turgescence, which is the increased fluid pressure being relieved by suckling. If the pain persists throughout the nursing, the situation demands attention.

Nipple pain was studied in 102 women in the first 96 hours postpartum, and engorgement was most closely associated with nipple discomfort, which may be enhanced by the general discomfort of the breast. Prenatal breast preparation was unrelated to soreness. Length of time spent suckling was also unrelated.[69] No record was kept on nonnutritive suckling, although others have found suckling without swallowing to be more stressful early in lactation. How the breast is presented to the infant is the most critical factor[40] (maternal hand position and infant squarely facing breast). This is the time to observe the feeding, looking for malpositioning or other abnormalities.

The most common cause of painful nipples in the first few days is positioning, and this should be reviewed in detail, being certain the areola is softened sufficiently to have the infant grasp adequately. Check infant's lower lip to be sure it is flanged around the breast and not drawn into the mouth, which can abrade the nipple.

If no abnormality is found, the pain may be due to a "barracuda baby" with a vigorous suck. The breast will gradually adapt to it, and it will not last indefinitely. Sometimes the maternal tissues are unusually tender and delicate. Dry heat may help between feedings. The mother should remove the waterproofing from her brassiere and expose her breasts to air or an electric lamp with a 60-watt bulb for 20 minutes four times per day. A lamp similar to the perineal lamp can be used in the hospital.

Even more effective is the use of an electric hair dryer, set on warm and fanned across the breast about 6 to 8 inches away. This brings remarkable comfort and can be done sitting, standing, or lying down. Many patients bring hair dryers to the hospital with them. The breast will be moist with milk right after a feeding. This should not be wiped away but allowed to dry. Many cultures treat irritation of the skin with human milk. The drying effect of the treatment will help counteract the increase in moisture experienced in the first days of lactation.

Stabbing pain that radiates through the breast so that mother feels the ducts are liquid fire is associated with candida infection of the breasts, usually seen after antibiotic treatment when the infant has thrush, and deserves special attention. It is discussed under mastitis.

Ointments. The routine application of ointments to the nipple, areola, or breast should be discouraged. Except in unusual cases of extremely dry skin, the tissue does not need to be oiled. Lanolin is most hazardous to anyone with a wool allergy. Some ointments and creams have irritants.[50] The sebaceous and Montgomery glands of the areola and nipple are easily plugged by repeated applications of oily substances. Preparations with vitamins A and D are innocuous but unnecessary; those with vitamin E or hormones are unsafe unless prescribed for a specific problem. Any irritation or rash should first be treated by discontinuing any ointments or other self-medicating material. This is the first step in the treatment of any dermatologic problem.

Nipple shields. A nipple shield is a device worn over the nipple and areola while the infant is suckling and has been made of rubber and synthetic materials. A makeshift shield of a nursing bottle nipple should never be used. Shields differ from the shells designed to evert nipples (see Fig. 8-12). Shells should never be worn while breastfeeding, and any milk that drips into them should not be saved to feed the infant because it is heavily contaminated and of lower quality. A study of the effect of a thin latex nipple shield on suckling showed no difference in length of suckling time and no difference in cortisol

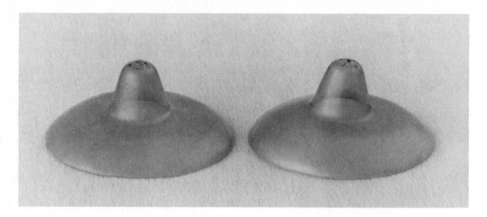

Fig. 8-12.   Nipple shield made of tasteless, odorless silicone in very thin flexible form referred to as "Mexican hat."

levels or prolactin levels (which were correlated with length of time suckling). There was no effect on prolactin levels by just wearing the shield without suckling. The amount of milk received by the infant was significantly reduced, however.

Nipple shields should not be used unless all else has failed, since it often becomes hard to wean the infant back. The infant becomes confused in learning his sucking routine. Glass or plastic with a rubber nursing nipple never works well, although the mother can see the milk through the glass or plastic. The effect of a traditional red rubber nipple shield referred to as "Mexican Hat" was compared to a new thin latex nipple shield. Normal mothers with no problems lactating nursed their infants using the shields.[114] The red rubber shield reduced the milk transfer by 58% and increased the infants' sucking rate and time spent resting. The thin latex shield reduced milk by 22% and had no effect on sucking patterns. These findings would suggest that new thin latex nipple shields could be used effectively when shields are absolutely necessary. Many lactation experts consider the use of a breast shield a sign of failure of proper lactation guidance and a preventable situation.

Small or flat nipples. When the nipples are small or flat, special attention to compress the breast and areola between two fingers to provide as much nipple as possible to the infant will assist him in getting a hold. Using the breast shell between feedings will help draw the nipple to greater prominence. Softening the areola before a feed to make it more compressible also helps. Rarely is it justified to use a nipple shield, but the thin pliable Sylastin shield is best. Try to remove it once the nipple is elongated to avoid having the infant adapt to it, since milk delivery is cut in half with a shield. Once engorgement is diminished and nursing is well established, small or flat nipples are usually no longer a problem.

Large nipples. Large nipples are occasionally a problem with a small infant or an infant with an indecisive suck. The shells may help the infant cope at first, but it is best just to work patiently with the infant. Manual expression, which softens the areola to make it more pliable before putting the infant to the breast, often helps.

Cracked nipples. Whenever the mother complains of nipple pain on nursing, the nipple should be examined in good light to look for cracks or subepithelial petechiae, which may be the precursor to cracking.[79] Taking a thorough history about care of the breast is important to identify the use of soaps, oils, ointments, or other self-prescribed treatments. Watching the nursing process may identify abnormal positioning at the breast.

If there are true cracks, however, therapy is indicated. In the precracked stage, dry heat between nursings will be most effective. When true fissures have developed, opening both sides of the nursing brassiere at feedings and beginning to nurse on the opposite side first will permit the initial let-down to occur "atraumatically"; then the infant can be put carefully to the affected breast. The heat treatments will assist in the therapy. When nursing has to be stopped on a given breast, it sets up a chain reaction of engorgement, reduced flow, and plugging of the ducts. A nipple shield should be tried before the nursing on a breast is stopped.

A very successful treatment described by Young,[117] which has now been adopted as a hospital routine in New Zealand, is the use of the mother's milk on the cracked nipple. A small amount is expressed and applied gently to the nipple and areola and allowed to dry on. Healing is rapid, and the success rate is excellent.*

A study comparing lanolin with drying on milk was conducted by Hewat and Ellis.[52] Mothers were instructed to use one treatment on one nipple and the other treatment on the opposite breast. They found no correlation with pain and frequency of feedings or with hair/skin color of mother. There was no difference between soreness and the two treatments. Many dermatologists feel applying two treatments to different parts on the same patient may lead to mixture of therapies and noncompliance rates higher than normal. A study of antiseptic sprays by Herd and Feeney[50] produced controversial results. Antiseptic sprays are rarely justifiable, given that there is a physiologic normal flora of the nipple and areola that should not be artificially altered.[58]

In cases of severe cracking of the nipple, the physician may wish to prescribe a 1% cortisone ointment to be applied after each feeding. With absorption and blotting onto clothing, there is no significant amount available to the infant. Usually 2-day treatment is adequate. It is important to treat the underlying cause of the original trauma to the nipple.

The application of any ointment that must be removed before nursing has disadvantages, since the removal is traumatic. A and D ointment, which does not have to be removed is occasionally effective. The indiscriminate use of ointment, however, can be the cause of nipple pain[79] and, as with many dermatologic problems, the initial treatment of the physician may be to discontinue previous treatments. Some ointments suggested as breast creams contain antibiotics, astringents, bismuth subnitrate, or petrolatum, all of which are contraindicated. These creams are available over the counter without a prescription.

Following is a summary of management of sore, painful, or cracked nipples:
1. Examine the breast, nipple, and nursing scene.
2. Conduct prefeeding manual expression.
3. Carefully position infant on breast.
4. Nurse on unaffected breast first with affected side exposed to air.
5. Let expressed breast milk dry on between feedings.
6. Apply dry heat 20 minutes, with a 60-watt bulb, 18 inches (45 cm) away, or with a hair dryer on low setting after feedings.
7. If necessary, use nipple shield while nursing, temporarily.
8. Rarely, temporarily stop nursing on affected side and replace it with manual expressing or pumping.
9. If necessary, give aspirin or codeine in short-acting preparation just before nursing (Chapter 11).

---

*Human milk has also been used in some cultures very successfully as eye drops in cases of bacterial ophthalmitis.

Infant in the hospital
Feeding characteristics

Infants have been aptly classified by their feeding characteristics by Barnes and colleagues[12] as barracudas, excited ineffectives, procrastinators, gourmets or mouthers, and resters.

These descriptions serve to demonstrate the fact that infants are different and the management of the nursing experience will vary accordingly. Therein lies the secret to appropriate counseling—recognizing the differences among infants and responding to them.

Barracudas. When put to the breast, barracudas vigorously and promptly grasp the nipple and suck energetically for 10 to 20 minutes. There is no dallying. Occasionally, this type of infant puts too much vigor into his nursing and hurts the nipple.

Excited ineffectives. Excited ineffective infants become so excited and active at the breast that they alternately grasp and lose the breast. They then start screaming. It is often necessary for the nurse or mother to pick up the infant and quiet him first, and then put him back to the breast. After a few days the mother and infant usually become adjusted.

Procrastinators. Procrastinators often seem to put off until the fourth or fifth post-partum day what they could just as well have done from the start. They wait until the milk comes in. They show no particular interest or ability in sucking in the first few days. It is important not to prod or force these infants when they seem disinclined. They do well once they start.

Gourmets or mouthers. Gourmets insist on mouthing the nipple, tasting a little milk, and then smacking their lips before starting to nurse. If the infant is hurried or prodded, he will become furious and start to scream. Otherwise, after a few minutes of mouthing he settles down and nurses very well.

Resters. Resters prefer to nurse a few minutes and then rest a few minutes. If left alone, they often nurse well, although the entire procedure will take much longer. They cannot be hurried.

Weight loss

Newborns usually lose some weight, and it tends to be a function of whether they are appropriate, large, or small for gestational age as well as how many kilocalories they ingest in the first few days. The infants of multiparas who are breastfeeding often lose little weight because the milk comes in so quickly. On the other hand, the normal primipara may not have a full supply for 72 to 96 hours. If the weight loss is over 5% (150 g in a 3 kg infant), evaluate the process to identify any problems before they become serious. A 10% weight loss is acceptable if all else is going well and the physical examination is negative, but it should be justified in the record, and the infant should be seen shortly after discharge from the hospital to assure resolution of the problem. If discharge home has taken place in 48 hours, it is imperative that the pediatrician's office keep in touch with the mother. Many have a nurse practitioner who makes the follow-up telephone calls or a home visit. Weighing before and after feedings produces tremendous anxiety in the mother and affords little information if it is inaccurate.

Weighing has been improved by the introduction of electronic digital read-out scales that are accurate to 1 g and are especially helpful in the intensive care nursery for infants under 1000 g.[21] Because of the cost and the sensitivity (fragility) of the equipment, these scales are not practical for home use yet. Their accuracy in before-and-after weighings has been verified by a number of investigators using comparison techniques.[108] When ordinary

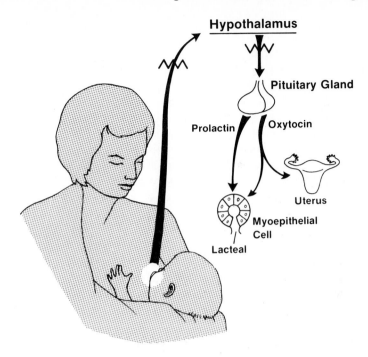

Fig. 8-13. Diagram of ejection reflex arc. When infant suckles breast, he stimulates mechanoreceptors in nipple and areola that send stimulus along nerve pathways to hypothalamus, which stimulates the posterior pituitary to release oxytocin. It is carried via bloodstream to breast and uterus. Oxytocin stimulates myoepithelial cell in breast to contract and eject milk from alveolus. Prolactin is responsible for milk production in alveolus. It is secreted by anterior pituitary gland in response to suckling. Stress such as pain and anxiety can inhibit let-down reflex. Sight or cry of infant can stimulate it.

scales are used, the margin of error has been shown to be greatest with the smaller volumes and is 20% in amounts less than 60 ml.

Vomiting blood

A breastfed baby who vomits blood should have the blood evaluated for fetal or adult hemoglobin by the Apt test. (Suspend blood in a small amount of saline solution and add an equal amount of 10% NaOH. Adult hemoglobin turns brown; fetal hemoglobin stays pink.) If it is adult hemoglobin, the nipple may be bleeding. Sometimes this bleeding is painless and unknown to the mother, and sometimes she is afraid to report it. If it is fetal hemoglobin, the infant demands evaluation.

Let-down reflex

The most important single function that affects the success of breastfeeding is the let-down reflex. A mother may produce the milk, but if she does not excrete it, further production is suppressed. Much has been written on this single reflex by physiologists, endocrinologists, biochemists, pathologists, anatomists, psychologists, psychiatrists, obstetricians, and pediatricians. Indeed, it is a complex function that depends on hormones, nerves, and glands, which can be inhibited most easily by psychologic block,[76] (Fig. 8-13).

The hormonal mechanism of milk ejection is described in Chapter 3. The reflex stimulation of milk ejection was meticulously studied by Caldeyro-Barcia[23] while he studied intramammary pressures. The more efficient stimulus for the milk-ejection reflex is suckling the nipple. The frequency of suckling is 70 to 120 strokes/min, and the mean pressure is between -50 and -150 mm Hg. The maximum recorded was -220 mm Hg. Within 1 minute of the onset of suckling, the first contraction of the mammary myoepithelium is recorded, but it may take 2 or more total minutes for full response. Further research by Cobo[27] has shown that, as in other species, the human response is undulating or spurtlike in release, although the level of oxytocin tends to reach a peak and plateau at 6 to 10 minutes during a feeding.[107] Some studies show no episodic secretion. When oxytocin levels are measured before the feeding, there is a response to the baby's crying or other anticipation of feeding. There is no prolactin response before actual suckling. A second release of oxytocin occurs when suckling begins.[31] There is not a direct correlation between levels of oxytocin and the volume of milk release at a given feeding.[74] The average pituitary gland contains 1000 mU of oxytocin, and only 0.5 U is required for the let-down reflex.

Uterine contractions are also stimulated by suckling. Amplitude and frequency may increase over time during nursing. Mechanical stimulation of the nipple can produce the same effect on the breast and uterus. The milk-ejection reflex is inhibited centrally by cold, pain, and emotional stress. Ejection response can be elicited by seeing the infant or hearing him cry.

The milk-ejection reflex can be at least partially blocked by large amounts of alcohol, which seems to have a central effect preventing the release of oxytocin, since the mammary gland and uterine response to injected oxytocin are not changed by alcohol. Studies on mothers with diabetes insipidus suggest that the patient retains the ability to synthesize and release oxytocin despite the fact that she is unable to produce ADH (vasopressin) in response to stimuli. Artificial cervical dilation postpartum will also cause milk ejection. Vaginal stimulus also initiates let-down in all species.

Injection of oxytocin reproduces the effect of suckling. A rapid series of injections of 1 to 10 mU intravenously will simulate suckling. A continuous drip is less effective. Use of Pitocin as a snuff or nasal spray is the best method for home use of oxytocin to initiate let-down.

The oxytocin concentration in the blood rises with suckling, which supports the hypothesis that suckling elicits the release of oxytocin.

The data on the question of ADH release during suckling are confused, but it would seem release of oxytocin and of ADH are independent.

The mammary myoepithelium is stimulated to contraction by oxytocin, and the milk-ejection reflex results in the contraction of the myoepithelium and the release, or let-down, of milk (Fig. 8-13). In the first weeks of lactation, the threshold dose of oxytocin is very low, averaging 0.65 mU from the fifth day. Thirty days after weaning it is 100 mU. Vasopressin is not as effective and requires 100 times the dosage of oxytocin to produce the same effect during lactation. Deaminooxytocin is 1.5 times as potent as oxytocin on the third postpartum day, but the difference disappears over time, probably because of the rapid breakdown of natural oxytocin by oxytocinase early in the postpartum period. Prostaglandins have been shown to have a number of physiologic effects, including an effect on mammary epithelium to increase mammary duct pressure.[103] In a blind crossover study, oxytocin, intravenous prostaglandin, and nasal prostaglandin were given and the intraductal pressures measured. The most effective intravenous prostaglandins were 16-phenoxy-PGE_2 and $PGF_{2\alpha}$ which were then tried nasally, but only $PGF_{2\alpha}$ was effective nasally. The potential

Table 8-1. Ejection reflex*

Maternal disturbance	Mean amount of milk obtained by infant (g)
No distractions (no injection)	168
Distraction (saline injection)	99
Distraction (oxytocin injection)	153

Modified from Newton M and Newton N: J Pediatr 91:1, 1977.
*Interrupted milk flow can be restarted with hormone injection.

for nasal $PGF_{2\alpha}$ treatment in engorgement and failure of let-down is possible but is as yet unexplored clinically.

Practical aspects of the milk-ejection reflex

When the nipple is stimulated, the receptors at the nipple and areola are stimulated and nervous impulses are transmitted to the hypothalamus via the somatic afferent nerves. The hypothalamus stimulates the pituitary gland to secrete prolactin, which induces the alveoli in the breast to secrete milk. The cell membranes release fat globules and protein into the lumen. This produces the hindmilk, which has a higher protein and fat content. Part of the foremilk has been present since the previous nursing and is released first. It is a more dilute, less fatty solution that empties into the lactiferous sinuses awaiting the next suckling. The ejection reflex induces the holocrine excretion of milk from the cells. The posterior pituitary gland secretes oxytocin, which stimulates the myoepithelial cells to contract and eject the milk from the ducts.

Early in lactation, if there is marked engorgement, the ejection reflex may be inhibited by the congested blood flow to the target organ, the myoepithelial cell. Therefore, when suckling is initiated and oxytocin is released into the bloodstream, it is delayed in reaching the myoethelial cell with the message due to congestion. Preparing the breast with warm soaks, gentle massage, and manual expression of a little milk may facilitate let-down.

Newton and Newton[76] have studied the ejection reflex and clearly show the effect of distraction to the let-down effect. Distractions included immersing feet in ice water (reported to be the worst); being asked mathematical questions in rapid series, which resulted in electric shock if a wrong answer was given; or having painful traction on the big toe (Table 8-1). In practice, for some mothers pain, stress, and mental anguish interfere with let-down. When simple adjustments such as making the mother more comfortable, playing soft music, or leaving the mother in a quiet room do not work, other techniques should be tried.

Gentle stroking of the breast may help to decrease anxiety and stimulate flow. Tactile warmth as opposed to cold may improve release. Ice should not be used to make the nipple erect, as ice interferes with let-down because cold is known to interrupt the reflex.[77]

The most direct therapy is oxytocin. When simple supportive measures fail, this can be prescribed at home as a nasal spray, most readily available as synthetic oxytocin (Syntocinon). It is packaged in 2 and 5 ml spray bottles. A mother almost never needs a second bottle. A bottle contains 40 USP units (IU) per milliliter of spray of synthetic oxytocin, a polypeptide hormone of the posterior pituitary gland. (A prescription is required.) It is destroyed in the gastrointestinal tract; therefore it must be sprayed nasally, where it is rapidly absorbed. One spray into one or both nostrils 2 to 3 minutes before putting the infant to the breast (or before pumping, in the case of collecting for an infant unable to nurse at the breast) is sufficient.

It has been suggested by Aono and colleagues[7] that sulpiride be given orally to mothers who produce less than 50 ml of total milk yield in first 48 hours of lactation. Sulpiride is known to stimulate secretion of prolactin. In a control study of 96 normal primiparas and multiparas with poor lactation, half were given 50 mg sulpiride twice daily from the fourth to the seventh day postpartum and half received a placebo. There was no difference in milk production in the multiparas, but there was a significant difference in the primiparas, who had higher milk yield, higher prolactin levels, and higher percentage still breastfeeding at 1 month in the treated group.

POSTNATAL, OR POSTHOSPITAL, PERIOD

When the family makes the transition from hospital to home, it can be stressful. The parents hear the infant, who has been passive and content, wake up and cry for the first time. Because of all the procedures necessary to discharge an infant from the hospital (discharge physicals, blood tests, etc.), the well-planned discharge is often delayed and everyone is frantic, including the infant. The mother should be reassured about this and not be alarmed if she has to feed the infant frequently the first day at home.

Feeding frequency

Many hospital schedules are on a 4-hour feeding program, based on the feedings of bottle fed infants whose slow emptying time of the stomach with formulas requires up to 4 hours. The emptying time for breast milk is about 1½ hours; thus frequent feedings are not unusual. Pediatric textbooks at the turn of the century described 10 to 12 feedings a day as normal.[64] Comparison of mammalian care patterns and composition of their milk shows an inverse relationship between protein content and frequency of feedings. From this it might be deduced that the human infant might well need to be fed more frequently than every 4 hours (Table 8-2).[70] Infants who sleep 5 to 6 hours at a stretch at night may make up for skipped feedings during the day.

When milk intake and feeding patterns of thriving exclusively breastfed infants were documented from birth for the first 4 months of life by Butte et al.,[22] two feeding patterns emerged. In one the authors describe the feedings as distributed throughout the 24-hour day, and in the other feedings were excluded from midnight to 6 AM, although all were feeding ad lib. Total intake was the same in 24 hours. Milk intake per feeding decreased over the day. Frequency and duration declined over the 4-month period. Weight gain was similar in the two groups.

The pattern of intake during a feeding is different between breastfed and bottle fed infants.[56] A bottle feeding infant sucks steadily in a linear pattern, receiving 81% of the feed in 10 minutes. A breastfed infant has a biphasic pattern, which includes the first 4 minutes on the first breast and the first 4 minutes on the second breast (between 15 and 19 minutes into the feed). He receives 84% of the total volume in those 8 minutes. In another study, 50% of the feed on each breast was consumed in 2 minutes and 80% to 90% by 5 minutes. Milk flow was minimal during the last 5 minutes. All these observations were made on the fifth to seventh day (Fig. 8-14).

Switch nursing is often suggested to increase total intake of an infant when milk production needs stimulating, especially if the infant is not gaining adequately (Fig.

Table 8-2. Mammalian care patterns and composition of species milk

	Species of mammal						
	Pinnipedia seal sea lion	Tree shrew	**Rabbit**	**Rat**	Black rhino*	Chimpanzee	**Human**
Infant care pattern	Return to ocean after birth	—	Cache	Carry, hiber-nate	—	Carry	?
Feeding interval	Once a week	48 hr	24 hr	Continuous	—	Continuous	?
Composition of milk							
Total solids (%)	62-65	20	33-40	21	8.1	11.9	12.4
Protein (%)	8-14	11	14-23	10	0.0	3.7	3.8
Fat (%)	53	6.5	18	8	1.4	1.2	1.2
CHO (%)	0-0.90	3.2	2.0	2.6	6.1	7.0	7.0

*The rhino has an anatomic variation in the stomach that provides four pouches that fill during a feeding and provide a constant trickle of milk to the central groove leading to the small intestine, thus creating a constant feed.

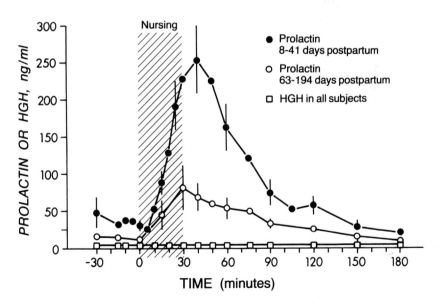

Fig. 8-14. Plasma prolactin and growth hormone concentrations during nursing in postpartum women. Eight women were studied 8-41 days postpartum and six women were studied 63-194 days postpartum. Prenursing prolactin levels in latter group were within normal range. Plasma growth hormone showed no change in any subjects during nursing. (From Noel GL, Suh HK, and Frantz AG: J Clin Endocrinol Metab 1974; 38:413-423 © 1974, The Endocrine Society.)

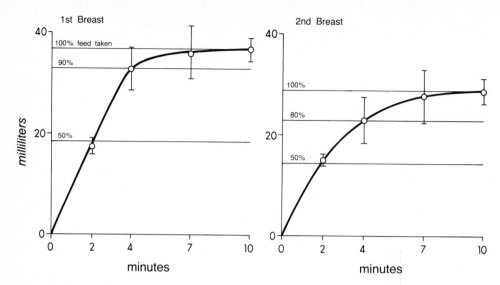

Fig. 8-15. Mother-infant pattern of milk flow. (From Lucas A, Lucas PJ, and Baum JD: Lancet 2:57, 1979.)

8-15), but this may be counterproductive. When mothers fed 10 minutes on each breast (10 × 10), they produced the same amount of milk as they did nursing 5 minutes on a side and switching back (5 × 5 × 5 × 5). The suckling-induced prolactin is similar with both patterns as well. The infants do not nurse for a full 20 minutes in some cases, and the nutritive feeding time was under 15 minutes. It is suggested that the duration of the feeding should be determined by the infant's response and not by time. This switching may prevent full hindmilk fat production and lower energy content. More high-calorie milk may be produced by nursing at only one breast per feeding.

The wide range in breast milk volume in well-nourished mothers was shown by Dewey and Lönnerdal[34] to be a variation in infant "demand" rather than an inadequacy of milk production. They stimulated milk production with postfeeding pumping for 2 weeks, but the infants failed to continue to take more than previously. Although milk production was augmented by pumping, the infants regulated their own intake.

New mothers are often most insecure and most concerned about lack of scheduling, especially if an ad lib program of feeding has been suggested. Other mothers seem to thrive on random scheduling. Some pediatricians continue to rigidly instruct mothers about adhering closely to a schedule designed for the bottle fed infant that can lead to failure of lactation unless the mother is sufficiently confident to follow her infants' demands and feed more frequently.[64]

Breastfed infants do not differ from bottle fed infants at 3 and 5 months of age in terms of the number of night feedings. At 3 months breastfed infants spend about 20 minutes less time at night sleeping and 20 minutes less time during the day according to studies by Alley and Rogers.[2]

When a mother expresses concerns about frequent feedings and worries about the adequacy of her milk (she is often disturbed that it looks so thin and blue after the luxurious color of colostrum), Jackson[12] would suggest she keep a record of feeding times and duration, as well as sleep and wakeful times. If a chart was kept, the mother was usually surprised to find how quickly her infant developed a schedule. Often the infant was sleeping longer than she thought. The chart is also reassuring to the physician, especially if weight gain is marginal. In some cases it will highlight a problem not previously identified, such as a poor gainer who sleeps all night, missing several feedings.

Adequate rest

If nursing is not going well, the most likely cause of problems is fatigue on the part of the mother. She may need to be ordered by her physician to nap and rest. She will have to learn to nap when the infant is napping. This becomes more difficult when there are other young children, but a simultaneous nap for all the little ones and mother may have to be engineered. Otherwise she may have to go to bed with the children at night and just concentrate on resting and feeding the infant. When the need for rest is acute, the father should be assigned infant care with the possible inclusion of a bottle feeding in extreme cases, while the mother sleeps undisturbed.

Sore breasts—caked breasts

Tender lumps in the breasts in a mother who is otherwise well are probably due to plugging of a collecting duct. Some women on high calcium diets have excreted grains of white sand that are thought to be calcium stones plugging a duct. The best treatment is to continue nursing. Manually massaging the area to initiate and assure complete drainage should be recommended. Hot packs before feedings may help. If the breast is especially tender, initiating nursing on the opposite breast first permits the affected breast to let-down without the pressure of suckling. The affected breast should be completely emptied by nursing or manual expression. The brassiere may be cutting off an alveolus from pressure of a narrow strap. Changing the infant's position may help also.

Repeated "caking"

When caking is recurrent, one needs to look for a major cause such as exhaustion and fatigue. Several women have come to my attention who have had repeated lumps in their breasts with poor flow of milk, often as if the ducts were plugged. The condition responded fairly well to manual expression before each feeding, often with the expulsion of small plugs. The condition dramatically improved by limiting the mother to polyunsaturated fats and adding lecithin to the diet. It was also necessary for subsequent pregnancies in all three cases. Lecithin is an oily substance that can be used as an oil on salads or taken by spoon, one tablespoon per day.

Galactocele

Milk-retention cysts are uncommon and, when found, are almost exclusively in lactating women. The contents at first are pure milk. Owing to absorption of the fluid they later contain thick, creamy, cheesy, or oily material. The swelling is smooth and rounded, and compression of it may cause milky fluid to exude from the nipple. Galactoceles are believed to be caused by the blockage of a milk duct. The cyst may be aspirated to avoid surgery but will fill up again. It can be removed surgically under local anesthesia without stopping the breastfeeding. Its presence does not require cessation of the lactation. A firm diagnosis can be made by ultrasound; a cyst and milk will appear the same, and a tumor will be distinguishable (Figs. 8-16 and 8-17).

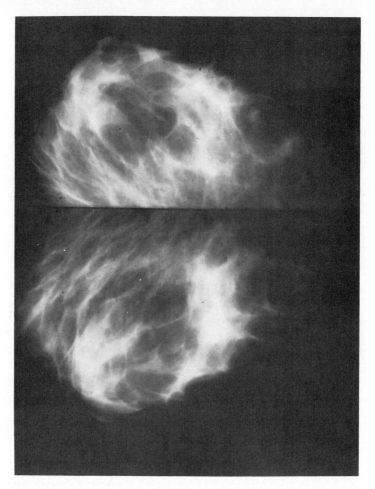

Fig. 8-16. Normal breast tissue by mammography. Tissue is one-third fat and appears cystic in nature. (Courtesy Dr. Wende Logan.)

Breast rejection

Infants have been observed to reject the breast intermittently, most often at 3 to 4 months, and then to go back after several feedings or a day or so. A bottle can be substituted. Total rejection of both breasts may be due to the return of menstruation. A mother will notice the infant will reject the breast for a day or so with each period. Other infants seem unaffected. Strong foods in the diet may cause rejection of milk, which usually occurs 8 to 12 hours after ingestion and disappears by 24 hours after ingestion.

Unilateral breast rejection

Some infants prefer one breast and even refuse the other. When this occurs, manual expression or softening the nipple for easier grasp may help, thus enticing the infant to suckle. Holding the infant in the same position (i.e., on same side in same direction, so-called football hold) for the other breast may lead the infant to take the second breast. Sometimes applying syrup to the rejected nipple or using a breast shield will help. Unilateral

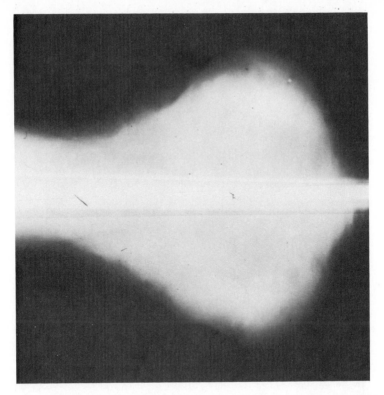

Fig. 8-17. Breast tissue during pregnancy and lactation by mammography. Fat is replaced by lactation tissue and presents solid appearance. Tumor would be easily distinguished by this procedure in lactating breast. It is a safe, noninvasive technique that does not interfere with nursing. (Courtesy Dr. Wende Logan.)

breastfeeding is a custom in some parts of China. Sodium and chloride levels may rise in milk after mastitis. It is wise to taste the milk or have SMA6 done on milk from both breasts if the problem persists to be sure there is not a reason for the rejection.

Goldsmith[43] reported five cases of lactating women whose infants suddenly rejected a single breast. Weeks or months later a mass was noted by the mother and biopsy revealed malignancy. It would be wise to examine any patient who complains of unilateral breast rejection that does not respond to simple measures to rule out a tumor. Ultrasound followed by a mammogram, if necessary, can be performed without discontinuing lactation.

Mastitis

Mastitis is an infectious process in the breast producing localized tenderness, redness, and heat, together with systemic reactions of fever, malaise, and sometimes nausea and vomiting. It no longer occurs in epidemics as seen in hospitals at one time before the common use of antibiotics and when hospital stays were prolonged for normal childbirth. The infection, however, may be hospital acquired if the mother or infant is colonized with a virulent bacteria before leaving the hospital.

Little appears in the medical literature about mastitis because women are rarely hospitalized for the problem and are treated at home and, in some cases, over the telephone.

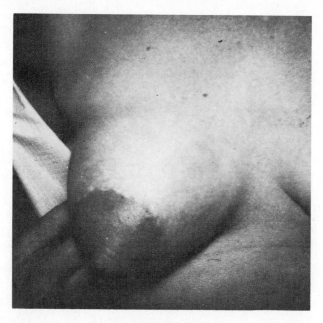

Fig. 8-18. Mastitis in medial upper quadrant. (From Marshall BR: JAMA 233:1377, 1975. Copright 1975, American Medical Association.)

When staphylococcal disease was a major problem on postpartum wards, lactating and nonlactating women alike developed mastitis; thus the differentiation of two types—acute puerperal mammary cellulitis, a nonepidemic mastitis involving interlobular connective tissue, and acute puerperal mammary adenitis, which was epidemic, associated with an outbreak of skin infections in infants. The current definition includes fever of 38.5° C or more, chills, flulike aching, systemic illness, and pink, tender, hot, swollen, wedge-shaped area of the breast[80] (Fig. 8-18). The significant differential points between mastitis and engorgement and plugged duct are listed in Table 8-3.

The portal of entry of the disease is through the lactiferous ducts to a secreting lobule, through a nipple fissure to periductal lymphatics, or through hematogenous spread. The common organisms involved include *Staphylococcus aureus, Escherichia coli,* and (rarely) *Streptococcus.* Tuberculus mastitis does occur, and the infant often develops tuberculosis of the tonsils. In populations where tuberculosis is endemic, it occurs in about 1% of cases.[46]

Factors predisposing the patient to mastitis include poor drainage of a duct and then of an alveolus, presence of an organism, and lowered maternal defenses such as those associated with stress and fatigue. Insufficient emptying and obstruction of ducts by tight clothing cause plugged ducts, which can be prevented from becoming mastitis if identified early and treated vigorously with local masasge, moist heat, and rest. Missing a feeding or having the infant suddenly sleep through the night may cause engorgement, plugging, and then mastitis.[90] Cracked or painful nipples may herald a problem, more because mother avoids complete emptying on the painful side than because bacteria suddenly gain access.

Devereux[33] describes 20 years of experience with 53 lactating patients who experienced 71 acute attacks of mastitis. The highest incidence was in the second and third weeks postpartum. No infant was weaned because of the mastitis. No infants were sick in as-

Table 8-3 Comparison of findings of engorgement, plugged duct, and mastitis

Characteristics	Engorgement	Plugged duct	Mastitis
Onset	Gradual, immediately postpartum	Gradual, after feedings	Sudden, after 10 days
Site	Bilateral	Unilateral	Usually unilateral
Swelling and heat	Generalized	May shift/little or no heat	Localized, red, hot, and swollen
Pain	Generalized	Mild but localized	Intense but localized
Body temperature	$<38.4°$ C	$<38.4°$ C	$>38.4°$ C
Systemic symptoms	Feels well	Feels well	Flulike symptoms

sociation with the mastitis. All but five mothers nursed subsequent infants. Six patients had mastitis with other pregnancies. Eight of 71 patients (11.1%) developed abscesses, six of which required incision and drainage. The bacterial cause was not stated. When treatment was delayed beyond 24 hours, the abscess rate increased.

Another series of 65 cases of mastitis, reported by Marshall et al.,[72] showed a 2.5% incidence of the disease among a population of 2534 lactating women. *S. aureus* was the offending organism in 23 of the 48 infected breasts that were cultured. In 19 normal (no mastitis) lactating women, only one grew this organism. Of the 65 women, 41 continued to nurse without difficulty for an average of 13 weeks longer. There were three breast abscesses for a rate of 4.6%, all in women who had chosen to wean. Onset was 5½ weeks postpartum (5 days to 1-year range). Of the 65, nine had missed feedings or acutely weaned, eight women had noticed a fissured nipple before the infection, and the others were unanticipated. Treatment included 41 with penicillin V, 12 with ampicillin, and 8 with other antibiotics. Mastitis recurred in four of the women who continued to nurse.

Half the patients in a series reported by Niebyl et al.[80] were due to *S. aureus* by culture. They were treated with antibiotics, continued nursing on both sides, and observed no abscesses or problems in the infant. Investigators in the Gambia[88] observed mastitis in 2.6% of women, with recurrence common. They noted the milk was deficient in IgA, C_3, and lactoferrin when comapred to that of other lactating mothers. The authors suggested these mothers were predisposed to mastitis. Coagulase-negative staphylococci isolated from the milk of mothers with mastitis has been shown to cause experimental acute mastitis when injected into mice and should be considered a possible etiologic agent in nursing women.[102]

While breastfed infants usually remain well during bouts of acute mastitis in their mothers, a case of scalded skin syndrome is reported by Katzman and Wald[63] in an infant fed by a mother with mastitis that did not respond to ampicillin for 14 days. The child responded to intravenous nafcillin. It is worthy of note that the mother had a lesion on her areola on the infected breast, and she was told to use breast shields, although she was to continue nursing. Breast shields have been shown to decrease breast emptying by half. This case points out the urgency of evaluating both the mother and the infant when mastitis or any breastfeeding problem occurs.

Using leukocyte counts and microbiologic counts, Thomsen et al.[101] have separated breast inflammations into three clinical states: milk stasis (counts $<10^6$ leukocytes and $<10^3$ bacteria per milliliter of milk), noninfectious inflammation (counts of $>10^6$ leukocytes and $<10^3$ bacteria), and infectious mastitis (counts $>10^6$ leukocytes and $>10^3$ bacteria). In a controlled study no treatment in all three groups led to recurrence, lactation failure, and abscesses in mastitis. Emptying the breast completely was sufficient in most cases of stasis and noninfectious inflammation; however, recurrence was inappropriately high. Mastitis clearly required antibiotics. Because cultures require time, when the bacteria count is finally available and the clinical course is clear, the noninfectious variety should be cleared already. These laboratory results are confirmatory; however, the skilled clinician can avoid the relapses and progression to abscess by close monitoring and selective aggressive treatment before the cultures are reported.

Unilateral breast dysfunction in lactating Gambian women is not an unusual finding.[85] It has been attributed to episodes of low-grade mastitis with the production of high-sodium milk, which the infant rejects. The unused breast involutes, and the functioning breast increases production. In subsequent pregnancies function returns to the involved breast.

The clinician should be sure to inform his patients of the need to contact him if any unusual symptoms occur so that proper management can be initiated early, since prevention is the most effective treatment. Inappropriately or inadequately treated cases of mastitis predispose the patient to chronic mastitis, which may last for months and require more antibiotics than would have been required initially. A mother should be instructed to contact her physician if there is local pain, heat, and redness, or whenever there is a fever while lactating. When proper treatment is initiated promptly, the course of the disease is usually brief; if it is delayed, prolonged antibiotics will become necessary.

The management regimen that has been most successful at the University of Rochester is as follows:

1. Continue to nurse on both breasts, but start the infant on the unaffected side while the affected side "lets down." Be sure to empty the affected side by feeding or pumping.
2. Insist on bed rest (mandatory). The mother can take the infant to bed and obtain assistance for the care of the rest of the family.
3. Choose an antibiotic that can be tolerated by the infant as well as the mother (avoid sulfa drugs when the infant is under 1 month). The decision should be based on local sensitivities and length of time since delivery or exposure to resistant flora. In florid staphylococcal disease, amoxicillin, dicloxacillin, and nafcillin maybe the drugs of choice. In streptococcal disease, penicillin is usully preferable. In uncomplicated mastitis after 1 month postpartum, penicillin, ampicillin, or erythromycin is preferable initially. Regardless of the course of the disease, the antibiotic should be given for at least 10 days. Shorter courses are associated with relapses.
4. Apply ice packs or warm packs to the breast, whichever provides the most comfort. Experience indicates that heat is better.
5. Provide plenty of fluids for the mother.
6. Give an analgesic such as aspirin or acetominophen.
7. The mother should wear a supporting brassiere that does not cause painful pressure.

Recurrent or chronic mastitis and monilial infection

Recurrent mastitis is usually caused by delayed or inadequate treatment of the initial disease. If antibiotics are initially started, they should be coninued for a minimum of 10 days. Often, because the mother feels better, she discontinues them on her own. At the first recurrence, cultures should be sent of the breast and the infant's nasopharynx and oropharynx. The patient should be seen and the circumstances completely reviewed. An aggressive course of rest, nourishment, stress management, and complete drainage of the breast should be initiated. The antibiotics should be carefully selected and maintained for 2 weeks. Fluids should be increased. Failure of the second treatment is usually due to failure to complete the entire treatment, which may mean failure to get adequate rest and build up maternal resistance.

A secondary complication of recurrent mastitis is invasion of the breast by yeast or fungus such as *Candida albicans* (Chapter 15), as is frequently seen postantibiotic treatment. Mothers describe incredible pain when the infant nurses, pain they describe as feeling like hot cords burning in their chest wall. This is usually fungal infection of the ducts. The best treatment is to massage nystatin cream (Mycostatin) or Mycolog, which contains cortisone, into the nipple and areola after each feeding. The infant should also be given oral nystatin simultaneously, or the mother will be reinfected. If the mother is known to have a recurrent vulvovaginitis, initiation of nystatin prophylactically should be considered when the antibiotics are begun. Although the infant may or may not have oral thrush or a diaper rash, he should be treated. The nipple may not look unusual despite exquisite pain.

Abscess formation

Abscess can also be a complication of mastitis and is usually the result of delayed or inadequate treatment. A true abscess will require surgical drainage but should be treated with antibiotics, rest, warm soaks, and complete emptying of the breast at least every few hours. The milk will remain clean unless the abscess ruptures into the ductal system. Usually it drains to the outside. Nursing can be maintained when the breast is surgically drained as long as the incision and drainage tube are sufficiently far from the areola so that they are not involved in feeding. In any event, the breast should be manually drained frequently to maintain the milk supply until feeding can resume (usually sufficient healing takes place in 4 days). The infant should always be monitored for infection.

Laboratory findings

Cultures of the breast milk, when indicated, should be done after the breast has been cleaned with water and the mother's hands have been thoroughly washed. The milk stream should be initiated by manual expression and the first 3 ml discarded to get a midstream clean-catch specimen. It has been suggested that antibody coating be looked for in the bacteria found in the milk to confirm its relationship to the disease.[100] It is important to remember that the normal cell count of normal uninfected human milk is 1000/mm^3 to 4000/mm^3. The presence of cells should not automatically be construed as infection.

The levels of sodium and chloride in milk from mastitic breasts have been reported in the literature to be extremely elevated (Na $\geq$100 mEq/L, Cl $\geq$80 mEq/L, K $\leq$10).[28] Usually, electrolyte abnormalities are associated with recurrent mastitis or chronic subclinical mastitis. The quickest screen for the problem is for the mother to compare the tastes of milk from each side.

Neonatal mastitis. Neonatal mastitis occurs infrequently, although it was a common event in the 1940s and 1950s when staphylococcal disease was rampant in the nursery. It occurs in full-term infants 1 to 5 weeks of age and in as many females as males, usually unilaterally. It is unrelated to maternal mastitis and usually occurs in bottle fed infants. Prior to the use of intravenous antibiotic therapy, surgical incision and drainage were common. Prognosis for cure is excellent. In recent years the rare cases that occur are seen in conjunction with manipulation of the neonatal breast.

Supplementary feedings

To supplement a breastfed infant continues to be controversial in pediatric circles. For the normal full-term infant, it is not necessary. Evaluation of serial blood glucoses in breastfed and bottle fed infants from birth reported by Heck and Erenberg[49] demonstrated a significant number of bottle fed infants with hypoglycemia presumed to be a rebound phenomenon from dextrose and water feeding early. Some breastfed infants had a value less than 40 on the second day. There were no significant differences in serum bilirubins and weight loss between supplemented and unsupplemented breastfed infants in Herrara's[51] study. At the age of 3 months a significant number of supplemented infants were no longer breastfeeding (still breastfeeding, 81% unsupplemented versus 53% supplemented). Even in hot, dry climates, water supplements were not found to be necessary.[3,11,42] Urine osmolarity remains within physiological ranges in unsupplemented breastfed infants studied by Goldberg and Adams.[42] This has been demonstrated by a number of other investigators. The supplementation with water did not influence the "coming-in" of mother's milk according to Schultzman et al. What they did observe, however, was that infants in the group being supplemented took very little water after nursing (less than 4 oz in the first 3 days).[92]

Many physicians suggest to mothers that a supplementary bottle can be added any time. Actually, when lactation is going well, it is not needed, and when it is not going well, a bottle may aggravate the problem. During hospitalizaiton, giving a substitute bottle may confuse a new infant, who may be having trouble sucking at first. Infants who are given water or glucose water in the hospital do less well and usually lose more weight. There is a significant relationship between supplements in the hospital and early discontinuation of breastfeeding. It is a marker of impending trouble and of insufficient milk production, which is best treated with frequent feedings at the breast and some intervention from an experienced support person.

In a study by Gray-Donald et al.[44] of the affect of formula supplementation on outcome of breastfeeding of the two nurseries, one was used as a control and one was supplemented. Mothers could request supplements in either group, and any baby put to the breast twice was called "breastfed." It was clear that mothers who requested formula in the hospital and requested a going home formula package were more likely to discontinue breastfeeding. They considered this early behavior a marker of high risk for failure.[44] These patients should receive follow-up and considerable support.

Use of complementary bottles, that is, those given after a breastfeeding to top off the feeding, is the beginning of a downhill course that may doom lactation to failure. It would be better to take the infant to breast more often or switch back to the first breast if the baby is hungry. If it is necessary for the mother to be away at feeding time, she can pump a feeding ahead of time and save it in the refrigerator or freezer for someone else to give by bottle. If this is not practical, a bottle of formula can be given. It can be made up from a formula powder more economically one feeding at a time, and there is no waste. Powder preparations have a long shelf life even when open and are better tolerated by the infant because lower temperatures are required to manufacture powders; thus there is no caramelizing of the sugars or denaturing of the proteins. A powder goes quickly into solution if the water is warm when mixing is attempted. (Prepare formula powder as follows: one scoop of powder to 2 oz of water gives 20 kcal/oz).

Solid foods

Successful nursing mothers are rarely impatient to start the baby on solid foods, as bottle feeding mothers frequently are. Milk, and especially human milk, supplies the appropriate nutrients. (Some physicians, however, prescribe vitamin D, 200 units [Chapter 9].) At about 6 months a normal infant begins to use his iron stores, and that is probably an appropriate time to start solid foods, especially iron-containing ones. This permits the entire process of weaning to cup and solid foods to be a gradual one. An infant does not need teeth to eat baby food, and, conversely, he does not have to be weaned from the breast because teeth have erupted. By 6 months the number of feedings usually has decreased, and the timing and volume are beginning to cycle to a schedule that resembles three meals a day and some snacks. A breastfed infant should start some solids by 6 months of age.

Carrying and holding

Carrying and holding young infants have been considered by some in the era of peak bottle feeding as predisposing to spoiling the infants. In many cultures around the world, infants are carried with the mother night and day. In Western cultures infants are tightly swaddled, i.e., wrapped up like a package and put down. In a randomized controlled study of primiparous breastfeeding women, Hunziker and Bass[57] showed that increased carrying reduces infant crying and colicky behavior. The authors concluded that the lack of carrying predisposes to crying and colic. A study among young mothers in New York City who were given infant carriers showed that carrying the infant was more apt to influence infant crying than breastfeeding.

Colic

Colic by definition is spasmodic contractions of smooth muscle, causing pain and discomfort. It can be experienced in many organs, such as the gatrointestinal or genitourinary tract, and at all ages. When the term *colic* is used in reference to infants, it usually means a syndrome in which the young infant has unexplained paroxysms of irritability, fussing, and crying for a prolonged period, often at the same time of day, in the early months of life. The infant usually draws his legs up as if in pain. There are a myriad of remedies directed at various possible causes, including allergy, hypertonicity, and hormone withdrawal.

The infant-feeding survey conducted on the Isle of Wight among all infants under 1 year in 1977 was studied to determine the prevalence of infant colic[53]; 16% of the 843 infants had colic, all but 10 of the 135 cases developing before 6 weeks of age. Almost half were free of symptoms by 3 months of age. Only 12% persisted after 6 months of age. Surprisingly, only 20% occurred most commonly in the evening. Colic occurred equally among breastfed and bottle fed infants but was more common if solid foods were started under 3 months of age. The authors found no relationship to parental allergies or feeding methods, but only to social class: 23% of the professional group, 16% of the skilled group, and only 7% of the unskilled group complained of colic in their infants. Pediatricians have made this observation for generations, but it may be a matter of parenting style and expectations that brings a parent to complain about colic. Colic does occur in premature infants but usually not until they reach 42 weeks gestation.

Infantile colic has been reported to occur equally among breastfed (20%), formula (19%), and mixed breastfed and formula (21%) in a study of almost 1,000 infants.[1] The fecal α_1-antitrypsin and fecal hemoglobins were not different in colicky infants. There was no evidence of dietary protein hypersensitivity in this series.[99]

Characteristically, the infant will cry and scream as if in pain from 3 to 4 hours at a stretch, usually between 6 PM and 10 PM at night. The infant will nurse frequently, then scream and pull away from the breast as if in pain, only to cry out a few minutes later. Sometimes the infant can be comforted by another adult such as his father or grandmother. The infant will respond to gentle rocking when held against a warm shoulder. If the infant is put down, the screaming starts up again. If the nursing mother holds the infant, he is frantic unless nursed and yet does not need to be fed. This may disturb a new mother who wonders why she cannot console her infant (Is her milk weak? Does it disagree with her infant? Is she an inadequate mother?). None of these options is true, but the fact that the infant smells her milk makes him behave as if he needs to nurse. Anyone who is not nursing can quickly quiet the infant. Picking the infant up does not spoil him, and rocking and cuddling are appropriate.

A carefully taken history and physical examination are always in order to rule out other pathologic conditions such as otitis media, anal fissure, or hernia before a diagnosis of colic is made. If true colic is diagnosed because of the consistency of the screaming for several hours each day at the same time, treatment is in order. Warm pressure is usually palliative. A warm bath or warm soaks to the abdominal wall or warm hot bottle or warm shoulder with some pressure or massage is comforting. Elixir of diphenhydramine (Benadryl) or pyribenzamine (1 to 2 tsp immediately and every 4 hours as necessary) is usually very effective. If the medicaiton is given 30 minutes before the anticipated colic begins, it works best. The elixir is sedating as well as having an "antiallergic" component. Spiritus fermenti or other forms of alcohol, such as 5 drops of whiskey in 1 tsp of warm water, may help the colic.

Adams and Davidson recommend 1 tsp of 20 proof wine or 1.5 ml of 80 proof liquor in two ounces of warm water with a little sugar. When wine or beer is suggested to the mother as an aperitif before dinner, it may serve to relax the frantic mother as well as the colicky infant. Beer and other forms of alcohol have been shown by several investigators to produce significant increases in prolactin levels within 30 minutes. In all studies beer was more effective than the same amount of alcohol in another form.[24,32,45] It is recognized that excessive alcohol while nursing can produce failure to thrive and hypoglycemia in the neonate, but when used in moderate dosage it may be very effective. The use of rhythmical incessant sounds or lights (i.e., the vacuum cleaner or the untuned TV) have variable success.

Influence of cow's milk in maternal diet

The literature is not straightforward on the issue of the effect of cow's milk in the maternal diet and infantile colic. Talbot[97] first published information on congenital sensitization to food (especially eggs and cow's milk) in humans in 1918, which was manifested as clinical allergy in the breastfed infant. Research techniques are far superior today, and information is accumulating. Gerrard and Shenassa[41] report sensitization caused by substances in breast milk thought to be due to two types of food allergy; one is IgE-mediated and triggered by trace amounts of antigen, and the other is not IgE-mediated and is triggered by large amounts of antigen. Gastrointestinal transport of macromolecules in the pathogenesis of food allergy is under investigation as is T cell–mediated immunity in food allergy. However, the present state of scientific knowledge has not resolved the issue of colic and cow's milk for the clinician.

Clinical studies have been done to test the association of dairy products in the mother with colic in some breastfed babies. Jakobsson and Lindberg[59] described a cause-and-effect relationship in a group of 18 mothers in 1978, which was criticized because it was not a double-blind study. Evans et al.[38] then reported that they found no such relationship when they did a double-blind crossover study in which mothers received cow's milk protein for 2 days and then a placebo for 2 days. Jakobsson and Lindberg[60] have repeated their work using a double-blind crossover study design in the mother-baby pairs in which the infants had colic; 35% of the infants improved on maternal diets free of cow's milk. A torrent of mail to the journals confirmed these conclusions in small clinical practice trials as well.

Jakobsson et al.[61] found bovine β-lactoglobulin in milk of 18 out of 38 mothers chosen at random. Three mothers had very high amounts, and their infants had colic that was relieved by a maternal diet free of bovine milk products.

In the face of a clinical picture of colic, a history of allergy in the family, especially to cow's milk, is suggestive. A diet free of cow's milk should be tried in any severe colic for at least a week (2 days rarely produces significant improvement). Usually a mother eliminates drinking milk, and for some babies that is enough. If not, all milk products are then eliminated. For the group of infants who have a cow's milk allergy, the treatment is impressive. Not all colic is due to cow's milk. It may be associated with other dietary items such as eggs or chocolate, or it may be totally unrelated to maternal food intake.

Acute 24-hour colic in a breastfed infant may be due to something in the maternal diet. When a strong vegetable like beans, onions, garlic, or rhubarb is taken for the first time and the infant starts to cry within a few hours and continues for 20 to 24 hours, this may be transient colic. This colic is self-limited and does not need any treatment. The colic-inducing foods are different for different infants. Some infants have no trouble. During the period of colic the infant may need frequent small feedings and much cuddling. Sometimes the infants overfeed, then vomit and settle down and go quietly to sleep, just as an overfed bottle infant does.

The distress or discomfort may be due to tension, and "colic" has been noted to be more common in the first infants of high-strung mothers. Colic has been associated with hormone withdrawal and has been treated with progesterone. In the breastfed baby this is a less likely cause because of the presence of hormones in breast milk. Allergy to cow's milk can be manifest by bouts of pain and crying, and switching to hypoallergenic milk may help the bottle fed infant. The breastfed infant may be reacting to something in the mother's diet, which can be easily eliminated after it is identified by association. Colicky breastfed infants who are weaned to formula are usually much worse. Weaning is not an appropriate treatment for the colicky breastfed infant in most cases. Colic usually diminishes in the third month of life, when the infant's gastrointestinal tract matures.

Another explanation for colic and failure to thrive has been suggested by Woolrich and Fisher[116] who note that when an infant is taken from the first breast and switched to the second, it may decrease the amount of fat and energy received. In addition, it will take more volume to get enough calories with symptoms of hunger with crying and fretfulness. Lower fat causes rapid gastric emptying with less digestion of lactose, thus producing diarrhea. It may be appropriate for such an infant to empty the first breast before switching.

REFERENCES

1. Adams LM and Davidson M: Present concepts of infant colic, Pediatr Ann 16:817, 1987.
2. Alley JM and Rogers CS: Sleep patterns of breast-fed and non breast-fed infants, Pediatr Nurs 12:349, 1986.
3. Almroth SG: Water requirements of breastfed infants in a hot climate, Am J Clin Nutr 31:1154, 1978.
4. Amado A, Lawrence RA, and Roghman K: Perinatal home care: a report on a Blue Cross and home care effort, Caring 2:27, 1983.
5. Amatayakul K, Vutyavanich T, Tanthayaphinant O et al: Serum prolactin and cortisol levels after suckling for varying periods of time and the effect of a nipple shield, Acta Obstet Gynecol Scand 66:47, 1987.
6. Anderson GC et al: Development of sucking in term infants from birth to four hours post birth, Res Nurs Health 5:21, 1982.
7. Aono T et al: Effect of sulpiride on poor puerperal lactation, Am J Obstet Gynecol 143:927, 1982.
8. Aono T et al: The initiation of human lactation and prolactin response to suckling, J Clin Endocrinol Metab 44:1101, 1977.
9. Ardran GM, Kemp FH, and Lind J: A cineradiographic study of bottle feeding, Br J Radiol 31:11, 1958.
10. Ardran GM, Kemp FH, and Lind J: A cineradiographic study of breast feeding, Br J Radiol 31:156, 1958.
11. Armelini PA and Gonzalez CF: Breastfeeding and fluid intake in a hot climate, Clin Pediatr 18:424, 1979.
12. Barnes GR et al: Management of breast feeding, JAMA 151:192, 1953.
13. Bentovim A: Shame and other anxieties associated with breast feeding: a systems theory and psychodynamic approach. In Ciba Foundation Symposium, no 45, Breast feeding and the mother, Amsterdam, 1976, Elsevier Scientific Publ Co
14. Blass EM and Teicher MH: Suckling, Science 210:15, 1980.
15. Bowen-Jones A, Thompson C, and Drewett RF: Milk flow and sucking rates during breastfeeding, Dev Med Child Neurol 24:626, 1982.
16. Brazelton TB: Effect of maternal medication on the neonate and his behavior, J Pediatr 58:513, 1961.
17. Bremme K, Eneroth P, and Kindahl H: 15-Keto-13, 14-dihydroprostaglandin F_{2a}, and prolactin in maternal and cord blood during prostaglandin E_2 or oxytocin therapy for labor induction, J Perinat Med 15:143, 1987.
18. Brenman HS et al: Multisensor nipple recording oral variables, J Appl Physiol 26:494, 1969.
19. Brown MS and Hurlock JT: Preparation of the breast for breastfeeding, Nurs Res 24:448, 1975.
20. Burke PM: Swallowing and the organization of sucking in the human newborn, Child Dev 48:523, 1977.
21. Butte NF et al: Evaluation of the deuterium dilution technique against the test-weighing procedure for the determination of breast milk intake, Am J Clin Nutr 37:996, 1983.
22. Butte NF, Wills C, Jean CA et al: Feeding patterns of exclusively breastfed infants during the first four months of life, Early Hum Dev 12:291, 1985.
23. Caldeyro-Barcia R: Milk ejection in women. In Reynolds M and Folley SJ, editors: Lactogenesis, Philadelphia, 1969, University of Pennsylvania Press.
24. Carlson HE, Wasser HL, and Reidelberger RD: Beer-induced prolactin secretion: a clinical and laboratory study of the role of salsolinol, J Clin Endocrinol Metab 60:673, 1985.
25. Chayen B, Tejani N, and Verma U: Induction of labor with an electric breast pump, J Reprod Med 31:116, 1986.
26. Christensen S, Dubignon J, and Campbell D: Variations in intra-oral stimulation and nutritive sucking, Child Dev 47:539, 1976.
27. Cobo E et al: Neurohypophyseal hormone release in the human. II. Experimental study during lactation, Am J Obstet Gynecol 97:519, 1967.
28. Conner AE: Elevated levels of sodium and chloride in milk from mastitic breast, Pediatrics 63:910, 1979.
29. Cross BA: Comparative physiology of milk removal, Symp Zool Soc 41:193, 1977.
30. Davis HV et al: Effects of cup, bottle, and breast feeding on oral activities of newborn infants, Pediatrics 2:549, 1948.
31. Dawood MY et al: Oxytocin release and plasma anterior pituitary and gonadal hormones in women during lactation, J Clin Endocrinol Metab 52:678, 1981.

32. DeRosa G, Corsello SM, Ruffilli MP et al: Pro-lactin secretion after beer, Lancet 2:934, 1981.

33. Devereux WP: Acute puerperal mastitis, Am J Obstet Gynecol 108:78, 1970.

34. Dewey KG and Lonnerdal B: Infant self-regulation of breast milk intake, Acta Paediatr Scand 75:893, 1986.

35. Drewett RF: Returning to the suckled breast: a further test of Hall's hypothesis, Early Hum Dev 6:161, 1982.

36. Elder MS: The effects of temperature and position on the sucking pressure of newborn infants, Child Dev 41:95, 1970.

37. Elliott JP and Flaherty JF: The use of breast stimulation to ripen the cervix in term pregnancies, Am J Obstet Gynecol 145:553, 1983.

38. Evans RW et al: Maternal diet and infantile colic in breast-fed infants, Lancet 1:1340, 1981.

39. Fisher SE, Painter M, and Milmor G: Swallowing disorders in infancy: symposium on pediatric otolaryngology, Pediatr Clin North Am 28:845, 1981.

40. Frantz K: Techniques for successfully managing nipple problems and the reluctant nurser in the early postpartum period. In Freier S and Eidelman A, editors: Human milk: its biological and social value, Amsterdam, 1980, Excerpta Medica.

41. Gerrard JW and Shenassa M: Sensitization to substances in breast milk: recognition, management and significance, Ann Allergy 51:1300, 1983.

42. Goldberg NM and Adams E: Supplementary water for breastfed babies in a hot and dry climate—not really a necessity, Arch Dis Child 58(1):73, 1983.

43. Goldsmith HS: Milk-rejection sign of breast cancer, Am J Surg 127:280, 1974.

44. Gray-Donald K, Kramer MS, Munday S et al: Effect of formula supplementation in the hospital on the duration of breastfeeding: a controlled clinical trial, Pediatrics 75:514, 1985.

45. Grossman ER: Beer, breastfeeding, and the wisdom of old wives (letter), JAMA 259:1016, 1988.

46. Gupta R, Gupta AS, and Duggal N: Tubercular mastitis, Int Surg 67:422, 1982.

47. Hall B: Changing composition of human milk and early development of an appetite control, Lancet 1:779, 1975.

48. Hauben DJ and Mahler D: A simple method for the correction of the inverted nipple, Plast Reconstr Surg 71:556, 1983.

49. Heck LJ and Erenberg A: Serum glucose levels in term neonates during the first 48 hours of life, J Pediatr 110:119, 1987.

50. Herd B and Feeney JG: Two aerosol sprays and nipple trauma, Practitioner 230:31, 1986.

51. Herreara AJ: Supplemented versus unsupplemented breastfeeding, Perinatol-Neonatol 8:70, 1984.

52. Hewat RJ and Ellis DJ: A comparison of the effectiveness of two methods of nipple care, Birth 14:41, 1987.

53. Hide DW and Guyer BM: Prevalence of infant colic, Arch Dis Child 57:559, 1982.

54. Hoffmann JB: A suggested treatment for inverted nipples, Am J Obstet Gynecol 66:346, 1953.

55. Horowitz M et al: Effect of modification of fluid intake on puerperium on serum prolactin levels and lactation, Med J Aust 2:625, 1980.

56. Howie PW et al: The relationship between suckling-induced prolactin response and lactogenesis, J Clin Endocrinol Metab 50:670, 1980.

57. Hunziker UA and Barr RG: Increased carrying reduces infant crying: a randomized controlled trial, Pediatrics 77:641, 1986.

58. Inch S and Fisher C: Antiseptic sprays and nipple trauma, Practitioner 230:1037, 1986.

59. Jakobsson I and Lindberg T: Cow's milk as a cause of infantile colic in breast-fed infants, Lancet 2:437, 1978.

60. Jakobsson I and Lindberg T: Cow's milk proteins cause infantile colic in breast-fed infants: a double-blind crossover study, Pediatrics 71:268, 1983.

61. Jakobsson I, Lindberg T, Benediksson B et al: Dietary bovine β-lactoglobulin is transferred to human milk, Acta Paediatr Scand 74:342, 1985.

62. Johnson P and Salisbury DM: Breathing and sucking during feeding in the newborn. In Bosma JF and Showacre J, editors: Development of upper respiratory anatomy and function, Bethesda, 1975, National Institutes of Health.

63. Katzmen DK and Wald ER: Staphylococcal scalded skin syndrome in a breastfed infant, Pediatr Inf Dis J 6:295, 1987.

64. Klaus MH: The frequency of suckling, Obstet Gynecol Clin North Am 14:623, 1987.

65. Kron RE, Stein M, and Goddard KE: Newborn sucking behavior affected by obstetric sedation, Pediatrics 37:1012, 1966.

66. Lipitz S, Barkai G, Rabinovici J, et al: Breast stimulation test and oxytocin challenge test in fetal surveillance: a prospective randomized study, Am J Obstet Gynecol 157:1178, 1987.

67. Lucas A, Lucas PJ and Baum JD: Differences in the pattern of milk intake between breast and bottle fed infants, Early Hum Dev 5:195, 1981.

68. Leonard EL, Trykowski LE, and Kirkpatrick BV: Nutritive sucking in high-risk neonates after perioral stimulation, Phys Ther 60:299, 1980.

69. L'Esperance CM: Pain or pleasure: the dilemma of early breastfeeding, Birth Fam J 7:21, 1980.

70. Lozoff B et al: The mother-newborn relationship: limits of adaptability, J Pediatr 91:1, 1977.
71. Maekawa K, Nara T, and Hoasti E: Influence of breastfeeding on neonatal behavior, Acta Paediatr Jpn 27:608, 1985.
72. Marshall BR, Hepper JK, and Zirbel CC: Sporadic puerperal mastitis, JAMA 233:1377, 1975.
73. Mashini IS, Devoe LD, McKenzie JS et al: Comparison of uterine activity by nipple stimulation and oxytocin, Obstet Gynecol 69:74, 1987.
74. McNeilly AS et al: Release of oxytocin and prolactin in response to suckling, Br Med J 286:257, 1983.
75. Neifert MR and Seacat JM: A guide to successful breastfeeding. Contemp Pediatr 3:26, 1986.
76. Newton M and Newton N: The let-down reflex in human lactation, J Pediatr 33:698, 1948.
77. Newton M and Newton N: The normal course and management of lactation, Clin Obset Gynecol 5:44, 1962.
78. Newton N: Nipple pain and nipple damage problems in the management of breast feeding, J Pediatr 41:411, 1952.
79. Newton N and Newton M: Relationship of ability to breast feed and maternal attitudes toward breast feeding, Pediatrics 5:869, 1950.
80. Niebyl JR, Spence MR, and Parmley TH: Sporadic (nonepidemic) puerperal mastitis, J Reprod Med 20:97, 1978.
81. Nowlis GH and Kessen W: Human newborns differentiate differing concentrations of sucrose and glucose, Science 191:865, 1976.
82. Nysenbaum AN, and Smart JL: Sucking behavior and milk intake of neonates in relation to milk fat content, Early Hum Dev 6:205, 1982.
83. Olsen A: Nursing under conditions of thirst or excessive ingestion of fluids, Acta Obstet Gynecol 20:313, 1939.
84. Pollitt E, Consolazio B, and Goodkin F: Changes in nutritive sucking during a feed in two-day and thirty-day-old infants, Early Hum Dev 5:201, 1981.
85. Prentice A and Prentice AM: Unilateral breast dysfunction in lactating Gambian women, Ann Trop Pediatr 4:19, 1984.
86. Prentice A, Prentice AM, and Lamb WH: Mastitis in rural Gambian mothers and the protection of the breast by milk antimicrobial factors, Trans Roy Soc Trop Med Hyg 79:90, 1985.
87. Raphael D: The tender gift: breast feeding, New York, 1976, Schocken Books, Inc.
88. Rayner CR: The correction of permanently inverted nipples, Br J Plast Surg 33:413, 1980.
89. Reiff MI and Essock-Vitale SM: Hospital influences on early infant feeding, Pract Pediatr 76:872, 1985.
90. Riordan J: A practical guide to breastfeeding, St. Louis, 1983, The CV Mosby Co.
91. Salisbury DM: Bottle-feeding: influence of teat hole size on suck volume, Lancet 1:655, 1975.
92. Schutzman DL, Hervada AR, and Branca PA: Effect of water supplementation of full term newborns on arrival of milk in the nursing mother, Clin Pediatr 25:78, 1986.
93. Skoog T: Surgical correction of inverted nipples, J Am Med Wom Assoc 20:931, 1965.
94. Smith WL, Erenberg A, and Nowark A: Imaging evaluation of the human nipple during breastfeeding, Am J Dis Child 142:76, 1988.
95. Smith WL, Erenberg A, Nowak A et al: Physiology of sucking in the normal term infant using real time, US Radiol 156:379, 1985.
96. Süsswein J: Zur Physiologie des Trinkens beim Säugling, Arch Kinder Heilkd 40:68, 1905.
97. Talbot FB: Eczema in childhood, Med Clin North Am 1:985, 1918.
98. Taylor RN and Green JR: Abruptio placentae following nipple simulation, Am J Perinatol 4:94, 1987.
99. Thomas DW, McGilligan K, Eisenberg LD et al: Infantile colic and type of milk feeding, AJDC 141:451, 1987.
100. Thomsen AC: Infectious mastitis and occurrence of antibody-coated bacteria in milk, Am J Obstet Gynecol 144:350, 1982.
101. Thomsen AC, Espersen T, and Maigaard S: Course and treatment of milk stasis, noninfectious inflammation of the breast, and infectious mastitis in nursing women, Am J Obstet Gynecol 149:492, 1984.
102. Thomsen AC, Morgensen SC, and Jepson FL: Experimental mastitis in mice induced by coagulase-negative staphylococci isolated from cases of mastitis in nursing women, Acta Obstet Gynecol Scand 64:163, 1985.
103. Toppozada MK, El-Rahman HA, and Soliman AY: Prostaglandins as milk ejectors: the nose as a new route of administration, Adv Prost Thrombox Leukotr Res 12:449, 1983.
104. Waldenstrom U, Sundelin C, and Lindmark G: Early and late discharge after hospital birth: breastfeeding, Acta Paediatr Scand 76:727, 1987.
105. Walsh M and McIntosh K: Neonatal mastitis, Clin Pediatr 25:395, 1986.
106. Weber F, Woolridge MW, and Baum JD: An ultrasonographic study of the organization of sucking and swallowing by newborn infants, Dev Med Child Neurol 28:19, 1986.
107. Weitzmen RE et al: The effect of nursing on neurohypophyseal hormone and prolactin secretion in human subjects, J Clin Endocrinol Metab 51:836, 1980.

108. Whitfield ME, Kay R, and Stevens S: Validity of routine clinical test weighing as a measure of the intake of breast-fed infants, Arch Dis Child 56:919, 1981.

109. Wolff PH: Sucking patterns of infant mammals, Brain Behav Evol 1:354, 1968.

110. Wolff PH: The serial organization of sucking in the young infant, Pediatrics 42:943, 1968.

111. Woolridge MW: Aetiology of sore nipples, Midwifery 2:172, 1986.

112. Woolridge MW: The "anatomy" of infant sucking, Midwifery 2:164, 1986.

113. Woolridge MW, Baum JD, and Drewett RF: Does a change in the composition of human milk affect sucking patterns and milk intake, Lancet 2:1292, 1980.

114. Woolridge MW, Baum JD, and Drewett RF: Effect of a traditional and of a new nipple shield on sucking patterns and milk flow, Early Hum Dev 4:357, 1980.

115. Woolridge MW et al: The continuous measurement of milk intake at a feed in breast-fed babies, Early Hum Dev 6:365, 1982.

116. Woolridge MW and Fisher C: Colic, "overfeeding," and symptoms of lactose malabsorption in the breast-fed baby: a possible artifact of feed management, Lancet 2:382, 1988.

117. Young D: Personal communication, 1978.

Diet and dietary supplements for the mother and infant

9

Lactation is the physiologic completion of the reproductive cycle, and the maternal body prepares during pregnancy for lactation not only by developing the breast to produce milk but also by storing additional nutrients and energy. For milk production the transition to fully sustaining the infant should not be complex or require major adjustments for the mother. After delivery mothers usually note an increase in appetite and thirst and a change in some dietary preferences. In simple cultures, anthropologists have noted that tradition prescribes upon the birth of a baby bringing gifts of special foods—usually high in protein, nutrients, and calories—for the mother to ensure she will make good milk for the infant. This tradition may have affected some early studies where relatively malnourished women were noted to produce milk comparable to that produced by well-nourished women in industrialized countries.

The Committee on Recommended Dietary Allowances of the Food and Nutrition Board[58] considers the question of diet for the lactating mother fully answered by saying the diet should supply somewhat more of each nutrient than that recommended for the nonpregnant female.* Most writings for the nursing mother regarding maternal diet during lactation set up complicated "rules" about dietary intake that fail to consider the mother's dietary stores and normal dietary preferences. Thus one barrier to breastfeeding for some women is the "diet rules" they see as too hard to follow or too restrictive.[31] Therefore the physician and nutritionist must understand the simple requirements and wide acceptable variations so that dietary guidelines make minimal demands on a woman's lifestyle. All over the world women produce adequate and even abundant milk on very inadequate diets.[42] Women in primitive cultures with modest but adequate diets produce milk without any obvious detriment to themselves and none of the fatigue and loss of well-being that some well-fed Western mothers experience.

IMPACT OF MATERNAL DIET ON MILK PRODUCTION

Although much has been learned about dietary requirements for lactation by studying women from many cultures[43] and various levels of poor nutrition, some of the information is conflicting principally because of varying sampling techniques and the improvement

---

*A Committee on Lactation of the Food and Nutrition Board is scheduled to report on these requirements for the first time in 1991.

over time in laboratory analysis. Extensive reviews of the current literature on various nutrients in human milk and the influence of maternal dietary intake have been referenced.[27,49,51,55,83] Those readers needing access to the original studies are referred to the bibliographies from these reviews, which include hundreds of items, a listing beyond the scope of this text.

Volume

The volume of milk produced varies over the duration of lactation from the first few weeks to 6 months and beyond but is remarkably predictable except for extreme malnutrition or severe dehydration. In periods of acute water deprivation manifest in the healthy mother by an acute bout of vomiting and diarrhea, the volume of milk will diminish only after the maternal urinary output has been significantly compromised (10% dehydration). Malnutrition, on the other hand, is complex, and single-nutrient deficiencies are rare. Malnutrition does seem to have an effect on the total volume of milk produced. In the extreme, when famine occurs, the milk supply dwindles and ceases, with ultimate starvation of the infant. The classic study is the report of Smith[71] on the effects of maternal undernutrition on the newborn infant in the Hunger Winter in Holland in 1944 to 1945. It was reported that the volume of milk was slightly diminished, but the duration of lactation was not affected. The latter is a testimony to courage rather than diet. Analysis of milk produced showed no significant deviations from normal chemical structure. Milk was produced at the expense of maternal tissue.

These data from the Dutch famine were reexamined by Stein et al.,[76] who pointed out that the women who had conceived during the famine did develop some maternal stores in anticipation of lactation that were not accounted for by the fetus, placenta, or amniotic fluid even though the fetus was a pound lighter at birth. They reported fetal weight down by 10% but maternal weight down by only 4%. This demonstrates the maternal body's strong commitment to preparing for lactation during pregnancy.

In countries where foods supplies vary with the season, milk supplies drop 1 dl/day during periods of progressively greater food shortage. Studies continue on lactation performance of poorly nourished women around the world, including Burma, The Gambia, New Guinea, and Ethiopia as well as among the Navajo. Results continue to reflect an impact on quantity, not quality, of milk.[9,18,46,60,69]

When food is supplemented, the volume output and protein content increase (Table 9-1). Edozien et al.[23] showed in a Nigerian village that the ultimate result of supplementing maternal diet with protein and kilocalories was an increased rate of weight gain in the infant. Sosa et al.[73] have shown a dramatic increase in milk volume by supplementing maternal diets in Guatemala (Fig. 9-1, *A*). The weight gain in these infants is shown in Fig. 9-1, *B*. Thus an inadequate diet seemed to affect volume and not the composition because the breast depleted the maternal stores of nutrients to maintain the proper composition of milk.

The interrelationship of milk volume, nutrient concentration, and total nutrient intake by the infant has to be considered. The reason for low protein content in a given sample may be lack of protein, lack of total energy content, or lack of vitamin B_6, a requirement of normal protein metabolism.

Of great concern, however, is the report of dietary supplementation of Gambian nursing mothers in which the lactational performance was not affected by increased calories (700 kcal/day).[63] The supplement produced a slight initial improvement in maternal body

Table 9-1. Effect of maternal dietary supplementation with protein on volume and protein content of breast milk and weight gained by baby (Nigeria)*

	Daily protein intake					
	50 g (initially, mean ± SD)	100 g (mean ± SD)	P	25 g (initially, mean ± SD)	100 g (mean ± SD)	P
Number of subjects	7	7		3	3	
Total milk solids (g/100 ml)	13.8 ± 1.3	13.4 ± 0.9		12.0 ± 0.6	11.9 ± 0.5	
Milk protein (g/100 ml)	1.61 ± 0.15	1.57 ± 0.19		1.20 ± 0.21	1.25 ± 0.23	
Milk lactose (g/100 ml)	8.1 ± 0.9	7.9 ± 1.0		7.3 ± 1.4	8.0 ± 1.8	
Milk produced (ml/day)	742 ± 16	872 ± 32	<0.05	817 ± 59	1059 ± 63	<0.05
Milk consumed (ml/day)	617 ± 15	719 ± 10	<0.05	777 ± 38	996 ± 74	<0.05
Weight gained by infant (g/day)	30.4 ± 3.6	45.7 ± 2.0	<0.05	10.5 ± 3.6	32.2 ± 10.1	<0.05

From Edozien JC, Rahim-Khan MA, and Waslien CI: J Nutr 106:312, 1976, Copyright © American Institute of Nutrition.
*Subjects were fed the initial diets for the first 14 days and then a diet providing 100 g protein/day for the next 14 days. Results for each subject represent the mean value for milk samples collected during days 8 to 14 (for initial diet) and days 21 to 28 (for diet providing 100 g protein/day). Duration of lactation for all subjects was between 30 and 90 days.

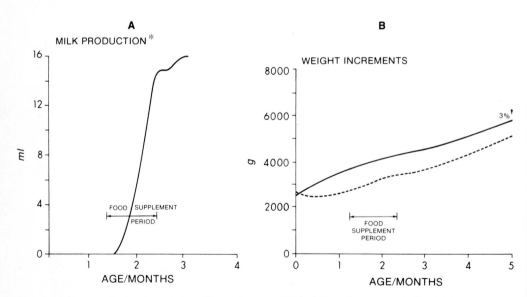

Fig. 9-1. **A,** Increments in milk production during maternal supplementation period. *Milliliters of milk obtained 1 hour after milk production. **B,** Weight increments of infants during maternal supplementation and follow-up period. †Boston growth curves. (From Sosa R, Klaus M, and Urrutia JJ: J Pediatr 88:668, 1976.)

Table 9-2. Comparison of milks of healthy and malnourished mothers

Factors	Apparently healthy		Clinically malnourished	
	Range	Mean	Range	Mean
Protein (g/100 ml)	0.95-1.36	1.09	0.76-1.32	0.93
Lactose (g/100 ml)	5.58-7.95	6.65	4.08-8.29	6.48
Fat (g/100 ml)	2.8-6.8	4.43	2.8-6.2	4.01
Calories (kcal/100 ml)	61-92	70.8	48-78	65.8
Amount (ml/day)	450-1290	922	180-1770	723
Protein (g/day)	4.3-15.0	10.02	1.6-14.9	6.65
Calories (kcal/day)	310-900	648	100-1080	475

Modified from Hanafy MM et al: J Trop Pediatr 18:188, 1972.

weight and subcutaneous fat but not in milk output. Whether the mothers utilized the increased energy to work harder farming or whether the infants did not stimulate increased milk production is unresolved. These observations suggest that other assessments are necessary before conclusions about supplementation are revised. The Committee on Nutrition of the Academy of Pediatrics suggests that the data in support of the value of protein supplements justify a recommendation that malnourished mothers receive additional supplements.[16]

Protein content

Since the work of Hambraeus et al.[35] has reestablished the norms for protein in human milk to be 0.8 to 0.9 g/100 ml in well-nourished mothers, figures from previous studies will have to be recalculated to consider the fact that all nitrogen in human milk is not protein (25% of the nitrogen is nonprotein nitrogen [NPN] in human milk, and 5% of the nitrogen is NPN in bovine milk). The protein content of milk from poorly nourished mothers is surprisingly high, and malnutrition has little effect on protein concentration. An increase in dietary protein increases volume but not overall protein content, given the normal variations seen in healthy well-nourished women.

Observations made over a 20-month period of continued lactation showed that milk quality did not change, although the quantity decreased slightly, which Von Mural[79] attributed to the decreasing demand of a child who is receiving other nourishment. Therefore the total protein available with the decreased volume of milk and increased weight of the child decreased from 2.2 g/kg of body weight to 0.45 g/kg. The need for additional protein sources for the child after 1 year of age becomes obvious.

A painstaking study by Hanafy et al.[36] comparing maternal nutrition and lactation performance demonstrates what most clinicians have believed must be true: The well-fed lactating mother is more likely to produce a healthy infant. The investigators compared two groups of urban mothers of a moderate to poor socioeconomic standard in Egypt. The groups were similar except for the state of nutrition. The comparison of their milks is presented in Table 9-2. The ultimate goal of lactation is a healthy, growing infant. One must recognize that the foundation for good nutrition in any infant is established in utero. Nonetheless, significant differences in growth were shown by the two groups (Table 9-3).

The effect of very low-protein (8% of energy) and very high-protein (20% of energy) diets on the protein and nitrogen composition of breast milk in three healthy Swedish

Table 9-3. Comparison of infants of healthy and malnourished mothers

Factors	Apparently healthy		Clinically malnourished	
	Range	Mean	Range	Mean
Age (mo)	1-10	5.0	1-12	4.7
Arm circumference (% of predicted)*	43-133	72	43-102	70
Weight (% of predicted)*	60-139	102	43-120	86
Height (% of predicted)*	87-106	94	76-106	93
Serum albumin (g/100 ml)	1.8-4.6	3.11	1.2-3.7	2.50
NSII†	55-119	83	45-101	70

Modified from Hanafy MM et al: J Trop Pediatr 18:189, 1972.
*Percent of predicted value.
†Nutritional state index of infants.

Table 9-4. Milk production over the first 4 months of lactation

	Mo 1 (n = 37)		Mo 2 (n = 40)		Mo 3 (n = 37)		Mo 4 (n = 41)	
Human milk* (g/day)	751	(130)†	725	(131)	723	(114)	740	(128)
Feedings (no/day)	8.3	(1.9)	7.2	(1.9)	6.8	(1.9)	6.7	(1.8)
Total nitrogen (mg/g)	2.17	(0.30)	1.94	(0.24)	1.84	(0.19)	1.80	(0.21)
Protein nitrogen (mg/g)	1.61	(0.24)	1.42	(0.17)	1.34	(0.15)	1.31	(0.17)
Nonprotein nitrogen (mg/g)	0.56	(0.28)	0.52	(0.20)	0.50	(0.13)	0.48	(0.14)
Fat (mg/g)	36.2	(7.5)	34.4	(6.8)	32.2	(7.8)	34.8	(10.8)
Energy (kcal/g)	0.68	(0.08)	0.64	(0.08)	0.62	(0.09)	0.64	(0.10)

*At the onset of the study, milk was estimated by deuterium dilution, a technique that was later determined to be inaccurate. For this reason, data are missing at 17 time points during the first 3 months.
†Mean (SD).

women "in full lactation" was significant.[29] High-protein diets produced higher production and greater concentrations of total nitrogen, true protein, and NPN. The increased NPN was due to increased urea levels and free amino acids. The 24-hour outputs of lactoferrin, lactalbumin, and serum albumin were not significantly higher. The practical significance, except as related to fad diets, of these results is limited because the diets were extreme and were maintained for only 4 days. The impact on human nutritional physiology, however, is significant.

Of practical significance for counseling the healthy woman in the industrialized world is the work of Butte and colleagues[10] investigating the effect of maternal diet and body composition on lactational performance. Forty-five healthy lactating women were followed for 4 months from delivery with detailed measurements of milk production, dietary intake, and maternal body composition. The overall mean energy intake was 2186 ($\pm$463) kcal/day. Milk production averaged 751, 725, 723, and 740 g/day for months 1, 2, 3, and 4. Average maternal weight reduction was from 64.6 kg to 59.3 kg. Energy was calculated to be sufficient for maintenance and activity, yet the mothers achieved gradual weight reduction. The authors conclude that energy intakes less than currently recommended by about 15% are compatible with full lactation, full activity, and gradual weight reduction to prepregnant weight (see Tables 9-4 and 9-5). Diets otherwise contained recommended daily allowances for lactation. Other investigators studying the impact of weight loss noted

Table 9-5. Anthropometric changes in mothers during lactation

Parameter	Postpartum	Mo 1	Mo 2	Mo 3	Mo 4
Wt (kg)	64.6 (9.1)*	61.3 (9.5)	60.7 (10.0)	60.2 (10.4)	59.3 (10.5)
Wt/ht (kg/cm)†	0.40 (0.04)	0.37 (0.05)	0.37 (0.05)	0.37 (0.05)	0.36 (0.06)
Wt/prepregnancy wt‡	1.16 (0.06)	1.08 (0.05)	1.07 (0.05)	1.06 (0.05)	1.05 (0.07)
Wt change (kg/mo)		-3.83 (2.26)	-0.59 (1.20)	-0.62 (1.12)	-0.80 (1.86)
Triceps (mm)	16.3 (5.1)	16.9 (4.6)	17.0 (4.7)	17.3 (5.3)	17.2 (5.2)
Subscapular (mm)	18.2 (7.1)	16.8 (6.4)	16.4 (7.4)	15.7 (7.2)	15.1 (7.3)
Biceps (mm)	7.8 (3.9)	6.9 (3.2)	6.9 (3.3)	7.3 (4.6)	6.8 (3.4)
Suprailiac (mm)	26.1 (8.5)	25.7 (6.9)	25.2 (7.6)	23.1 (8.1)	22.2 (8.0)
Sum skinfolds (mm)	68.4 (20.2)	66.3 (18.9)	65.5 (20.6)	63.4 (22.9)	61.7 (21.8)
Midarm circumference (cm)	26.9 (3.5)	26.7 (2.6)	26.8 (3.2)	26.6 (2.9)	26.7 (3.6)

From Butte NF et al: Am J Clin Nutr 39:296, 1984.

*Mean (SD).

†Maternal ht = 163.0 (6.3 cm).

‡Prepregnancy wt gain = 14.4 (3.3 kg).

that the rate of postpregnancy weight loss affected the level of elaidic acid in milk and of trans-fatty acid level.[13] This is explained by the mobilization of fatty acids from adipose tissue.

Fat and cholesterol

Considerable interest has been focused on the impact of dietary fat and cholesterol on the composition of human milk. Fat is the main source of kilocalories in human milk for the infant. The fatty acid composition of the triglycerides, which make up over 98% of the lipid compartment of human milk, can be affected by maternal diet. Diets with different lipid composition, caloric content, proportion of calories from fat, and fatty acid composition have been studied. In a classic work that was carefully controlled, Insull et al.[41] fed a lactating woman in a metabolic ward diets that differed in caloric content, proportion of calories from fat, and fatty acid composition. Neither milk volume nor total milk fat was affected by diet. When the high-calorie, no-fat diet was fed, milk triglycerides were higher in 12:0 and 14:0 and lower in 18:0 and 18:1, which indicated that when fatty acids were synthesized from carbohydrate, there were more intermediate-chain fatty acids. When the low-calorie, no-fat diet was fed, the fatty acid composition of the milk resembled the maintenance diet and the depot fat. When corn oil was the fat source, milk levels of 18:2 and 18:3 were higher, with a major increase in linoleic acid, than when lard or butter was used. Multiple studies have shown that medium-chain fatty acids, lauric and myristic acid (12:0 and 14:0), are not affected by diet, indicating synthesis by the mammary gland.[26,51,55]

Trans-fatty acids are produced in hydrogenation reactions and appear in human milk as a reflection of dietary intake, so that women who eat margarine rather than butter have high levels in their milk. Elaidic acid (18:1 trans) is found in margarine, for instance. Because of the high level of trans-fatty acids in hydrogenated vegetable oils such as margarine, the milk of U.S. women is high in trans-fatty acids, whereas the milk of West German women is low in trans-fatty acids.[26] There is considerable controversy about the biologic effects. In mammals, trans-isomers have been noted to alter permeability and fluidity of membranes, inhibit a number of enzyme reactions of lipid metabolism, and impair synthesis of arachidonic acid and prostaglandins.

The concern about fat composition in terms of the polyunsaturated fatty acid (PUFA) to saturated fatty acid ratio (P/S ratio) and the high level of cholesterol normally found in breast milk have led to monitoring mothers on altered lipid intakes. Potter and Nestel[62] studied lactating women who were placed on one of two experimental diets after a period of a study of their normal Australian diet, which includes 400 to 600 mg of cholesterol/day and fat that is rich in saturated fatty acids. Following this baseline study, the mothers were either given diet A, with 580 mg cholesterol and a high level of saturated fats, or diet B, with 110 mg cholesterol and a higher level of polyunsaturated fats from vegetable oils. A second study was carried out with the two diets high in either saturated or unsaturated fats, but the cholesterol remained the same, 345 to 380 mg/day.

The low-cholesterol diets lowered the maternal blood cholesterol but not the triglyceride levels. The cholesterol level of the milk, however, was unaffected in any diet combination. The increase in PUFA in the diet rapidly increased the levels of linoleate in the milk to twice the previous level at the expense of myristate and palmitate. Protein levels remained the same in the milk throughout the study. Infant plasma cholesterol levels decreased in response to an increase in the concentration of linoleate in the milk. The

Table 9-6. Lipid concentrations of mature human milk

	Diet			Lipid concentration in milk		
Study	Plan	Saturation of fat*	Cholesterol (mg/day)	Cholesterol (mg/100 ml)	Triglyceride (g/100 ml)	Phospholipid (mg P/100 ml)
I (n = 7)	A	S	580	18.1 ± 2.7†	3.42 ± 0.61	4.04 ± 0.71
	B	P	110	19.3 ± 3.6	3.57 ± 0.82	4.18 ± 0.91
II (n = 3)	C	S	380	23.3 ± 2.3	4.11 ± 0.42	
	D	P	345	21.3 ± 2.4	4.12 ± 0.56	

From Potter JM and Nestel PJ: Am J Clin Nutr 29:54, 1976.
*S, rich in saturated fatty acids (P/S ~ 0.07); P, rich in polyunsaturated fatty acids (P/S ~ 1.3).
†Mean ± SEM.

significant dietary change seemed to depend on the consumption of high PUFA and low cholesterol to alter the levels in the milk and thus in the infant's plasma (Table 9-6).

Cholesterol levels remain relatively stable throughout at least 16 weeks of lactation. The presence or absence of phytosterols influences both the accuracy of analysis (i.e., overestimate level of cholesterol) and the physiologic significance of cholesterol. During a given feeding, the concentration of cholesterol in the milk may increase over 60%, although the total for the feeding is constant. The effect of maternal diet on cholesterol and phytosterol levels in human milk was measured by Mellies et al.,[56] who reported no change in cholesterol but a dramatic increase in phytosterols on high-cholesterol and/or phytosterol diets. The level of phytosterol in infant plasma did not change, however. These observations further confirm that cholesterol is synthesized at least in part in the mammary gland, while phytosterol is not. Phytosterols are those sterols derived from plant sources. They are distinguishable from cholesterol, which is of animal origin.

The synthesis of fatty acids up to the carbon number of 16, as well as the direct desaturation of stearic acid into oleic acid, can take place in the mammary gland, while longer-chain fatty acids come directly from plasma triglycerides (see Chapter 4). The intake of both carbohydrate and fat must be taken into account when evaluating maternal diet because high-carbohydrate diets increase lauric acid and myristic acid, and moderate levels of carbohydrate influence linoleic acid.

When serum lipids are measured in African women accustomed to a low fat intake, the levels are relatively low and the women are virtually free of coronary heart disease.[1] Among long-lactating (1 to 2 years minimum) African mothers, the amount of fat in their daily milk is of the same order as that ingested in their habitual diet. Despite this, they are not significantly hypolipidemic when compared with nonlactators.

Guthrie and associates[34] have provided data on the fatty acid patterns of human milk in correlation with the current American diet, which has a high P/S ratio. Compared with previous studies in 1953, 1958, and 1967, there was a shift toward higher levels of C18:2 fatty acids, linoleic acid, and C18:3 linolenic acid. Depot fat reflects dietary fatty acid patterns and thus the pool for mammary gland synthesis of milk fats. The mammary gland can dehydrogenate saturated and monosaturated fatty acids.

The habitual diet of healthy primiparas in Finland was associated with breast milk containing 3.8% fat.[80] Their diet was 16% protein, 39% fat, and 45% carbohydrate. Half the fatty acids of the diet and the milk were saturated, and one third were monoenoic. PUFAs were 15% of the diet and 13% of the breast milk, with a P/S ratio of 0.3 for both.

Table 9-7. Effect of various carbohydrate diets on milk composition

Milk components	Carbohydrate level in diet (g/kg body weight)		
	5-6	6-7	7-8
Protein (g/100 ml)	1.168	1.146	1.177
Fat (g/100 ml)	4.09	4.40	4.67
Lactose (g/100 ml)	7.30	7.38	7.38

Modified from Hytten FE and Thomson AM: Nutrition of the lactating woman. In Kon SK and Cowie AT, editors: Milk: the mammary gland and its secretion, vol 2, New York, 1961, Academic Press, Inc.; and Morrison SD: Technical communication bulletin no 18, London, 1952, Commonwealth Bureau of Animal Nutrition.

The maternal diet had no effect on total fat content of the milk except for the low level of oleic acid, which is apparently peculiar to Finnish breast milk.

A word of caution on the lowering of fats in the diet inordinately—evaluation of the effects of a low-fat maternal diet on neonatal rats by Sinclair and Crawford[70] is pertinent. They made the distinction between two types of lipid in animals—storage and structural. This is correlated with histologic findings of visible and invisible fats. Visible fats are triglycerides found in body depots. Invisible or structural fats include phosphoglycerides, sphingolipids, and some neutral lipids, including cholesterol. The structural fats are key constituents of cellular membranes, certain enzymes, and myelin. The brain contains more structural lipids than protein.

Sinclair and Crawford[70] found that neonatal rats born to mothers raised on low-fat diets had a higher mortality, and survivors had smaller body, brain, and liver weights than controls. The lipid content of the body, brain, and liver was significantly less than controls. During life, the rat pups had depended entirely on their mother's milk for nutrition.

Docosahexaenoic acid (DHA), a long-chain fatty acid $22:6 \omega 3$ has attracted attention, since deficiency has been associated with visual impairment in offspring of rhesus monkeys.[55] Human milk contains consistent levels; formulas contain little or none. DHA can be synthesized from linoleic acid, but high levels of linoleic acid suppress production. An excellent dietary source of DHA is fish oil, and women who consistently eat fish have higher levels in their milk. Vegetarians have higher DHA levels in their milk than omnivore controls.[26]

Lactose

Of all the nutrients in human milk, lactose is least likely to be affected by maternal diet or the level of blood glucose from which it is synthesized. The lactose level is recognized as being reasonably stable in human milk, which may be a function of the fact that lactose is a determinant of volume. Changes in the carbohydrate levels in the diet have been studied. Comparison of mothers on diets with three different levels of carbohydrate shows that the amounts of protein, fat, and carbohydrate in their milk are similar (Table 9-7).

Water

No data support the assumption that increasing fluid intake will increase milk volume. Conversely, restricting fluids has not been shown to decrease milk volume.[39,59] Forcing fluids, on the other hand, has been shown by Dusdieker et al.[21] to negatively affect milk production in a controlled crossover–design study of breastfeeding mothers. Thus, women taking excessive fluids produced less milk, suggesting that drinking to thirst and heeding body cues is more physiologic than prescribing a specific amount of fluid a day. This observation was first demonstrated in a 1939 study by Olsen, who concluded, "Forced, excessive drinking is therefore neither necessary nor beneficial as far as the nursing is concerned and may even be harmful."[59] He had studied great variations in quantity of fluids taken and also noted that "hypogalactia cannot be arrested by forced drinking beyond the natural dictates of thirst." Urinary output in these studies was proportional to intake. Illingworth and Kilpatrick[40] did a similar study in 210 postpartum mothers, half of whom drank ad lib, taking an average of 69 oz daily; the other half was forced to take 6 pints and averaged 107 oz daily. The mothers forced to drink beyond thirst produced less milk, and their babies gained less well.

From a practical standpoint, mothers have an increased thirst, which usually maintains a need for added fluid intake. When fluids are restricted, mothers will experience a decrease in urine output, not in milk. On the other hand, sharply decreasing fluids to prevent engorgement in the mother who is not lactating is ineffectual and only adds another inconvenience and discomfort.

Kilocalories

The caloric content, sample by sample, of milk from well-nourished mothers does vary somewhat but averages about 75 kcal/100 ml. Since fat is the chief source of kilocalories, the fat content has the greatest impact on total kilocalories, with lactose and protein also contributing to the total. Thus, in malnourished mothers the caloric content may be reduced.

Body fat increases during pregnancy and decreases during lactation. Changes in the adipose depot are primarily due to change in fat cell size, not number. Adipose tissue fatty acid synthesis remains low throughout lactation, as does lipoprotein lipase activity. Mammary lipoprotein lipase activity, on the other hand, increases and remains high during lactation.[77]

How does this correlate with the caloric needs of the mother to produce milk? The calculations for energy requirement have been made by comparing the energy intakes of nursing mothers and nonnursing mothers who were matched for other variables. English and Hitchcock[24] found that nursing mothers consumed 2460 kcal daily and nonnursing mothers consumed 1880 kcal, a net difference of 580 kcal.

Lactation will not produce a net drain on the mother if the amount of energy available and the requirement of any given nutrient are replaced in the diet. There is small energy cost of milk production, although the breast does work at remarkable efficiency. During pregnancy, fat and other nutrients are stored for the fetus and in preparation for lactation. Lactation is subsidized, as is fetal growth, by maternal stores, even though the diet on any given day may be relatively deficient in a specific nutrient. This can be clarified by Fig. 9-2, which shows that diet and stores are available for milk, as well as for maintenance of the mother.

Although the recommended daily allowance published by the National Research Council[58] for lactation is set at baseline plus 500 to 1000 kcal or 2600 kcal total, calculations of actual intakes in well-nourished women are less than this. Similar surveys among poorly nourished, fully lactating women report 1600 to 1800 kcal intakes. A study of 26 healthy, normotensive, nonsmoking, euthyroid women—12 of whom were breastfeeding, 7 bottle feeding, and 7 nonpregnant, nonlactating controls—was reported by Illingworth et al.[39]

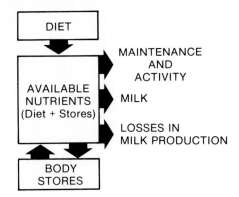

Fig. 9-2. Energy utilization in lactation, showing availability of body stores and dietary sources.

Energy expenditure at rest and in response to a meal and to an infusion of noradrenaline was measured. During lactation the resting metabolic rate was unaltered, but there was a reduced response to infusion of noradrenaline and to a meal. These responses returned to normal control values in these women postlactation. Bottle feeders were similar to controls. The metabolic efficiency of the individual is greatly enhanced during lactation and results in a reduction in the nonlactational component of maternal energy expenditure (Fig. 9-3).

The maternal energy requirement can be calculated by determining the caloric content of the milk itself, plus an allowance for the energy cost of production. Using this formula, if there is 850 ml of milk with 600 kcal and the production efficiency is estimated at 60%, then the additional caloric need each day will be 1000 kcal minus 250 kcal to be used from extra body stores accrued during pregnancy.

Vitamins
Water-soluble vitamins

Water-soluble vitamins move with ease from serum to milk; thus, their dietary fluctuation is more apparent. Levels of water-soluble vitamins in milk are raised or lowered by change in the maternal diet. The body's requirement for vitamin C increases under stress, including lactation. Furthermore, the vitamin C content of human organs at autopsy is much higher in the neonate than at any other time of life. This is true of all the major organs, including the brain.

The influence of maternal intake of vitamin C on the concentration of vitamin C in human milk and on the intake of vitamin C by the infant was carefully measured by Byerley and Kirksey[11] in 25 well-nourished lactating women. Supplements ranged from 0 to 1000 mg (ten times the RDA) vitamin C daily. Concentrations in milk ranged from 44 to 158 mg/L and were not correlated significantly with maternal intakes, which ranged from 156 (0 mg supplement) to 1123 (1000 mg supplement). Dietary vitamin C had no effect on the volume of milk produced. Maternal excretion of vitamin C in urine was correlated with maternal intake. Regardless of the level of maternal intake of vitamin C, the mean vitamin C concentration in breast milk was twice that recommended for infant formula. Vitamin C levels in milk did not increase in response to increasing maternal intake despite tenfold increases, whereas urinary excretion did suggest that mammary tissue becomes saturated. A regulatory mechanism is postulated by the investigators to prevent an elevation

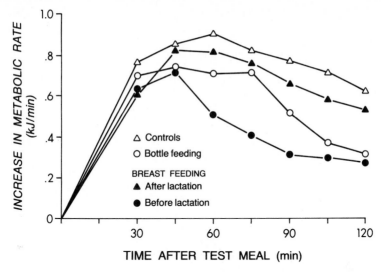

Fig. 9-3. Metabolic response to test meal while breastfeeding compared to response of bottle feeders and nonpregnant controls. (From Illingworth PJ, Jung RT, Howie PW et al: Br Med J 292:437, 1986.)

in concentration of vitamin C beyond a certain level in milk. Vitamin C levels were at the same or higher levels in exclusively breastfed infants at 6 months and 9 months of age than levels of supplemented bottle fed controls. Levels were dependent on maternal nutrition and vitamin C levels in milk. Byerley and Kirksey[11] found 6% of well-nourished healthy mothers had low levels of vitamin C. In malnourished women, tissue stores may take time to replenish, which explains why 35 mg/day supplementation failed to increase low plasma levels. Data from multiple studies suggest that there is a level above which further vitamin C supplementation will not affect milk vitamin C levels.[55]

The level of B vitamins, also water soluble, reflects dietary intake. The levels are affected acutely by maternal diet. Infantile beriberi is not unheard of in seemingly normal infants nursed by apparently well-nourished mothers with thiamin-deficient diets. The influence of maternal diet has been pointed out dramatically in the reported case of megaloblastic anemia and methylmalonic aciduria and homocystinuria in the breastfed infant of a strict vegetarian. Vitamin B_{12} exists in all animal protein but not in vegetable protein. A strict vegetarian would require B_{12} supplements during pregnancy and lactation. B_{12} deficiency in infants has also been seen in New Delhi, where mothers had B_{12}-deficient milk. These infants also had megaloblastic anemia.[18]

Thiamin (B_1) has been studied infrequently, but maternal supplementation does not increase milk levels beyond a certain limit. Urinary excretion of thiamin is significantly higher in supplemented compared to unsupplemented women. In malnourished women, there is evidence that supplementation does increase thiamin levels in milk.

Riboflavin (B_2) requirements of lactating women in The Gambia in a controlled study showed the minimum to be 2.5 mg/day to maintain normal biochemical status in the mother and adequate levels of B_2 in her milk.[7] This level is higher than that recommended in the United States and the United Kingdom. The pantothenic acid content of human milk does not vary appreciably with dietary variations in well-nourished mothers, but the overall intake over time does influence milk levels.[44]

Niacin (B_3) content of human milk has been reported to parallel dietary intake. In unsupplemented diets, low B_3 levels usually parallel low levels of other B vitamins and low protein intakes.

Pyridoxine (B_6) intake and milk levels were studied in healthy lactating women by West and Kirksey.[82] There were marked diurnal variations of B_6 levels, with peaks occurring in those mothers taking supplements 3 to 5 hours after a dose. Those taking less than 2.5 mg/day had much lower milk levels (129 μg/L).

When lactating mothers received supplements of B_6 ranging from 0 to 20 mg pyridoxine HCl, the levels of B_6 measurable in the milk paralleled the intake, with levels peaking 5 hours after ingesting the supplement.[2] When maternal intakes of vitamin B_6 approximated 20 mg/day, breastfed infants were unlikely to receive the current RDA of 0.3 mg vitamin B_6 per day when intake was calculated from morning B_6 level in milk and daily volume was assumed to be 850 cc. The Academy of Pediatrics Committee on Nutrition[16] recommends a minimum of 35 mg vitamin B_6/100 kcal milk from birth to 12 months. There was no significant effect on the plasma prolactin levels in lactating women supplemented with 0.5 to 4.0 mg/day B_6 daily from 1 day postpartum through 9 months of lactation.[78]

Pantothenic acid levels in milk are strongly correlated with maternal intake for the preceding day. It has been suggested by Johnston et al.[44] that some pantothenic acid is stored in the body. Studies of malnourished women show increased levels in milk following supplementation.

Biotin is reported in few studies, but the findings are consistent that levels range 5 to 12 mg/L, with supplementation even up to 250 mg/day having little effect except when levels are significantly below this range.[63,65]

Folate supplementation in well-nourished women does not affect the level of folate in the milk, although studies involving women with low folate (less than 60% RDA) show they responded to supplementation with an increased level in their milk. Differences in assay methods have produced inconsistencies among studies. Milk levels normally range between 40 and 70 mg/L and increase slightly in the early weeks of lactation. Supplementation is 0.8 to 1.0 mg/day.[55]

Deodhar and Ramakrishnan[18] studied the effect of the stage of lactation on levels of vitamins B_1, B_2, B_3, B_6, B_{12}, and ascorbic acid. The values remained fairly constant throughout, except for those of B_3, which increased slightly over time. The relationship to socioeconomic group showed an increase in B_3 and B_6 levels with increased status. B_1 was higher in poorer mothers. The effect of diet on vitamin levels in maternal milk is summarized in Tables 9-8 and 9-9.

Fat-soluble vitamins

There are some significant changes in the information, and therefore changes in the recommendations about the fat-soluble vitamins are in order. Fat-soluble compounds are generally transported into milk via the fat, and levels are less easily improved by dietary change. Because A and D are stored in tissues, the impact of dietary supplement is more difficult to measure. Milk levels do not change until a certain level is achieved in the stores. High dietary levels of β carotene do not appear to result in excessive levels of either vitamin A or β carotene. Increase in vitamin A in the diet of undernourished women does increase its level in milk.

Vitamin D was considered to be at a stable level in milk; however, studies involving maternal supplementation have demonstrated increased milk levels.[38] When mothers were

Table 9-8.   Water-soluble vitamins in human milk

Vitamin	Recognizable clinical deficiency in infant	Effect of maternal supplements		Effect of dietary intake on milk content
		In malnourished	In well-nourished	
Ascorbic acid (C)	Rare	Yes	No	Limited
Thiamin (B_1)	Yes	Yes	Limited	Yes
Riboflavin (B_2)	Yes	Yes	Yes	Yes
Niacin (B_3)	Unknown	Yes	Yes	Yes
Pantothenic acid	Unknown	Yes	No	Yes
Pyridoxine (B_6)	Yes	Yes	Yes	Limited
Biotin	Yes	Yes	No	Limited
Folate	Unknown	Yes	No	No
Cyanocobalamin (B_{12})	Rare	Yes	No	Yes

Modified from the Committee on Nutrition, American Academy of Pediatrics: Pediatrics 68:435, 1981, Copyright American Academy of Pediatrics, 1981.

Table 9-9.   Fat-soluble vitamins in human milk

Vitamin	Recognizable clinical deficiency in infant	Effect of maternal supplements		Effect of dietary intake on milk content
		In malnourished	In well-nourished	
D	Yes	Yes	Unknown	Unknown
K	Yes	Unknown	None	None
A	Unknown	Unknown	Yes	Yes
E	Unknown	Unknown	Yes	Unknown

From the Committee on Nutrition, American Academy of Pediatrics: Pediatrics 68:435, 1981, Copyright American Academy of Pediatrics, 1981.

given 0, 500, and 2500 IU ergocalciferol daily, they produced milk with 39, 218, and 3040 mg/ml vitamin D. The effect on levels of 25-hydroxy vitamin D was less dramatic. The physiological significance to the infant is disputed, however, since the major source of antirachitic sterols seems to be sunlight, not milk. The role of water-soluble vitamin D in human milk has not been confirmed.

Dark-skinned infants reared in climates where sunlight is minimal may be at significant risk for rickets when breastfed unless attention is given to the possible need for supplements of vitamin D.[5] It has been estimated by Specker et al.[75] that 30 minutes of sunlight per week wearing only a diaper or 2 hours a week fully clothed (no hat) would maintain serum 25-OHD concentrations above lower limits of normal.

Vitamin E has not been the focus of study of maternal dietary supplements except in the report by Kramer[49] that sunflower oil replacing lard in the diet resulted in a 50% increase in vitamin E levels in the milk. On the other hand, the liberal use of vitamin E creams by health enthusiasts may well expose an infant to large doses by maternal absorption as well as directly when the creams are applied to the breast. α-Tocopherol levels are highest in the colostrum when the neonate is most dependent on its physiologic effect as an antioxidant and in the prevention of hemolytic anemia attributed to vitamin E deficiency.

The most critical time for vitamin K is during the birth process and in the first few days of life when the risk of bleeding, especially intracranial bleeding, is greatest. Maternal dietary intake is most critical during the end of gestation. It has been established that all newborns require vitamin K at birth. No studies are available to correlate diet and milk levels.

While dietary supplements improve the milk quality and quantity in malnourished women, a balanced diet without excessive supplementation is the most physiologic and economic way to assure good milk. Nutrients, especially vitamins, are only excreted when taken in excess.

Minerals
Calcium

Calcium has been associated with bone growth, and concern has been expressed because the total calcium in breast milk is low. The available information is inadequate to determine the requirement for lactation. Studies with radioactive calcium in the nonpregnant adult have shown that there are losses into the gut and through the kidney. Absorption and retention also depend on the reserves in the body. Long-term shortage causes economy of utilization, and the apparent requirement is lower. In lactation, the absorption and retention are greater but not as great as during pregnancy. Atkinson and West[4] showed by scanning transmission techniques that lactating women mobilize about 2% of their skeletal calcium over 100 days of nursing. The calcium content of milk appears to be maintained despite markedly deficient intake, probably because of skeletal stores. The milk calcium levels are the same in mothers of rachitic and nonrachitic infants.

The additional requirement for calcium in the lactating women's diet in 400 mg daily over normal or 1200 mg totally, which is not easily achieved without milk products and may require special attention on the part of the physician.[32] When dietary calcium intake is greater than the RDA for lactating women, bone mineral content is not diminished during the first 6 weeks of lactation at least.

Sodium

The concentration of sodium is the most variable of all the minerals, fluctuating as much as tenfold during normal lactation and diurally, separate from the effects of mastitis or involution. There is no immediate influence of maternal sodium or potassium intake, either high or low, on postprandial milk sodium or potassium concentrations. Dietary potassium may influence milk potassium more significantly. With increasing numbers of women with cardiac and renal disease wishing to lactate, potassium levels in the diet would be of significance in addition to concerns about necessary medications.[45]

Chlorine

It is believed that chlorine level in the breast milk is not affected by maternal diet. Chlorine deficiency reported in a breastfed infant was associated with normal maternal serum and milk levels and dietary intake.[3]

Iron

The iron content of milk is not readily affected by the iron content of the diet or the maternal serum iron level. Increases in dietary iron that increase serum levels do not increase iron in the milk. It is important, however, for the mother to replace her iron stores postpartum.[61] It has not been established that increases in tissue iron are advantageous. Iron that is added to human milk will bind to lactoferrin and may interfere with its function.

Table 9-10. Minerals in human milk

Mineral	Concentration throughout lactation	Facilitated bioavailability	Effect of maternal mineral intake on milk content
Sodium	Varies	Unknown	None
Calcium	Unchanged	Unknown	None
Iron	Unchanged	Facilitated	None
Zinc	Declines	Facilitated	None
Copper	Unchanged	Unknown	None
Manganese	Declines	Unknown	Yes
Selenium	Unknown	Unknown	None
Iodine	Declines	Unknown	Yes
Fluoride	Stable	Unknown	Yes

Modified from the Committee on Nutrition, American Academy of Pediatrics: Pediatrics 68:435, 1981, Copyright American Academy of Pediatrics, 1981.

Phosphorus, magnesium, zinc, and copper

Phosphorus, magnesium, zinc, and copper levels in milk are not affected by dietary administration of these elements. Again, however, it is important for the mother to replenish her stores.[61]

Iodine

Iodine in milk does depend on dietary content. The breast is able to raise the concentration of iodine in the milk above that in the blood, and thus there is an increased danger in giving radioactive iodine to the lactating woman. With iodized salt, bread dough conditioners, and common usage of iodine-containing cleaners, there is actually a risk of excessive iodine intake. Milk iodine concentrations are higher now than were reported in the 1930s. Mean breast milk iodide levels ranged from 29 to 490 ng/L, averaging 178 ng/L, above the recommended daily allowance for infants.[33]

Fluorine

Human milk contains $16 \pm$ μg fluoride/L and reflects in some degree the level in the water supply. The risk of excessive fluoride has been pointed out by Walton and Messer,[82] who report dental mottling and milk fluorosis in supplemented breastfed infants. The Committee on Nutrition of the Academy of Pediatrics has stated therefore, "It may not be necessary to give fluoride supplements to breastfed infants who are living in an area where water is adequately fluoridated."[17]

The effects of diet on mineral levels in maternal milk are summarized in Table 9-10.

MATERNAL NUTRITION AND IMMUNOLOGICAL SUBSTANCES AND LEUKOCYTE ACTIVITY

Substances in colostrum and mature milk confer important infection protection on the breastfed infant. Maternal malnutrition was associated with lower IgG and IgA in a group of Columbian women studied by Miranda et al.[57] The colostrum contained only one-third the normal levels of IgG and less than half the normal albumin. Significant reductions in IgA and complement (C_4) were observed in colostrum, but lysozyme, C_3 complement, and IgM were normal. Titers against respiratory syncytial virus were unaffected by nutritional status. The protective deficiencies improved in mature milk over time and with improvement of nutritional status. The total leukocyte concentrations as well as their bactericidal capacity were similar in well-nourished and undernourished women. Breast milk antimicrobial factors of rural Gambian mothers were measured by Prentice et al.[64] The concentrations and daily secretions of all immuno proteins, except lysozyme, decreased during the first year and then remained steady. Compared to Western women, levels of IgG, IgM, C_3, and C_4 were higher in the Gambia; IgA and lactoferrin were similar; and lysozyme was lower in the Gambia. Dietary supplement in the Gambia did not raise the breast milk immunoproteins in this study. The relationship of diet to these immune factors continues under investigation.

RECOMMENDATIONS FOR NUTRITIONAL SUPPORT DURING LACTATION

In the previous section it was noted that the quantity, protein content, and calcium content of milk are relatively independent of maternal nutritional status and diet. Amino acids, lysine and methionine, certain fatty acids, and water-soluble vitamin contents vary with intake. It is important to point out that stores of calcium, minerals, and fat-soluble vitamins need to be replenished. Much of the data collected have varied, depending on the method used in collection. The daily intakes believed necessary for infants were determined by feeding infants processed human milk in a bottle, which is not a physiologic standard. It is known, for example, that putting the entire sample in one container removes the natural variation in fat from beginning to end of the feeding.

The Committee on Recommended Dietary Allowances of the Food and Nutrition Board[28] has recommended a balanced diet comparable to one for the nonlactating postpartum patient, with a few additions. Although the calculated caloric cost of producing 1 L of milk is 940 kcal, it should be noted that during pregnancy most women store 2 to 4 kg of extra tissue in the physiologic preparation for lactation. It is probably necessary therefore to add only 500 kcal to the diet, except in women with known high metabolic rates.

Table 9-11. Recommended dietary allowances for lactation

Age	Body weight (kg)	Energy* (kcal)	Energy* (mega j)	Protein*† (g)	Vitamin A‡,§ (µg)	Vitamin D‖,# (µg)
Adult woman (moderately active)	55.0	2200	9.2	29	750	2.5
Pregnancy (later half)		+350	+1.5	38	750	10.0
Lactation (first 6 months)		+550	+2.3	46	1200	10.0

*Energy and Protein Requirements. Report of a Joint FAO/WHO Expert Group, FAO, Rome, 1972.
†As egg or milk protein.
‡Requirements of vitamin A, thiamin, riboflavin and niacin. Report of a Joint FAO/WHO Expert Group, FAO, Rome, 1965.
§As retinol.
‖Requirements of ascorbic acid, vitamin D, vitamin B_{12}, folate and iron. Report of a Joint FAO/WHO Expert Group, FAO, Rome, 1970.
#As cholecalciferol.

Preparation for lactation begins in pregnancy, if not before. The major daily increases for pregnancy are 300 kcal, 20 g of protein, a 20% increase in all vitamins and minerals except folic acid, which is doubled, and a 33% increase in calcium, phosphorus, and magnesium. It should be noted in comparing the RDA for lactating women to nonlactating adult women that the increases suggested should provide ample nutrition and replace stores (Table 9-11).

When dietary supplements are suggested (Table 9-12), there is concern about increased costs. Cost increases are modest for the standard diet and minimal for the low-budget diet, as demonstrated by Worthington-Roberts.[86] Although one rarely chooses breast-feeding or bottle feeding on the basis of cost, one needs to consider far more than the price of a few extra maternal kilocalories, and the cost of formula feeding makes a reassuring comparison. Hypoallergenic formulas are even more costly.

Malnutrition
Special supplementation for the lactating woman

It has been suggested that supplementing the diet of malnourished mothers with a special formula would be the best way to achieve nourishment for mother and child. The infant will then gain the additional advantages of human milk, such as protection against infection. Such formulas have been devised. Sosa et al.[73] have tried this approach in Guatemala.

With the ready availability of well-balanced nutrition supplements today in both supermarkets and drugstores in the form of stable powders, it should not be difficult to initiate a high-protein, vitamin-enriched diet supplementation that is also palatable for the occasional mother who is at nutritional risk. With the inclusion of breastfeeding as a goal in the Women, Infants, and Children (WIC) program, dietary counseling and supplementation are available for mothers at poverty level to encourage these mothers to breastfeed and give them nutritional support while doing so. Infants in the WIC programs will receive the greatest benefit from being breastfed.

Since studies have revealed a negative effect of malnutrition on infection protection properties as well as on galactopoietic hormones (corticosteroids are markedly increased

Thiamin‡ (mg)	Ribo-flavin‡ (mg)	Niacin‡ (mg)	Folic acid‖ (μg)	Vitamin B₁₂‖ (μg)	Ascorbic acid‖ (mg)	Calcium** (g)	Iron‖,†† (mg)
0.9	1.3	14.5	200	2.0	30	0.4-0.5	14-28
+0.1	+0.2	+2.3	400	3.0	50	1.0-1.2	‡‡
+0.2	+0.4	+3.7	300	2.5	50	1.0-1.2	‡‡

**Calcium requirements. Report of a Joint FAO/WHO Expert Group, FAO, Rome, 1961.
††On each line the lower value applies when over 25% of calories in the diet come from animal foods, and the higher value when animal foods represent less than 10% of calories.
‡‡For women whose iron intake throughout life has been at the level recommended in this table, the daily intake of iron during pregnancy and lactation should be the same as that recommended for nonpregnant, nonlactating women of childbearing age. For women whose iron status is not satisfactory at the beginning of pregnancy, the requirement is increased, and in the extreme situation of women with no iron stores, the requirement can probably not be met without supplementation.

Table 9-12. Extra daily nutrient allowances for lactation over baseline

Nutrient	Nonpregnant, nonlactating	Lactating	Increase
Energy (kcal)	2100	2600	500
Protein (g)	44	64	20
Retinol (μg)	800	1200	400
Vitamin D (μg)	7.5	12.5	5
Vitamin E (mg)	8	11	3
Vitamin C (mg)	60	100	40
Riboflavin (mg)	1.3	1.8	0.5
Nicotinic acid (mg)	14	19	5
Vitamin B_6 (mg)	2.0	2.5	0.5
Folate (μg)	400	500	100
Thiamin (mg)	1.1	1.6	0.5
Calcium (mg)	800	1200	400
Iron (mg)	18	18	18
Zinc (mg)	15	25	10

National Research Council: Recommended daily allowances, ed 9, Washington DC, 1980, National Academy of Sciences.

and prolactin decreased), nourishing the mother is the most effective way of benefitting the infant rather than supplementing the infant to meet growth standards.[55]

Allergy

In families with a strong history of allergy, a hypoallergenic diet avoiding the common allergens such as wheat and eggs should be recommended. Further details are described in Chapter 15. An allergy prophylaxis scheme is described in Appendix K.

Vegetarian diet

The growing interest in vegetarianism has necessitated the clinician's having a better understanding of the several types of diets and their potential for adequate nutrients and growth as well as the motivation for these diets (Table 9-13). In general, serious vegetarians usually have a greater knowledge of and commitment to good nutrition.[14] Reports of malnutrition among breastfed infants of vegetarians usually focus on the very strict groups such as vegans and those on macrobiotic diets. The dietary risks involved are chiefly with the B vitamins because these vitamins are usually associated with protein, which is also proportionally lower from vegetable sources. An additional concern is the availability of various amino acids in specific concentrations to utilize them for protein synthesis. The net protein utilization (NPU) of a food may be considerably lower than total protein content; therefore, it is important when using vegetable sources of protein to use foods with "complementary protein" at the same meal. Vegetarian cookbooks emphasize this.[66] Throughout history, culturally traditional meals have assured complementary proteins. As noted previously, vegetarians had higher levels of DHA.

B_{12} deficiency has been described in vegans because of the absence of animal protein.[87] It is advisable in these cases to supplement diets of the pregnant or lactating woman, as well as of an infant or growing child, with up to 4 mg/day of B_{12}. It has been shown that fermented soybean foods do contain B_{12}, as do the single-cell proteins such as yeast.

Table 9-13. Vegetarianism and associated risks

Type of vegetarian	Diet includes	Diet avoids	Risks
Semivegetarian	Vegetables, milk products, seafood, poultry	Red meat	Minerals*
Ovo-lacto-vegetarian	Vegetables, milk products, eggs	Flesh foods (meat, seafood, poultry)	Minerals* esp. zinc
Lacto-vegetarian	Vegetables, milk products	Flesh foods, eggs	Minerals* esp. zinc and protein†
Ovo-vegetarian	Vegetables, eggs	Flesh foods, milk products	Minerals* esp. iron and zinc, protein,† riboflavin, vitamin D, B_{12}
Vegan	Only vegetables	Flesh foods, milk products, eggs	Minerals,* protein,† riboflavin, vitamin D, B_{12}
Macrobiotic	Gradual progression to a diet of only cereals		Advanced stage nutritionally inadequate

*Excessive dietary phytates and dietary fiber inhibit absorption of minerals such as iron, zinc, and calcium. Phytates are organic chemicals present in many vegetables and unleavened bread that bind with minerals.
†Diets not using complementary proteins may be deficient in net protein because the NPU is low.

Reports of growth curves in vegetarian children over the first few years show them to be shorter and leaner than standard, with the greatest effect among the most restricted diets.[22] Breastfed vegetarian infants are usually on the norms for growth with the exception of those receiving minimal vitamin D and calcium as reported in dark-skinned mothers in cloudy climates. Among 34 breastfed infants at 7 months in the Tufts study, three infants were below the tenth percentile for height and weight, one had low weight for length, and three had high weight for length, whereas of the 51 who were not breastfed, six were below the tenth percentile, two had low weight for length, and four had high weight for length.[30]

Four vegetarian children between 8 months and 24 months of age were reported by Hellebostad et al.[37] to have vitamin D–deficient rickets (three with tetany and seizures) and vitamin B_{12} deficiency. All the infants were initially breastfed by mothers whose diets were low in vitamin D, high in fiber and phytate (which interferes with enterohepatic circulation of vitamin D), and low in calcium and phosphate.

General recommendations for lactating vegetarian women are as follows:

1. Supplement with soy flour, molasses, and nuts.
2. Use complementary protein combinations.
3. Avoid excessive phytates and bran.
4. Watch protein, iron, calcium, vitamins D, B_{12}, and riboflavin to assure adequate intake.

Supplementing the breastfed infant's diet

For the newborn infant, human milk is the ideal food containing all the necessary nutrients. In establishing dietary norms for infants fed cow's milk, many nutrients identified as being needed in the diet were found to exist in greater amounts in cow's milk than in human milk. This does not consider the probability that the nutrient may be in a more bioavailable form in human milk. The specific items in question are protein, sodium, iron, vitamin D, and fluorine.

The Committee on Nutrition of the Academy of Pediatrics[15] has noted that iron deficiency is rare in breastfed infants and attributes this to increased absorption and the absence of microscopic blood loss into the gastrointestinal tract, which is seen in bottle fed infants. The committee recommends a source of iron in solid foods (fortified infant cereal) by 4 to 6 months of age for breastfed infants.

Since rickets have been described in breastfed infants, consideration should be given to the maternal intake of vitamin D and the exposure of the infant to sunshine as discussed previously. Fomon[27] cautions, however, against reliance on sunshine in the first year of life and advises providing infants with 400 IU of vitamin D. Individual discretion is appropriate, since infants of healthy mothers have not been observed to have rickets.

The Academy of Pediatrics no longer recommends fluoride supplements in all breastfed infants.[17] Many breastfed infants have done without fluorine supplementation and have had no adverse dental problems, but the decision should be based on individual determinants, including family dental history and level of fluoride in the water supply, which is ideally between 0.7 and 1.0 ppm. If the level is less than 0.3 ppm, 0.25 mg of daily fluoride should be given.

Exercise while breastfeeding

There are usually no contraindications, but the greatest deterrent to exercise while breastfeeding is lack of time. Any mother with a new baby will have time problems, so ingenuity in combining other activities with exercise (taking the baby for a walk in the carriage) will be essential. Women who exercise excessively, especially jogging, have had trouble maintaining milk supply. It may be the excessive motion of the breasts while jogging without a firm brassiere. Relationship to later sagging of the breasts is not established.

Dieting while breastfeeding

If one eats a balanced diet of nutritious food, one need not gain weight while nursing. If 940 kcal are used to nourish an average 3-month-old infant, then a mother could lose weight while nursing by not increasing her caloric intake. Weight loss by this method would require attention to selecting nourishing foods and avoiding junk food. With elimination of the "empty calorie" part of a diet, the infant will be provided with adequate nutrients. Fad diets are inappropriate. The high-protein low-carbohydrate diet is apt to increase a mother's blood urea nitrogen level, which would be passed into the milk. Since dieting involves mobilizing fat stores, it should not be pursued if there is a chance there are PBCs, DDT, or any other environmental toxin stored in the fat. No reduction diet during lactation should be recommended by the clinician without careful consideration and design.

Foods to avoid

The concern about gassy foods causing gas in the breastfed baby has no scientific basis. The normal intestinal flora produce gas from the action on fiber in the intestinal tract. Neither the fiber nor the gas is absorbed from the intestinal tract nor do they enter the milk, even though they may afford the mother some discomfort. The acid content of the maternal diet does not affect the milk either because it does not change the pH of the maternal plasma. There are essential oils in such foods as garlic, and some spices that have characteristic odors and flavors may indeed pass into the milk, and an occasional infant objects to their presence.

Some infants do not tolerate certain foods in the mother's diet, predominantly specific vegetables and fruits. Garlic and onions may cause colic in some infants. Cabbage, turnips, broccoli, or beans may also bother others, making them colicky for 24 hours. The same has been said of rhubarb, apricots, and prunes. If a mother questions the effect of a food, she should avoid it or document its effect carefully by watching for colic in the 24 hours following ingestion. In the summer, a heavy diet of melons, peaches, and other fresh fruits may cause colic and diarrhea in the infant. Chocolate rarely lives up to its reputation and can be consumed in moderation without causing colic, diarrhea, or constipation.

Color of milk and maternal diet

Although the color of mature human milk is bluish white and the color of colostrum is yellow to yellow-orange, mothers will occasionally report changes in the color of their milk. Most of these reports can be traced to pigments consumed in the diet. The infant's urine may also turn color.

Pink or pink-orange milk

Pink-orange milk was traced to Sunkist orange soda, which contains red and yellow dyes. A case of a breastfed infant with pink to orange urine was reported by Roseman.[67] This combination of food dyes is also used in other brands of soda, fruit drinks, and gelatin desserts.

Green milk

Several cases of green milk have been reported to us. A careful search of the diet for the offending substance was made in each case. The effect of ingestion of the identified culprit and avoidance of it were then tested to confirm the association with the color in the milk. Several items have been clearly identified. Gatorade (the green beverage), kelp and other forms of seaweed, especially in tablet form, and natural vitamins from health-food sources each have been associated with one or more cases of green milk and usually green urine.

Black milk

Minocycline hydrochloride therapy was associated with black milk in galactorrhea in a 24-year-old who had received the compound for postulocystic acne for 4 years.[6] Examination of the fluid revealed that the macrophages contained hemosiderin, thus causing the black color. This drug is known to cause black pigmentation of the skin.

REFERENCES

1. Alexander RP et al: Serum lipids in long-lactating African mothers habituated to a low-fat intake, Atherosclerosis 44:175, 1982.
2. Andon MB, Howard MP, Moster PB et al: Nutritionally relevant supplementation of vitamin B_6 in lactating women: effect on plasma prolactin, Pediatrics 76:769, 1985.
3. Asnes R, Wisotsky DH, Migel PF et al: The di-
etary chloride deficiency syndrome occurring in a breastfed infant, J Pediatr 100:923, 1982.
4. Atkinson PJ and West RR: Loss of skeletal calcium in lactating women, J Obstet Gynecol Br Commonwealth 77:555, 1970.
5. Bachrach S, Fisher J, and Parks JS: An outbreak of vitamin D-deficiency rickets in a susceptible population, Pediatrics 64:871, 1979.

6. Basler RS and Lynch PJ: Black galactorrhea as a consequence of minocycline and phenothiazine therapy, Arch Dermatol 121:417, 1985.

7. Bates CJ et al: Riboflavin requirements of lactating Gambian women: a controlled supplementation trial, Am J Clin Nutr 135:701, 1982.

8. Bhaskaram P and Reddy V: Bactericidal activity of human milk leukocytes, Acta Paediatr Scand 70:87, 1981.

9. Butte NF, Calloway DH, and Van Dozen JI: Nutritional assessment of pregnant and lactating Navajo women, Am J Clin Nutr 34:2216, 1981.

10. Butte NF, Garza C, Stuff JE et al: Effect of maternal diet and body composition on lactational performance, Am J Clin Nutr 39:296, 1984.

11. Byerley LO and Kirksey A: Effect of different levels of vitamin C intake on the vitamin C concentration in human milk and vitamin C intakes of breastfed infants, Am J Clin Nutr 41:665, 1985.

12. Byrne J, Thomas MR, and Chan GM: Calcium intake and bone density of lactating women in their late childbearing years, J Am Diet Assoc 87:883, 1987.

13. Chappell JD, Clandinin MT, and Kearney-Volpe C: Trans fatty acids in human milk lipids: influence of maternal diet and weight loss, Am J Clin Nutr 42:49, 1985.

14. Christoffer K: A pediatric perspective on vegetarian nutrition, Clin Pediatr 20:632, 1981.

15. Committee on Nutrition, Academy of Pediatrics: Iron supplementation for infants, Pediatrics 58:765, 1976.

16. Committee on Nutrition, Academy of Pediatrics: Nutrition and lactation, Pediatrics 68:435, 1981.

17. Committee on Nutrition, American Academy of Pediatrics: Fluoride supplementation, Pediatrics 77:758, 1986.

18. Deodhar AD and Ramakrishnan CV: Studies on human lactation, part II. Effect of socioeconomic status on vitamin content of human milk, Indian J Med Res 47:352, 1959.

19. Dewey KG, Finley DA, and Lönnerdal B: Breast milk volume and composition during late lactation (7-20 months), J Pediatr Gastroenterol Nutr 3:713, 1984.

20. Duckman S and Hubbard JF: The role of fluids in relieving breast engorgement, Am J Obstet Gynecol 60:200, 1950.

21. Dusdieker LB, Booth BM, Stumbo PJ et al: Effect of supplemental fluids on human milk production, J Pediatr 106:207, 1985.

22. Dwyer JT et al: Preschoolers on alternate lifestyle diets, J Am Diet Assoc 72:264, 1978.

23. Edozien JC, Khan MAR, and Waslien CI: Human protein deficiency: results of a Nigerian village study, J Nutr 106:312, 1976.

24. English RM and Hitchcock NE: Nutrient intakes during pregnancy, lactation and after the cessation of lactation in a group of Australian women, Br J Nutr 22:615, 1968.

25. Ereman RR, Lönnerdal B, and Dewey KG: Maternal sodium intake does not affect postprandial sodium concentration in human milk, J Nutr 117:1154, 1987.

26. Finley DA, Lönnerdal B, Dewey KG et al: Breast milk composition: fat content and fatty acid composition in vegetarians and non-vegetarians, Am J Clin Nutr 41:787, 1985.

27. Fomon SJ: Breastfeeding and evolution, J Am Diet Assoc 86:317, 1986.

28. Food and Nutrition Board, National Research Council: Recommended dietary allowances, ed 9, Washington, DC, 1984, National Academy of Sciences.

29. Forsum E and Lönnerdal B: Effect of protein intake on protein and nitrogen composition of breast milk, Am J Clin Nutr 33:1809, 1980.

30. Fulton JR, Hutton CW, and Sitt KR: Preschool vegetarian children, J Am Diet Assoc 76:260, 1980.

31. Gabriele A, Gabriele KR, and Lawrence RA: Cultural values and biomedical knowledge choices in infant feeding: analysis of a survey, Soc Sci Med 23:501, 1986.

32. Greer FR, Tsang RC, Levin RS et al: Increasing serum calcium and magnesium concentrations in breast-fed infants: longitudinal studies of minerals in human milk and in sera of nursing mothers and their infants, J Pediatr 100:59, 1982.

33. Gushurst CA, Mueller JA, Green JA et al: Breast milk iodide: reassessment in the 1980s, Pediatrics 73:354, 1984.

34. Guthrie HA, Picciano MF, and Sheehe D: Fatty acid patterns of human milk, J Pediatr 90:39, 1977.

35. Hambraeus L: Proprietary milk versus human breast milk in infant feeding: a critical approach from the nutritional point of view. In Neumann CG and Jelliffe DB, editors: Symposium on nutrition in pediatrics, Pediatr Clin North Am 24:17, 1977.

36. Hanafy MM et al: Maternal nutrition and lactation performance, J Trop Pediatr 18:187, 1972.

37. Hellebostad M, Markestad T, and Halvorsen KS: Vitamin D deficiency rickets and vitamin B_{12} deficiency in vegetarian children, Acta Paediatr Scand 74:191, 1985.

38. Hollis BW, Pittard III WB, and Reinhardt TA: Relationships among vitamin D, 25-hydroxy vitamin D, and vitamin D-binding protein concen-

trations in the plasma and milk of human subjects, J Clin Endocrinol Metab 62:41, 1986.

39. Illingworth PJ, Jung RT, Howie PW et al: Diminution in energy expenditure during lactation, Br Med J 292:437, 1986.

40. Illingworth RS and Kilpatrick B: Lactation and fluid intake, Lancet 2:1175, 1953.

41. Insull W, Hersch J, James T et al: The fatty acids of human milk. II. Alterations produced by manipulation of caloric balance and exchange of dietary fats, J Clin Invest 38:443, 1959.

42. Jelliffe DB and Jelliffe EFP: Human milk in the modern world, New York, 1978, Oxford University Press.

43. Jelliffe EFP: Maternal nutrition and lactation. In Ciba Foundation Symposium, no 45, Breast feeding and the mother, Amsterdam, 1976, Elsevier Scientific Publ. Co.

44. Johnston L, Vaughn L, and Fox HM: Pantothenic acid content of human milk, Am J Clin Nutr 34:2205, 1981.

45. Keenan BS et al: Diurnal and longitudinal variations in human milk sodium and potassium: implications for nutrition and physiology, Am J Clin Nutr 35:527, 1982.

46. Khin-Maung-Naing, Tin-Tin-Oo, Kywe-Thein, and Nwe-New Hlaing: Study on lactation performance of Burmese mothers, Am J Clin Nutr 33:2665, 1980.

47. Kliewer RL and Rasmussen KM: Malnutrition during the reproductive cycle: effects on galactopoietic hormones and lactational performance in the rat, Am J Clin Nutr 46:926, 1987.

48. Koletzko B, Gwosdz M, and Bremer HJ: Trans isomeric fatty acids in human milk lipids in West Germany. In Schaub J, editor: Composition and physiological properties of human milk, Amsterdam, 1985, Elsevier Science Publ. Co.

49. Kramer M, Szöke K, Lindner K, et al: The effect of different factors on the composition of human milk and its variations. III. Effect of dietary fats on the lipid composition of human milk, Nutr Diet 7:71, 1965.

50. Krebs NF, Hambidge KM, Jacobs MA et al: The effects of a dietary zinc supplement during lactation on longitudinal changes in maternal zinc status and milk zinc concentrations, Am J Clin Nutr 41:560, 1985.

51. Lammi-Keefe CJ and Jensen RG: Lipids in human milk: a review. 2. Composition and fat-soluble vitamins, J Pediatr Gastroenterol Nutr 3:172, 1984.

52. Lammi-Keefe CJ, Jensen RG, Clark RM et al: Alpha tocopherol total lipid and linoleic acid contents of human milk at 2, 6, 12, and 16 weeks. In Schaub J, editor: Composition and physiological properties of human milk, Amsterdam, 1985, Elsevier Science Publ. Co.

53. Levander OA, Moser PB, and Morris VC: Dietary selenium intake and selenium concentrations of plasma, erythrocytes, and breast milk in pregnant and post partum lactating and non-lactating women, Am J Clin Nutr 46:694, 1987.

54. Lipsman S, Dewey KG, and Lönnerdal B: Breastfeeding among teenage mothers: milk composition, infant growth, and maternal dietary intake, J Pediatr Gastroenterol Nutr 4:426, 1985.

55. Lönnerdal B: Effects of maternal dietary intake on human milk composition, J Nutr 116:499, 1986.

56. Mellies MJ, Ishikawa TT, Gartside P et al: Effects of varying maternal dietary cholesterol and phytosterol in lactating women and their infants, Am J Clin Nutr 31:1347, 1978.

57. Miranda R, Saravia NG, Ackerman R et al: Effect of maternal nutritional status on immunological substances in human colostrum and milk, Am J Clin Nutr 37:632, 1983.

58. National Research Council: Recommended dietary allowances, ed 9, Washington DC, 1980, National Academy of Sciences.

59. Olsen A: Nursing under conditions of thirst or excessive ingestion of fluids, Acta Obstet Gynecol Scand 20:313, 1940.

60. Paul AA, Muller EM, and Whitehead RG: The quantitative effects of maternal dietary energy intake on pregnancy and lactation in rural Gambian women, Trans Roy Soc Trop Med Hygi 73:686, 1979.

61. Picciano MF, Calkins EJ, Garrick JR et al: Milk and mineral intakes of breastfed infants, Acta Paediatr Scand 70:189, 1981.

62. Potter JM and Nestel PJ: The effects of dietary fatty acids and cholesterol on the milk lipids of lactating women and the plasma cholesterol of breast-fed infants, Am J Clin Nutr 29:54, 1976.

63. Prentice AM et al: Dietary supplementation of Gambian nursing mothers and lactational performance, Lancet 2:886, 1980.

64. Prentice A, Prentice AM, Cole JJ et al: Breast milk anti-microbial factors of rural Gambian mothers. I. Influence of stage of lactation and maternal plane of nutrition, Acta Paediatr Scand 73:796, 1984.

65. Prentice AM, Roberts SB, Prentice A et al: Dietary supplementation of lactating Gambian women. I. Effect on breast milk volume and quality, Hum Nutr 37C:53, 1983.

66. Robertson L, Flinders C, and Godfrey B: Laurel's kitchen: a handbook for vegetarian cookery and nutrition, Petaluma Calif, 1976, Nilgiri Press.

67. Roseman BD: Sunkissed urine (letter to the editor), Pediatrics 67:443, 1981.

68. Salmenpera L: Vitamin C nutrition during prolonged lactation: optimal in infants while marginal in some mothers, Am J Clin Nutr 40:1050, 1984.

69. Schutz Y, Lechtig A, and Bradfield RB: Energy expenditures and food intakes of lactating women in Guatemala, Am J Clin Nutr 33:892, 1980.

70. Sinclair AJ and Crawford MA: The effect of a low-fat maternal diet on neonatal rats, Br J Nutr 29:127, 1973.

71. Smith CA: Effects of maternal undernutrition upon newborn infants in Holland (1944-1945), J Pediatr 30:229, 1947.

72. Sneed SM, Zane C, and Thomas MR: The effects of ascorbic acid, vitamin B_6, vitamin B_{12} and folic acid supplementation on the breast milk and maternal nutritional status of low socioeconomic lactating women, Am J Clin Nutr 34:1338, 1981.

73. Sosa R, Klaus M, and Urrutia JJ: Feed the nursing mother, thereby the infant, J Pediatr 88:668, 1976.

74. Specker BL, Tsang RC, and Hollis BW: Effect of race and diet on human milk vitamin D and 25 hydroxy vitamin D, Am J Dis Child 139:1134, 1985.

75. Specker BL, Valanis B, Hertzberg V et al: Sunshine exposure and serum 25-hydroxy vitamin D concentration in exclusively breastfed infants, J Pediatr 107:372, 1985.

76. Stein ZA, Susser MW, Saenger G et al: Famine and human development: the Dutch hunger winter of 1944-45, New York, 1975, Oxford University Press.

77. Steingrimsdottir L, Brasel JA, and Greenwood MRC: Diet, pregnancy, and lactation: effects on adipose tissue, lipoprotein lipase, and fat cell size, Metabolism 29:837, 1980.

78. Styslinger L and Kirksey A: Effects of different levels of vitamin B_6 supplementation on vitamin B_6 concentrations in human milk and vitamin B_6 intakes of breastfed infants, Am J Clin Nutr 41:21, 1985.

79. Von Muralt A: Maternal nutrition and lactation. In Ciba Foundation Symposium, no 45, Breast feeding and the mother, Amsterdam, 1976, Elsevier Scientific Publ. Co.

80. Vuori E et al: Maternal diet and fatty acid pattern of breast milk, Acta Paediatr Scand 71:959, 1982.

81. Walker ARP, Walker F, Bhamjee D et al: Serum lipids in long-lactating African mothers habituated to a low fat intake, Atherosclerosis 44:175, 1982.

82. Walton JL and Messer LB: Dental caries and fluorosis in breast-fed and bottle-fed children, Caries Res 15:124, 1981.

83. West KD and Kirksey A: Influence of vitamin B_6 intake on the content of the vitamin in human milk, Am J Clin Nutr 29:961, 1976.

84. Whitehead RG: Pregnancy and lactation; nutrition and growth, aging and physiologic stress. In Shils ME and Young VR: Modern nutrition in health and disease, ed 7, Philadelphia, 1988, Lea & Febiger.

85. World Health Organization: Handbook on human nutritional requirements, Geneva, 1974, World Health Organization.

86. Worthington-Roberts BS: Lactation, human milk, and nutritional considerations. In Worthington-Roberts BS, Vermeersch J, and Williams SR, editors: Nutrition in pregnancy and lactation, ed 4, St Louis, 1988, The CV Mosby Co.

87. Zmora E, Gorodescher R, and Bar-Ziv J: Multiple nutritional deficiencies in infants from a strict vegetarian community, Am J Dis Child 133:141, 1979.

Weaning

10

What does *weaning* mean? The textbooks on pediatrics and the mother's manuals all imply that it is the process by which one changes from one method of feeding to another. Raphael[23] states that the very first introduction of solid foods is the true beginning of weaning. The term weaning is derived from the Anglo-Saxon *wenian,* which means "to become accustomed to something different." It does not mean the total cessation of breast-feeding but adding other things.[24] If one consults the dictionary, however, one learns that to wean is to transfer the young of any animal from dependence on its mother's milk to another form of nourishment or to estrange from former habits or associations. A weanling is a child or animal who is newly weaned. If one likens breastfeeding to the continuation of intrauterine life, then weaning is a "second birth." Weaning from a physiologic point of view is a complex process involving nutritional, microbiologic, immunologic, biochemical, and psychologic adjustments. Boys tend to be weaned earlier than girls, possibly because the energy intakes of boys at all ages are greater and the male rate of growth is more rapid.

INFANT'S NEED

When discussing the process of weaning the human infant, one might say it is the transfer of the infant from dependence on mother's milk to other sources of nourishment. If one were to determine the appropriate time for this to take place, it would be based on nutritional needs and developmental goals. Observations among other mammals suggest achievement of a degree of maturity that allows the pup to forage for himself. When weaning time is correlated with birth weight in placental mammals, a ratio of 3:1 is noted, that is, weaning takes place when birth weight has tripled. As a general rule, the smaller the animal, the shorter the time required for both gestation and maturation of the young. The weaning process is a gradual one, terminating after a time approximately equal to the period of gestation. The elephant's gestational period is 20 to 21 months, and the young are totally weaned at about 2 years of age. Other species gradually introduce other foods and teach their offspring how to obtain them on their own. Usually the mother of most species makes the determination for final termination and no longer permits the young to nurse. Studies on the milk-borne factors that might cue the initiation of weaning in other species have not shown any cause and effect. In the rat there is a "weaning crisis" during which the anatomy of the gut changes; some enzymes appear and others disappear. The enzymatic adaptations of the human infant are discussed in the chapter on physiology.

Among humans many cultural influences mandate weaning time and process. Public and social pressure have influenced weaning for some families in industrialized society. Very few traditional societies wean under 1 year, and some do not begin until 2 years of age. In the Moslem world, especially Africa and the Sudan, however, weaning of children is by the teaching of the Koran, which advises complete weaning by 2 years of age. The average time of complete cessation worldwide is 4.2 years.

Nutritionally, it is appropriate to begin iron-containing foods at 6 months, since that is the time the stores from birth are being diminished. The requirement at this age exceeds that supplied by human milk. An additional source of protein becomes necessary toward the end of the first year of life because the grams of protein per kilogram of body weight supplied by milk drop as the infant grows heavier. The content of protein in the milk begins to drop slightly after 9 months of lactation. A human infant also needs bulk, or roughage, in the diet. The exact time this need becomes apparent is not known, but it is certainly by the end of the first year.

Developmentally, he is ready to learn to chew solids instead of suckle liquids at about 6 months. Illingworth and Lister have suggested that there may be a "critical period of development" during which infants can and must learn to chew.[19] Chewing is an entirely different motion of the tongue and mouth from sucking. The sucking fat pads in the cheeks begin to disappear at the end of the first year. The rooting reflex has been lost. Even though the teeth are not all in, the development of good dentition requires chewing exercise.

ROLE OF DEVELOPMENT IN INITIATION OF WEANING

While the developmental milestones of infant behavior are noted to influence the introduction of weaning foods, the development of the gastrointestinal tract plays an equal role. Even the taste buds, which have been identified at the seventh week of fetal life as collections of elongated cells on the dorsal surface of the tongue, over the next weeks are fully innervated. The fetus is known to suck and swallow in utero; sucking is discussed in Chapter 8.

When taste becomes a factor in feeding is not known, although a lack of discrimination has been noted in the first weeks of life as infants have consumed formula with high salt or absence of chloride with morbid results. Because of the variation in the composition of mother's milk over a feeding, over a day, and from time to time according to maternal dietary intake, the breastfed infant has had a richer range of experience in tasting than the formula-fed infant. Breastfed infants are therefore more accustomed to new taste experiences. Similarly, feeding problems in infants are rare in breastfed infants.[3,5,14,24,27,28]

Both sucking and chewing are complex, having reflex as well as learned components. The development of the chew-swallow reflex is necessary for the successful introduction of solids. It has been hypothesized by Schmitz and McNeish that this skill develops sequentially with neuronal development, then is a learned behavior conditioned by oral stimulation.[24] Prior to this point, when a spoon is introduced, the infant purses his lips and pushes the tongue against the spoon. By 4 to 6 months, the tongue is depressed in response to the spoon and the food accepted, and by 7 to 9 months rhythmic biting movements occur regardless of the presence of teeth. Biting and masticatory strength and efficiency progress through infancy. If a stimulus is not applied when the neural development is taking place, Merchant and others[21a] feel that the chewing reflex will not develop and the infant will always be a poor chewer. There is a relationship between prolonged sucking without solids and poor eating. The clinical model for this is the child sustained on parenteral feedings or gastrostomy beyond a year who has tremendous difficulty accepting solids.

For the human infant, there is also the role of nursing as a comfort and emotional support, a mechanism often referred to as "comfort nursing" or as nonnutritive suckling. This need may last several years for some children, just as the need for the nursing bottle or pacifier may last through the toddler years.

In summary, the infant is ready to explore new feeding experiences around 6 months. Feeding is an important social as well as nutritional encounter. Eating solids and learning to drink from a cup are important social achievements as well. That does not mean the infant is taken from the breast, but his diet is expanded and now includes solid foods, other liquids, and breast milk. While there are a range of qualitative, quantitative, and temporal practices, the optimal approach matches the needs and requirements of a given child with the functions and capacities of his body.

Introduction of solids

The Academy of Pediatrics Commitee on Nutrition[7] made recommendations on the feeding of supplemental foods to infants. They described three overlapping stages of infant feeding: the nursing period, during which breast milk or infant formula is the source of nutrition; a transitional period, during which solid foods are introduced; and the modified adult period, during which most of the nutrition is similar to the family's. They further stated that no nutritional advantage results from the introduction of supplemental foods prior to 4 to 6 months of age. Similar statements have been made by the World Health Organization, the Canadian Pediatric Society, the Paediatric Society of New Zealand, and similar groups in England and Scotland.[5,8] They all emphasize weaning is not the termination of breastfeeding but the addition of solids.

When new foods are added to the breastfed infant's diet, this is called *complementary feeding*. The appropriate timing was studied by a consultation group on Maternal and Young Child Nutrition of the UN/ACC Sub-committee on Nutrition.[27] Although practice depends on many biological, cultural, social, and economic factors, when mother's milk fails to meet the energy and nutrient needs of an infant, inadequate growth and development threaten the health and survival of the child. In general, the committee declared that children who are not receiving complementary feeding beyond 6 months do not maintain adequate growth but should not receive it before 4 months. In his extensive review of the world literature and careful recalculation of infant requirements, Whitehead states that a typical volume of breast milk of 800 ml/day is sufficient to meet the needs of a female infant to 16 weeks of age[29] (not the 8 weeks reported by 1973 FAO/WHO recommendations). Many mothers produce 1000 ml/day, and this would sustain an average female infant to age 24 weeks and a very large male to 12 weeks. He finds these calculations compatible with introducing solid foods at 4 to 6 months while continuing to breastfeed fully.

MOTHER'S RIGHTS

In practice, mothers are often the determinants of weaning time as seen in other species. Some mothers want to nurse for a few weeks and wean to a bottle to go to work. Other mothers wean at 3 months to be free again. Certainly any time spent breastfeeding is to the infant's advantage. The critical point in weaning is to make it a gradual adjustment for both the mother and infant. The health goals for the United States have recommended that mothers nurse at least 6 months.[22]

WEANING PROCESS

Gradually replacing one feeding at a time with solids or a bottle or cup, depending on the infant's age and stage of development, is usually preferable.[2] After the adjustment has been made to one substitute feeding, then a second feeding is replaced with a substitute, usually at the opposite time of day. This process is continued until only the morning and night feedings remain. Then these two are gradually stopped. The morning and night feedings can be maintained for some months, and often an infant may be nursed beyond the second year, especially at these times. Mothers who wish to wean partially as early as 3 months may continue the morning and night nursing. This is especially suited to the working mother. The decline in lactation and the regression of the mammary gland occur slowly with gradual weaning.

The composition of milk during abrupt weaning, carefully analyzed by Hartmann and Kulski,[15] revealed that the secretory capability of the mammary gland of women changed dramatically after complete cessation of breastfeeding but that the involuting gland remained partially functional for 45 days. After termination that occurred in 1 day, sample collections were attempted for each breast by manual expression at the same time on days 1, 2, 4, 8, 16, 21, 31, 42, and 45. The concentrations of lactose and potassium decreased, while sodium, chloride, fat, and total protein increased progressively over 42 days. The increase in protein was related to increases in the concentrations of lactoferrin, IgA, IgG, IgM, albumin, lactalbumin, and casein. Concentrations from each breast were similar throughout. One woman in the study breastfed for 39 days; six women fully lactated an average of 332 days (251 to 443 range).

The involution in other species is rapid. There is complete resorption in 7 days in cows, for instance. The threshold dose of oxytocin required to elicit milk ejection was shown by Caldeyro-Barcia[4a] to increase progressively for at least 30 days after termination of breastfeeding. It is believed that a psychologic nursing stimulus contributes to this effect in humans because they continue contact with their infants, whereas other species are separated. Experimental animals given oxytocin postweaning also show a delay in involution.

Emergency weaning

Occasionally there is a need for sudden weaning because of severe illness in the mother or some prolonged separation of mother and infant. (Sudden illness in the infant does not require weaning, and, in fact, weaning would be contraindicated.) This is difficult for both. After abrupt weaning, the mammary glands remain partially functional for over a month.

Depending on the infant's age and flexibility, it may take a patient surrogate mother a feeding or two to switch the infant to a bottle. In other cases the infant may take only solids and refuse other liquids for days. The mother may have considerable discomfort. Engorgement may be significant if it is only 4 to 6 weeks postpartum. The mother may experience milk fever at any time there is abrupt weaning. This illness is characterized by fever, chills, and malaise, resembling a flulike syndrome. It is believed to be due to the sudden resorption of milk products into the system. Milk fever usually lasts 3 to 4 days and should not be confused with more serious illness.

The hormonal change resulting from sudden weaning early in lactation is more definitive because the prolactin levels from suckling are higher immediately postpartum

(Chapter 3). The hormone-withdrawal syndrome may be more marked with early weaning. Prolactin has been associated with a feeling of well-being; thus its decrease may be associated with relative depression. Patients with psychiatric disorders have been observed to cope by compensation postpartum until they wean the infant from the breast. It is important to provide an adequate support system during weaning for the mother who is prone to depression.

The normal, well-adjusted mother may experience some depression and sadness at the reality of the last feeding. It may be very difficult to face this experience. It is important to recognize this as a physiologic phenomenon as well as an emotional one. If a mother is forced by circumstances beyond her control to wean early, she may need a lot of understanding and encouragement to cope with the disappointment. If she has had pressure from friends or relatives to breastfeed, she may need to face what she considers failure and recognize that one can bottle feed and still mother very well.

Historically, weaning has varied from strict to permissive schedules with cultural styles. Rigid feeding schedules were associated with early weaning. Weaning has varied from early denial to slow and gentle withdrawal. In this century, the time considered proper for weaning has gradually shortened from as much as 2 or 3 years to as little as 6 to 8 months, or less. Public opinion has overlooked the infant's needs in favor of what are considered the mother's rights. It is not necessary to have clearly in mind a specific plan for weaning in the early weeks of nursing unless there are some constraints on the mother's time. Weaning should be done with the infant's needs as a guide. If an infant under 1 year of age rejects the breast, it is unusual but not abnormal and should not be considered by the mother as a personal rejection. Some bottle fed infants throw down the bottle at 9 months also.

Studies of weaning practices are few. In a study of primigravidas, they introduced solids because their infant seemed hungry and less satisfied and woke more frequently. The average time to introduce nonmilk food in bottle fed infants was 3 months; in breastfed, 5 months. Most observations are done on duration of feeding when the success rate is low. Jackson and associates[21] studied weaning times in mothers participating in the rooming-in project from 1942 to 1951 as compared with mothers who received traditional postpartum care at the New Haven Hospital during the same period. Rooming-in meant mother and infant were together in a special unit designed to accommodate both mothers and infants and managed as a pair by the same nursing staff. Infants were with their mothers as much as each mother wished. The rooming-in mothers nursed significantly longer.[20] They averaged 3.5 to 3.8 months, whereas the controls weaned at 1.8 to 2.5 months postpartum. The incidence of breastfeeding decreased as the difficulty of the delivery increased. The number who breastfed their infants did not differ by age, education, or race. Older mothers, better-educated mothers, and black mothers who breastfed, however, nursed longer.

The reasons given why women in Dunedin, New Zealand, elected to wean their infants early included concern about their milk supply and other maternal problems.[18] One of the most significant factors in lactation termination was mismanagement of breastfeeding by health professionals, according to the authors. A similar study in Sweden reported that 66% of the mothers weaned because they thought their milk was drying up.[25]

The patterns of weaning were studied in southern Brazil by Sousa et al.[26] Brazil was also experiencing a decline in breastfeeding. The study was undertaken to understand the causes of early weaning to develop better means of encouraging longer breastfeeding and delaying weaning. The bottle was introduced at birth by 24%, by 2 months by 72.6%, and by 6 months by 88.0%. The main reasons given for weaning are shown in Table

Table 10-1. Main reasons for premature weaning

Reason	N	%
Not enough, inadequate, or "weak" milk	307	30.9
Child refused breast	177	17.8
Illness of child	159	16.0
Mother needed to go to work	149	15.0
"Correct age for bottle feeding"	139	14.0
Other reasons	64	6.3
TOTAL	995	100.0

Table 10-2. Reasons for "milk inadequacy"

Reason	N	%
Milk is weak, thin, translucent	189	61.0
Infant cries after being breastfed	59	18.7
Infant needs to be fed very often	35	11.2
Breast not adequately full	24	9.1
TOTAL	307	100.0

10-1. A third of the mothers believed their milk was weak. The reasons the mothers thought their milk was thin are shown in Table 10-2. The researchers believed these data supported the hypothesis that the mothers did not understand the value of human milk and were influenced by advertisements about formulas and therefore compared their milk with formulas. In general most studies of weaning practices indicated that most weaning is mother initiated, most commonly because she thinks her milk is no longer adequate. The primary cause of failing milk supply reported by most investigators is inadequate help or instructions about milk production from medical personnel. Those who breastfeed longer tend to be older than 25 years, be well-educated middle class and self-educated about lactation, and enjoy breastfeeding.

Infant-initiated weaning

Infant-initiated weaning the first year of life was investigated by Clarke and Harmon,[6] who studied 50 healthy breastfed infants who were totally weaned; 46% of the group of infants initiated the weaning. This is often mistakenly referred to as self-weaning. The onset was usually between 5 to 9 months of age, with a median age of 6 months. Mothers described the behavior as an increased interest in exploring the environment and in other foods with a decreased interest in breastfeeding. Brazelton described a similar phenomenon and reported that there are three ages in the first year during which the infant exhibits a lagging interest in breastfeeding as a direct or indirect result of developmental events; 4 to 5 months, 7 months, and 9 to 12 months.

The duration of the infant-initiated weaning is about 1 month and is an interactive process that requires "at a minimum maternal complicity."[11] It can lead to relatively easy mutual weaning.

Refusal to breastfeed: "nursing strike"

Sudden onset of refusal to nurse can occur at any time and often is taken as a personal rejection by the mother, who promptly follows through by weaning completely. Often these mothers consider it to mean that they do not have enough milk or that something is wrong with their milk. This behavior has been called "nursing strike" and has been noted to be temporary.[16] The various causes associated with this abrupt behavior include the following:

1. Onset of menses in the mother
2. Dietary indiscretion by the mother
3. Change in maternal soap, perfume, or deodorant
4. Stress in the mother
5. Earache or nasal obstruction in the infant
6. Teething
7. Episode of biting with startle and pain reaction of mother

If a reason is identified that is possibly associated and it can be changed, nursing will resume. It may take extra effort to reestablish the relationship. Suggestions that may be made to the mother include the following:

1. Make feeding special and quiet, with no distractions and no other people.
2. Increase amount of cuddling, stroking, and soothing the baby.
3. Offer the breast when the infant is very sleepy.
4. Do not starve the child into submission.
5. If simple remedial steps do not result in a return to nursing, the physician should see the child to rule out otitis media, fever, infection, thrush, and so on.

Weanling diarrhea and malnutrition in weanling

Most writings on weaning refer to the problems in underdeveloped countries when infants are weaned early to overdiluted cow's milk or formulas that cost money but do not contain the anti-infective properties of human milk for the human infant. Weanling diarrhea is well described by Gordon and Ingalls[13] as the clinical syndrome (weanling diarrhea is a collection of diseases) associated with weaning from the breast. In 1900 in New York City, the death rate from dysentery, diarrhea, and enteritis in children in the first year of life was 5603/100,000 infants. This was largely attributed to weaning from the breast. Diarrheas are strongly associated with weaning not only because of the introduction of other foods but also because of the loss of the protective properties of human milk. The diarrheas themselves contribute to the malnutrition seen in underdeveloped countries because of the resultant lack of appetite and increased metabolic losses. In Third World countries morbidity and mortality in infancy rise sharply at the time of weaning from human milk because of the rapid onset of infections. Malnutrition is also a major threat to the weanling in the developing world. Rickets, iron deficiency, and protein energy malnutrition are the three major threats according to Wharton.[28] Close behind are the risks of zinc deficiency, allergy, and obesity, which affect a wider group of children.[28] In well-nourished mothers and their infants, diarrhea does not occur from controlled gradual weaning unless there is a milk allergy or metabolic disorder in the infant.

Changes in milk composition during gradual weaning

Changes in the nutrient composition of human milk during gradual weaning were studied by Garza et al.[10] in six fully lactating women recruited at 5 to 7 months postpartum

Table 10-3. Nutrient density (mg/100 kcal) of milk during weaning

	Week								
	0	2	4	6	8	10	12	PTM*	R†
Protein	1.5	1.2	1.3	1.0	1.3	1.2	1.9	1.8	2.7
Na	24.0	17.0	20.0	13.0	24.0	25.0	46.0	25.0	53.0
Ca	38.0	30.0	33.0	21.0	30.0	26.0	38.0	34.5	140.0
Zn	0.21	0.17	0.19	0.09	0.10	0.10	0.11	3.8	0.5

From Garza C et al: Am J Clin Nutr 37:61, 1983.
*Nutrient densities of milk from delivering premature infants.
†Nutrient densities calculated to achieve intrauterine growth rates assuming that the caloric requirements of low-birth-weight infants is 130 kcal/kg.

(Table 10-3). The weaning consisted of decreasing the frequency and duration of breast-feeding by one third each month for a period of 3 months. Milk was collected at 2-week intervals. Volume decreased to 67%, 40%, and 20% of baseline each month. The concentrations of protein and sodium were increased to 142% and 220% of baseline, respectively, by the twelfth week of weaning. Changes in fat composition were linear through the tenth week but at the twelfth week were similar to baseline. Iron was increased 172%, calcium was unchanged, and zinc fell to 58%. Similar observations have been made in bovine milk. Milk produced during either rapid or gradual weaning is characterized by a decreasing concentration of lactose. Fat accounts for an increasing percentage of calories (up 80%) and protein a stable 6% of calories.

The immunologic components in human milk were also measured, and the concentrations of certain components of the immunologic system are maintained during gradual weaning.[12] The effect of gradual weaning differs from that of abrupt weaning, in which the concentrations of all components rise dramatically. Measurements at 4 weeks, 8 weeks, and 12 weeks showed a decrease in the milk volume of 67%, 40%, and 20% as the levels of IgA and secretory IgA rose slightly. Lysozyme and lactoferrin rose slightly.

Studies in other species suggest that gut maturation observed at normal weaning time is not dependent on components in the milk but is triggered by thyroxine and corticosterone in the plasma of the offspring.[17] The anatomic changes in the breast during weaning are discussed in Chapter 2.

Physician's role in weaning

The physician's responsibility is the initiation of the appropriate solid foods, which probably should begin at 6 months of age.

Introduction of a cup as a developmental step should usually begin by 7 months.

Eating finger foods and learning to feed himself are the next steps for the child.

None of the above means the termination of breastfeeding but rather the gradual developmental progression of feeding. As other foods are introduced and feeding begins to cluster into three meals and some "snacks," breastfeedings will be decreased eventually to two or three per day.

The nourishment value is not a key issue after 1 year if other foods are adequate. The physician's role is to assure adequate nutrition.

There is no known detriment to nursing and some indication that nursing a few times a day or during times of stress is beneficial to the mother-infant relationship when the child is over a year of age. The objections raised are usually based on custom or personal taste. It is important for the clinician to avoid judgmental counseling based only on personal biases. Lay publications on the subject may help the mother who is nursing a toddler.

The physician may need to help the mother work through her own feelings about nursing her infant beyond the first year. Many women have been overwhelmed by friendly advice from lay experts about the infant who nurses for several years. Beyond a year, weaning is rarely child initiated until age 4. The child may not lose interest, so that the final steps in termination may require maternal intervention. A mother is not a poor parent if she begins to feel resentful toward nursing. Planning appropriate alternatives to the breastfeeding session that is to be eliminated is helpful in turning the child's attention toward the new event instead of toward the loss of an old and cherished one, a feeding at the breast. The mother may need to be helped to see how to avoid situations that easily predispose to nursing. She needs to know that it is acceptable to set some rules and to have some limitations and control over the breastfeeding.

If mother becomes pregnant, she will want to decide when she wishes to wean or whether she will continue to nurse right through pregnancy and then tandem nurse the new baby (see Chapter 17). For the child, it is important to avoid abrupt weaning or weaning to make room for the new baby who will now take his place. Weaning well before delivery is usually less traumatic for the child.

WEANING AND THE WORKING MOTHER

Some mothers return to work. Whether the reason is money, career, or personal satisfaction is not relevant to management. It takes tremendous commitment to work and breastfeed, but it can be done, it has been done, and it will be done. Usually the biggest problem a mother faces is coping with people who do not understand why she bothers. An understanding physician who provides the reassurance and support necessary to manage is a great asset. A mother may go home for a feeding in the middle of the day, pump milk to leave for the infant to have from a bottle, or give a substitute bottle. If there are occasional bottles of formula, the powder preparations are more economical and require only warming the water before adding the powder to assure rapid solution. Suggestions for collecting milk are in Chapter 19. Some infants quickly learn the mother's schedule and will sleep while she is away and feed more frequently during the evening and night to make up for it. It takes some personal adjustment to plan ahead and a babysitter who is patient and cooperative. A mother needs to be alert to the infant's needs as well and may need to leave feedings ready when she is away even if she had hoped the infant would sleep through the day. If a mother works long hours or an inflexible schedule, it may be necessary to wean the infant to morning and night feedings at the breast. However, this arrangement still provides the special benefits of human milk as well as the closeness that an infant needs; thus it is worth the effort. Employment is discussed in Chapter 13.

WEANING TIMES AND LEGAL OVERTONES

In the present turmoil of family life where parents are separating when the children are still young, several custody cases have been based on weaning times or, more accurately, on the time breastfeeding is totally terminated. Three separate cases in the United States have come to the author's attention where the father has sought custody on the basis of prolonged breastfeeding where the child nursed for comfort to about age 4. In two cases the judge found in favor of the mother. In one case in Rochester, NY, the judge found in favor of the father when an expert witness, a local psychologist, declared that "you have to be crazy to nurse that long." It would seem appropriate that judges review the entire case and qualifications of the respective parents and refrain from basing their decision on personal biases and emotional testimony. It is also advisable for expert witnesses to be fully informed on a subject about which they will testify. Developmental psychologist Ainsworth[1] has studied the maturation of the child and summarized the literature, which shows that infants with a strong attachment to mother are psychologically independent at 2 years of age. These children have more mastery of themselves at age 5 and less anxiety entering school.

REFERENCES

1. Ainsworth MA: The development of infant-mother attachment. In Caldwell BM and Ricciuti HN, editors: Review of child development research 3:1-94, Chicago University Press 1973.
2. Barnes GR et al: Management of breast feeding, JAMA 151:192, 1953.
3. Birkbeck JA, Chairman: The age of weaning: a statement of the infant nutrition subcommittee of the Paediatric Society of New Zealand, NZ Med J 95:584, 1982.
4. Brazelton TB: Infants and mothers: differences in development, New York, 1969, Delacorte Press.
4a. Caldeyro-Barcia R: Milk ejection in women. In Reynolds M and Folley SJ, editors: Lactogenesis: the initiation of milk secretion at parturition, Philadelphia, 1969, University of Pennsylvania Press.
5. Canadian Pediatric Society Nutrition Committee: Infant feeding: a statement, Can J Pub Health 70:376, 1979.
6. Clarke SK and Harmon RJ: Infant-initiated weaning from the breast in the first year, Early Hum Dev 8:151, 1983.
7. Committee on Nutrition, American Academy of Pediatrics: On the feeding of supplemental foods to infants, Pediatrics 65:1178, 1980.
8. Department of Health and Social Security: Present day practice in infant feeding: studies on health and social subjects, London, 1977, DHSS.
9. Finberg L, Kiley J, and Luttrell CN: Mass accidental salt poisoning in infancy, JAMA 184:121, 1963.
10. Garza C et al: Changes in the nutrient composition of human milk during gradual weaning, Am J Clin Nutr 37:61, 1983.
11. Goldfarb J and Tibbetts E: Breastfeeding handbook, Hillside, NJ, 1980, Enslow Publishers.
12. Goldman A et al: Immunologic components in human milk during weaning, Acta Paediatr Scand 72:133, 1983.
13. Gordon JE and Ingalls TH: Weaning diarrhea, Am J Med Sci Prev Med Epidemiol 245:345, 1963.
14. Gunn TR: The incidence of breastfeeding and reasons for weaning, NZ Med J 97:360, 1984.
15. Hartman PE and Kulski JK: Changes in the composition of the mammary secretion of women after the abrupt termination of breastfeeding, J Physiol 275:1, 1978.
16. Helsing E and King FS: Breast-feeding practice, New York, 1980, Oxford University Press.
17. Henning SJ: Role of milk-borne factors in weaning and intestinal development, Biol Neonate 41:265, 1982.
18. Hood LU et al: Breast feeding and some reasons for electing to wean the infant: a report from the Dunedin Multidisciplinary Child Development Study, NZ Med J 88:273, 1978.
19. Illingworth RS and Lister J: The critical or sensitive period, with reference to certain feeding problems in infants and children, J Pediatr 65:839, 1964.
20. Jackson EB: Pediatric and psychiatric aspects of the Yale Rooming-In Project, Conn State Med J 14:616, 1950.
21. Jackson EB, Wilkins LC, and Auerbach H: Statistical report on incidence and duration of breast feeding in relation to personal-social and hospital maternity factors, Pediatrics 17:700, 1956.
21a. Merchant SM: Neural development for sucking, swallowing and chewing. In Ballabriga A and Rey J: Weaning: why, what, and when? Workshop Series, vol 11, New York, 1987, Raven Press.
22. National Health Goals: Am J Pub Health Suppl 43:142, 1978.
23. Raphael D: The tender gift: breastfeeding, New York, 1976, Schocken Books.
24. Schmitz J and McNeish AS: Development of structure and function of the gastrointestinal tract: relevance for weaning. In Ballabriga A and Rey

J, editors: Weaning: why, what and when, Workshop Series, vol 11, New York, 1987, Raven Press.

25. Sjölen S, Hofvander Y, and Hillervik G: Factors related to early termination of breast feeding, Acta Paediatr Scand 66:505, 1977.

26. Sousa PLR et al: Patterns of weaning in South Brazil, J Trop Pediatr 21:210, 1975.

27. Underwood BA and Hofvander Y: Appropriate timing for complementary feeding for the breastfed infant, Acta Paediatr Scand Suppl 294: I-24, 1982.

28. Wharton BA: Food for the weanling: the next priority in infant nutrition, Acta Paediatr Scand Suppl 323:96, 1986.

29. Whitehead RG: Infant physiology, nutritional requirements, and lactational adequacy, Am J Clin Nutr 41:447, 1985.

30. World Health Organization: Joint WHO/UNICEF meeting on infant and young child feeding, Geneva, 1979, WHO.

Drugs in breast milk 11

$\mathbf{D}$espite the overwhelming advantages of human milk and the advantages of being breastfed, there are times when the physician must consider the risk of a maternal medication to the nursing infant. Even when the data about the medication include the milk-plasma ratio, the physician has to consider several factors related to this infant and this situation before deciding if breastfeeding can be initiated or continue. The more complicated the mother's medical problems, the greater the possibility that the infant also has complications of prematurity or illness that will alter the ability to excrete medication. This is a situation that requires scientific information and experienced clinical judgment to appraise the situation and determine the therapeutic regimen. The clinician must determine the risk-benefit ratio of continued breastfeeding. The data are still meager and sometimes conflicting, yet maternal medication is the single most common problem in managing breastfeeding patients.

There are a number of general reviews of drugs in breast milk and dozens of articles about the effect of a specific medication in a particular infant.* The Committee on Drugs of the American Academy of Pediatrics[15] has published a list of drugs and other chemicals that transfer into human breast milk. The list is divided into those which are contraindicated, those which require temporary interruption of breastfeeding, and those which are compatible with breastfeeding. Concern about this issue of drugs in breast milk has spread. The Department of Health and Human Services and the Food and Drug Administration have proposed a standard warning on all nonprescription drugs that are absorbed by the body. The warning states, "As with any drug, if you are pregnant or nursing a baby, seek professional advice before using this product." Since studies of pregnant women have shown that they take five to eight medications on their own during pregnancy and postpartum, the education by the clinician of these patients needs to continue. It is not appropriate to substitute wishful thinking for specific knowledge, yet it is equally inappropriate to discontinue breastfeeding when it is not medically neccessary.

Consideration of some of the pharmacokinetics will contribute to the understanding of the problems involved. Some data reported have been extrapolated from experiments performed on cows, goats, and rodents. Bovine experiments have been conducted using continuous infusions, which provide data on the passage of a drug into milk under certain circumstances of pH and plasma level. In an effort to explain and clarify the issues involved, the literature has oversimplified the problem so that individuals lacking a background in

---

*See references 2, 9, 10, 11, 23, 28, 38, 39, 58, 77, and 82.

pharmacology or pediatrics have misused the published data in drawing unwarranted conclusions.

Factors that influence the passage of a drug into the milk in humans include the size of the molecule, its solubility in lipids and water, whether it binds to protein, the drug's pH, and diffusion rates. Following is a summary of these factors:

I. Drug
   A. Route of administration: oral, IM, or IV
   B. Absorption rate
   C. Half-life or peak serum time
   D. Dissociation constant
   E. Volume of distribution
II. Size of molecule
III. Degree of ionization
IV. pH of substrate (plasma 7.4, milk 6.8)
V. Solubility
   A. In water
   B. In lipids
VI. Protein binding more to plasma than to milk protein

Passive diffusion is the principal factor in the passage of a drug from plasma into milk. The drug may appear in an active form or as an inactive metabolite. The route of administration to the mother, the drug's half-life, and drug dissociation constants are also to be considered.

Finally, a factor that has received relatively little attention is the infant. Will the infant absorb the chemical from the intestinal tract? If the infant absorbs the chemical, can the infant detoxify and excrete it, or will minimal amounts in the milk build in the infant's system? Is the infant premature, small for gestational age, or a high-risk infant due to complications of the pregnancy or delivery? Is the drug a material that could be safely given to an infant directly and at what risk? What dosages and blood levels are safe? These latter two questions are more critical than the pharmacokinetic theory. The ultimate question faced by the physician is, Can this infant be safely exposed to this chemical as it appears in breast milk without a risk that exceeds the tremendous benefits of being breastfed? Almost any drug present in mother's blood will appear to some degree in her milk.

CHARACTERISTICS OF THE DRUG
Protein binding

Drugs entering the circulation become protein bound or remain free in the circulation. The protein-bound component of the drug serves as an inactive reservoir of the drug that is in equilibrium with the free drug. Most drugs enter the mammary alveolar cells in the unbound form (Fig. 11-1).

At term, plasma proteins may be reduced and the fatty acid and hypoprotein fraction slightly increased in the mother, which results in the displacement of some drugs from plasma proteins.[20] It has been demonstrated during the postpartum period for 5 to 7 weeks that the free fraction of some drugs increases and therefore more readily crosses into milk (e.g., salicylate, phenytoin, and diazepam).

For most drugs there will be more drug found in the plasma than in the milk. Only the small free fraction of drug can cross the biologic membrane. The total concentration

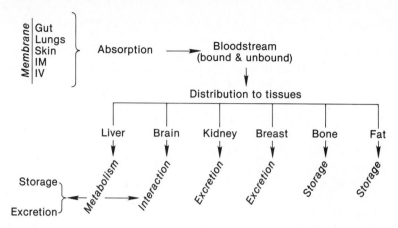

Fig. 11-1. Distribution pathways for drugs, once absorbed during lactation. (Modified from Rivera-Calimlim L: The significance of drugs in breast milk. In Lawrence R, editor: Breastfeeding, Clinics in Perinatology 14:51, 1987.)

in milk is only minimally influenced by binding of drugs in milk proteins (milk protein concentration is 0.9% in mature milk). Only those drug molecules which are free in solution can pass through the endothelial pores, either by diffusion or by reversed pinocytosis. Pinocytosis is the process whereby drug molecules dissolved in the interstitial fluid attach to receptors located at the surface of the cell membrane.[60,61] The cell membrane invaginates at the site of the drug attachment, bringing the drug into the cell. The membrane is pinched off, and the drug, surrounded by membrane, remains in the cell. Then the membrane is dissolved, leaving the drug molecule free in the cell. Reverse pinocytosis is the process by which the apical membrane evaginates after fusion of the intracellular membrane-bound secretion granules with the plasma membrane. The granules include lipids, proteins, lactose, drug molecules, and other cellular constituents. The evagination of the plasma membrane is pinched off and released into the alveolar lumen. Within the extravascular space, the drug may be bound to proteins in the interstitial fluid. Some agents in free solution can pass into the alveolar milk directly by way of the spaces between the mammary alveolar cells. These paracellular areas account for a major portion of the fluid changes across the epithelium. These spaces between adjacent alveolar cells serve to carry water-soluble drugs from the tissue into the milk.

These junctions are "open" at delivery as lactation is being established and gradually "tighten" over the next few days. The amount of drug passed into milk on day 1 is higher than on day 3 or later. The composition of the milk changes as well from colostrum to mature milk, altering the amount of protein and fat that could also influence milk levels of the drug. It is always important to know when plasma and milk samples were measured in relationship to the onset of lactation. Furthermore, some studies have been done on nonlactating women by pumping enough milk to measure the drug. These "weaning samples" provide only misinformation.

Ionization

Drugs that are nonionized are excreted in the milk in greater amounts than are ionized compounds. Depending on the pH of the solvent and the drug dissociation constant (pK_a),

Table 11-1. Association between milk/plasma ratios and pK_a of sulfonamides

Sulfonamide	Milk/plasma ratio	pK_a
Sulfacetamide	0.08	5.4
Sulfadiazine	0.21	6.5
Sulfathiazole	0.43	7.1
Sulfamethazine	0.51	7.4
Sulfapyridine	0.85	8.4
Sulfanilamide	1.00	10.4

Modified from Lein EJ, Kuwahara J, and Koda RT: from Gaginella TS: US Pharm 3:39, 1978.

many weak electrolytes are more or less ionized in solution. Blood plasma and interstitial fluid are slightly alkaline (pH 7.4). Drugs that are weak acids are ionized to a greater extent in alkaline solution and are more extensively bound to protein. The amount of drug excreted from plasma (pH 7.4) to milk (pH 6.8 to 7.3, average 7.0) depends on the pH of the compound. Thus, a weakly acidic compound has a higher concentration in plasma than in milk. Conversely, weakly alkaline compounds are in equal or higher levels in the milk than in the plasma. The degree of drug ionization changes with the pH of the plasma and milk. Weak bases become more ionized with decreasing pH; thus, the ionized component will increase in milk. The concentration in plasma and milk for the nonionized fraction will be the same, but the total amount of drug in the milk will be greater than in plasma. The sulfonamides demonstrate the effect of the pK_a on the concentration of drug that reaches the milk. Sulfacetamide, with a low pK_a, has a low milk/plasma (M/P) ratio, whereas sulfanilamide has a pK_a of 10.4 and an M/P ratio of 1.00 (Table 11-1).

The studies done in cows and goats with constant infusions demonstrate this principle more dramatically because the pH of bovine plasma is 7.4 to 7.5 and of bovine milk, 6.5. Under normal circumstances, however, concentrations of drugs are rarely constant, and there is a delay in achieving a new equilibrium. During periods of rapidly decreasing blood levels there is some back diffusion into the plasma, according to Catz and Giacoia.[11]

Molecular weight

The passage of molecules into the milk also depends on the size of the molecule, or the molecular weight (mol wt). Water-filled membranal pores permit the movement of molecules of less than 200 mol wt. Owing to action similar to the limitation of transport of certain large molecular chemicals across the placenta, insulin and heparin are not found in human milk, presumably because of the size of the molecule.

Solubility

The alveolar epithelium of the breast is a lipid barrier that is most permeable in the first few days of lactation, when colostrum is being produced. The solubility of a compound in water and in lipid is a determining factor in its transfer. Un-ionized drugs, which are lipid soluble, usually dissolve and descend in the lipid phase of the membrane.[77,78] The solubility is closely linked to the manner in which the drug crosses the membranes (Table 11-2). The membrane of the alveolar epithelial cells is composed of lipoprotein, glycolipid, phospholipid, and free lipids, as described in Chapter 3. The transfer of water-soluble

Table 11-2. Predicted distribution ratios of drug concentrations in milk and plasma

	Milk/plasma ratio
Highly lipid-soluble drugs	~1
Small (mol wt <200) water-soluble drugs	~1
Weak acids	≤1
Weak bases	≥1
Actively transported drugs	>1

From Gaginella TS: US Pharm 3:39, 1978.

drugs and ions is inhibited by this hydrophobic barrier. Water-soluble materials pass through pores in the basement membrane and paracellular spaces. Low lipid solubility of an un-ionized compound will diminish its excretion into milk.

Lipid solubility affects the profile of the drug in the milk and plasma. A drug with high lipid solubility will have parallel elimination curves in the plasma and the milk. A drug with low lipid solubility will clear the plasma at a constant rate, but the clearance curve for the milk will peak lower and later, and the drug will linger in the milk. A prolonged terminal elimination phase may exist when there is a long time between feedings.[20]

Mechanisms of transport

Drugs pass into milk by simple diffusion, carrier-mediated diffusion, or active transport. Following is a summary of the methods of transport:

Simple diffusion—concentration gradient decreases
Carrier-mediated diffusion—concentration gradient decreases
Active transport—concentration gradient increases
Pinocytosis
Reverse pinocytosis

Pharmacokinetic principles relate to the specific variation with time of the drug concentration in the blood or plasma as a result of its absorption, distribution, and elimination. Ultimately, by extrapolation of these factors, one determines the effect of the drug. The most elementary kinetic model is based on the body as a single compartment. Distribution of the drug in the compartment is assumed to be uniform and rapidly equilibrated. In the single-compartment model, the volume of distribution of a drug is considered to be the same as that of the plasma, assuming a rapid uniform distribution.[24] The volume of distribution is

$$V_d = \frac{\text{Total amount of drug in body}}{\text{Concentration of drug in plasma}}$$

The absorption and elimination are considered to be exponential or first-order kinetics. A two-compartment model of drug kinetics takes into account the phase of decreasing drug concentration as drug distributes into the tissues. There is an initial rapid fall in concentrations as the drug distributes, then first-order elimination follows. When considering the pharmacokinetics of drugs in breast milk, one has to consider also that elimination in the breast is then by two potential routes: one excreted with the milk to the infant and the other by back diffusion into the plasma to reequilibrate with the falling level in the plasma.

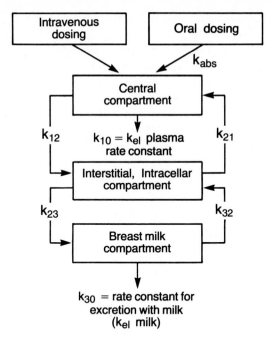

Fig. 11-2. Three-compartment model. (Modified from Wilson JT: Drug Metab Rev 14:619, 1983.)

With access to the volume of distribution of the drug in question, the amount of the dose, the weight of the mother, the concentration of drug in breast milk could be theoretically calculated:

$$\text{Concentration in breast milk} = \frac{\text{Dose}}{\text{Volume of distribution}}$$

The average total body store of drug at the plateau is approximately equal to 1.5 times the amount administered per one-half time of elimination.[59] The effect of a single dose of the drug is characterized by latency, time of peak effect, magnitude of peak effect, and duration. As dosage is increased, latency is reduced, and peak effect is increased without changing the time. Repeated dosage is usually calculated on one-half times of elimination, assuming four half-times are required for complete elimination. When the drug is given in less time, then the drug accumulates. Accumulation continues, in first-order kinetics, until the rate of elimination equals the rate of administration. A constant fraction of the drug is eliminated per unit of time. In general terms, maximal accumulation occurs after four half-times, and at this time the rate of elimination is equal to the rate of administration.[84]

Three-compartment model

To account for the relationship of the maternal body, the breast, the milk, and the infant, Wilson and his colleagues[82,83,84] have proposed a three-compartment model of kinetics to describe the drug excretion in breast milk. In this model there is a deep compartment—the third compartment—the breast (Fig. 11-2). When the infant is feeding, the rate constant is zero-order kinetics, and when there is no milk being removed, drug accumulates in the deep compartment and begins to transfer back. Compartment 1 represents the central compartment, which receives the drug directly following dosing. This compartment connects to compartment 2, as seen in two-compartment models by a reversible transport process of interstitial and intracellular water. The breast milk, which is compartment 3, is in equilibrium with compartment 2. Drug is eliminated from the mother's body at a constant rate (K_{10}) and from the breast milk by an infant-modulated rate constant (K_{30}). It is zero order during feeding, and therefore the rate is feeding dependent. Between feedings, however, K_{30} is zero, i.e., no drug leaves via the milk. The drug therefore accumulates in the third compartment, the breast. The drug can be transferred back to compartment 2 during this period between feedings. The rate constants differ for different drugs.

The concentration of the drug in the circulation of the mother depends on the mode of administration—oral, intramuscular, or intravenous. Absorption through the skin, the lungs (inhalants), or vaginally may also need to be considered. The curves produced by bolus intravenous medication peak high and early and taper sharply, thus making avoiding peak plasma levels more feasible. Absorption from intramuscular dosing is less rapid but follows a similar but less sharp curve. Oral dosing is dependent on other factors such as taking medication between or during meals. Depending on the curve of uptake and removal of drug from the plasma, the area under the curve varies. Single doses are simple area-under-the-curve calculations, but multiple doses or chronic use vary with the steady state of the drug in the body.

Nonelectrolytes such as ethanol, urea, and antipyrine enter the milk by diffusion through the lipid membrane barrier and may reach the same concentrations in the milk as in the plasma, irrespective of the pH. The main entrance site of molecules is at the basement laminal membrane, where water-soluble materials pass through the alveolar pores. Un-ionized drugs cross the membrane more easily than ionized ones because of the structure of the membrane. The un-ionized drugs pass through the membrane by diffusion. When simple diffusion takes place, the ratio between the concentration in the milk and in the plasma (the M/P ratio) is 1.0. Passive diffusion provides the same ratio regardless of the plasma concentrations of the drug or the volume of milk secreted. Different M/P ratios depend on the binding to protein and are a measure of the protein-free fraction. The dissimilar ratios for the sulfa drugs (Table 11-1) are partially due to the difference in protein binding.

Large molecules depend on their lipid solubility and ionization to cross the membrane, since they pass in a lipid-soluble nonionized form. The M/P ratio is determined when there is equilibrium in the amount of un-ionized drug in the aqueous phase on both sides of the membrane. When drugs are only partially ionized, the un-ionized fraction determines the concentration that crosses the membrane. The drugs whose un-ionized fraction is not very lipid soluble will pass only in limited degree into breast milk.

Passive drug transport may occur in the form of facilitated diffusion. The active compound is transported across the cell membrane by a carrier enzyme or protein. The gradient is toward a lesser or equal concentration in both simple diffusion and facilitated diffusion and is controlled by chemical activity gradients. Facilitated diffusion usually involves a water-soluble substance too large to pass through the membrane pores.

Active transport mechanisms provide a process whereby the gradient is "uphill," or higher, in the milk. The process is similar to facilitated diffusion except that metabolic energy is required to overcome the gradient. Examples of substances actively transported include glucose, amino acids, calcium, magnesium, and sodium. Pinocytosis and reverse pinocytosis, as described previously, are involved in the transport of very large molecules and proteins. Chloride ions are secreted into milk via an active apical membrane pump, whereas sodium and potassium are diffused by electrical gradient. Since the level of sodium is kept low, there may be an active return of sodium into the plasma.

A summary of the steps in the passage of drugs into breast milk follows:[78]

1. Mammary alveolar epithelium represents a lipid barrier with water-filled pores and is most permeable for drugs during colostral phase of milk secretion (first week postpartum).
2. Drug excretion into milk depends on the drug's degree of ionization, molecular weight, solubility in fat and water, and relation of pH of plasma (7.4) to pH of milk (7.0).
3. Drugs preferably enter mammary cells basally in the un-ionized, non-protein-bound form by diffusion or active transport.
4. Water-soluble drugs of mol wt below 200 pass through water-filled membranal pores.
5. Drugs leave mammary alveolar cells apically by diffusion or active transport.
6. Drugs may enter milk via spaces between mammary alveolar cells.
7. Most ingested drugs appear in milk; drug levels in milk usually do not exceed 1% of ingested dosage and are independent of milk volume.
8. Drugs are bound much less to milk proteins than to plasma proteins.
9. Drug-metabolizing capacity of mammary epithelium is not understood.

EFFECT ON THE NURSING INFANT
Absorption from the gastrointestinal tract

Although there is concern about the amount of a given agent in the breast milk, of greater importance is the amount absorbed into the infant's bloodstream. There is no accurate way to measure this because other factors also affect the level in the infant's bloodstream. The tolerance of the chemical to the pH of the stomach and the enzymatic activity of the intestinal tract are significant. The volume of milk consumed is a factor as well.

Infant's ability to detoxify and excrete the agent

Any drug given to an infant by any route has to be evaluated according to the infant's ability to detoxify or conjugate the chemical in the liver and/or excrete it in the urine or stool. Some compounds that appear in milk in very low levels are not well excreted by the infant and therefore accumulate in the infant's system to the point of toxicity.

Drugs that depend on the liver for conjugation, such as acetaminophen, are theoretic risks because of the limited reserve of the neonatal hepatic detoxification system. When actual measurements were made of neonates given acetaminophen, they were noted to handle it well because they conjugate it in the sulfhydral system as an alternative pathway used only to a small extent in adult metabolism of acetaminophen. When a single dose of a drug is given to a mother and the level is measured in her milk and in her infant, it does not give a clear picture of the potential for accumulation in the infant's system. The competition for binding a drug to protein is also important. Some drugs such as sulfadiazine compete for binding sites that might normally bind bilirubin in the first week or so of life. This puts the infant in jeopardy of kernicterus at a given bilirubin level because of an increase in the fraction of bilirubin left unbound for lack of binding sites. The indirect

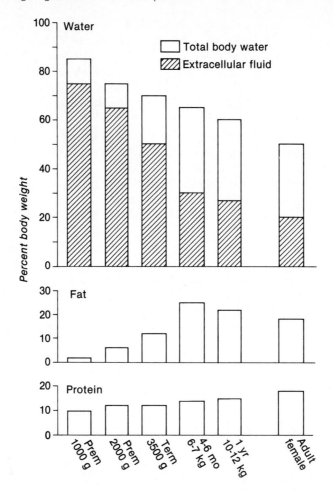

Fig. 11-3.   Comparative body composition of infants and adults. (Redrawn from Pencharz P B: Body composition and growth. In Walker WA and Waktins JB, editors: Nutrition in pediatrics, basic science and clinical application, Boston, 1985, Little, Brown.)

bilirubin level may even appear to be below the dangerous level. Some other compounds that displace bilirubin from albumin-binding sites include salicylic acid (aspirin or acetyl-salicylic acid breaks down to salicylic acid), furosemide, and phenylbutazone.

The maturity of the infant at birth is an extremely important factor during the first few months of life; thus the gestational age at birth should be established.[43] Clearly, the less mature the infant, the less well-tolerated the drug, not only because of the immaturity of the organ systems but also because of differences in body composition (Fig. 11-3). The less mature the infant, the greater the water content of the body and the proportion of extracellular water. Although the percentage of body weight taken up by protein is similar for all newborns, i.e., 12%, the absolute amount of protein for binding is less the smaller the infant. The amount of body fat is also low, by percent of body weight and in absolute values. The distribution of highly lipid-soluble drugs therefore will be more apt to deposit in the brain of a 1000 g infant with 3% body fat by weight than in a 3500 g full-term infant with 12% body fat. This may explain the more sedating effect of a drug on the central nervous system the younger and less mature the infant. The relative lack of plasma protein-binding sites in the small premature compared to the more mature and the older infant results in more free (unbound) active drug in circulation. Complications of premature birth such as acidosis and hypoxia also contribute to the unavailability of albumin binding sites and thus result in more unbound drug. The immaturity of the liver contributes to hyperbilirubinemia, and the increased bilirubin competes for albumin binding sites and increases the potential for kernicterus. The inability of the liver to metabolize drugs effectively results in the accumulation of some compounds that might be readily cleared by an older infant. At about 42 weeks conceptual age, an infant's liver is able to metabolize most drugs competently. Renal clearance similarly is less effective with decreasing maturity, which increases the risk of drug accumulation. The need to dose a premature only once or twice a day is common to many drugs, such as antibiotics, caffeine, and theophylline, and is testimony to the fact that a small premature does not clear drugs well.

Drugs that compete for albumin binding sites, such as sulfa drugs, may not be safe for a premature or even a full-term infant in the first weeks of life, when there is additional circulating bilirubin needing binding sites. Special problems in the neonate in addition to the presence of jaundice or low serum albumin may require special consideration. Low Apgar scores at birth signifying some degree of stress, hypoxia, or acidosis may alter binding-site availability but may also alter metabolism and excretion of a drug. Continuing respiratory distress requiring ventilatory support, sepsis, and renal failure are some of the neonatal stresses that require consideration when determining if a sick neonate can receive his mother's milk when she is being treated with certain medications. Prescribing in such a mother should be done in consultation with the neonatologist if the woman is lactating.[43]

The age of the infant makes a difference in the total volume of milk consumed, and in the older child there are other items in the diet so that milk does not comprise the total intake. Age makes a difference because the more mature infant can metabolize drugs more effectively; thus sulfa drugs, for instance, can be given to infants after the first month of life.

If the agent is fat soluble, the fat content of the milk may be a significant variable. The fat content at any feeding increases over time; thus the so-called foremilk is low in fat and the hindmilk is four to five times richer in fat toward the end of a feeding. The total amount of fat in a given feeding is less in the morning, peaks at midday, and drops off in the evening even though the total amount of fat will be about the same each 24-hour period. The coefficient of lipid solubility for an un-ionized drug determines both its penetration of the biologic membrane to gain entrance to milk and its concentration in milk fat, according to Wilson.[82] Sulfonamides with low fat solubility are in the aqueous and protein fraction of milk, whereas many barbiturates are in the lipid fraction. There is an inverse relationship between a drug's lipid solubility and the amount that appears in the skim fraction. The concentrations in fat differ for each member of the barbital family. Pentobarbital and secobarbital are found in the lipid phase, whereas phenobarbital is found in the aqueous phase.

The agent may appear in low levels in a mother's serum, but mammary blood flow during lactation is 500 ml/minute and a mother produces between 60 and 300 ml of milk/hour. The agent that appears in minimal concentrations in the milk may present a significant problem when one considers that 1000 ml of milk may be consumed in a day by an infant. During the colostral phase of lactation, the breast is more permeable to drugs.

BREAST MILK/PLASMA RATIO FOR DRUGS

The milk/plasma ratio for drugs has been measured and reported as the single most valuable piece of information necessary for the clinician to use in making a decision about a medication during lactation.[83] By definition, it is the concentration of the drug in the milk versus the concentration in maternal plasma (serum) at the same time. It presumes that the relationship between the two concentrations remains constant, which in most cases it does not. If it were a constant, it would allow the estimation of the amount of drug in the milk from any given plasma level in the mother. An inaccurate ratio or one determined under variable circumstances produces erroneous estimates of the amount of drug in the milk as pointed out by Wilson et al.,[84] who state that a pharmacokinetic model is a requisite foundation for studies of drugs in breast milk. A single-point-in-time M/P ratio or an average ratio calculated with single-dose, area-under-the-curve data does not work for all drugs. Neither ratio accounts for the importance of time-dependent variations of drug concentration in milk. Dose strength, duration of dosing, maternal variation in drug disposition, maternal disease, drug interactions and competition of additional drugs for metabolism or binding sites, and racial variations in drug metabolism all influence the M/P interpretation. The characteristics of the drug and the dosing pattern are essential to the interpretation of the M/P ratio.[84]

EVALUATING DATA ABOUT A GIVEN DRUG

The paucity of carefully controlled studies on large enough samples to validate the results when such a large number of variables are active has been lamented by many authors. Some data collected are not pharmacokinetically sound. The clinician needs to understand these variables as well as pharmacokinetic principles so that a reasonable judgment about a given case can be made.

Although it should be theoretically possible to determine how much of a specific drug reaches the infant in his mother's milk by knowing all the properties of the drug—including its volume of distribution, pH, pK_a, lipid solubility, protein-binding activity, and rate of detoxification in the maternal system—there is sufficient variation in the levels that reach the infant and how he deals with the agent to make it necessary to have specific data about a specific drug. Thus a few simple steps in the decision-making process are helpful in determining risk.

Safety for the infant

Is this a drug that can be given to the infant directly if necessary? Antibiotics such as penicillin, for instance, that one could give the infant are in this category, whereas an antibiotic such as chloramphenicol, which one would not give the infant under ordinary circumstances, should be avoided in the nursing mother. The toxicity of chloramphenicol in the infant is dose related and associated with an unpredictable accumulation of the drug. There is also an idiosyncratic reaction that occurs with chloramphenicol, which is unrelated to dose but is capable of causing pancytopenia.

If the drug in question can be given to the infant, is there any risk to the infant in the amount in the milk? Phenobarbital can be given to infants for various reasons; thus the question is whether enough will reach the infant to cause difficulty. The infant should be watched for symptoms of depression, such as a change in feeding or sleeping pattern.

If the infant is sleeping long periods and feeding less than usual (specifically, fewer than five or six times a day), then the medication may be at fault. Phenobarbital is a significant drug for the mother with seizures; therefore, a careful review of the risk-to-benefit ratio to the mother as well as to the infant should be undertaken. Barbiturates vary in their effect in young infants because the newborn does not handle the short-acting barbiturates well. They are readily detoxified in the adult liver, whereas phenobarbital depends more on the kidney for excretion.

If the drug was taken during pregnancy, as in epilepsy, the infant already has the drug in his system via the placenta at a steady state that the infant will have to begin to excrete on his own.[57] On the other hand, enzyme induction may have taken place in the neonate due to exposure to the drug in utero; this will hasten maturation of the liver.[62] Enzyme induction of the hepatic oxygenase system by phenobarbital, phenytoin, primidone, and carbamazepine is well established. Valproate does not induce enzyme activity. If one can safely give the drug to an infant, then it is a question of watching for any symptoms of excessive accumulation that might develop. The age of the infant is critical also.

When the drug in question is one not normally given to an infant of his particular age, weight, or degree of maturity, then a decision is more difficult. Specific information about the amount of the drug that appears in the milk is essential in decision making. Often conflicting information is available. Many lists of drug-milk levels have perpetuated the same errors in calculation; thus, having more than one reference may not provide confirmed information.

If the medication will have to be taken for weeks or months, as is the case with the cardiovascular drugs, the drug has greater potential impact than when it will only be taken for a few days. If the drug exposure has gone on for 9 months in utero already, some feel it is less of a problem; on the other hand, it may compound the problem.

To determine the dose delivered to the infant, the following formula is used:

Dose delivered to the infant:

Dose/24 hours = Concentration of drug in milk $\times$ Wt (kg) of Baby $\times$
Amount of milk ingested in 24 hours

$$\text{Dose/24 hours} = C_{milk} \times \text{Weight} \times \text{Volume/kg}$$

Sensitization

Is there risk of sensitization, even in the small dosages of a drug that might pass into the milk? This question arises most frequently around the use of antibiotics, and use of penicillin is most frequently questioned. Certainly if there is a strong history of drug sensitization in the family, it should be considered. In that case, however, it should be questioned for the mother as well. Whether infants are put at risk of developing resistant strains of bacteria in their systems by small amounts of antibiotic in their feedings is a serious question and, of course, is pertinent for the dairy and meat industry as well as for the humans who consume these products.

Correlation of drug safety in pregnancy and lactation

Very rarely is valid information on the appearance of a drug in milk available on the package insert, since the pharmaceutical companies usually merely indicate that it should not be taken during pregnancy and lactation. Agents that may be safe in pregnancy may not be so in lactation because during pregnancy the maternal liver and kidney are serving as detoxification and excretion resources for the fetus via the placenta, whereas during lactation the infant has to handle the drug totally on his own once it has reached his circulation. The infant in utero receives the drug in greater quantity via the circulation, whereas the nursing infant receives only what reaches the milk. One should be cautious about translating data pertaining to these two states back and forth.

Oral bioavailability

The dose of a drug via the milk to the infant is significantly affected by the oral bioavailability, which is the percentage of the drug absorbed into the infant's system via the gut.[64] These values are provided in Table E-1, Appendix E. If a compound is poorly absorbed, it is of less concern than one with 100% bioavailability.

MINIMIZING THE EFFECT OF MATERNAL MEDICATION

If a mother needs a specific medication and the hazards to the infant are minimal, the following important adjustments can be made to minimize the effects:

1. Do not use the long-acting form of the drug because the infant has even more difficulty excreting such an agent, which usually requires detoxification in the liver. Accumulation in the infant is then a genuine concern.
2. Schedule the doses so the least amount possible gets into the milk. Check the usual absorption rates and peak blood levels of the drug. Having the mother take the medication immediately after breastfeeding is the safest time for the infant in most, but not all, drugs.
3. Watch the infant for any unusual signs or symptoms such as change in feeding pattern or sleeping habits, fussiness, or rash.
4. When possible, choose the drug that produces the least amount in the milk (Tables 11-1 and 11-2).

Classification systems

A Swedish classification system for drug information regarding drug use during pregnancy and breastfeeding was devised in 1978 by the National Swedish Board of Health with the help of the drug manufacturers' trade organizations.[5,67] The system classifies drugs into categories regarding pregnancy (Categories A, B, C, or D) and the following four groups to describe drugs during lactation:

Group I   Active ingredients do not enter the milk.
Group II   Active ingredients enter the milk but in such small amounts that there is no risk to the infant.
Group III Active ingredients enter the milk in sufficient quantities to represent a risk to the child even at therapeutic levels.
Group IV   Not known whether active ingredients enter the milk.

Of 960 drugs registered and reviewed, 5% were in Group I, 32% in Group II, 12% in Group III, and 50.8% in Group IV.

In 1983 the American Academy of Pediatrics published a list of the transfer of drugs and other chemicals into human breast milk.[15] This list was also divided into four categories with very opposing definitions to the Swedish ratings:

1. Drugs contraindicated during breastfeeding

2. Drugs requiring temporary cessation of breastfeeding
3. Drugs usually compatible with breastfeeding
4. Food and environmental agents affecting breastfeeding

Only compounds about which there is information are listed. Most compounds are given a "3" by this coding, although there is conflicting information about many items in the third group. There is little or no debate about items in categories 1 and 2.

SPECIFIC DRUG GROUPS

Information available about specific individual drugs has been provided in Appendix E. Table E-1 provides information about the oral bioavailability for the infant, the peak serum time in the mother (and peak milk time when available), the volume of distribution for the drug, the available information about levels in milk, the Academy of Pediatrics' classification number (1, 2, 3, 4), the Swedish classification (I, II, III, IV), and the references. With this information the physician should be able to adjust dose, time, and associated breastfeeding.

Analgesics

Drugs such as heroin have been known for decades to appear in milk, and at one time withdrawal symptoms in the neonate were prevented or treated by breastfeeding and then gradual weaning. Codeine, meperidine (Demerol), and pentazocine (Talwin) appear in milk at low levels. Individual variation is common, and neonates can be depressed by the medication; therefore care should be taken to monitor the infant carefully. For example, a breastfed newborn was transferred to the special-care nursery at Rochester because of unusual floppiness and poor muscle tone. His mother was taking dextropropoxyphene (Darvon) every 4 hours. Temporarily stopping the nursing until the mother's drug level dropped and discontinuing use of the drug produced dramatic improvement, which persisted when the infant went back to nursing. Diazepam (Valium) when taken in multiple doses has caused sleepiness, mild depression, and decreased intake in some infants and has a tendency to accumulate in the neonate, especially in the first weeks. An occasional Diazepam is not contraindicated.

The dose schedule for analgesics is usually single dose, especially in the postpartum period. A mother should not be subjected to great discomfort when a dose or two of analgesics would improve her well-being. Aspirin on a single-dose schedule is quite safe, although it is known to pass into her milk. The case of metabolic acidosis reported in a nursing infant occurred when the mother took 10 grains of aspirin every 4 hours for arthritis.[13] A serum salicylate in the infant on the third day of hospitalization with no breastfeeding was still 24 mg/100 ml. This demonstrates the tendency of salicylate to accumulate in the neonate. Acetylsalicylic acid, not the metabolite salicylate, is responsible for the platelet aggregate abnormalities, so there should be no concern about aspirin in this regard, since it is the metabolite that appears in the milk. Acetaminophen is remarkably well tolerated by the neonate, as noted earlier in this chapter, and can be given to a nursing mother, although it does reach the milk in small amounts.

Antibiotics

Levels in milk vary with the pH of the drugs and their pK_a. The risks vary among groups of antibiotics. Penicillins are not usually toxic but theoretically can cause sensitivity.

Sulfa drugs should not be used in the first month of life because they can interfere with the binding of bilirubin to protein. The risk diminishes with age, and infants are given sulfa drugs directly at 6 to 8 weeks of age. Infants with G_6PD deficiency should never receive sulfa drugs directly or via the breast milk. Chloramphenicol is contraindicated in nursing very young infants because of the risk of accumulation of the drug even from small amounts in milk and the potential for idiosyncracy. Tetracycline causes staining of teeth and abnormalities of bone growth when given directly to children for a week or more. Infants breastfed by mothers taking tetracycline for mastitis may have stained and mottled first and second teeth when therapy exceeds 10 days. The amount in milk is half that in the mother's plasma. Tetracycline should only be given mothers for life-threatening infections.

Erythromycin appears in higher amounts in milk than in plasma. When given intravenously to the mother, the levels are 10 times higher. When the infant is old enough to receive erythromycin directly, the mother can take it as well.

Aminoglycosides are common constituents of postpartum antibiotic therapy and are given parentally. They readily appear in the milk but, like kanamycin, are not readily absorbed from the gastrointestinal tract; therefore, under usual circumstances they pose no problem to the neonate, who will not absorb them.

Metronidazole (Flagyl) does appear in milk at levels equal to those in serum. Most researchers consider the risk to the infant sufficient to suggest alternative therapy for the mother. Symptoms include decreased appetite and vomiting and, occasionally, blood dyscrasia.

An alternative treatment regimen is 2 g metronidazole in a single dose. When milk concentrations are measured with a 2 g dose, the highest concentrations are found at 2 and 4 hours post-ingestion and decline over the next 12 hours to 19.1 μg/ml and to 12.6 μg/ml at 24 hours.[19,27] The dose to the infant is calculated to be 21.8 mg over the first 24 hours and only 3.5 mg in the second 24 hours. It has been recommended that the single-dose regimen be used in nursing mothers, which necessitates that a mother pump and discard milk for only 24 hours. Metronidazole is often the only drug that works in a serious trichomoniasis, giardiasis, or amebiasis infection[19] when all other treatments have failed.

Amoxicillin, cephalexin, and cefadroxil, when given orally in a single dose, peak in the milk at 4 to 6 hours.[33] Cephalothin, cephapirin, and cefotaxime, when given in a bolus IV injection, peak at 2 hours. Cefadroxil reached the highest levels (1.64 ± 0.73 μg/ml) at 6 hours.

The serum half-lives of parenterally administered cephalosporins are three to four times longer in the neonate than the serum half-lives in the mother. The half-life of ceftriaxone in the milk is 12 to 17 hours compared to the maternal serum half-life of 6 hours. The milk/plasma ratio at 8 hours was 0.05 and at 24 hours, 0.1. Moxalactam concentrations in milk with multiple doses are 3.24 ± 1.7 ng/ml, which would provide the neonate with 1.8 mg/day.[52]

Chloroquine, oxacillin, and para-aminosalicylic acid are reported by O'Brien[57] to be safe because they are not excreted in milk. Additional antibiotics are listed in Appendix E.

Anticholinergics

Anticholinergic drugs include atropine, scopolamine (hyoscine), and synthetic quaternary ammonium derivatives, some of which are available in over-the-counter medications. Some atropine does enter the milk. Infants are particularly sensitive to this drug; therefore the infant involved should be watched for tachycardia and thermal changes, which are more easily measured in infants. There may be a decrease in milk secretion in the mother, and constipation and urinary retention may occur in the infant. The quaternary anticholinergics should not appear in milk in any degree because, as cations, they do not pass into the acidic milk. Mepenzolate methylbromide (Cantil) has been reported by both O'Brien[57] and Gaginella[23] not to appear in milk.

Cimetidine (Tagamet), a potent H_2-receptor antagonist, is used for conditions associated with acid peptic digestion in the gastrointestinal tract. Cimetidine excretion into breast milk has resulted in concentrations higher than in the corresponding plasma sample.[72] Levels were highest at 1 hour after a single dose. Chronic-dose studies revealed variable M/P ratios, all of which were higher than the single-dose ratio. The authors suggest an active transport mechanism for this medication. The maximum amount of cimetidine ingested by an infant was calculated at 6 mg for 1 L of milk (or 1.5 mg/kg). Caution is recommended in nursing with this medication until more is known of its side effects, especially the antiandrogenic features. It has been listed by Feldman and Pickering as contraindicated during lactation.[20] Classification is 1 (AAP) and III (Swedish System).

Sulfasalazine treatment of ulcerative colitis and Crohn's disease during breastfeeding has been widely discussed on theoretic grounds because the compound splits to sulfapyridine and 5-aminosalicylic acid (5-ASA). The sulfapyridine is absorbed from the colon and is metabolized in the liver. The 5-ASA is partly absorbed and rapidly excreted in the urine, so serum concentrations are low. The sulfapyridine and its metabolites do appear in the milk in lower concentrations than in the serum. A dose of 2 g/day of drug to the mother would produce 4 mg/kg of sulfapyridine in the milk, about 40% of maternal levels.[32] It is felt the risk of recurrent ulcerative colitis if medication is withdrawn outweighs the risk of sulfasalazine to the infant.[36]

Anticoagulants

Heparin does not pass into milk, but it is not a drug that can be given orally to the mother or without close monitoring of prothrombin times. Anticoagulants had been reported to appear in breast milk and to prolong prothrombin times not only in the mother but also in the infant. Infants nursed by these mothers had been sustained with 1 mg of vitamin K daily. Because of the competition for conjugation in the glucuronidase system, extra vitamin K is not recommended in the first few weeks of life except for the initial dose at birth. Knowles[39] has reviewed the literature on anticoagulant drugs thoroughly and specifically bis-3′:3′-(4-oxycoumarinyl) ethyl acetate (Tromexan). Although infants nursed by mothers taking the drug had been observed to hemorrhage, they had improvement of their prothrombin times. Infants given the drug directly in milk had poorer prothrombin times. It is believed the drug is altered by maternal metabolism. The drug has also been observed to cause changes in capillary resistance, especially when there has been previous vascular damage. Vitamin K has no effect on the hemorrhagic tendencies in these infants. When the mother was taking phenindione (an indanedione derivative), hemorrhaging in the nursing newborn has been associated with trauma. Ethyl biscoumacetate has also been found in mother's milk by Illingworth and Finch.[30]

Analysis of the milk of mothers using warfarin by Orme et al.,[58] however, did not reveal any drug in the milks or in the infants. The infants' prothrombin times remained normal. This has been further confirmed by McKenna et al.,[49] who followed two breastfed infants whose mothers were anticoagulated prior to delivery and maintained on warfarin postpartum. They found no immediate or delayed biologic effect on coagulation in 56 and 131 days of follow-up. From this it has been suggested that warfarin is the drug of choice in the lactating mother who requires anticoagulant therapy and wishes to continue breast-feeding. If surgery is contemplated or unusual trauma occurs, a review of the coagulation status of the infant is indicated as a precautionary measure.

Antithyroid drugs

Iodide has been known for generations to pass into the milk and has been recorded to cause symptoms in infants when used not only for hyperthyroidism but also in asthma preparations and cough medicines. Iodides have been noted to be goitrogenic and to sensitize the thyroid gland to other drugs such as lithium, chlorpromazine, and methylxanthines.

Thiouracil is actively transported into the milk and appears in higher concentration in milk than in blood or urine, being reported at three to twelve times higher in milk than blood. It has the potential of causing goiter-suppressing thyroid activity or agranulocytes.

Methimazole (Tapazole) presents risks to the nursing infant similar to those seen with thiouracil, that is, thyroid suppression and goiter. Giving 0.125 grain of thyroid extract to an infant may not adequately protect him, and careful monitoring of neonatal thyroid function is mandatory. Measurement of amounts of methimazole in milk and serum when a mother received 2.5 mg every 12 hours by Tegler and Lindström[76] were found to be similar. They found 7% to 16% of the maternal dose in the milk; thus a dose of 5 mg, four times daily, might provide the infant with 3 mg daily. Studies of carbimazole using ^{38}S-labeled compound show a similar trend, with 0.47% of the dose appearing in the milk. Studies were done on a single dose of 10 mg carbimazole.

Propylthiouracil (PTU) has been investigated by several groups with similar results reported, showing that little of the compound is excreted in the milk (0.025% to 0.077% of total dose) in single-dose studies.[34,48] An infant followed 5 months on maternal doses of 200 to 300 mg PTU daily showed no neonatal thyroid symptoms and normal triiodo-thyronine (T_3), thyroxine (T_4), and thyroid-stimulating hormone (TSH). On the strength of these reports, others have proceeded to use PTU and permit breastfeeding. The availability of microdeterminations for T_3, T_4, and TSH improve the quality of monitoring, and all infants given PTU via the milk should be followed closely.

Caffeine and other methylxanthines

Caffeine ingestion has been singled out for discussion because it is a frequent concern, yet the data provided in most reviews are misleading. Although with a given dose of caffeine that is comparable to that in a cup of coffee the level in the milk is low (1% of level in mother) and the level in the infant's plasma is also low, caffeine does accumulate in the infant. Before the availability of the laboratory test for caffeine, cases were managed on clinical symptoms alone. It had been recognized by many clinicians and documented in the Rochester series[42] of nursing mothers that wakeful, hyperactive infants were often the victims of caffeine stimulation. If a mother drank more than 6 to 8 cups of any caffeine-containing beverage in a day's time, her infant could accumulate symptomatic amounts of caffeine. Often soft drinks such as colas and other carbonated drinks (such as Mountain Dew) contributed to the caffeine buildup. When the situation was identified—a wide-eyed, active, alert infant who never slept for long—it was suggested that the mother try caffeine-free beverages, both hot and cold drinks. Often the infant settled down to a reasonable sleep pattern after a few days with no caffeine. Since information on milk and plasma levels has become available, researchers[43] have identified three cases of caffeine excess in breastfed infants, one of which Rivera-Calimlin[63] reported. The infants all had measurable levels of caffeine in the plasma, which disappeared over a week's time after the caffeine was discontinued. The corresponding milk levels were as previously reported, about 1% of the mother's level, which supports the hypothesis that caffeine accumulates in the infant. The infants do not need to be hospitalized, and verification of blood caffeine levels is helpful but not mandatory, since clinical trial will suffice. Smoking has been observed to augment the caffeine effect.

With an increasing number of women with asthma wishing to breastfeed, a question arises about the impact of theophylline. The methylxanthines have also been used in apnea of prematurity so that information has been generated around dose, clearance, and toxicity in the neonate.[6] In addition, microdeterminations of blood levels are readily available.

Several studies of theophylline in mothers on regular doses have shown that the serum levels are lowest just before the oral dose and that M/P ratio is 0.60 to 0.73, with milk levels paralleling serum levels.[7,73] It has been estimated that the infant receives 1% of the maternal dose. Data on IV and oral medication are similar in terms of M/P ratio. Maximum exposure was estimated at 7 to 8 mg/24 hours.

Dyphylline is a compound introduced clinically as a bronchodilator because of its lack of side effects.[31] It is excreted renally with little biotransformation. The milk serum ratio was determined to be 2.08 ± 52, and the biologic half-life was 3.21 hours. Although this is considerably greater than theophylline, it is not yet known how this would affect the infant.

Theobromine, which occurs in chocolate and cocoa, has been studied as well to evaluate its possible cumulative effects when taken with caffeine or theophylline.[6] A very small amount was detected in the milk, with a potential dose to the infant after one chocolate bar (1.2 oz) of 0.44 to 1.68 mg. No theobromine was found in the infant's urine.[7]

Herbs and herbal teas

There has been an increase in the use of herbs and herbal teas, especially among those interested in natural foods. As is well known to all students of pharmacology, many of today's effective medications originated in these natural products. In the early part of the century many compounds were still being dispensed in their natural form, including foxglove leaves for digitalis. The natural product was unpredictable because one leaf or plant contains more or less active principle than another, so that careful dose control was impossible and results were often unpredictable. Much of the interest in herbal teas has evolved as individuals seek a beverage that does not contain caffeine; what they get is another compound instead, often one more potent and much of the time one about which considerably less is known (Table 11-3).

Herbal teas are available that are prepared carefully, using herbs only for essence (Celestial Seasonings brand tea) and avoiding heavy doses of herbs with active principles. The strength of any tea depends on how it is made, however. An ordinary teabag with hot water run over it will contain little caffeine and theobromine; however, when it is steeped for 5 minutes the potency is increased tenfold. Some of the preparations are benign or even nutritious, such as rose hips tea, which contains a large amount of vitamin C. Other teas are made from plants known to the toxicologist as poisonous. Isolated reports of toxicity from these preparations are appearing in the medical literature; many others probably go undiagnosed.[68] Use of these preparations is certainly an important part of a medical and dietary history.

Mother's milk tea is a blend of plants handed down for many generations as a galactagogue; it contains a mixture of fennel seeds, coriander seeds, chamomile flowers,

Table 11-3. Psychoactive substances used in herbal preparations

Labeled ingredient	Botanical source	Pharmacologic principle	Suggested use	Reported effects
African Yohimbe bark; yohimbe	*Corynanthe yohimbe*	Yohimbe	Smoke or tea as stimulant	Mild hallucinogen
Broom; scotch broom	*Cytisus* spp	Cytisine	Smoke for relaxation	Strong sedative-hypnotic
California poppy	*Eschscholtzia californica*	Alkaloids and glucosides	Smoke as marihuana substitute	Mild euphoriant
Catnip	*Nepeta cataria*	Nepetalactone	Smoke or tea as marihuana substitute	Mild hallucinogen
Cinnamon	*Cinnamomum camphora*	?	Smoke with marihuana	Mild stimulant
Damiana	*Turnera diffusa*	?	Smoke as marihuana substitute	Mild stimulant
Hops	*Humulus lupulus*	Lupuline	Smoke or tea as sedative and marihuana substitute	None
Hydrangea	*Hydrangea paniculata*	Hydrangin, saponin, cyanogenes	Smoke as marihuana substitute	Stimulant
Juniper	*Juniper macropoda*	?	Smoke as hallucinogen	Strong hallucinogen
Kavakava	*Piper methysticum*	Yangonin, pyrones	Smoke or tea as marihuana substitute	Mild hallucinogen
Kola nut; gotu kola	*Cola* spp	Caffeine, theobromine, kolanin	Smoke, tea, or capsules as stimulant	Stimulant

From Siegel RK: JAMA, 236:473, 1976, Copyright 1976, American Medical Association.

lemongrass, borage leaves, blessed thistle leaves, star anise, comfrey leaves, and fenugreek seeds.[75] It is promoted as containing no caffeine. Some of the things it does contain are shown in Table 11-4. Although not all the constituents have pharmacologic actions, several do and were used medicinally for centuries. These popular teas have the same potential for problems as do the common popular beverages coffee and cola. The euphoric effects are the most prominent.

A hemorrhagic diathesis was described in a woman who drank quarts of herbal tea that contained tonka beans, melilot (sweet clover), and woodruff, all of which contain natural coumarins.[29] She narrowly avoided gynecologic surgery for excessive hemorrhaging before the history was obtained. The tea also included hawthorn, which contains cardioglucosides that cause hypotension.

Table 11-3. Psychoactive substances used in herbal preparations—cont'd

Labeled ingredient	Botanical source	Pharmacologic principle	Suggested use	Reported effects
Lobelia	*Lobelia inflata*	Lobeline	Smoke or tea as marihuana substitute	Mild euphoriant
Mandrake	*Mandragora officinarum*	Scopolamine, hyoscyamine	Tea as hallucinogen	Hallucinogen
Mate	*Ilex paraguayensis*	Caffeine	Tea as stimulant	Stimulant
Mormon tea	*Ephedra nevadensis*	Ephedrine	Tea as stimulant	Stimulant
Nutmeg	*Myristica fragrans*	Myristicin	Tea as hallucinogen	Hallucinogen
Passion flower	*Passiflora incarnata*	Harmine alkaloids	Smoke, tea, or capsules as marihuana substitute	Mild stimulant
Periwinkle	*Catharanthus roseus*	Indole alkaloids	Smoke or tea as euphoriant	Hallucinogen
Prickly poppy	*Argemone mexicana*	Protopine, bergerine, isoquinilines	Smoke as euphoriant	Narcotic-analgesic
Snakeroot	*Rauwolfia serpentina*	Reserpine	Smoke or tea as tobacco substitute	Tranquilizer
Thorn apple	*Datura stramonium*	Atropine, scopolamine	Smoke or tea as tobacco substitute or hallucinogen	Strong hallucinogen
Tobacco	*Nicotiana* spp	Nicotine	Smoke as tobacco	Strong stimulant
Valerian	*Valeriana officinalis*	Chatinine, velerine alkaloids	Tea or capsules as tranquilizer	Tranquilizer
Wild lettuce	*Lactuca sativa*	Lactucarine	Smoke as opium substitute	Mild narcotic-analgesic
Wormwood	*Artemisia absinthium*	Absinthine	Smoke or tea as relaxant	Narcotic-analgesic

Sassafras contains an aromatic oil, safrole, which has been shown to cause cancer in mice; it is therefore no longer permitted as a commerical flavoring, but it appears in herbal teas. It causes central nervous system symptoms in mice including ataxia, ptosis, and hypothermia.[68] It is also thought to interfere with the action of other medications. Belladonna alkaloids are common in some teas used to create euphoria or ease pain.

Pyrolizidine alkaloids have been identified in an herbal tea used in the Southwest that was responsible for several deaths in children given the tea when they were ill. The alkaloid is excreted within 24 hours, but symptoms may not start for several days or weeks. Death is due to liver failure.

The clinician needs to inquire about all foods and beverages when taking a history. If an excessive amount of any herbal product is being consumed, its contents should be

Table 11-4. Ingredients and effects of mother's milk tea

Plant	Constituents	Effects	Toxicity
Fennel seed	Volatile oil, anisic acid	Weak diuretic stimulant	"Disturbs CNS"
Coriander seed	Volatile oil, coriandrol	Increases flow of saliva and gastric juice	
Chamomile flower	Volatile oil, bitter glycoside	Sudorific; antispasmodic; used to lighten hair	Vomiting and vertigo
Lemongrass	Lemon flavor		
Borage leaf	Volatile oil, tannin, mineral acids	Diuretic, sudorific, euphoric	Possible
Blessed thistle leaf	Volatile oil, bitter principle	Appertif, galactagogue, diaphoretic	Strongly emetic
Star anise	Volatile oil, anethole, resin, tannin	Stimulant, mild expectorant	
Comfrey leaf	Protein, vitamin B_{12}, tannin, allantoin, choline	Used as mucilage to knit bones, weak sedative, demulcent, astringent	
Fenugreek seed (Greek hay) (coffee substitute and natural dye)	Mucilage, trigonelline, physterols, celery flavor		
Other beverages			
Coffee plant	Volatile oil, caffeine, tannin	Stimulant, diuretic, coloring	Insomnia, restlessness
Blue cohosh	Saponin, "glucoside that affects muscles"	Oxytocic, potent, acts on voluntary and involuntary muscles	Irritant, causes pain in fingers and toes

checked. The regional poison control center may be able to identify active principles if the plant constituents of the tea are known.

Cardiovascular drugs and diuretics

Digitalis is given to infants, but only for serious reasons. Measurements of digitalis in the milk in mothers maintained on digitalis throughout pregnancy and lactation showed concentrations of 0.825 nmol/L, which was 59% of the maternal plasma level in one study[12] and 75% in another.[21] If one calculates the predicted level of digitalis using the volume of distribution which is high, 7.5 L/kg, the infant would receive 1.1 ng/ml in the milk with a 60 kg mother receiving 0.5 mg dose of digoxin.[59] Authors agree that digoxin levels would be low and the dosage to the infant low, but the long-range effects are not known.[12,21,48] There is sufficient experience accumulated to date to conclude that mothers taking sustaining doses of digitalis preparations may nurse their infants without any harm to the infant.

Propranolol was found in the milk of mothers but does not appear to accumulate in the infant. Thus experienced cardiologists have permitted mothers taking propranolol to nurse their infants without any ill effect observed in the infants. In 1973, Levitan and Manion[44] reported significant quantities of propranolol in breast milk. Propranolol and its major metabolites were measured in milk and found by Smith et al.[71] to provide the infant with a maximum dose of less than 0.1% of the maternal dose or approximately 7μg/100 ml. The half-life of elimination from the milk was over 6 hours.[4] β-Adrenergic blockade effects, including hypoglycemia, have been described in an infant breastfed by a mother taking propranolol. Since the reports are conflicting, it would be necessary to monitor the breastfed infant carefully when the mother is taking propranolol. Monitoring plasma levels of the infant may be helpful if there is any question.

The antihypertensive drugs atenolol (Tenormin), metoprolol (Lopressor), and nadolol (Corgard, Corzide) have been evaluated in human milk.[17,18,50] Metoprolol had a peak level in the blood of 713 ng/100 ml at 1.1 hours and in the milk of 4.7 ng/100 ml at 3.8 hours. The data suggest that metoprolol appears minimally in milk and is probably safe for the breastfeeding neonate.[18] Nadolol appears in serum at 77 ng/100 ml and in milk at 357 ng/100 ml.[17] Atenolol levels in milk are also higher than in the maternal serum.[50] These drugs are rated 3 (AAP) and II (Swedish System). Serum levels of atenolol in one breastfed infant reached 0.16 μmol/L.

Reserpine, on the other hand, has been reported to cause nasal stuffiness, bradycardia, and respiratory difficulty with increased tracheobronchial secretion and is contraindicated in both pregnancy and lactation.

Most diuretics are weak acids and little passes into milk. Use of diuretics, however, requires careful observation because they have the potential for causing a diuresis in the neonate that could be markedly dehydrating. Although diuretics such as furosemide (Lasix) are given to neonates, this is done only when fluid and electrolyte levels can be followed closely. Oral diuretics were used to suppress lactation in a study by Healy[26] in 40 postpartum women who chose not to breastfeed. Bendroflumethiazide (Naturetin) was used, 5 mg twice daily for 5 days. He found it more effective than estrogens, with fewer side effects. Reports have also appeared documenting the interaction of three diuretics with bilirubin-albumin complexes.[79] Chlorothiazide presented the greatest risk for producing free bilirubin, with ethacrynic acid and furosemide producing considerably less. The latter two are clinically effective in lower doses as well. The levels of chlorothiazide and hydro-chlorothiazide in milk are less than 100 ng/ml.[51,53] For most infants these are safe; however, these findings certainly suggest caution is necessary if the infant is jaundiced or very immature. Chlorthalidone (Hygroton) appears in milk.[80] A term baby might receive 180 μg per day. The half-life is 60 hours. Furosemide has been shown by several techniques not only to displace bilirubin from albumin in the newborn but also to be slowly excreted by the newborn, with only 84% excreted in 24 hours.

A mother who is lactating may actually require substantially less medication, particularly diuretics. Close monitoring of the mother during lactation to try to reduce her medications may provide a therapeutic balance that is good for the mother and safe for the infant.

Central nervous system drugs

Phenobarbital can be given to infants and is usually safe, but careful observation of the infant for variation in sleeping and feeding habits is important.

Phenytoin in the breast milk has been associated with vomiting, tremors, rash, blood dyscrasia (rarely), and methemoglobinemia, but not with drowsiness and lethargy. Many

Table 11-5. Anticonvulsant concentrations in maternal serum and milk

Drug	Maternal serum (μg/ml)	Milk (μg/ml)	Day 1	Milk/serum Day 7	Day 30
Diphenylhydantoin (half-life in neonate 9-56 hrs)	3.0	0.7	18 ± 15	19 ± 4	13 ± 6
Phenobarbital (half-life in neonate 156 ± 29 hrs)	12.0	5.0	30 ± 16	36 ± 7	30 ± 5
Primidone (half-life in neonate 23 ± 8 hrs)	4.0	2.1	141 ± 9	56 ± 15	46 ± 7
Carbamazepine (half-life in neonate 13-36 hrs)	4.0	1.8	41 ± 16	38 ± 8	—
Valproic acid (half-life in neonate 47 hrs)	123 μmol/L	3 μmol/L	0.01 to 0.16	—	—

Adapted from Kaneko S, Suzuki K, Sato T et al: In Janz D, Dam M, Richens A et al, editors: Epilepsy, pregnancy, and the child, New York, 1982, Raven Press.

mothers have nursed without apparent incident while taking phenobarbital and phenytoin.[74] Phenytoin levels in milk of mothers treated for epilepsy have been measured, and levels in the infant have been calculated to provide less than 5% of the calculated therapeutic dose for infants.[56] Valproic acid in maternal milk is low (3% of maternal serum concentrations), but the mean half-life is 47 hours, four times that in adults, so there is risk of accumulation (Table 11-5).[55,74]

Poor weight gain after birth of infants whose mothers received antiepileptic medication during pregnancy has been reported by Kaneko et al.[35] They also report inadequate suckling and a high incidence of vomiting immediately after birth with difficulty establishing lactation. The drug continues to be provided through the milk, and the poor suckling becomes protracted. Levels of drug in the milk are shown in Table 11-5. The authors suggest avoiding breast milk or giving mixed feedings for the first few days postpartum until the level of drug in the milk drops and the infant is able to clear the drug that was in his system from birth. The clinician should observe these infants closely to be sure they receive adequate calories until they can suck vigorously. The mother should be sure to supplement the infant's suckling with a pump. With proper management in the first few days, the adjustment can be smooth and the infant can go on to nurse effectively and safely.[8] When infant plasma level determinations are available, it might be advisable to check the plasma level after 1 or 2 weeks of nursing, providing an opportunity to evaluate possible accumulation.

Psychotherapeutic agents

Lithium is the one drug in the psychotherapeutic group with a clear risk of toxicity in the neonate as well as clear evidence that it reaches the breast milk. Lithium is contraindicated in pregnancy as well as in lactation. Infants have been reported to be hypotonic, flaccid, and "depressed" when the nursing mother is taking lithium.

Chlorpromazine or phenothiazine appears in the milk in small amounts even at doses of 1200 mg, but does not appear to accumulate. Doses of 100 mg/day do not appear to cause symptoms in the infants. Diazepam (Valium) has been detected in milk and in breastfed infants' serum and urine. It has caused depression and poor feeding with weight loss in the infant. Chlordiazepoxide (Librium) and clorazepate (Tranxene) do reach the milk and may cause drowsiness and poor suckling. These substances' metabolites are also active, and therefore the half-life of therapeutic activity is prolonged. Meprobamate (Miltown, Equanil) has an M/P ratio greater than 1 and has been identified in milk. Infants whose mothers are taking meprobamate may become drowsy, but dosage adjustment may be indicated if there is significant benefit for the mother to breastfeed.

Tricyclic antidepressants such as imipramine are lipid soluble and have been identified in the breast milk;[38] thus cautious use may well be appropriate.[39] Amitriptyline (Elavil) was not found in milk according to Ayd.[3] The Committee on Drugs of the American Academy of Pediatrics[14] has reviewed psychotropic drugs in lactation and concluded that most drugs are found in the milk but the concentration is usually low; therefore, there is little likelihood of an effect on the infant. The infant should be observed for overt signs of drug effect as well as long-term effects on the developing nervous system, even with low doses.

Pesticides and pollutants

Human milk has been known to contain insecticides. Chlorinated hydrocarbons such as DDT and its metabolites dieldrin, aldrin, and related compounds are the best known. The major reason these compounds appear in breast milk is that they are deposited in body lipid stores and move with lipid. It has been pointed out that the fetus receives his greatest dose in utero and that adult body fat has approximately 30 times the concentration in milk.

Polychlorinated biphenyls (PCBs) in heavily contaminated pregnant Japanese women produced small-for-gestational-age infants who had transient darkening of the skin ("cola babies"). Polybrominated biphenyls (PBBs) are similar compounds associated with a heavy exposure to farm animals and contaminated cattle fed in the lower Michigan Peninsula. The women in the United States who have the greatest risk of high exposure to PCBs or PBBs are those who have worked with or eaten in excess (i.e., at least once a week) fish that was caught by sports fishing in contaminated waters. Others at high risk are those who live near a waste disposal site or have been involved in environmental spills. Unless there is heavy exposure, however, there is no contraindication to breastfeeding. When there is a question, the state health department can be consulted for specific advice or to measure plasma and milk levels. The epidemiologists are usually aware of the risks in a given geographic area and whether it is necessary to measure milk levels once lactation is fully established. If this sampling is planned for in advance during the pregnancy, little time need be lost. Unless there is a unique and excessive exposure, the infant could breastfeed until levels are returned from the laboratory.

In most cases, the levels of pesticides in human milk have been less than those in cow's milk. The accumulated amounts have not usually exceeded safe allowable limits. There are several extensive reviews published about the dilemma of pollutants in human milk.[65,66,81,85] It has been suggested that the body burden at birth can be added to by exposing the infant to small levels in the milk that may indeed exceed the exposure limits allowable for daily intake set by the World Health Organization. Human milk levels are used epidemiologically as markers of human exposure in a community exposure because there is a close correlation of milk levels to the levels in the fat stores. Unselected mothers in the Great Lakes region were tested by the State of New York in 1978, and there was no chemical (PCB, PBB) in any milk in random sampling of residents. Thus, unless the circumstances are unusual, breastfeeding should not be abandoned on the basis of insecticide contamination.

Agent Orange, the best known of the dioxins, was identified in Vietnam as a powerful teratogen. Dioxin has been found in human milk from pooled samples from high-risk women with known exposure. There is no evidence that the population at large is at risk. Women working in dry-cleaning plants, viscose rayon plants, photographic laboratories, and chemical industries where proper precautions are not taken have been noted to absorb tetrachloroethylene, carbon disulfide, and bromides.[69]

Heavy metals that have been found in milk include lead, mercury, arsenic, and cadmium. Whenever there has been a maternal exposure, the breastfed infant and the milk should be tested. It has been shown that lead and mercury are more rapidly absorbed from human milk than formula or other foods.[69] Levels in milk of these heavy metals, however, are lower than would be predicted from maternal levels (see Appendix E). Most common air pollutants are not found in human milk.

Psychologic impact of toxin in the milk

The psychologic reactions of a group of nursing mothers from the lower Michigan Peninsula whose breast milk was contaminated with a toxic fire-retardant chemical, PBB, were studied.[25] Every tenth woman who had had her milk tested for PBB was contacted for the study (a sample of 200 women); 139 responded and received a questionnaire, and 97 (70%) filled out the questionnaire. The subjects knew their own level and that the range for all mothers was from undetected to 0.46 ppm with an average of 0.1 ppm. The testing was voluntary and cost $25. Of those tested, 96% had measurable amounts.

The data were collected in a six-page questionnaire that included demographics, facts and attitudes about pregnancy and breastfeeding, what the respondent knew about PBB, why she had her milk tested, her feelings about the contamination, a section consisting of three projective tests to tap less conscious attitudes, and any medical problems that had occurred since the contamination. Two modes of coping emerged: denial and mastery. In general, the findings indicated that the greater the level of toxic contamination of PBB reported in a mother's milk, the greater the denial, to the point of not having correct information even about her own level. Those in the denial group were less able to allow unconscious conflicts about nursing to surface. The entire study group was a select group, of course, because the majority of Michigan's nursing mothers chose not to have their milk tested at all, thus electing to remain uninformed. Those who handled the PBB situation by mastery changed their breastfeeding patterns or their food buying or even moved away. These individuals tested to be more consciously aware of what they were feeling as well as the behaviors they wished to change. This group was also more knowledgeable about the facts in general.

In response to a question about what they would advise someone else to do, they were decisive: 77% would suggest testing, 52% would suggest stopping breastfeeding, and 10% more would suggest at least shortening the breastfeeding. Ambivalence toward nursing was correlated with guilt in both groups (only 15% discontinued breastfeeding). The "draw-a-baby" test showed an unusual amount (94%) of distortion and expressions of anguish. These findings were consistent throughout all the test modalities; thus they were not thought to be a function of personality.

Radioactive materials

Because of the increasing number of diagnostic tests available today with radioactive materials, it is not uncommon for a nursing mother to face such a procedure.

Radioactive iodine (^{125}I and ^{131}I) passes into milk at levels as high as 5% of the dose. When this is used for diagnostic purposes, breastfeeding should be discontinued for 24 hours. The excretion by the breast may alter the validity of the test result. If radioactive iodine is to be used therapeutically, breastfeeding must be discontinued until the iodine has cleared the system, which may be 1 to 3 weeks. A carefully collected sample of milk can be tested for radioactivity so that the period that the infant is off the breast is not unnecessarily long. If more than a 30 μci dose of ^{131}I is used, nursing should not be resumed until the milk is clear. If the infant is older and getting other foods, time can be altered accordingly.

^{67}Gallium citrate appears in significant amounts in the milk. It does clear the body quickly and is relatively safe for use in patients. Breastfeeding should be discontinued for at least 72 hours.

^{99m}Technetium is reported to clear the milk in 6 to 48 hours. The stage of lactation, whether the breast is emptied prior to receiving the dose, and the method of clearing the breast may well be responsible for the inconsistent results. Discontinuing breastfeeding for at least 24 hours is advisable.

With the advent of ultrasound examination, CT scanning, magnetic imagery, and other techniques, there are alternatives to use of radioactive material during lactation.

IMMUNIZATIONS
Immunizing the breastfed infant

Questions often arise as to whether a breastfed infant should be immunized on a different schedule because of the protective maternal antibodies that might interfere with the infant's response to antigen stimulation. Following are some brief guidelines on the more common situations of concern:

1. Diphtheria-pertussis-tetanus (DPT) vaccination is not altered by breastfeeding, and the regular schedule should be followed for the infant.[16]
2. Since oral poliovirus vaccine (OPV) is an oral live virus vaccine, there was concern that the maternal antibodies would inactivate the live virus. The recommendation of the Centers for Disease Control is, however, that the same schedule be followed. They state that the current scientific literature indicates that for infants older than 6 weeks (which is the earliest age of vaccination recommended), there is no indication for withholding breastfeeding in relationship to OPV administration, nor is there need for extra doses of vaccine.[16]
3. Rubella, mumps, and measles vaccines should be given at the regularly scheduled times.[16]
4. Hemophilus influenza B vaccine (HBPV) is available for infants 18 months or older. At this age diet is mixed, and protection with antibodies should not influence effectiveness of vaccine. When a vaccine becomes available for the fully breastfed infant (6 months or younger), consideration will have to be given to giving an additional dose postbreastfeeding.

Immunizing the nursing mother
Smallpox

Smallpox vaccination is inadvisable for the mother of any infant under 1 year of age, nursing or not. It is the personal contact, not the breastfeeding, that causes the risk; therefore there is no advantage to weaning if vaccination is necessary.

Rh immune globulin

Only rare trace amounts of anti-Rh are present in colostrum and none in mature milk of women given large doses of Rh immune globulin immediately postpartum. No adverse response was noted, even with these high dosages. It has been thought that any Rh antibodies in the mother's milk were inactivated by the gastric juices. Rh immune globulin or Rh sensitization is not a contraindication to breastfeeding.

Rubella

Following is the recommendation of the American College of Obstetrics and Gynecology with respect to rubella:

1. In the adult female population, approximately 85% to 90% of the individuals are thought to have a high level of naturally acquired immunity, and only 10% to 15% are considered to be susceptible to rubella infection.
2. Vaccination of pregnant women is contraindicated under all circumstances.
3. No woman of childbearing age should be vaccinated without having been first tested for immunity.
4. If the test is negative, the woman may be vaccinated if there is reasonable assurance that she will not become pregnant for at least 2 months.

The rubella virus was found in the milk of 69% of the women immunized with live attenuated rubella (HPV-77 DE5 or RA 27/3 strains).[45,46] A virus-specific IgA antibody response was seen in milk of all the women. Infectious rubella virus or virus antigen was recovered from the nasopharynx and throat of 56% of the breastfed infants and none of the nonbreastfed infants. No infant had disease in this study, but 25% of the breastfed group had seroconversion transiently.[46] Infants given early strains of the virus via the milk were reported to develop mild symptoms.[9,37,41,46] Although the attenuated virus may appear in the milk, this should not dissuade one from vaccinating a breastfeeding mother at the safest time, that is, immediately postpartum.

REFERENCES

1. Aranda JV et al: Metabolism and renal elimination of furosemide in the newborn infant, J Pediatr 101:777, 1982.
2. Arena JM: Drugs and breast feeding, Clin Pediatr 5:472, 1966.
3. Ayd F: Excretion of psychotrophic drugs in human breast milk, Int Drug Ther Newsletter 8:33, 1973.
4. Bauer JH et al: Propranolol in human plasma and breast milk, Am J Cardiol 43:860, 1979.
5. Berglund F, Flodh H, Lundborg P et al: Drug use during pregnancy and breastfeeding, Acta Obstet Gynecol Scand Suppl 126, 1984.
6. Berlin CM: Excretion of methylxanthines in human milk, Semin Perinatol 5:389, 1981.
7. Berlin CM and Daniel CH: Excretion of theobromine in human milk and saliva, Pediatr Res 15:492, 1981.
8. Bossi L: Neonatal period including drug disposition in newborns: review of the literature. In Janz D, Dam M, Richens A et al, editors: Epilepsy, pregnancy and the child, New York, 1982, Raven Press.
9. Bowes WA, Jr: The effect of medications on the lactating mother and her infant, Clin Obstet Gynecol 23:1073, 1980.
10. Briggs GG et al, editors: Drugs in pregnancy and lactation, Baltimore, 1983, Williams & Wilkins.
11. Catz CS and Giacoia GP: Drugs and breast milk, Pediatr Clin North Am 19:151, 1972.
12. Chan V, Tse TF, and Wong V: Transfer of digoxin across the placenta and into breast milk, Br J Obstet Gynecol 85:605, 1978.
13. Clark JH and Wilson WG: A 16-day-old breastfed infant with metabolic acidosis caused by salicylate, Clin Pediatr 20:53, 1981.
14. Committee on Drugs, American Academy of Pediatrics: Psychotropic drugs in pregnancy and lactation, Pediatrics 69:241, 1982.
15. Committee on Drugs, American Academy of Pediatrics: The transfer of drugs and other chemicals into human breast milk, Pediatrics 72:375, 1983.
16. Committee on Infectious Disease: Report of the Committee on Infectious Disease, ed 21, Evanston Ill, 1988, American Academy of Pediatrics.

17. Devlin RG, Duchin KL, and Fleiss PM: Nadolol in human serum and breast milk, Br J Clin Pharmacol 12:393, 1981.
18. Devlin RG and Fleiss PM: Captopril in human blood and breast milk, J Clin Pharmacol 21:110, 1981.
19. Erickson SH, Oppenheim GL, and Smith GH: Metronidazole in breast milk, Obstet Gynecol 57:48, 1981.
20. Feldman S and Pickering LK: Pharmacokinetics of drugs in human milk. In Howell RR, Morriss FH, and Pickering LK, editors: Springfield Ill, 1986, Charles C Thomas Publisher.
21. Finley JP et al: Digoxin excretion in human milk, J Pediatr 94:339, 1979.
22. George DI and O'Toole TJ: A review of drug transfer to the infant by breastfeeding: concerns for the dentist, J Am Dent Assoc 106:204, 1983.
23. Gaginella TS: Drugs and the nursing mother-infant, U S Pharm 3:39, 1978.
24. Gilman AG, Goodman LS, and Gilman A, editors: Goodman and Gilman's the pharmacological basis of therapeutics, ed 6, New York, 1980, Macmillan Publishing Co.
25. Hatcher SL: The psychological experience of nursing mothers upon learning of a toxic substance in their breast milk, Psychiatry 45:172, 1982.
26. Healy M: Suppressing lactation with oral diuretics, Lancet 1:1353, 1961.
27. Heislerberg L and Branebjerg PE: Blood and milk concentrations of metronidazole in mothers and infants, J Perinat Med 11:114, 1983.
28. Hervada AR, Feit E, and Sagraves R: Drugs in breast milk, Perinat Care 2:19, 1978.
29. Hogan RP, III: Hemorrhage diathesis caused by drinking an herbal tea, JAMA 249:2679, 1983.
30. Illingworth RS and Finch E: Ethyl discoumacetate (Tromexan) in human milk, J Obstet Gynecol Br Empire 66:487, 1959.
31. Jarboe CH et al: Dyphylline elimination kinetics in lactating women blood to milk transfer, J Clin Pharmacol 21:405, 1981.
32. Järnerot G and Into-Malmberg MB: Sulphasalazine treatment during breast feeding, Scand J Gastroenterol 14:869, 1979.
33. Kafetzis DA et al: Passage of cephalosporins and amoxicillin into breast milk, Acta Paediatr Scand 70:285, 1981.
34. Kampmann JP et al: Propylthiouracil in human milk, Lancet 1:736, 1980.
35. Kaneko S, Suzuki K, Sato T et al: The problems of antiepileptic medication during the neonatal period: is breastfeeding advisable? In Janz D, Dam M, Richens A et al, editors: Epilepsy, pregnancy, and the child, New York, 1982, Raven Press.
36. Khan AKA and Truelove SC: Placental and mam-

37. mary transfer of sulphasalazine, Br Med J 2:1533, 1979.
37. Klein EB, Byrne T, and Cooper LZ: Neonatal rubella in a breast-fed infant after postpartum maternal infection, J Pediatr 97:774, 1980.
38. Knowles JA: Excretion of drugs in milk: a review, J Pediatr 66:1068, 1965.
39. Knowles JA: Breast milk: a source of more than nutrition for the neonate, Clin Toxicol 7:69, 1974.
40. Kuhnz W, Koch S, Helge H et al: Primidone and phenobarbital during lactation period in epileptic women: total and free drug serum levels in the nursed infants and their effects on neonatal behavior, Dev Pharmacol Ther 11:147, 1988.
41. Landes RD et al: Neonatal rubella following postpartum maternal immunization, J Pediatr 97:465, 1980.
42. Lawrence R: Unpublished data.
43. Lawrence RA: Drugs in breast milk, Neonatal Intensive Care, 1989 (in press).
44. Levitan AA and Manion JC: Propranolol therapy during pregnancy and lactation, Am J Cardiol 32:247, 1973.
45. Losonsky GA et al: Effect of immunization against rubella on lactation products. I. Development and characterization of specific immunologic reactivity in breast milk, J Infect Dis 145:654, 1982.
46. Losonsky GA et al: Effect of immunization against rubella on lactation products. II. Maternal-neonatal interactions, J Infect Dis 145:661, 1982.
47. Loughnan PM: Digoxin excretion in human breast milk, J Pediatr 92:1019, 1978.
48. Low LCK, Lang J, and Alexander WD: Excretion of carbimazole and propylthiouracil in breast milk, Lancet 2:1011, 1979.
49. McKenna R, Cole ER, and Vasan V: Is warfarin sodium contraindicated in the lactating mother? J Pediatr 103:325, 1983.
50. Melander FA et al: Accumulation of atenolol and metoprolol in human breast milk, Eur J Clin Pharmacol 20:229, 1981.
51. Miller ME, Cohn RD, and Burghart PH: Hydrochlorothiazide deposition in a mother and her breast-fed infant, J Pediatr 101:789, 1982.
52. Miller RD, Keegan KA, Thrupp LD et al: Human breast milk concentrations of moxalactam, Am J Obstet Gynecol 148:348, 1984.
53. Mulley BA et al: Placental transfer of chlorthalidone and its elimination in maternal milk, Eur J Clin Pharmacol 13:129, 1978.
54. Nation RL and Hotham N: Drugs and breastfeeding, Med J Aust 146:308, 1987.
55. Nau H et al: Valproic acid and its metabolites: placental transfer, neonatal pharmacokinetics, transfer via mother's milk and clinical status in neonates of epileptic mothers, J Pharmacol Exp Ther 219:768, 1981.

56. Nau H, Rating D, Hauser I et al: Placental transfer at birth and postnatal elimination of primidone and metabolites in neonates of epileptic mothers. In Janz D, Dam M, Richens A et al, editors: Epilepsy, pregnancy, and the child, New York, 1982, Raven Press.

57. O'Brien TE: Excretion of drugs in human milk, Am J Hosp Pharm 31:844, 1974.

58. Orme ML et al: May mothers given warfarin breast-feed their infants? Br Med J 1:1564, 1977.

59. Peterson RG and Bowes WAJ: Drugs, toxins and environmental agents in breast milk. In Neville MC and Neifert MR, editors: Lactation, physiology, nutrition, and breast-feeding, New York, 1983, Plenum Press.

60. Rasmussen F: Mammary excretion of benzyl penicillin, erythromycin and penethamate hydriodide, Acta Pharmacol Toxicol (Kbh) 16:194, 1959.

61. Rasmussen F: Mammary excretion of antipyryne ethanol and urea, Acta Vet Scand 2:151, 1961.

62. Rating D, Jäger-Roman E, Koch S et al: Enzyme induction in neonates due to antiepileptic therapy during pregnancy. In Janz D, Dam M, Richens A et al, editors: Epilepsy, pregnancy, and the child, New York, 1982, Raven Press.

63. Rivers-Calimlim L: Drugs in breast milk, Drug Ther 2:20, 1977.

64. Rivera-Calimlim L: The significance of drugs in breast milk, Clin Perinatol 14:51, 1987.

65. Rogan WJ, Bagniewska A, and Damstra T: Pollutants in breast milk, N Engl J Med 302:1450, 1980.

66. Rogan WJ and Gladen B: Monitoring breast milk contamination to detect hazards from waste disposal, Environ Health Perspect 48:87, 1983.

67. Sannerstedt R, Berglund F, Flodh H et al: Medication during pregnancy and breastfeeding: a new Swedish system for classifying drugs, Int J Clin Pharmacol Ther Toxicol 18:45, 1980.

68. Segelman AB et al: Sassafras and herb tea, JAMA 236:477, 1976.

69. Seifert WE and Caprioli RM: Chemical contaminants in human milk. In Howell RR, Morriss FH, and Pickering LK, editors: Springfield Ill, 1986, Charles C Thomas Publisher.

70. Siegel RK: Herbal intoxication: psychoactive effects from herbal cigarettes, tea and capsules, JAMA 236:473, 1976.

71. Smith MT et al: Propranolol, propranolol glucuronide, and naphthoxylactic acid in breast milk and plasma, Ther Drug Monit 5:87, 1983.

72. Somogyi A and Gugler R: Cimetidine excretion into breast milk, Br J Clin Pharmacol 7:627, 1979.

73. Stec GP et al: Kinetics of theophylline transfer to breast milk, Clin Pharmacol Ther 28:404, 1980.

74. Steen B et al: Phenytoin excretion in human breast milk and plasma in nursed infants, Ther Drug Monit 4:331, 1982.

75. Stuart M, editor: The encyclopedia of herbs and herbalism, New York, 1979, Crescent Books.

76. Tegler L and Lindström B: Antithyroid drugs in milk, Lancet 2:591, 1980.

77. Vorherr H: Drug excretion in breast milk, Postgrad Med 56:97, 1974.

78. Vorherr H: The breast, morphology, physiology and lactation, New York, 1974, Academic Press, Inc.

79. Wennberg RP, Rasmussen LF, and Ahlors CE: Displacement of bilirubin from human albumin by three diuretics, J Pediatr 90:647, 1977.

80. Werthmann MW and Krees SV: Excretion of chlorothiazide in human breast milk, J Pediatr 81:411, 1981.

81. Wichizer TM and Brilliant LB: Testing for polychlorinated biphenyls in human milk, Pediatrics 81:781, 1972.

82. Wilson JT: Drugs in breast milk, Balgowlah, Australia, 1981, Adis Press.

83. Wilson JT: Determinants and consequences of drug excretion in breast milk, Drug Metab Rev 14:619, 1983.

84. Wilson JT, Brown RD, Hinson JL et al: Pharmacokinetic pitfalls in the estimation of the breast milk/plasma ratio for drugs, Ann Rev Pharmacol Toxicol 25:667, 1985.

85. Wolff MS: Occupationally derived chemicals in breast milk, Am J Ind Med 4:259, 1983.

86. Yurchak AM and Jusko WJ: Theophylline secreted into breast milk, Pediatrics 57:518, 1976.

Normal growth, failure to thrive, and obesity in the breastfed infant

NORMAL GROWTH

The growth of exclusively breastfed infants has become the focus of much interest among pediatricians, researchers, and nutritionists. A number of long-range follow-up studies have been initiated to address the issues of growth during the critical first year of life when brain growth is greater than it ever will be again in postnatal life. An interest in height and weight increments and ratios is only part of the concern about obesity and the long-range issues of adiposity. Does breastfeeding protect against adult obesity? Does human milk protect against cholesterol "intolerance" in adult life? The questions are clear, but the answers are not unless one assumes the teleologic approach: Human milk is ideal for the human infant with its low protein, controlled calories, and persistent unchangeable cholesterol. The question is actually; Is it safe to overfeed an infant with formula? Is it safe to deprive an infant of cholesterol during a period of critical brain growth when brain growth is dependent upon cholesterol? When infants are deprived of cholesterol in early infancy, are they less able to tolerate it later?

Antiquated data and anthropometric standards have led to the expression of doubt about the growth curves and tables of normal height and weight that do not reflect the growth of most healthy, well-fed breastfeeding infants. During several decades of formula feeding, "normal" growth curves were developed based only on formula-fed infants. Furthermore, whole cow's milk is fortunately almost totally abandoned, and the recommendations for introduction of solid food beyond 4 or even 6 months have been universally adopted by nutrition-conscious physicians and parents. New growth curves are being developed based on breastfed or formula-fed infants on delayed solids.

Bottle fed infants gain more rapidly in weight and length during the first months of life than do breastfed infants. Therefore, evaluating an infant's physical growth by standards set by bottle fed infants predisposes one to the diagnosis of failure to thrive. Fomon et al.[21] reported a longitudinal study of breastfed and bottle fed infants during the first few months of life that demonstrated that the tenth and ninetieth percentile values for weight and length of the two groups were similar at birth, and the tenth percentile values of the two groups were similar at age 112 days. The significant difference was in the values for the ninetieth percentile, which showed the bottle fed infants to be substantially greater.

These differences were attributed to caloric intake rather than the difference in composition of the diet. Fomon et al.[21] have shown that not only did the bottle fed infant gain more in weight and length but he also gained more weight for a unit of length. This reflects the overfeeding of the bottle fed infants. Whether this contributes to subsequent obesity is an important issue.

Most studies of growth in breastfed infants have been plagued with the problem of variation in supplementation and the occurrence of partial weaning. The growth of the exclusively breastfed infant was investigated in 1980 by Ahn and MacLean,[1] who conducted a retrospective study of enthusiastic and successful La Leche League mothers and their babies in the Baltimore–Washington, DC area. Mothers who had exclusively breastfed for 6 months or longer were randomly selected and all agreed to participate. They were educated, middle-income, married women. Growth records were obtained from the mothers from their pediatricians' records. The weight and length curves of these infants remained above the fiftieth percentile of the National Center for Health Statistics through at least the sixth month. In those infants who were exclusively breastfed longer, all were above the twenty-fifth percentile through the ninth and tenth month of life. Vitamin and mineral supplements were taken by 75% of all mothers and given to 35% of the infants. This study does demonstrate that under optimal circumstances exclusive breastfeeding does indeed support growth in the first 6 months or longer that matches norms set by formula-fed infants. When the growth of healthy exclusively breastfed infants was evaluated in the first 6 months of life in Australia, the weight increments in the first 3 months compared favorably with standards from the Ministry of Health in Great Britain.[29] The weight increment for the second 3 months was significantly less. The data from Great Britain had been accumulated from a mixed sample of breastfed and bottle fed infants in the 1950s, when most infants were fed cow's milk with a high solute load.

The growth pattern of full-term infants in the United States followed prospectively from birth showed no significant differences in mean growth measurements (weight, crownrump length, head circumference, and skinfold thickness) between infants fully breastfed and those fed whey-predominant formula. Plasma amino acid concentrations, including those for taurine, were similar at 3 days and 2, 8, and 16 weeks of age in both groups.[53]

The effects on growth of specific protein and energy intake in 4- to 6-month-old infants who were either breastfed or formula-fed with high and low protein were measured by Axelsson et al.[4] No significant differences were found in the rate of growth of crownheel length and head circumference or weight gain. The differences in protein intake between breastfed and formula-fed infants without differences in growth indicate that the formulas may provide a protein intake in excess of the needs, the authors concluded. When milk intake and growth in 45 exclusively breastfed infants were carefully documented in the first four months by Butte et al.,[9] energy and protein intakes were substantially less than current nutrient allowances. Infant growth progressed satisfactorily compared to the National Center for Health Statistics Standards despite the fact that energy dropped from 110 ± 24 kcal/kg/day at 1 month to $71 \pm$ kcal/kg/day at 4 months.[43] Similarly, protein intake decreased from 1.6 ± 0.3 gm/kg/day at 1 month to 0.9 ± 0.2 gm/kg/day at 4 months. The authors urge reevaluation of protein and energy requirements as they are currently set.[4]

Weight-for-length and weight gain were significantly correlated with total energy intake but not with activity level during the first 6 months of life in breastfed infants studied by Dewey and Lönnerdal.[14] Energy intake was considerably lower than recommended— 85 to 89 kcal/kg/day—when compared to the 115 kcal/kg/day recommended allowances of the National Academy of Sciences in 1980. Those infants who consumed the most breast milk became the fattest.

The physical growth of normal, healthy, breastfed and formula-fed infants from birth to 2 years was reported by Czajka-Narins and Jung[13] at a university hospital in the Midwest. Although breastfed males were lighter at 6 and 12 months, at 24 months the differences were not significant. Using height-to-weight indices, fewer infants who were breastfed longer were categorized as obese. These data suggest that longer breastfeeding affects weight but not length. One hundred twenty-eight breastfed and 3084 formula-fed infants were followed from birth through infancy and again at 3 to 12 years by Pomerance.[49] A comparison of the two groups, both given additional foods with similar timing, revealed no significant differences in growth velocity for weight or for length/height, either during the first 3 years or during the period from age 3 to age 12.

When patterns of growth are examined in the infants of marginally nourished mothers, weight gain is comparable to a reference population but does not permit recovery of weight differential at birth, which was significantly small for gestational age.[8] The intakes of energy and protein by individual infants were reflected in their weight gain but were indeed below internationally recommended norms. Maternal milk alone, when produced in sufficient amounts, can maintain normal growth up to the sixth month of life. Exclusive breastfeeding in Chilean infants of low-middle and low socioeconomic families produced the highest weight gain and practically no illness or hospitalization.[31]

While recognizing the importance of genetic metabolic and environmental influences in producing significant differences in growth patterns, Barness[5] suggests that recommendations for nutrition of healthy neonates may be too high for some and too low for others, but the benchmark for nutritional requirements of the full-term infant remains milk from the infant's healthy, well-nourished mother. Dietary energy intakes are substantially lower than most recommendations, according to Whitehead and Paul,[56] who reviewed infant feeding practices. Diet-related growth faltering in breastfed infants rarely occurs in developing countries until later than would be suggested by growth standards currently in use, they state.

Gain in physical growth is not as critical as gain in brain growth, but measurements of brain growth are only indirectly implied from growth of the head. In evaluating any infant's progress, head circumference is an important consideration, especially in the first year of life. Deceleration in the rate of increase in head circumference occurs over the first year. The head circumference increases about 3 inches in the first year of life and another 3 inches in the next 16 years of life. When growth failure includes failure of head growth, the failure is severe. Many other factors independent of body growth influence head growth, however.

Initially after birth, the normal infant loses 5% of body weight before starting to gain, whether breastfed or bottle-fed. In a study of infants at the University of Rochester, it was noted that breastfed infants who were given added water or added formula to force fluids in the first few days of life lost more weight and were less likely to start gaining prior to discharge than infants who were entirely breastfed or who were bottle-fed.

According to the National Center for Health Statistics, birth weight is doubled between the 50th and 75th percentiles at 4 months of age and tripled at 12 months. When doubling and tripling times were studied by type of feeding as well as birthweight, sex, and race by Czajka-Narins and Jung,[13] they concurred with doubling time but found tripling time to be 412 days for black males and 484 days for white females with no significant difference between breast or bottle feeders. They found obese infants with higher weight-to-length ratios tripled their weight sooner, suggesting that rapid tripling time may be an indicator of obesity. Black infants in general doubled and tripled their weights sooner, but more blacks were bottle-fed in this study.

Development

Cognitive development in the first 7 years of life was related to breastfeeding practices in a birth cohort of New Zealand.[17] The researchers took into account maternal intelligence, maternal education, maternal training in child rearing, childhood experiences, family socioeconomic status, birth weight, and gestational age. The breastfed children had slightly higher test scores on the Peabody Picture Vocabulary Test, the 5-year measure on the Stanford Binet Intelligence Scale, and the 7-year measure on the Weschler Child Intelligence Scale. Measures of language development were equally influenced. This very small improvement in scores persisted when all variables were taken into account. The scores were also influenced by length of breastfeeding below and above 4 months.

An additional study on the same birth cohort was done to assess breastfeeding and subsequent social adjustment in 6- to 8-year-old children. Fergusson et al.[18] studied prospectively 1024 children who were part of the Christ Church Child Development Study. They used the maternal and teacher ratings of childhood conduct disorders. There was a statistically significant tendency for conduct disorder scores to decline with increasing duration of breastfeeding, i.e., breastfed children were less prone to conduct disorder than bottle fed children. Breastfed children, however, tended to come from slightly more socially advantaged, economically privileged homes, that tended to be more stable. The analysis failed to examine early mother-infant interaction patterns, however.

Another group of children was followed in New Zealand to evaluate the effects of infant feeding, birth order, paternal occupation, and socioeconomic status on speech in 6-year-old children. Controlling for the demographic effects, the association of breastfeeding with clear speech was different for the sexes, being negligible for girls and strongly positive for boys.[17]

The relationship of infant-feeding practices and dependent variables to the subsequent cognitive abilities were reported by Young et al.[59] from the Yale Harvard Research Project in Tunisia. Within the underprivileded group they found that breastfeeding promoted not only physical growth but also sensory motor development as assessed by Bayley motor and mental scales. There were no great differences in the ability to sit alone or to take first steps, but especially among males in the lower socioeconomic group there was significant superiority of breastfed infants at 8, 14, and 16 months of age in Bayley mental scales.

FAILURE TO THRIVE
Definition

The term *failure to thrive* has been loosely used to describe all infants who show some degree of growth failure. It is a syndromic classification that has been used to describe infants whose gain in weight or length or both fails to occur in a normal progressive fashion. For the breastfed infant, it may be a matter of comparing a slower gainer to the excessive weight-gain patterns of the bottle fed infant. The definition offered by Fomon[20] states that "failure to thrive [should] be defined as a rate of gain in length and/or weight less than the value corresponding to two standard deviations below the mean during an interval of at least 56 days for infants less than five months of age and during an interval of at least three months for older infants." Fomon further suggests that infants gaining in length and weight at rates less than the tenth percentile values be suspected of failing to thrive. Certainly in managing the breastfed infant, more careful and frequent medical evaluation should be provided for the infant who drops to the tenth percentile for weight, fails to gain weight, or continues to lose after the tenth day of life, rather than waiting for 56 days to establish the trend unquestionably. In our work in Rochester, it is defined as failure to thrive or slow weight gain when the infant continues to lose weight after 10 days of life, does not regain birth weight by 3 weeks of age, or gains at a rate below the tenth percentile for weight gain beyond 1 month of age. Unlike the bottle fed infant, who can then be placed in the hospital where professionals can feed him, the breastfed infant needs to be evaluated in the home setting, nursing at the breast.

As more and more women breastfeed, increasing numbers of cases of failure to thrive appear in the literature, although it is a rare phenomenon. No statistical data on incidence rates are available because there has been no large prospective study. Only extreme cases are hospitalized, but the number of these is increasing as well, partially due to a failure to recognize the disorder.

Diagnosis

The problem of slow or inadequate weight gain has confounded even the physicians most committed to breastfeeding. It should be approached with the same orderly diagnostic process that one uses to attack any medical problem. Thus a complete history, a physical examination of the infant, an examination of the maternal breast, observation of the feeding, and appropriate laboratory work are indicated. Organizing the data amassed by this process will help identify the facts that do appear under maternal and infant causes separately.

Slow gaining versus failure to thrive

There are some helpful distinctions between the breastfed infant who is slow to gain weight and the infant who is failing to thrive while breastfeeding.[34,35] These parameters should be included in the routine "well baby" evaluation of all breastfed infants, beginning with the first visit a week to 10 days after discharge home (Table 12-1).

The feeding pattern of the infant with slow weight gain is usually frequent feedings with evidence of a good suck. The mother's breasts are full before feeding, and she can describe a let-down during the feeding. There are at least six wet diapers a day, and urine is pale and dilute; stools are loose and seedy. Weight gain is slow but consistent. If the infant is gaining painfully slowly but is alert, bright, and responsive and developing along the appropriate level, he is a "slow gainer." In contrast, the infant with true failure to thrive is usually apathetic or weakly crying with poor tone and poor turgor. There are few wet diapers (none are every soaked) and "strong" urine. Stools are infrequent and scanty. Feedings are often by schedule but always fewer than eight per day and brief. There are no signs of a good let-down reflex. True failure to thrive is potentially serious; early recognition is essential if the integrity of both brain growth and breastfeeding is to be safely preserved.

A schema for classifying failure to thrive at the breast is suggested in Fig. 12-1. Here the causes associated with infant behavior and problems are distinguished from those due to problems in the mother. The causes in the infant can be further evaluated by looking at net intake, which may be associated with poor feeding, poor net intake due to additional losses, or high energy needs. The maternal causes can be divided into poor production of milk and poor release of milk. When a poor let-down reflex acts long enough, it will eventually cause a decrease in milk production. There may be several factors affecting the outcome, thus more than one management change may be indicated.

Evaluation of infant

Examination of the infant should suggest any underlying physical problems such as hypothyroidism, congenital heart disease, or mechanical abnormalities of the mouth such as cleft palate, or major neurologic disturbances.[6] The infant's ability to root, suck, and

Table 12-1. Parameters for evaluation of breastfed infants

Infant who is slow to gain weight	Infant with failure to thrive
Alert healthy appearance	Apathetic or crying
Good muscle tone	Poor tone
Good skin turgor	Poor turgor
At least 6 wet diapers/day	Few wet diapers
Pale, dilute urine	"Strong" urine
Stools frequent, seedy (or if infrequent, large and soft)	Stools infrequent, scanty
8 or more nursings/day, lasting 15–20 minutes	Fewer than 8 feedings, often brief
Well-established let-down reflex	No signs of functioning let-down reflex
Weight gain consistent but slow	Weight erratic—may lose

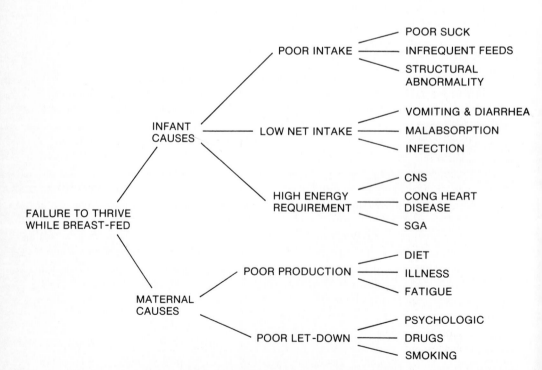

Fig. 12-1. Diagnostic flow chart for failure to thrive.

coordinate swallowing should be observed. There is a greater risk today of missing subtle structural problems because infants spend much of their hospital life out of the newborn nursery away from the watchful eyes of experienced nurses and then are discharged before problems become manifest. The first office visit for breastfeeding infants should be at 1 week following discharge home or earlier and include a complete inspection whether there are complaints from the parents or not. A small number of infants will be identified with physical abnormalities that need medical attention (Table 12-2).

Small-for-gestational-age infant. The small-for-gestational-age (SGA) infant will be identified if gestational age and birth weight are scrutinized. This infant is small at birth despite full gestation time in utero. The SGA infant has a large nutritional deficit to make up from his intrauterine failure to grow. The cause of his intrauterine problem should be assessed (placental insufficiency, maternal disease, toxemia, heavy smoking, or intrauterine infection such as toxoplasmosis). SGA infants are difficult to feed initially by any method and often require tube feedings for a few days. Their caloric needs parallel the needs of an infant of appropriate weight for gestation rather than their actual low weight. The SGA infant should be placed on frequent feedings, every 2 to 3 hours by day and every 4 hours at night. He should be awakened for feedings if he sleeps long periods of time. If he has not been nursing well, the breast has not been stimulated to produce to its full capability. The mother may need to express milk manually or mechanically pump milk to enhance her production. Her milk may then be given by a passive means such as a tube, a dropper, or a lactation supplementing device (see Appendix F). An infant who is sufficiently starved in utero may have a degree of inanition that prevents active suckling at first, predisposing him to further starvation. The successful nursing of an SGA infant may require extended effort on the part of the mother to assure adequate growth. On the other hand, such effort

Table 12-2. Conditions associated with or causing disorders of sucking and swallowing

Absent or diminished suck	Mechanical factors interfering with sucking	Disorders of swallowing mechanism (not including esophageal abnormalities)
Maternal anesthesia or analgesia	Macroglossia	Choanal atresia
Anoxia or hypoxia	Cleft lip	Cleft palate
Prematurity	Fusion of gums	Micrognathia
Trisomy 21	Tumors of mouth or gums	Postintubation dysphagia
Trisomy 13-15	Temporomandibular an-	Palatal paralysis
Hypothyroidism	kylosis or hypoplasia	Pharyngeal tumors
Neuromuscular abnormalities		Pharyngeal diverticula
Kernicterus		Familial dysautonomia
Werdnig-Hoffmann disease		
Neonatal myasthenia gravis		
Congenital muscular dystrophy		
Infections of the CNS		
Toxoplasmosis		
Cytomegalovirus infection		
Bacterial meningitis		

Modified from Gryboski J: Philadelphia, 1975, WB Saunders Co. From Behrman RE, Driscoll JM Jr and Seeds AE, editors: Neonatal-perinatal medicine: diseases of the fetus and infant, ed 2, St Louis, 1977, The CV Mosby Co.

is well worth the trouble if one considers the impact of intrauterine growth failure on the central nervous system (CNS). It would be to the infant's advantage to have the critical amino acids such as taurine and the lipids of human milk with which to "catch up" brain growth.

Jaundice. Hyperbilirubinemia is discussed in Chapter 13, but an infant with an elevated bilirubin level from any cause may be depressed and lethargic and therefore may not nurse well. If the infant appears jaundiced, laboratory evaluation in search of the cause and its appropriate treatment should be undertaken. When an infant is taken from the breast at 2 or 3 days of age because of jaundice, it interferes with the establishment of lactation at a critical time, especially for a primipara. Management of the jaundiced infant is dependent on adequate calories and the active passage of stools, which is the means by which the body excretes the bilirubin in meconium. "Breast-milk jaundice" does not develop until the infant is 3 or more days old, so other causes must be sought. In addition, care must be taken to help the mother continue to stimulate production with manual expression or pumping to avoid inducing iatrogenic lactation failure.

Metabolic screen. Most hospitals provide, often because the law mandates it, screening for metabolic disorders including galactosemia, phenylketonuria, maple sugar urine disease, and disorders of metabolism of other amino acids. If these simple screening tests were not performed or their validity is in doubt, they should be done again. Usually the service is available in the state or county laboratory. Thyroid screening for abnormal thyroxine (T_4) and/or thyroid-stimulating hormone (TSH) should also be performed. Mass screening programs for neonatal thyroid disease have identified cases of deficiency that, even in retrospect, show none of the characteristic findings of hypothyroidism such as thick, coarse features, hoarse cry, slow pulse, macroglossia, umbilical hernia, or jaundice. In the neonate hypothyroidism is often associated with failure to thrive, if undiagnosed.

Galactosemia. Galactosemia, which is a hereditary disorder of the metabolism of galactose-1-phosphate, is manifested by renal disease and liver dysfunction following the ingestion of lactose. The lack of galactose-1-phosphate uridyl transferase may be relative or partial. The clinical symptoms may be fulminating with severe jaundice, hepatosplenomegaly, vomiting, and diarrhea or may be more subtle. Cataracts are not invariably present. In mild cases, failure to thrive may be the presenting symptom. A screen of the urine for reducing substances (by Clinitest and not just Dextrostix, which will only identify glucose) should be done on all infants who fail to thrive, especially if there is hepatomegaly or jaundice. The definitive diagnosis is the identification of absence or near absence of galactose-1-phosphate uridyl transferase in red blood cell hemolysates. A screen of the urine should be considered even though an initial metabolic screen for galactosemia was done on the second or third day of life by hospital routine. The treatment is a lactose-free diet, which would mandate prompt weaning from breast milk to prevent further insult to the liver and kidneys. This is one of the few indications for prompt weaning from human milk. A formula free of lactose such as Isomil or Nutramigen is indicated. (Refer to pediatric texts on neonatal metabolic disorders for a full description of the disease; see Chapter 14.)

Vomiting and diarrhea. Vomiting and diarrhea are very unusual in a breastfed infant. Spitting up small amounts of milk after feedings is sometimes observed in otherwise normal infants and is of no consequence if it does not affect overall weight gain. Although pyloric stenosis is reportedly less common in breastfed infants, this phenomenon should be ruled out in any infant who vomits consistently after feeding, has diminished urine and stools, shows no weight gain or actually loses weight, and has reverse peristalsis. Usually these infants do well initially, and then the vomiting becomes progressive.

Vomiting may be a presenting symptom for various metabolic disorders. Thus metabolic disorders should be considered in the differential diagnosis. The usual causes of vomiting, as well as the causes peculiar to breast milk, should be considered. Maternal diet should be checked for unusual foods. In families at high risk for allergy, intake by the mother of known family food allergens may cause symptoms in the infant. Diarrhea may be due to foods in the mother's diet or the use of cathartics by the mother such as phenolphthalein (Ex-Lax).

Infection. Chronic intrauterine infection, which predisposes an SGA infant to intrauterine growth failure, may continue to cause problems of growth in the presence of adequate kilocalories. Chronic viral infections include CMV (cytomegalovirus), hepatitis, AIDS, or other less common viruses.

Acute infections. An infant who is not growing well may have an infection in the gastrointestinal tract; therefore, the nature of the stools is important. The urinary tract may be another site of infection not readily identified. If, however, the initial evaluation includes a urinalysis with microscopic evaluation and a white blood cell count and differential count, this can usually be ruled out.

High energy requirements. When the metabolic rate of the infant is increased, the weight gain will be diminished or absent. When the infant is hyperactive with a strong startle reflex and sleeps poorly, consideration should be given to stimulants present in the milk as well as to neurologic disorders. When a mother drinks coffee, tea, including herbal teas, cola, or other carbonated beverages with added caffeine, the accumulated caffeine may be sufficient to make the infant very irritable and hyperactive. The best treatment is to replace the caffeine-containing beverages (Chapter 11). Some CNS disorders are associated with hyperactivity. Infants with severe congenital heart disease are constantly exercising to breathe and oxygenate and have markedly increased metabolic rates. For management of these special infants at the breast, see Chapter 14.

Observation of nursing process

When it has been established that there are no obvious physical or metabolic reasons for the failure to gain weight, the infant should be observed suckling at the breast. Does the infant get a good grasp and suck vigorously? If not, what interferes? A receding chin, a weak suck, lack of coordination, the breast obstructing breathing, and mouthing of the nipple or other ineffectual sucking techniques are some of the possibilities. If the problem is the suckling process, the infant may need assistance. This cause is more common with infants who have had some experience with bottles or rubber nipples or who use a pacifier. Small or slightly premature infants who were started on bottle feedings have trouble relearning the proper sucking motion with the tongue (Figs. 8-6 to 8-9). Bottle feedings and pacifiers may have to be discontinued until the infant is more experienced at the breast. This will require a program of manually expressing milk to soften the areola, having milk at the nipple to entice the infant, and gently offering the nipple and areola well compressed between two fingers. If the infant has a receding chin or a relaxed jaw, it may help to have the mother hold the lower jaw forward by supporting the angle of the jaw with her thumb.

It may be necessary to assist both mother and baby. If the infant by 2 weeks of age cannot maintain the breast in his mouth without the mother holding it there, it is an indication of improper suckling. In that situation, the infant may need to be repositioned with his ventral surface squarely facing the mother's chest wall and the breast presented with thumb on top and fingers below breast. (See discussion in Chapter 8.) A good check of adequate let-down is to observe the opposite breast as the baby nurses to see if milk flows or to interrupt nursing abruptly. If there has been a good let-down, milk will continue to flow, at least drop by drop, for a few moments from the breast being suckled. The mother can also be trained to listen for the infant's swallowing. During proper sucking, the masseter muscle is in full view and is contracting visibly and rhythmically. Occasional infants do not suck vigorously at the breast but use rapid shallow sucks occasionally called "flutter sucking." These infants can be gradually taught to suck effectively. Correct positioning of the breast directly in the infant's mouth and holding the breast firmly in position with all the fingers under the breast and only the thumb above allow the infant to grasp properly without sucking the tongue or lower lip. Nipple shields make the situation worse and should be avoided.

The most productive part of the diagnostic workup is often observation of the baby at the breast. For this reason, this critical responsibility should not be passed on to others but should be performed personally by the physician.

The five general types of nursing patterns described in Chapter 8 should be kept in mind. If the mother understands that it is acceptable for the infant to drop off to sleep and snack later, she may not hesitate to follow his lead, thus providing a more adequate feeding.

Some infants will not settle down and nurse well if there is too much activity or noise. Some need to be tightly swaddled; others fall asleep and need to be unwrapped and stimulated to provide adequate suckling time. Frequent feedings, using both breasts, may be the answer in some cases. In others there may be too many ineffective feedings, which are wearing the mother out; a change that lengthens the time between feedings but also lengthens the time at the breast may help.

Nonorganic failure to thrive

When an infant does not have an organic disorder that explains the growth failure, the patient is diagnosed as having nonorganic failure to thrive (NOFTT). The typical psychosocial and nutritional pattern reported in NOFTT includes evidence of a chaotic family life, emotional deprivation, and inadequate nutrition as pointed out by Weston et al.[55] These authors reported four children ages 13 to 19 months with NOFTT who were breastfeeding. They had exclusively breastfed for at least 12 months, reportedly refusing solid foods. Failure to gain was noted at 9 months, followed by weight loss increasing at 12 months. Children were all from middle-class families, and parents had at least high school educations or more. The children all were first-born and scored "advanced" on the Bayley scales. They were active and alert but difficult to control. They all separated only briefly from their mothers in the clinic and initiated nursing for comfort when anxious. Total dietary energy intakes were below levels for growth. These children were not typical NOFTT in any of their demographics but had missed a critical developmental task of learning to eat according to the authors, who interpreted it as being a need on the part of these mothers to keep the child close. Treatment included having someone else teach these children to eat solids. Prolonged exclusive breastfeeding may occasionally result in a unique deficit in the developmental process of eating.[55] Exclusive breastfeeding is not nutritionally adequate in the second half of the first year, especially beyond 12 months, although nursing can safely continue for several years with a good diet.[47]

Parental misconception and health beliefs concerning what constitutes a normal diet for infants has been reported by Pugliese et al.[50] as a cause for NOFTT as well. They report seven infants from 7 to 22 months of age with poor weight gain and linear growth who

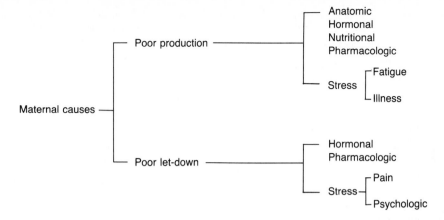

Fig. 12-2.   Maternal causes of failure to thrive.

received only 60% to 90% of minimum caloric intake for their age and sex. The parents explained that they wanted to avoid obesity, atherosclerosis, or junk food habits. It has also been shown that parental health beliefs and expectations have led to short stature and delayed puberty in older children.

Maternal causes of failure to thrive

Questions about the mother's health, her dietary habits, sleep pattern, smoking habits, medication intake, the events that occur during nursing, and the psychosocial atmosphere in the home are an important part of the history (Fig. 12-2).

Anatomical causes

Lactation failure due to insufficient glandular development of the breast has been described by Neifert et al.,[45] who report three cases in which the breast tissue was asymmetric. Transillumination confirmed little active gland. One family showed a history of similar failure. All three women benefited psychologically from the diagnosis and chose to continue to breastfeed and supplement. The authors have since identified 14 more women who had anatomic deficiency but normal prolactin levels and failed to respond to a thorough team approach to lactation support.[44] Retained placenta as described in Chapter 4 is also a cause of early lactation failure that is quickly identified by a complete history of postpartum breast change and patterns of lochia that the obstetrician associates with retained tissue.

Poor milk production

Diets. Although it has been demonstrated that malnourished mothers can produce milk for their infants, marginal diets in Western cultures do affect some mothers' ability to nourish an infant. If the mother is restricting intake deliberately or inadvertently, she should be instructed to meet the dietary requirement for lactating women (Chapter 9). One does not have to drink milk, but the necessary dietary constituents should be in the diet through cheese, eggs, ice cream, or other sources of calcium and protein. It may not be the nutrition itself but the calming effect of a nourishing beverage while breastfeeding that facilitates nursing. Studies of hormones triggered while eating have shown that more milk is produced if a mother eats just before or during breastfeeding. Prescribing brewer's yeast as a dietary supplement has been observed to provide improvement in milk production beyond that accounted for by mere addition of the same nutrients. Some mothers report a feeling of well-being from taking yeast that they do not obtain from taking daily vitamins. Concern has been expressed regarding the effect of increased vitamin B$_6$ on prolactin production, but doses that suppress lactation are 60 times the therapeutic dose.

Maternal illness. The presence of infection or other illness in the mother may affect milk production, and the cause of the illness should be identified and treated. Urinary tract infection, endometritis, or upper respiratory infection may need treatment with antibiotics. The antibiotic prescribed should be appropriate for the infant as well, since it will pass into the milk. Metabolic disorders such as thyroid disease should also be considered.

Fatigue. The most common cause of inadequate milk supply is fatigue. Fatigue may be lack of sleep because the infant demands considerable attention at night, but generally it is more subtle. The pressures of the rest of the family for meals or services or the self-inflicted demands of a job, career, or social commitments may be the cause. The mother must be placed on a medically mandated strict rest regimen that is respected by family and friends. In the first month, while lactation is being established, fatigue is devastating to milk production. The infant then becomes hungry more often, cries, and demands more frequent feeding; thus the vicious cycle is established. In later months of lactation, a mother becomes quickly aware of the impact of protracted fatigue on the nursing experience and usually will take steps to increase her rest.

Poor release of milk. Interference with the let-down reflex may cause a well-nourished lactating mother to fail to satisfy her infant. The collecting ducts may be full, but if the let-down or ejection reflex is not triggered, the process will be at a standstill. The infant becomes frustrated and pulls away crying or screaming. Interference with the ejection reflex is predominantly iatrogenic and rarely hormonal (see Fig. 8-13).

Smoking may interfere with the let-down reflex, and if this is the case, a mother who wants to smoke while nursing should wait to light up until the infant is sucking vigorously and the ejection is well established. Actually, mothers should be discouraged from ever smoking in the same room with the infant because of the occurrence of early and frequent respiratory infections in infants of smokers. Smokers are less likely to breast-feed, and if they do choose to breastfeed, they tend to wean earlier due to insufficient milk. Trouble with milk production may be related to the nicotine itself.

Experimentally, alcohol has been shown to interfere with oxytocin release in laboratory animals, but the dosage used collates with moderate to heavy drinking in humans. Therapeutically, alcohol has been recognized as an excellent adjunct to nursing if used judiciously. A glass of wine, a mug of beer, or a cocktail, especially in the early evening when some mothers may be under tension to feed the infant and family, will provide the relaxation necessary to permit adequate let-down response. In countries where wine and beer are common beverages, they have been recognized for centuries as important tonics for lactation. Alcohol's medical uses have been obscured by the concern for the disease of alcoholism, but the small amount of alcohol that would reach the milk is a sedative and muscle relaxant for the frantic infant.*

---

*An alternative treatment for colic is a few drops of alcohol in warm water or via the breast milk. An elixir is 25% alcohol, and it is often the elixir, not the drug for which it serves as the vehicle, that sedates the infant. Thus elixir of phenobarbital is more sedating to the infant than the same dose of phenobarbital alone.

Medications that the mother may be taking should be evaluated. Although L-dopa and ergot preparations are known to inhibit prolactin release, other medications less well identified may have the same effect (see Chapter 11).

The most common cause for the failure of the ejection reflex is psychologic inhibition. In a few cases the cause of the psychologic stress may be obvious, such as a husband or mother who openly disapproves of breastfeeding, but in most cases the nursing mother has already considered this possibility and reassures the physician that she is relaxed and calm. It will require carefully taking the mother's history to "tease out" the source of stress. This is the time when a home visit by the nurse practitioner from the physician's office or an experienced public health nurse will be valuable. The nurse may observe what is overlooked by the mother: construction of a new building next door, incessant barking from the neighbor's dog, or marital discord.

No obvious cause

Even though no obvious cause for failure to thrive is identified, the treatment may have to include establishing a positive attitude. Jelliffe[30] has often referred to nursing as a "confidence game." It becomes necessary to instill confidence rather than fear in the mother. Threatening the mother with stopping breastfeeding and switching to formula does not instill confidence. The physician should prescribe a positive plan for number and length of feedings, suggest diet and rest for the mother, and set reachable goals for growth.

If the let-down reflex is the crux of the problem and simple adjustments have not changed the ejection quality, oxytocin as a nasal spray (Pitocin), described in Chapter 8, should be prescribed. It is available only by prescription and should be used under the physician's guidance, although it is not dangerous. It does not affect the milk or the infant. It is contraindicated only in pregnancy or hypersensitivity.

Seven mothers whose infants were contented but starving breastfed infants were given metoclopramide (or chlorpromazine in one) in various dosages. In only one case did the mother feel it was not helpful. The authors did not describe how effective appropriate breastfeeding supportive management was and when the medication was started or how long it was maintained.[25] All the infants gained weight, and breastfeeding was continued for 2 to 12 months.

Measurement of levels of prolactin are readily available in most laboratories, but the appropriate clinical protocol has not been confirmed by controlled study. Given the information about baseline and response to stimuli (Chapter 4), it would be advisable to obtain a baseline level, which should be above normal for the laboratory and a second value after 15 minutes of breastfeeding. Using a heparin lock with venous line placed well before feeding would assure the least disturbance to lactation. The intrafeeding value should show an increase over baseline (twice baseline).

A group of women diagnosed with lactational insufficiency by history were given thyrotropin releasing hormone (TRH). Four received 5 mg every 12 hours for 5 days. There was a consistent 50% increase in prolactin concentrations. Both milk production and let-down were increased. Nine women received 20 mg twice a day, and basal prolactin was significantly elevated. The women all reported subjective and objective increases in breast engorgement and milk let-down, and all returned to full nursing according to the authors. Two women were given 40 mg TRH daily for 5 days and developed clincial signs of thyrotoxicosis by the seventh day, which disappeared by the tenth day. The investigators had previously given TRH to fully lactating women in a controlled study to demonstrate prolactin response, which did occur within 60 minutes. There was no change in the milk volume or quality in these fully lactating women and no side effects. When Hall and Kay[26] gave 200 μg TRF and followed prolactin and milk production for 6 hours, they did not have dramatic changes in milk production, although the prolactin levels rose. There is no indication that the mothers received more than one day's dose.

The rare infant who does not respond to this management protocol may have a malabsorption or metabolic disease as yet undiagnosed that will not become overt until cow's milk is introduced. Infants with a strong family history of cystic fibrosis, milk allergy, or malabsorption should have a careful diagnostic workup before abandoning human milk, which may be the most physiologic feeding available for the infant.

Dehydration, hypernatremia, or hypochloremia

A few cases of severe disease have been reported in the literature.* These infants have been hospitalized because of dehydration and evidence of more severe metabolic disturbance. They serve to illustrate the outcome if anticipatory care or palliative home management is unsuccessful. The mothers are usually but not always primiparas, new at breastfeeding and child rearing. Often it is seen when the record is reviewed that the early danger signs were present at discharge from the hospital. There may be a history of difficult delivery or of maternal medication for pain that leads to a less vigorous baby and, secondarily, inadequate stimulus for lactation. Supplementary bottles of water or milk are initiated in the hospital instead of directing attention toward the lactation process.

As a precautionary measure, the physician should see all breastfeeding dyads at 10 days to 2 weeks of age. At this visit review of the weight, feeding history, number of wet diapers, stool pattern, and physical findings should alert the physician to impending difficulties. A new problem in monitoring breastfed infants is the use of ultra absorbent diapers that makes it impossible to detect the number of voidings or volume of urine passed. No specimen can be rung from the diaper for specific gravity or other analysis. It is recommended that infants under 2 months not use ultra absorbent diapers, especially when breastfed, until a better monitoring device is developed. If, on the other hand, the patient is not seen in the office until there is significant dehydration, it is urgent that laboratory studies be obtained including sodium, chloride, potassium pH, BUN, and hematocrit (bilirubin when indicated). An assessment of the degree of dehyration should be made based on skin and tissue turgor and tone. When the breastfed infant has abnormal electrolyte levels, the physician should also obtain levels of sodium, chloride, and potassium from mother's milk, being certain to sample each breast separately. Collecting a few milliliters before and after the feeding and mixing the two samples from a single breast is a good technique. There may be occult loss of electrolyte in the infant such as that seen in abnormal renal wasting or retention, cystic fibrosis, hyperaldosteronism, or pseudohyperaldosteronism. The simplest approach is to measure milk electrolytes and infant urine levels to rule out high milk sodium.

In the cases reported in the literature, infants with hypernatremic failure to thrive are no different at initial presentation from infants with normal sodium levels.[10,35] They may even have a negative neonatal history. At home, they develop a poor suck, sleep for long intervals, cry infrequently, and feed infrequently. When observed at the breast they may be labeled as having a sucking disorder. On examination, however, the lethargy, dehydration, and malnutrition are obvious to the skilled clinician. In the extreme, there

---

*See references 2, 3, 10, 23, 24, 28, 47.

may be cardiovascular collapse with hypothermia and hypoglycemia. Elevated serum BUN, creatinine, and hematocrit and urinary specific gravity confirm the diagnosis. Hypernatremia has been observed in approximately half the reported cases of severe dehydration.[51,52] Although milk sodium levels were not reported in all cases, several cases of elevated milk sodium are reported. Sodium, chloride, and lactose are the prime constituents that control the osmolarity of the milk. Because the sodium chloride and lactose have a reciprocal relationship, inadequate lactose production ultimately results in elevated sodium levels.

Elevated sodium in the milk may be a cause or an effect of insufficient milk. When the breast is inadequately stimulated, it begins to involute and produces "weaning milk," which is high in sodium. Milk pumped from nonlactators in the postpartum period has high sodium. On the other hand, maternal sodium intake excesses do not result in elevated sodium levels in the milk.[16] Sodium enters the milk by a controlled mechanism independent of maternal levels in normal women.

Hypernatremic dehydration is an emergency that requires hospitalization.[34,35] The mother should room-in if at all possible. Most pediatric units provide this option. It is preferable to maintain lactation in most cases. The treatment of the illness after the dehydration has been treated with intravenous fluids depends on the etiology of the hypernatremia. The sodium of the infant's serum and mother's milk should be followed until stable. In decreasing maternal output with appropriate lactation counseling, including mechanical pumping between feedings to increase volume usually normalizes the sodium. The oral feedings for the infant should be limited to breastfeeding while the intravenous fluids are tapered. To provide increased caloric resources to the infant and an appropriate sodium load, the Lact-Aid supplementer may also be used (see Chapter 8 and Appendix F).

Chloride deficiency has received attention because of a highly publicized formula-manufacturing error. This syndrome is characterized by failure to thrive with anorexia, hypochloremia, and hypokalemic metabolic alkalosis. Chloride deficiency syndrome has also been reported in an infant whose mother had only 2 mEg/L chloride in her milk (normal is 8 mEg/L).[28] The mother had successfully nourished her previous five infants. The infant had done well until 3 months of age and then had gradually slipped below the third percentile for weight at 6 months. The infant was severely dehydrated and hypotonic with plasma sodium of 123 mEg/L, chloride of 72 mEg/L, potassium of 2.9 mEq/L, and blood pH of 7.61. There were no abnormal urinary losses. When there is clincial dehydration in the infant who is breastfeeding, it is important to check not only the sodium but also the chloride content of infant's serum, infant's urine, and mother's milk.

Human infants younger than 3 weeks of age do not respond to inappropriate solutions by not suckling. This finding is also observed in studies in other species in which pups continue to suck when the solution is unphysiologic.[7] A natural experiment occurred in a newborn nursery in the 1960s, when six infants died of hypernatremia after receiving many feedings of formula made from salt rather than sugar.[19] The infants who were less than 1 week old did not reject the feedings.

Lactation failure

In occasional situations failure to thrive is actually due to lactation failure. Historically, sudden complete cessation of lactation was described in the late 1800s after coaching accidents and other great trauma. Advocates of breastfeeding have tended to dismiss this as a possibility and struggle frantically to reverse the situation. There are women who cannot make milk; some of these women have primary hypoprolactinemia, and others have secondary hypoprolactinemia as in Sheehan's disease (see Chapter 15). Because it is now possible to identify these women by obtaining prolactin levels[54] that confirm the diagnosis, when reasonable efforts at stimulation are ineffective and the mother is unable to do without the Lact-Aid providing almost a full feeding volume, evaluation of the mother is appropriate. Some mothers prefer to discontinue efforts to breastfeed before they have been totally stripped of their egos by total failure.

If one explores the animal literature, one finds a similar situation in other species. Lactation failure in nursing animals is rare because it is not a trait that is transmitted from generation to generation, since the offspring do not survive. Interferences with milk ejection can be identified and treated in other mammals. There is a syndrome in sows of agalactia associated with mastitis and metritis.[12] Mammalian lactation failure is attributed to nutritional, pharmacologic, and "emotional stress" causes in animals. Aside from gross dietary deficiency, there is depression or inhibition of the anterior pituitary gland, which is responsible for synthesis in the alveolar cells, and inhibition of transport and discharge of synthesized products from alveolar cells to the lumen. Certain plant alkaloids have been noted in other species to inhibit lactation. Ergot derivatives are best known, but colchicine, vincristine, and vinblastine are also causative. Some plant lectins such as concanavalin interfere with transport and discharge phases of milk production. Understanding lactation failure is increasing among clinicians as the diagnostic resources expand.[54]

OBESITY

Discussion of the impact of adiposity is rarely undertaken without including a discussion of cholesterol levels. Obesity and atherosclerosis in developed societies is a major public health issue. Does breastfeeding in infancy protect against obesity and atherosclerosis in adult life? This remains an open question. Energy requirements for infants have been overestimated.[9] Breastfed infants require and receive 110 kcal/kg/day at 1 month and 70 kcal/kg/day at 4 months. The low energy intakes are not due to limitations in maternal milk production as previously assumed but represent physiologically regulated intakes. Breastfed infants deposit less fat than formula-fed infants despite the fact that the two diets appear similar on paper. Although the breastfed infant appears protected against obesity in infancy, the effect appears to be lost after 3 years of age.[27]

A prospective cohort study of 462 healthy full-term infants was observed from birth to 12 months by Kramer et al.[33] Their goal was to overcome methodologic defects in previous studies of the etiologic determinants of childhood obesity that failed to control for confounding factors. At 6 and 12 months, measurements of height, weight, body mass index (weight/height^2), and skinfold were taken and correlated with duration of breastfeeding, introduction of solids, and parental heights and weights. Significant determinants of body mass index were birth weight, duration of breastfeeding, and introduction of solid foods. Breastfeeding and delayed introduction of solid foods offered some protective effect against obesity at 1 year.

The effect of breastfeeding on plasma cholesterol and weight in young adults was studied longitudinally by Marmot and Page[39] in a sample of people born in 1946. The infant feeding history was obtained. At age 32, women who had been breastfed had significantly lower mean plasma cholesterol than women who had been bottle fed. The difference for men was smaller, and the breastfed male had higher mean weight and skinfold thickness (Fig. 12-3). Multiple studies, both short- and long-range, with small populations and conflicting results have been reported in humans, although animal studies strongly suggest

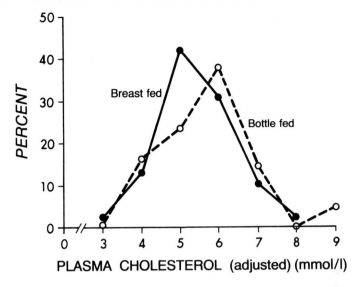

Fig. 12-3. Plasma cholesterol in adults according to infant feeding type. (From Marmot MG and Page CM: J Epidemiol Comm Health 34:164, 1980.)

that species-specific milk makes a difference in obesity and cholesterol. The subject of dietary cholesterol effects on serum cholesterol and atherosclerosis in humans has been reviewed by McGill.[40] The report of the conference on Blood Lipids in Children: Optimal Levels for Early Prevention of Coronary Artery Disease thoroughly reviews the question.[57] Indices of fatness and serum cholesterol at age 8 years in relation to feeding and growth during early infancy were reported by Fomon et al.[22] from their detailed longitudinal nutrition project involving 469 children born between 1966 and 1971. In infancy the formula-fed children had more rapid gains in height and weight, which were attributed to greater food intake. At age 8 there was no difference in indices of fatness related to mode of feeding during infancy nor were there significant differences in serum cholesterol concentrations. Fomon suggests that childhood and adolescence are too early to detect possible beneficial effects of breastfeeding on cholesterol homeostasis in later life in the human.[22]

Serum cholesterol may be too insensitive a quantitation to detect early changes and quantitation of lipoprotein classes, and apoprotein concentrations may be necessary.[27] The effects of breastfeeding versus formula feeding are not attributable to differences in cholesterol intake according to Mott[42] because varying the cholesterol content of infant formulas has not reduced long-lasting differences in serum cholesterol or lipoprotein concentrations or in cholesterol metabolism. Lack of control of genetic differences and sampling under uncontrolled dietary conditions have limited the interpretation of many human studies. Mott[41,42] performed a long-term study with 83 baboons to determine the effects of infant diet (breastfeeding versus formula feeding and the level of cholesterol in the formula). The type of dietary fat and level of dietary cholesterol as well as sex and heredity were reviewed. The progeny of 6 sires and 83 dams were randomly assigned to diet groups of breastfeeding or formula with 2, 30, or 60 mg, respectively, of cholesterol/dl. The 30 mg/dl milk resembled baboon milk. They were weaned to controlled juvenile diets. The differences in cholesterol content of the formula did not lead to later differences in serum cholesterol, lipoprotein concentrations, or cholesterol metabolism. Breastfeeding (species-specific milk), however, affected the subsequent cholesterol metabolism, with absorption of a higher

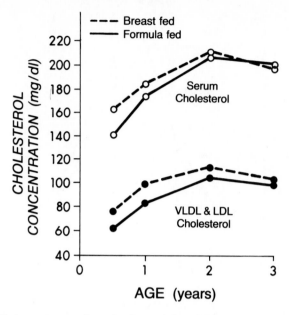

Fig. 12-4. Cholesterol, very low density and low-density lipoprotein in baboons: breastfed vs. formula fed. Open circle, serum cholesterol; closed circle, VLDL + LDL cholesterol; solid line, formula fed; dashed line, breastfed. (From Mott GE: Deferred effects of breastfeeding versus formula feeding on serum lipoprotein concentrations and cholesterol metabolism in baboons. In Report of the 91st Ross Conference on Pediatric Research: the breastfed infant: a model performance, Columbus Ohio, 1986, Ross Laboratories. Reprinted with permission of Ross Laboratories, Columbus, Ohio.)

percentage of cholesterol and lower cholesterol production rates as juveniles. The baboons were bred for high or low serum cholesterol concentrations, and in both groups the breastfed animals had higher very-low-density and low-density lipoprotein cholesterol levels from 6 months to 3 years than formula-fed animals and higher serum cholesterol from 6 months to 2 years (Fig. 12-4). Baboons are vegetarian and the weaning diet was not, however.

Overfeeding was a variable in a study of preweaning food intake influences on the adiposity of young adult baboons reported by Lewis et al.[37] Overfeeding did not have a major effect on the fat cell number. Overfed male baboons had a greater fat mass in four of ten fat depots at necropsy at age 5. Overfed female baboons had markedly greater fat depot mass in general primarily because of fat cell hypertrophy. Underfeeding in the preweaning period did not affect body weight or adipose mass in either sex in the juveniles.

In guinea pigs, stimulation of cholesterol catabolism by feeding cholestiramine after birth rather than cholesterol feeding can influence the response to dietary cholesterol in the adult. The efficient handling of dietary cholesterol in the cholestiramine-fed guinea pigs is directly associated with markedly higher levels of cholesterol 7 α-hydroxylase as sensitive to high dietary cholesterol during lactation.[38] Mott suggests that the long-term effects of breastfeeding on cholesterol metabolism are not likely to be due to the differences in neonatal cholesterol intake but to other components of breast milk, such as fatty acid composition, immunoglobulins, and hormones that might affect cholesterol metabolism.[42]

The best definition of obesity should be based on the percentage of body weight accounted for by fat. What percentage would be detrimental and how it could easily be measured is not known. Fomon[20] suggests, however, that until that is possible a clinical

Table 12-3. Tentative definition of obesity*

	Males		Females	
Age (mo)	Length (cm) less than	Weight (kg) more than	Length (cm) less than	Weight (kg) more than
1	51.8	4.2	51.5	4.0
	53.0	4.5	52.2	4.3
	54.2	4.7	53.5	4.6
	55.2	5.1	54.6	4.8
3	58.0	6.0	57.1	5.6
	59.2	6.4	58.0	5.9
	60.2	6.9	59.2	6.2
	61.5	7.3	60.5	6.6
6	65.6	7.7	63.3	7.5
	66.5	8.2	65.2	8.0
	67.8	9.0	66.3	8.4
	69.2	9.6	67.8	8.9
9	70.0	9.1	68.2	8.9
	70.9	9.7	69.5	9.4
	72.3	10.7	71.1	9.9
	73.6	11.2	73.1	10.4
12	73.6	10.2	72.5	9.9
	74.7	10.9	73.2	10.5
	76.4	11.6	75.1	11.1
	78.0	12.5	76.9	11.6
18	80.0	11.6	78.7	11.1
	81.7	12.6	80.2	11.8
	83.2	13.3	82.0	12.7
	85.3	14.4	84.2	13.2
24	85.0	12.8	84.2	12.3
	87.3	13.9	85.8	13.1
	88.8	14.5	87.5	14.2
	90.9	16.0	90.3	14.9
36	93.4	14.8	92.1	14.3
	95.3	15.7	94.2	15.3
	97.3	16.8	96.2	17.0
	100.6	18.6	99.0	17.7

From Fomon SJ: Infant nutrition, ed 2, Philadelphia, 1974, WB Saunders Co.
*The table is based on data of Fomon et al. (1970, 1971, 1973) for ages 1 and 3 months, and on the data of Karlberg et al. (1968) for subsequent ages. At each age, the values for length for each sex are the 10th, 25th, 50th and 75th percentiles, while the values for weight are the 50th, 75th and 90th percentiles, and the mean +2 standard deviations.

definition that circumvents clinical impressions would be useful. He suggests that "values greater than +2 standard deviation value for triceps and subscapsular skin-fold thickness be considered evidence of obesity." Foman also recognizes the difficulty of obtaining skinfold measurements on young infants and offers as a less satisfactory alternative the relation of body weight to stature (Table 12-3). The infant with a heavy bone structure and musculature but without excessive fat may appear to be obese based on this table. Infants who are overfed also grow in height and may well be in an advanced percentile for height. The infant who is born with a weight in the eightieth percentile (weight for age) and remains there may not be obese, but the infant who is born with a weight in the fiftieth percentile and crosses percentiles over time to the eightieth percentile may be at risk for long-term obesity. Therefore, some discretion is advised when using these criteria for obesity.

There are no benefits from infantile obesity. The concern for obesity rests with the long-range outcome as an obese adult. There is a problem that obesity in infancy predisposes the child to immobility and inactivity; thus an obese infant lags on the developmental curve or at least has delayed gross motor skills. The question of whether obesity in infancy predisposes the child to obesity in adult life has not been resolved satisfactorily. Retrospective studies support both sides of the question. A prospective study of 403 newborns in Canada was done measureing weight, length, and subcutaneous fat, but an infant was considered "breastfed" if he received any breastfeeding for 2 months and early solids.[32] Food feeding was defined as beginning solids by 2 months of age. The authors felt they refuted the hypothesis of bottle fed obesity in their 18-month follow-up. Most students of this subject would question the population definitions. A study of adolescents retrospectively tested the question of whether breastfeeding and delayed introduction of solids protect against subsequent obesity. The author concluded that breastfeeding does, but delayed solids alone do not protect against obesity.[58]

Breastfed infants are rarely obese. The usual cause of obesity in these infants is the early addition of solids. Solids often provide excessive kilocalories. The obese breastfed infant should have his diet and the feeding pattern scrutinized. If necessary, some restriction of prolonged feeding should be suggested. In the normal course of a breastfeeding, the fat content of the milk increases over the duration of the feeding and satisfies the infant after 10 to 15 minutes of nursing.

Since there is general agreement that, once established, childhood obesity often becomes chronic and resistant to treatment,[39] it is appropriate to focus attention on prevention and early intervention. The physician can counsel a family whose breastfed infant meets the criteria for obesity (above the eighty-fifth percentile for weight for length). The routine use of skinfold measurements as part of well baby care will increase the ability to diagnose obesity at it distinguishes the constitutionally bigger body frame from the fat infant.

Recommendations that will help taper unusual weight gain include the following:

1. Limit excessive feedings that are being provided on the mistaken belief that all the infant's needs are nutritional.
2. Encourage nonnutritive cuddling. If feeding is a response to all distress signals, the infant may expect feeding inappropriately, causing disassociation between appetite and energy need.
3. Use exclusive breastfeeding, i.e., no solids for 4 to 6 months.
4. Increase activity and energy utilization by encouraging movement rather than containing or restricting the infant in carriers or swaddlings. For the older infant, encourage play activity and crawling and minimize sitting.
5. If there is a persistent growth excess, it is appropriate to obtain a sample of maternal milk to rule out the rare case of hyperlipidemia with a "creamatocrit." See p. 476.

REFERENCES

1. Ahn CH and MacLean WC: Growth of the exclusively breast-fed infant, Am J Clin Nutr 33:183, 1980.
2. Anard SK et al: Neonatal hypernatremia associated with elevated sodium concentration of breast milk, J Pediatr 96:66, 1980.
3. Asnes RS et al: The dietary chloride deficiency syndrome occurring in a breast-fed infant, J Pediatr 100:923, 1982.
4. Axelsson I, Borulf S, Righard L et al: Protein and energy intake during weaning. I. Effects on growth, Acta Paediatr Scand 76:321, 1987.
5. Barness LA: Nutrition for healthy neonates. In Gracy M and Falkner F, editors: Nutritional needs and assessment of normal growth, New York, 1985, Vevey/Raven Press.
6. Behrman RE, Driscoll JM Jr, and Seeds AE, editors: Neonatal-perinatal medicine: diseases of the fetus and infant, ed 2, St Louis, 1977, The CV Mosby Co.
7. Blass EM and Teicher MH: Suckling, Science 210:15, 1980.
8. Brown KH, Robertson AD, and Akhtar NA: Lactational capacity of marginally nourished mothers: infant's milk nutrient consumption and patterns of growth, Pediatrics 78:920, 1986.
9. Butte NF, Garza C, Smith EOB et al: Human milk intake and growth in exclusively breast fed infants, J Pediatr 104:187, 1984.
10. Clarke TA et al: Hypernatremic dehydration resulting from inadequate breastfeeding, Pediatrics 63:931, 1979.
11. Committee on Dietary Allowances, Food and Nutrition Board, National Research Council: Recommended dietary allowances, Washington DC 1980, Natioanl Academy of Sciences.
12. Cowie AT, Forsyth IA, and Hart IC: Hormonal control of lactation monographs on endocrinology, Heidelberg-New York, 1980, Springer Verlag.
13. Czajka-Narins DM and Jung E: Physical growth of breastfed and formula fed infants from birth to age two years, Nutr Res 6:753, 1986.
14. Dewey KG and Lönnerdal B: Milk and nutrition intake of breastfed infants from 1 to 6 months: relation to growth and fatness, J Pediatr Gastroenterol Nutr 2:497, 1983.
15. Duncan B, Schafer C, Sibley B et al: Reduced growth velocity in exclusively breast-fed infants, AJDC 138:309, 1984.
16. Ereman RR, Lönnerdal B, and Dewey KG: Maternal sodium intake does not affect postprandial sodium concentrations in human milk, J Nutr 117:1154, 1987.
17. Fergusson DM, Beautrais AL, and Silva PA: Breastfeeding and cognitive development in the first seven years of life, Soc Sci Med 16:1705, 1982.
18. Fergusson DM, Horwood LJ, and Shannon FT: Breastfeeding and subsequent social adjustment in six to eight year old children, J Child Psychol Psychiatr 28:378, 1987.
19. Finberg L, Kiley J, and Luttrell CN: Mass accidental salt poisoning in infancy: a study of a hospital disaster, JAMA 184:187, 1963.
20. Fomon SJ: Infant nutrition, ed 2, Philadelphia, 1974, WB Saunders Co.
21. Fomon SJ et al: Growth and serum chemical values of normal breast fed infants, Acta Paediatr Scand (suppl) 202:1, 1970.
22. Fomon SJ, Rogers RR, Ziegler EE et al: Indices of fatness and serum cholesterol at age eight years in relation to feeding and growth during early infancy, Pediatr Res 18:1233, 1984.
23. Gilmore HE and Rowland TW: Critical malnutrition in breast-fed infants, Am J Dis Child 132:885, 1978.
24. Ghishan FK and Roloff JS: Malnutrition and hypernatremic dehydration in two breast-fed infants, Clin Pediatr 22:592, 1983.
25. Habbick BF and Gerrard JW: Failure to thrive in the contented breastfed baby, Can Med Assoc J 131:765, 1984.
26. Hall DM and Kay G: Effect of thyrotrophin-releasing factor on lactation, Br Med J 1:777, 1977.
27. Hamosh M: Does infant nutrition affect adiposity and cholesterol levels in the adult? J Pediatr Gastroenterol Nutr 7:10, 1988.
28. Hill ID and Bowie MD: Chloride deficiency syndrome due to chloride-deficient breast milk, Arch Dis Child 58:224, 1983.
29. Hitchcock NE, Gracey M, and Owles EN: Growth of the healthy breast-fed infants in the first six months, Lancet 2:64, 1981.
30. Jelliffe DB and Jelliffe EFP: Human milk in the modern world, Oxford, 1978, Oxford University Press.
31. Juez G, Diaz S, Casado ME et al: Growth pattern of selected urban Chilean infants during exclusive breastfeeding, Am J Clin Nutr 38:462, 1983.
32. Kramer MS: Do breast-feeding and delayed introduction of solid foods protect against subsequent obesity? J Pediatr 98:883, 1981.
33. Kramer MS, Barr RG, Leduc DG et al: Determinants of weight and adiposity in the first year of life, J Pediatr 106:10, 1985.

34. Lawrence RA: Successful breastfeeding, Am J Dis Child 135:595, 1981.

35. Lawrence RA: Infant nutrition, Pediatr Rev 5:133, 1983.

36. Lawrence R: Maternal factors in lactation failure. In Hamosh M and Goldman AS, editors: Human lactation. II. Maternal and environmental factors, New York, 1986, Plenum Press.

37. Lewis DS, Bertrand HA, McMahan A et al: Preweaning food intake influences the adiposity of young adult baboons, J Clin Invest 78:899, 1986.

38. Li JR, Bale LK, and Kottke BA: Effect of neonatal modulation of cholesterol homeostasis on subsequent response to cholesterol challenge in adult guinea pig, J Clin Invest 65:1060, 1980.

39. Marmot MG et al: Effect of breast-feeding on plasma cholesterol and weight in young adults, J Epidemiol Commun Health 34:164, 1980.

40. McGill HC Jr: The relationship of dietary cholesterol to serum cholesterol concentration and to atherosclerosis in man, Am J Clin Nutr 32:2664, 1979.

41. Mott GE: Deferred effects of breastfeeding versus formula feeding on serum lipoprotein concentrations and cholesterol metabolisms in baboons. In Report of the 91st Ross Conference on Pediatric Research. The breastfed infant: a model performance, Columbus Ohio, 1986, Ross Laboratories.

42. Mott GE, Jackson EM, McMahan CA et al: Cholesterol metabolism in juvenile baboons: influences of infant and juvenile diets, Arteriosclerosis 5:347, 1985.

43. National Center for Health Statistics: Trends in breastfeeding: advance data from vital and health statistics, Washington DC, 1980, DHHS pub no 59.

44. Neifert MR and Seacat JM: Mammary gland anomalies and lactation failure. In Hamosh M and Goldman AS, editors: Human lactation, II. Maternal and environmental factors, New York, 1986, Plenum Press.

45. Neifert MR, Seacat JM, and Jobe WE: Lactation failure due to insufficient glandular development of the breast, Pediatrics 76:823, 1985.

46. Oliva-Rasbach J and Neville MC: Longitudinal growth patterns of a reference population of breastfed infants, Fed Proc 45:362, 1986.

47. Paneth N: Hypernatremic dehydration of infancy, Am J Dis Child 134:785, 1980.

48. Podratz RO, Broughton DD, Gustafson DH et al: Weight loss and body temperature changes in breast-fed and bottle-fed neonates, Clin Pediatr 25:73, 1986.

49. Pomerance HH: Growth in breast-fed children, Hum Biol 59:687, 1987.

50. Pugliese MT, Weyman-Daum M, Moses N et al: Parental health beliefs as a cause of nonorganic failure to thrive, Pediatrics 80:175, 1987.

51. Roddey OF et al: Critical weight loss and malnutrition in breastfed infants, Am J Dis Child 135:597, 1981.

52. Rowland TW et al: Malnutrition and hypernatremic dehydration, JAMA 247:106, 1982.

53. Volz VR, Book LS, and Churella HR: Growth and plasma amino acid concentratioans in term infants fed either whey-predominant formula or human milk, J Pediatr 102:27, 1983.

54. Weichert CE: Lactational reflex recovery in breast-feeding failure, Pediatrics 63:799, 1979.

55. Weston JA, Stage AF, Hathaway P et al: Prolonged breast-feeding and nonorganic failure to thrive, AJDC 141:242, 1987.

56. Whitehead RG and Paul AA: Growth charts and the assessment of infant feeding practices in the Western world and in developing countries, Early Hum Dev 9:187, 1984.

57. Wissler RW and McGill HC Jr, chairman: Conference on blood lipids in children: optimal levels for early prevention of coronary artery disease, Pre Med 12:868, 1983.

58. Yeug DL et al: Infant fatness and feeding practices: a longitudinal assessment, J Am Diet Assoc 79:531, 1981.

59. Young HB et al: Milk and lactation: some social and developmental correlates among 1000 infants, Pediatrics 69:169, 1982.

Maternal employment   13

Maternal employment has been cited by many authors as the major reason for the decline in breastfeeding worldwide.[6,34] The international data do not actually support this contention. For the individual mother who wishes to return to work and breastfeed there are significant constraints, regardless of the statistical data. The physician should be knowledgeable about the principles and practice of this dual role and minimize the influence of his own biases when counseling about maternal employment.[45] Much of the literature is plagued with personal bias, glib generalizations, and anecdotal reports.

HISTORICAL PERSPECTIVE

In modern culture there has been a stigma attached to a mother's earning money while her children are young but no such stigma associated with leaving her children for social interaction, personal reasons, or a volunteer job. All women work when work is defined as expending energy for a purpose, but not all women are employed when it is defined as earning money for labor. Before industrialization, the working mother was the rule and not the exception. Home and work were separated by industrialization, making parenting a separate role for women. Women's work has been described by Sanday[38] as domestic or productive, public or private, traditional or modern. Domestic work, when performed for the family, is unpaid and thus is undervalued and not counted as productive work. Domestic work is performed in the private domain, and productive work is associated with the public domain. Women had previously worked in agriculture and cottage industries as well as in small-scale marketing, whereas today they participate in formal work including clerical, factory, and professional jobs predominantly in urban settings.

More women are employed outside the home today than previously in this century.[41] In 1900, 20% of the labor force was women; in 1950, 29%; and in 1985, almost 50%. Women with children under 6 years old are the fastest-growing segment of the female work force. Even more critical is the fact that the number of employed mothers with infants under 1 year has escalated to 48% of all women in 1985. This means that for many more women the decision about infant feeding methods includes the early return to work. Married women continue to carry at least 70% to 80% of the child care and household duties when both parents work. Census reports for 1980 for the United States indicate that 60% of women are employed, including 55% of all mothers with children under 18 years of age, and 45% of mothers with preschool-aged children. Sixty-two percent of the women between 24 and 34 years of age, the traditional childbearing years, have jobs. Women with children under 6 years of age, representing 6 million mothers, tripled from 1950 to 1978, and in 1985 reached 40 million. Three generations ago, the woman who worked violated the Victorian norms of role definition. Even when forced to work by sheer necessity, she was accused of neglecting her primary responsibility to her children. The new ethic proclaims work a cardinal virtue for the liberated woman, so that the woman who can and does stay home begins to feel inadequate.

Why women enter the work force is important to understanding the trend.[26] Before 1970 the need to earn money motivated 3 million women either because the mother was a single parent or husband-fathers were unable to earn an adequate income. For women whose husbands earned "enough" there was the need to provide a higher standard of living or provide the father with greater freedom of career choice.[46] There were few who sought careers for careers' sake because need for income was the only socially acceptable, defensible reason for a mother to work outside the home.

Since that time many women have found that the full-time care of a home leads only to higher standards of cleanliness with no greater sense of achievement or completion.[16] The exclusive investment of energy and emotion in the rearing of one to three children involves a considerable hazard not only to a mother but also to her children's ultimate achievement and ability to form a variety of responsive and satisfying personal relationships.[26,33] Women are responding to the pressures of an inflationary economy, to the costs of higher education, to the opportunities for personal fulfillment, and to the growing market for service occupations. Married women continue to carry at least 70% to 80% of the child care and household duties when both parents work.

ATTITUDES OF PROFESSIONALS TOWARD WORKING MOTHERS

Professional[7,20] and lay books[29,39] alike on child rearing have viewed working negatively except for economic necessity, thus enhancing the working mother's guilt and providing little substantial advice.

The Committee on Psychosocial Aspects of Child and Family Health of the Academy of Pediatrics wrote "The Mother Working Oustide the Home."[3] It is summarized by the statement: "Many mothers work outside the home and most have concerns about substitute child care. In addition to providing advice to individual parents, pediatricians can make an important contribution by supporting subsidized parental leaves after birth of a newborn infant, by encouraging the active participation of fathers in child and household care, and by having the knowledge to aid parents in access to high quality substitute child care."

The American College of Obstetrics and Gynecology[4] has acknowledged the current trend to work throughout pregnancy and to return to work promptly after delivery by preparing a physician's guide to patient assessment and counseling. There is also a patient occupational questionnaire provided the practitioner. This forms a basis of discussion with the patient and provides an opportunity to counsel the patient and her husband about plans to maintain a healthy environment and any special needs for child care. It is stated that with few exceptions, "the normal woman with an uncomplicated pregnancy and a normal fetus in a job that presents no greater potential hazards than those encountered in normal daily life in the community may continue to work without interruption until the onset of labor and may resume working several weeks after an uncomplicated delivery." Frederick and Auerbach[14] put it in more practical terms when they suggest that the obstetrician has a role in facilitating continued breastfeeding after the return to work or school. This includes counseling regarding pumping and storing milk and avoiding exhaustion.

Attitudes of pediatricians toward mothers working outside the home have been measured by mail survey, since attitudes seem to determine advice given.[19] The majority of pediatricians responding felt that the children of working and nonworking women were similar; that the mother could return to work at any age of the child; that it did not make any difference. Many respondents said they did not give advice about working (Tables 13-1 and 13-2). Only half the respondents provided special considerations such as evening hours for employed mothers.

Bias against employed mothers did exist, however, among some respondents. Bias was related to the age and sex of the respondent and to whether the respondent's spouse

Table 13-1. Responses for reasons to recommend work

	Frequency	
	No.	%
Economic reasons	1709	25
Never recommend mother work	1566	22
Mother's emotional needs	1220	18
Mother's fulfillment	1059	15
Child is better off without mother	644	9
Reassure mother	270	4
Adequacy of child care	266	4
Child's age	170	2
Mother does important work	64	1
TOTAL	6964	

From Heins M et al: Pediatrics 72:283, 1983. Copyright American Academy of Pediatrics 1983.

Table 13-2. Responses for reasons to recommend against working

	Frequency	
	No.	%
Child's physical health	1724	24
Child's mental health	1445	20
Never recommend against work	1318	18
Inadequate child care	701	10
Child's age	591	8
Mother feels guilty	540	7
No economic need	459	6
Usually say "Do not work"	72	1
Other	402	6
TOTAL	7252	

From Heins M et al: Pediatrics 72:286, 1983. Copyright American Academy of Pediatrics 1983.

worked. Those whose spouses did not work outside the home, those in older age groups, and male pediatricians in general held more traditional attitudes toward maternal employment. The researchers felt that a substantial number might give advice or cues that maternal employment might be detrimental to children, producing maternal conflict and guilt. The physician plays an important role in guiding parents with information about quality and availability of child-care facilities, as well as with advice about coping strategies.[13] As family counselor, the physician can help support mothers and fathers seeking to fulfill parental, occupational, and personal needs in a rapidly changing society.

OUTCOME OF CHILDREN WHOSE MOTHERS ARE EMPLOYED

Numerous studies since the early 1930s have looked at the effects of maternal employment. Assessment of infant behavior, school achievement and adjustment, children's attitudes, adolescence, and delinquency have all been used as outcome measures. Annotated bibliographies covering the range of research in areas of medicine, psychology, sociology, and education are available.* The four major considerations are the variables that facilitate or impede maternal employment, the effect of maternal employment on children during the four developmental stages, the effects on the family, and the effects on society in general.

It has been emphasized that the presence of the mother in the home does not guarantee high-quality mothering.[16] It has also been shown that well-educated (college) mothers, including those who are employed, spend time with their children at the expense of their own personal needs. Because employed mothers encompass a large group of women with different educations, different reasons for working, and different opportunities for employment, it is difficult to generalize about effects. Literature reviews have emphasized critical factors that are more important than maternal employment, such as good substitute care, maternal role satisfaction, family stability, paternal attitude toward maternal employment, and the quality of time spent with the children.[23] Despite the abundance of research on school-age children, there is still little reported about preschoolers because there are no school records or test results available to use in large-population analysis. To date there is no direct effect of nonexclusive mothering per se. In studies of infants of adolescent mothers it has been shown that the children do better socially and academically if there are multiple caregivers instead of the adolescent alone.[30] No uniformly harmful effects on family life or on the growth and development of children have been demonstrated. Maternal employment may jeopardize family life when the conditions of the mother's employment are demeaning to self-esteem, when others are strongly disapproving of her work away from the home, or when arrangements for child care are not adequate.[38]

Questions of the impact of separation of mother and infant and the timing of this separation have been raised.[9] Resumption of full-time employment when the child is under 1 year has sparked studies. Using the Ainsworth "Strange Situation" validated techniques, no relationship between maternal work status and the quality of the infants' attachments to their mothers is reported.[1,2] Early resumption of employment may not impede development of a secure infant-mother attachment.[10] A significantly higher proportion of insecure attachments to fathers in employed-mother families is reported for boys but not for girls.

*See references 6, 16, 25, 27, 38, 40, 41.

Boys are more insecurely attached than girls in most studies. It is believed that an infant's attachment relationship to mother emerges at about 7 months.[15] Other studies suggest that maternal employment can have a positive effect on girls but not boys. Whether breastfeeding accounts for some of the variability in these studies is not stated.[11,22-25,43] One of the strategies suggested is to advocate for infant care centers that provide breastfeeding facilities in the workplace, schools, and other locations serving working women.

BREASTFEEDING AND EMPLOYMENT

An important distinction must be made between work that separates the mother and infant for blocks of time and work that does not. In rural settings, women's work is usually compatible with all aspects of child care, including breastfeeding. Work in or around the home is usually flexible. If there are provisions for infants at the workplace, even formal urban work is compatible with child care and breastfeeding. The higher the education of the mother and the more advanced the job, the more opportunity there is for flexible arrangements that permit breastfeeding. Among the strategies available is pumping and saving milk while on the job to be fed to the baby by the baby-sitter the next day.

Dismissal from employment of nursing mothers demonstrates the unique problems for working women in certain jobs. Overall, the breastfeeding rates for working women do not show that breastfeeding and employment are mutually exclusive.[46] In Finland, the incidence of mothers breastfeeding at 1 month is 78% among nonworking and 80% among working mothers. The duration is also unaffected; 29% of nonworking and 32% of working mothers are breastfeeding at 3 months and 8% and 7% at 6 months.[42] Similar statistics are reported from Nigeria, the Philippines, and Chile.

The figures for the United States have been reported by Martinez and Dodd[31] (Table 13-3), who conducted a mail and telephone survey of new mothers in 1981, as described in Chapter 1. The survey has been conducted since 1955, but data on employment were not collected until 1981, so no trends are available. When the infant was 6 months of age, 20% of the respondents were employed full-time outside the home. The higher incidence of employment was among mothers who were college educated, upper income, and primiparous. The incidence of breastfeeding was not significantly influenced by employment, but the duration was negatively influenced. In 1987, Ryan and Martinez conducted another study of the impact of employment on breastfeeding as part of the annual Ross Laboratories Mother's Survey exploring infant feeding practices.[37] There were 38,985 questionnaires returned (54%). Those mothers at 6 months who were employed full-time numbered 22,316 (26.6%), part-time 12,186 (14.5%), and 49,483 (58.9%). The same proportion of employed mothers (55%) as not employed were breastfeeding when they left the hospital. On the other hand, only 10% of full-time employed mothers were breastfeeding at 6 months compared to 24% of those who were not employed. The highest incidence of breastfeeding at birth and at 6 months was among the over-30-year-old mother who is well educated and in a higher socioeconomic group. The continuance rate (see Table 13-4) for all mothers was 18% breastfeeding among those employed and 44% among those not employed. Not surprisingly, working mothers also used more supplementary bottles.

When the factors influencing the duration of breastfeeding were examined by West[44] by postal questionnaire at 6 months in Edinburgh, only 5 mothers of 116 listed "return to work" as a reason for discontinuing.

Table 13-3. Percentage of infants breastfed by maternal employment status, 1981*

Maternal employment status	Infant age			
	In hospital	2 mo	4 mo	6 mo
Full-time employment				
Breastfed alone	45.1	24.8	8.5	3.6
Breastfed with bottle	5.8	8.3	8.3	6.6
Total	50.9	33.1	16.8	10.1
Milk, bottle supplementation as % of total	11.4	25.1	49.4	65.4
% still breastfeeding among those breastfeeding in hospital	100.0	65.0	33.0	19.8
Not employed				
Breastfed alone	53.4	41.1	30.8	22.9
Breastfed with bottle	6.1	6.4	6.5	6.9
Total	59.5	47.4	37.3	29.8
Milk, bottle supplementation as % of total	10.3	13.5	17.4	23.2
% still breastfeeding among those breastfeeding in hospital	100.0	79.7	62.7	50.1

From Martinez GA and Dodd DA: Pediatrics 71:169, 1983. Copyright American Academy of Pediatrics 1983.
*Employment status was not elicited in second quarter of 1981. Data represent first, third, and fourth quarters only. Some totals do not add due to rounding.

A comparison by Martinez and Stahle[32] of low-income mothers who were receiving assistance from the Women's, Infants and Children's (WIC) Program showed that of the 38% who planned to work full-time and left the hospital breastfeeding, only 8.8% were breastfeeding at 6 months, whereas of the 42.4% who had no plans for employment on leaving the hosptial, 17.1% were still breastfeeding at 6 months.

Although work has been listed as a primary cause of early weaning, women seldom give employment as a reason for terminating breastfeeding. Review of the world literature documenting reasons for weaning, starting bottle feeding, or not initiating breastfeeding rarely mentioned employment.[42] In studies of the effect of mother's employment on the nutritional status of her children, poverty, not mother's work, was associated with poor nutrition.

The effect of employment on the duration of breastfeeding may be influenced by the fact that breastfeeding can be carried out while the mother performs other tasks around the house so that it is easier to breastfeed when she is home.[21] Many studies have found that employment has little or no effect on the duration of breastfeeding especially where cottage industry was prevalent. The greatest problems are the difficulties encountered finding a place to pump and store the milk on the job. Those women who work outside the home must schedule and plan carefully and are motivated to continue once the complex schedule is established. They also are more able to accommodate themselves to the stresses. A national study among women who responded to an advertisement in popular parenting magazines about working and breastfeeding found a relationship between work and breast-feeding success.[5] The timing of the return to work and the number of hours worked, not the type of work, influenced the duration of breastfeeding. Most of the respondents, however, were well educated and were motivated to respond to the advertisement and to retrospectively fill out a lengthy questionnaire. Results showed that mothers who pumped

Table 13-4. Percentage of infants breastfed* in hospital, and at 6 months, and continuance rate† by working status and selected demographic characteristics, 1987

Variables	Breastfed in hospital (%)		Breastfed at 6 months (%)		Continuance rate†	
	Employed full-time	Not working	Employed full-time	Not working	Employed full-time	Not working
All mothers	54.5	54.5	10.0	24.3	18.3	44.6
Maternal age						
<20 years	38.4	33.4	4.5	7.5	11.7	22.5
20-24 years	47.9	49.6	5.8	17.7	12.1	35.7
25-29 years	57.5	63.2	9.7	31.0	16.9	49.1
30-34 years	61.1	68.4	14.5	39.3	23.7	57.5
35+ years	61.1	66.1	20.0	40.4	32.7	61.1
Family income						
<$7,000	34.3	31.0	5.6	8.3	16.3	26.8
$7,000-$15,000	40.5	49.4	6.4	19.2	15.8	38.9
$15,001-$25,000	49.7	62.4	8.1	29.1	16.3	46.6
>$25,000	63.1	72.9	12.5	38.2	19.8	52.4
Maternal education						
High school or less	43.8	46.0	5.7	17.7	13.0	38.5
College	67.6	75.9	15.3	41.1	22.6	54.2
Parity						
Primiparous	58.1	54.4	10.1	20.7	17.4	38.1
Multiparous	49.1	54.7	9.8	27.6	20.0	50.5
Ethnicity						
White	58.9	62.3	10.7	28.7	18.2	46.1
Black	32.7	21.2	6.0	7.6	18.3	35.8
US census region						
New England	56.5	59.0	10.6	27.1	18.8	45.9
Middle Atlantic	48.5	48.3	9.5	22.0	19.6	45.5
East North Central	50.8	48.7	8.9	22.0	17.5	45.2
West North Central	57.5	58.7	8.6	25.3	15.0	43.1
South Atlantic	47.5	45.8	7.7	20.4	16.2	44.5
East South Central	39.2	38.0	7.1	15.1	18.1	39.7
West South Central	50.1	49.9	7.4	19.5	14.8	39.1
Mountain	71.3	75.5	15.5	37.2	21.7	49.3
Pacific	73.7	72.7	16.5	33.5	22.4	46.1

From Ryan AS and Martinez GA: Pediatrics 83:524, 1989. Reproduced by permission of Pediatrics.

*Includes supplemental bottle feeding, i.e., formula, in addition to human milk.

†The breastfeeding continuance rate was calculated using the following formula:

$$1.0 - \frac{\% \text{ breastfed in hospital} - \% \text{ breastfed at 6 months}}{\% \text{ breastfed in hospital}}$$

or hand expressed (86% of the respondents) while at work continued to breastfeed longer than the small percentage who did not pump at work.

Counseling the breastfeeding mother who wishes to work

Part of the physician's counseling session before the birth of a baby should include inquiry about mother's plan to work postpartum. Open discussion about work, breast-feeding, child-care arrangements, and general stress so incurred will be helpful. Most well-educated women who plan to return to a career have thought out the entire process carefully but may wish some reassurance or alternative suggestions. The physician should know what services are available locally. It may be helpful to have a list of other working mothers who are willing to share experiences and knowledge of resources. It is often helpful for a women to know a real person who has experienced similar career choices.

Some women have no experience with newborns and are totally unrealistic about the new responsibility and what it entails. The pediatrician may have to recommend a more realistic view of parenting and urge the parents to plan carefully and practically for working and parenting. The new mother needs to appreciate that events occur around children that cannot be totally controlled. If a women has been an efficient career woman in total control of her destiny, an infant with normal needs may be overwhelming. Women who have jobs that are rigid from the standpoint of work hours and workplace will not find a few glib remarks in a pamphlet very helpful when she wants to maintain her milk supply.

The physician may need to discuss specific issues of child care and feeding the infant while the mother is working.

Child care:

1. Child-care arrangements should be sought that permit sufficient time for feeding an infant inexperienced with a bottle and sufficient time for extra cuddling an infant who is used to a closer relationship with his "feeder." The child-care specialist should be familiar with breastfeeding and sympathetic to the philosophy.
2. The advantages and disadvantages of child care in the infant's home, in the sitter's home, with or without the sitter's children, and with or without other children should be discussed. Is day care a good arrangement for this family, and what centers take young infants and will work with breastfeeding mothers? In spite of low cost, nursery warehousing is to be avoided.
3. Are there child-care facilities available close to the workplace so that mother could leave work on her breaks to breastfeed?

Feeding the infant while mother is working:

1. Plans for feeding depend on the age of the child and his feeding pattern. If the infant is totally breastfed and under 6 months of age, feeding will be mother's milk (a) if his mother can actually breastfeed him because she can leave work and go to the infant or he can be brought to the workplace, (b) mother's milk in a bottle. If mother cannot leave work to nurse, then she may wish to pump her milk at work and save it for the following day. This necessitates having a rea-sonably sanitary place to pump, such as a lounge or clean locker room. It also necessitates having a means of storing the milk until she gets home, either in a refrigerator at work or by placing the milk in a portable refrigerator system. Mothers have used Styrofoam containers with ice or dry ice for the container of milk. If no such arrangement for chilling can be made, the milk can be stored in a sterile container a few hours without refrigeration. A woman who is away from

her breastfeeding infant past feeding time for any reason may need to pump to maintain her milk supply or simply for comfort. Techniques for pumping and storing milk are reviewed in Chapter 19.

A mother may also anticipate the infant's needs before she returns to work and practice pumping and actually store in her home freezer a small amount daily for several weeks so that mother's milk is available.

The mother should be instructed to introduce the baby to the bottle and an alternate caregiver before the first day of work. Developing a plan of organization and practicing it prior to the first day of work may avoid initial disaster. Also returning to work part-time at first may help minimize the adjustment.

The pediatrician may wish to consider that if the infant is over 6 months of age, other foods can be introduced, and the feeding given by the caregiver can be the solids by spoon and liquids from a cup so that no breastfeeding is actually missed. The professional can anticipate these issues and tailor feeding counseling accordingly. Some infants quickly learn the mother's schedule and may adjust their sleep pattern to allow a long stretch while mother is away. This may result in feedings during the night instead, but if the mother is informed of this phenomenon she may be less anxious if it occurs. It has been suggested in some studies that infants of mothers who work have more infections and illnesses, which is a reason to encourage a mother to continue breastfeeding, especially during the first weeks of adjustment to transient recurrent separation.

Maternal considerations

Counseling the breastfeeding family when the mother returns to work should also include attention to mothering the mother. Fatigue is a significant problem for all postpartum women and many nursing mothers and can easily become a major stress when the mother adds outside employment to her schedule. Any time there is a major change in anyone's schedule, there are several days or more of adjustment. If during this time the mother can be encouraged to focus on a few essential concerns—her infant, her job, and her own well-being, as opposed to the housework, fancy meals, or a social schedule—she will weather this transition without despair. The first casualty of fatigue may be breastfeeding, unless some anticipatory caution is taken. Once the schedule has been adjusted and a routine established, breastfeeding may offer tremendous satisfaction for both mother and infant in terms of a sustained relationship as well as a reaffirmation for the mother of the quality of her parenting. One of the most difficult adjustments to motherhood for an efficient career women is the need to set priorities and eliminate some chores of lesser urgency. The physician needs to reinforce this when the mother returns to work. If a mother continues to breastfeed, holding and cuddling her baby cannot become a lower priority. Mother's nourishment is also important, and nourishment for herself can be consumed during the time spent pumping.

Day care

Infants in day care have created a special concern for parents, pediatricians, social scientists, and policymakers. The published information to date does not discuss the impact of breastfeeding prior to or during the infant's involvement with day care. Haskins and Kotch have reviewed the literature (172 articles) in a monograph "Day Care and Illness: Evidence, Costs, and Public Policy."[18] The authors conclude that "children in day care, especially those under three years old and sometimes their teachers and household contacts have higher rates of diarrhea, hepatitis A, meningitis and possibly also otitis media than children not in day care." The data are less clear for respiratory illnesses and cytomega-lovirus. An extremely valuable but unavailable piece of data would be the relationship to breastfeeding and illness in and out of day care. Revisions of state regulatory policy regarding health practices in day care are necessary. Parents choosing day-care facilities for their children need to select them with consideration for health and safety. Currently more than 60% of the children under 6 years of age of women who work are in out-of-home care, approximately 4.7 million in the United States. This figure is projected to reach 6.3 million children by 1990.

In addition to health risks, it has been suggested that there is also considerable risk for developmental deficits, personality flaws, less intellectual development, and an increased sense of social isolation. There is no empirical support for these presumptions in studies available. This concern certainly deserves the attention of the pediatrician for his patients that should result in some involvement in assuring quality day care in the local community. In addition, for the infant in the age appropriate for breastfeeding, it would suggest that one possible preventive measure would be to encourage a continuation of breastfeeding where possible. Furthermore, it would suggest day-care policy and procedure should encourage and facilitate breastfeeding.

Resources for parents. The popular press has been inundated with books on child care and child rearing with a significant number on breastfeeding, specifically breastfeeding and employment. These volumes can be extremely helpful to young parents, providing detailed information about how to manage. Many recognize that mothers, fathers, infants, jobs, child-care arrangements, and support resources are all different. A disturbing number, however, are dogmatic and singleminded, imbuing the reader with the impression that there is only one recipe for successful lactation and that is how the author succeeded. The pediatrician should become familiar with a few of these guide books and certainly not recommend any without reading them first. A few have taken the opportunity to instill a little guilt in the working women about leaving her infant.

Women in health care head the list of authors, as many women physicians (especially residents), nurses, and hospital employees return to work while breastfeeding and then share their experiences in print.[17] Even the worst setup in a hospital may surpass the resources available to the women working in industry. Certainly hospitals and health care centers should provide models for other work places in supporting optimal day-care sources and making it possible for a mother-employee to return to work and maintain her milk supply.[28]

Responding to parental needs, T. Berry Brazelton has written a book about working parents.[8] He captured the quintessential challenge to parents in the title and the text *Working and Caring*. It is possible for parents to both work and care! Freud pointed out that the two most powerful requirements for human existence are "love" and "work." Our culture had suggested that men work and women love in relation to family obligations. Today it is possible not only for a mother to love her children and work but also for a father to work and love his children. Although the book was written for parents in his usual style of live reports of representative families, it also contains valuable guidance for the health care professional who counsels parents who work.

Surgeon General's Workshop

In the report of the Surgeon General's Workshop on Breastfeeding and Human Lactation, it is clearly enunciated that strategies need to be developed to reduce the barriers to breastfeeding while employed.[35] All six categories address the issue in some capacity. Category 1—The World of Work—states: A national breastfeeding promotion initiative directed to all those who influence the breastfeeding decisions and opportunities of women involved in school, job training, professional education, and employment is needed. Along with data collection, education, and change in institutional policy, it is suggested that legislation related to federal, state, and local tax incentives might be provided for institutions that successfully implement breastfeeding programs at work or at school. It also recommended the development of appropriate support services in the world of work such as prenatal care, social and nutritional services, paid maternity leave, child care, and alternate types of work arrangements such as flextime and job sharing.

The Workshop report also states that successful initiation and continuation of breastfeeding will require a broad spectrum of support services involving families, peers, care providers, employers, and community agencies and organizations.

Maternal benefits and breastfeeding

In 1919 the International Labor Organization established the Maternity Protection Convention for working women.[36] This document provided for two half-hour nursing breaks per day. It also recommended that employers provide creches or day care when more than a given number of women are employed, but few countries hold to its tenets today. Maternity benefits vary from country to country and may include maternity leave with or without pay, nursing breaks, provision of day-care facilities, and prohibition of dismissal. Physicians who care for mothers and infants should take a leadership role in ensuring that mothers can continue breastfeeding even when the mother is employed.

The physician can help support fathers and mothers alike who are faced with fulfilling the roles of parent, employee, and citizen in a rapidly changing society.

REFERENCES

1. Ainsworth MDS: The development of infant-mother attachment. In Caldwell BM and Ricciuti HN, editors: Review of child development research, Chicago, 1973, University of Chicago Press.
2. Ainsworth MDS, Blehar MC, Waters E et al: Patterns of attachment, Hillsdale NJ, 1978, Erlbaum.
3. American Academy of Pediatrics Committee on Psychosocial Aspects of Child and Family Health: The mother working outside the home, Pediatrics 73:874, 1984.
4. American College of Obstetricians and Gynecologists: Guidelines on pregnancy and work, Chicago, 1987, ACOG Publications.
5. Auerbach KG and Guss E: Maternal employment and breast feeding: a study of 567 women's experiences, Am J Dis Child 138:958, 1984.
6. Baden C: Work and family—an annotated bibliography 1978-1980, Boston, 1981, Wheelock College Center for Parenting Studies.
7. Brazelton TB: Toddlers and parents, New York, 1974, Delta Books.
8. Brazelton TB: Working and caring, Reading Mass, 1985, Addison-Wesley Publishing Co.
9. Bronfenbrenner U and Crouter AC: Work and family through time and space. In Kamerman SB and Hayes CD, editors: Families that work: children in a changing world, Washington DC, 1982, National Academy Press.
10. Chase-Lansdale PL and Owen MT: Maternal employment in a family context: effects on infant-mother and infant-father attachments, Child Dev 58:1505, 1987.
11. Easterbrooks MA and Goldberg WA: Effects of early maternal employment on toddlers, mothers, and fathers, Dev Psychol 21:774, 1985.
12. Eiger MS and Olds SW: The complete book of breastfeeding, ed 2, New York, 1987, Workman Publishing Company.
13. Eisenberg L: Caring for children and working dilemmas of contemporary womanhood, Pediatrics 56:24, 1975.
14. Frederick IB and Auerbach KG: Maternal-infant separation and breastfeeding: the return to work or school, J Reprod Med 30:323, 1985.
15. Freud A and Dann S: An experiment in group upbringing, Psychoanal Study Child 6:127, 1961.

16. Ginsberg E: The changing pattern of women's work, Am J Orthopsychiatr 28:313, 1969.
17. Grams M: Breastfeeding success for working mothers, Carson City Nev, 1985, National Capitol Resources, Inc.
18. Haskins R and Kotch J: Day care and illness: evidence, costs, and public policy, Pediatrics 77(suppl):951, 1986.
19. Heins M et al: Attitudes of pediatricians toward maternal employment, Pediatrics 72:283, 1983.
20. Helsing E and King FS: Breast-feeding in practice: a manual for health workers, Oxford, 1982, Oxford University Press.
21. Hirschman C and Sweet JA: Social background and breastfeeding among American mothers, Soc Biol 21:39, 1974.
22. Hock E: Working and nonworking mothers and their infants: a comparative study of maternal caregiving characteristics and infant's social behavior, Merrill-Palmer Q 46:79, 1980.
23. Hoffman L: The professional woman as mother, Ann NY Acad Sci 208:209, 1973.
24. Hoffman LW: Effects of maternal employment on the child: a review of the research, Dev Psychol 10:204, 1974.
25. Hoffman LW: Increased fathering: effects on mother. In Lamb M and Sagi A, editors: Fatherhood and family policy, Hillsdale NJ, 1983, Erlbaum.
26. Howell MC: Employed mothers and their families, Pediatrics 52:252, 1973.
27. Hurst M and Zambrana RE: Determinants and consequences of maternal employment, Washington DC, 1981, Business and Professional Women's Foundation.
28. Katcher AL and Lanese MG: Breastfeeding by employed mothers: a reasonable accommodation in the work place, Pediatrics 75:644, 1985.
29. La Leche League: The womanly art of breastfeeding, ed 4, Franklin Park Ill, 1988, La Leche League.
30. Lawrence RA: Early mothering by adolescents. In McAnarney ER, editor: Premature adolescent pregnancy and parenthood, New York, 1983, Grune & Stratton.
31. Martinez GA and Dodd DA: 1981 milkfeeding patterns in the United States during the first 12 months of life, Pediatrics 71:166, 1983.
32. Martinez GA and Stahle DA: The recent trend in milk feeding among WIC infants, Am J Pub Health 72:68, 1982.
33. Mead M: A cultural anthropologist's approach to maternal deprivation. Public Health Papers no 14, Deprivation of maternal care, Geneva, 1962, World Health Organization.
34. Popkin BM: Time allocation of the mother and child nutrition, Ecol Food Nutr 9:1, 1980.
35. Report of the Surgeon General's Workshop on Breastfeeding and Human Lactation: Lawrence RA, chairman, DHHS Pub no HRS-D-MC 84-2.
36. Richardson JL: Review of the international legislation establishing nursing breaks, J Trop Pediatr 21:249, 1975.
37. Ryan AS and Martinez GA: Breastfeeding and the working mother: a profile, Pediatrics 83:524, 1989.
38. Sanday P: Female status in the public domain. In Rosaldo M and Lamphere L, editors: Woman, culture and society, Stanford, 1974, Stanford University Press.
39. Spock B: Baby and child care, New York, 1977, Pocket Books.
40. U.S. Department of Labor: Manpower report of the president, Washington DC, 1974, US Government Printing Office.
41. U.S. Department of Labor, Office of the Secretary: Facts on women workers, Washington DC, 1980, Women's Bureau.
42. Van Esterik P and Greiner T: Breastfeeding and women's work: constraints and opportunities, Stud Fam Plan 12:184, 1981.
43. Vaugh BE, Gove FL, and Egeland B: The relationship between out-of-home care and the quality of infant-mother attachment in an economically disadvantaged population, Child Dev 51:1203, 1980.
44. West CP: Factors influencing the duration of breast feeding, J Biosoc Sci 12:325, 1980.
45. Winikoff B and Baer E: The obstetrician's opportunity: translating "breast is best" from theory to practice, Am J Obstet Gynecol 138:105, 1980.
46. Zambrana RE, Hurst M, and Hite RL: The working mother in contemporary perspective: a review of the literature, Pediatrics 64:862, 1979.

Breastfeeding the infant with a problem

14

A normal full-term infant can usually be breastfed with only minor adjustment, even without the support of medical expertise. The infant with a medical or surgical problem presents special concerns that cannot be conquered simply by a strong-willed mother who is determined to overcome all obstacles to breastfeed. An understanding of the medical problem of the infant, his special nutritional needs, and the mechanical obstacles to feeding and nutritional absorption will be necessary before a rational judgment can be made about breastfeeding. When the infant cannot nurse directly at the breast, would providing mother's milk be appropriate? What is the overall prognosis for ever feeding at the breast or, perhaps, for survival itself? Parents are so awed by the medical staff of special and intensive care nurseries that they are often afraid to bring up the subject of breastfeeding. In addition, the nursery staff may be so busy balancing electrolytes and adjusting ventilators and monitors that they have not thought to ask what plans the mother might have had for feeding before the infant developed a problem. There are absolute contraindications to breastfeeding infants with certain problems. These problems are few and rare. In this chapter, each medical problem will be dealt with separately. General information on establishing a milk supply without the stimulus of the infant's suckling is provided in Chapter 17.

LOW BIRTHWEIGHT INFANTS

Infants who are born weighing less than average, or less than 2500 g, will be referred to as low birthweight (LBW) infants. If the infants are less than 37 weeks of gestation, they are premature; if they are full term and low birth weight, they are small for gestational age (SGA).

Very low birthweight (VLBW) is an infant weighing less than 1500 g. The probability of survival has changed dramatically in all weight ranges. With the availability of surfactant for respiratory distress, infants between 500 and 1000 g are surviving in great numbers, too. The problems of nutrition, however, pose new challenges to the neonatologist. The feedings appropriate for a 2000 g premature vary only in volume and frequency from the full-term infant in most cases. Feedings for a VLBW infant must address the advantages and disadvantages of human milk at this point in the growth curve (see boxed material on p. 320).

Milk of mothers who deliver preterm

Level increased in preterm	*Level unchanged in preterm*
Total nitrogen	Volume
Protein nitrogen	Calories
Long-chain fatty acids	Lactose (? less)
Medium-chain fatty acids	Fat (?) by creamatocrit
Short-chain fatty acids	Linolenic acid
Sodium	Potassium
Chloride	Calcium
Magnesium (?)	Phosphorus
Iron	Copper
	Zinc
	Ozmolality
	Vitamin $B^{(1-12)}$

The advantages of human milk for the LBW infant include the physiologic amino acid and fat profile, the digestibility and absorption of these proteins and fats, and the low renal solute load.[148] The presence of active enzymes enhances the maturation and supplements the enzyme activity of this underdeveloped gut. The anti-infective properties and living cells protect the immature infant from infection and may even protect against necrotizing enterocolitis (NEC). The physiologic benefit to the mother who can participate in her infant's care by providing her milk is a less tangible but no less important advantage.

The disadvantages are the gap in certain nutrients required for adequate growth, which include the volume of total protein and macro minerals, especially calcium and phosphorus.[54,55,67] Much of the attention to the shortcomings has been based on work done using pooled milk samples collected from women whose infants are full term and many months old. The source of the human milk and processing—freezing or pasteurizing—are all significant to the question of nutritional adequacies. In the last decade many scientists and clinicians have studied the questions posed here and provided hundreds of reports regarding the nutrition and nurturance of the LBW and VLBW infant. Only a fraction of the resources can be referenced here.[73,76,140-142] The reader is especially directed to the overview and extensive bibliography prepared by Steichen, Krug-Wispe and Tsang.[148]

Optimal growth for the premature infant

Optimal growth for an infant born prematurely is considered to be the growth curve he would have followed had he remained in utero[57] (Fig. 14-1 and Tables 14-1 and 14-2). Achieving this goal utilizing the immature intestinal tract poses the added requirement that the nutrients are digestible and absorbable and will not impose a significant metabolic stress on the other immature organs, especially the kidney. Although human milk provides the ideal nutrients, it would require an inordinate unphysiologic volume to achieve adequate amounts of some without calculated supplementation. To fill these growth needs, one can just use an artificial or chemical formula or use human milk as a base with all its advantages and add the deficit nutrients to it.

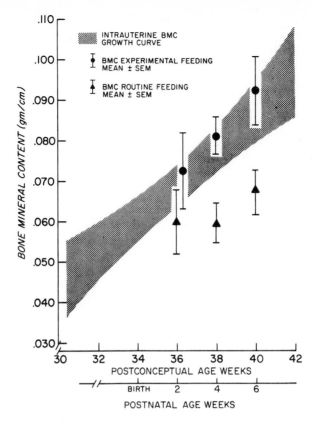

Fig. 14-1. Postnatal bone mineral content (MBC) in 33 to 35 weeks appropriate for gestational age preterm infants compared to the intrauterine bone mineralization curve (IUBMC). The regression curve and the 95th percentile confidence limits for the regression for BMC of infants born at different gestational ages (30-42 weeks' gestational age) represents the IUBMC. Infants fed routine cow's milk formula (closed triangles) had significantly lower BMC than infants fed standard formula supplemented with calcium and phosphorus (closed circles). In these infants BMC was not different from IUBMC at 4 and 6 weeks' postnatal age. (From Steichen JJ, Gratton TL, and Tsang RC: J Pediatr 96:528–534, 1980. With permission.)

Special properties of preterm milk

The identification of special quantitative differences in nutrients in the milk of mothers who delivered prematurely brought new interest in the use of human milk for prematures (see boxed material). Many investigators have contributed to the pool of knowledge after the initial revelations by Atkinson et al. in 1978, who reported the nitrogen concentrations of milk from mothers of premature infants to be greater than that of milk from mothers delivering at term.[15,16] Preterm milk is higher in protein content during the first months of lactation, containing between 1.8 and 2.44 g/dl. Preterm milk contains similar fat in quality and quantity, although Anderson et al.[9] reported increased values for preterm milk over term milk. Lactose in preterm milk averages 5.96 g/dl to 6.95 at 28 days, whereas term milk is 6.16 and 7.26, respectively. Preterm milk has higher energy than term milk, 58 to 70 kcal/dl, compared to 48 to 64 over the first month postpartum. The macro nutrients,

Table 14-1. Estimated requirements and advisable intakes for protein by infant's weight as derived by factorial approach

Ranges	Tissue increment (per day)	Dermal loss (per day)	Urine loss (per day)	Intestinal absorption (% intake)	Estimated requirement (per day)	Advisable intake Per day	Advisable intake Per kg*	Advisable intake Per 100 kcal[†]
800 g to 1200 g birth weight	2.32 g	0.17 g	0.68 g	87 g[†]	3.64 g	4.0 g	4.0 g	3.1 g
1200 g to 1800 g birth weight	3.01 g	0.25 g	0.90 g	87 g	4.78 g	5.2 g	3.5 g	2.7 g

From Ziegler EE, Biga RL, and Fomon SJ: Nutritional requirements of the premature infant. In Suskind RM, Textbook of pediatric nutrition, New York, 1981, Raven Press.
*Assuming body weight of 1000 g and 1500 g, respectively for 800 g to 1200 g infant and 1200 g to 1800 g infant, respectively.
[†]Assuming caloric intake of 120 kcal/day.

Table 14-2. Accumulation of various components during the last trimester of pregnancy

Component	Accumulation during various stages of gestation				
	26-31 wk	31-33 wk	33-35 wk	35-38 wk	38-40 wk
Body weight (g)*	500	500	500	500	
Water (g)	410	350	320	240	220
Fat (g)	25	65	85	175	200
Nitrogen (g)	11	12	12	6	7
Calcium (g)	4	5	5	5	5
Phosphorus (g)	2.2	2.6	2.8	3.0	3.0
Magnesium (mg)	130	110	120	120	80
Sodium (mEq)	35	25	40	40	40
Potassium (mEq)	19	24	26	20	20
Chloride (mEq)	30	24	10	20	10
Iron (mg)	36	60	60	40	20
Copper (mg)	2.1	2.4	2.0	2.0	2.0
Zinc (mg)	9.0	10.0	8.0	7.0	3.0

Modified from data of Widdowson, reproduced with permission from Heird WC and Anderson TL: Nutritional requirements and methods of feeding low birth weight infants. In Gluck L et al, editors: Current problems in pediatrics, vol 7, no 8, Chicago, 1977, Year Book Medical Publishers, Inc., Copyright © 1977.
*Body weight of the 26-week fetus is 1000 g; that of the 40-week fetus, 3000 g.

calcium and phosphorus, are slightly higher in preterm milk (14 to 16 mEq/L vs 13 to 16 calcium) and 4.7 to 5.5 mM/L vs 4.0 to 5.1 mM/L phosphorus). Neither term nor preterm milk has adequate calcium and phosphorus for the VLBW. Magnesium levels in preterm milk are 28 to 31 mg/L, dropping to 25 at 28 days, and term are 25 to 29 mg/L to 25. Zinc levels are higher in preterm milk, beginning at 5.3 mg/L and dropping to 3.9, whereas term milk begins at 5.4 and drops to 2.6 mg/L. Sodium levels in preterm milk are higher (26.6 mEq/L to 12.6 mEq/L) whereas term milk is 22.3 mEq/L to 8.5 mEq/L at 28 days.[142] Chloride has a similar average (preterm 31.6 to 16.8 mEq/L and term 26.9 to 13.1 mEq/L).

Requirements for growth in the premature infant

The whey protein in human milk is an advantage for all infants but especially the premature. It includes the nine amino acids known to be essential to all humans and taurine, glycine, leucine, and cystine, which are considered essential for the premature.[140] The premature lacks all the necessary enzymes for metabolism and has been noted to accumulate unphysiologic levels of methionine, tyrosine, phenylalanine, blood urea, and ammonia.[74] The protein requirement for the LBW infant based on intrauterine accretion rates is 2.5 g/100 kcal according to Fomon[54] or 325 mg/kg/day. Metabolizable energy requirement is 109 kcal/kg/day. The requirement for fat is based on the essential fatty acid proportion as 3% of total caloric intake. Human milk has high levels of linoleic acid (9% of lipids) and adequately meets this requirement. Human milk fat is more readily absorbed in the presence of milk lipase and other enzymes in milk. It is reported that infants under 1500 g absorb 90% of human milk fat and 68% of cow-milk-base formula fats.

Fat digestion is very efficient in LBW infants who receive their own mother's milk fresh and untreated. Fat absorption is decreased by calcium supplementation, however, and by sterilizing the milk.[34] If human milk is supplemented with lipids changing the vitamin E to polyunsaturated fatty acids (PUFA) ratio, vitamin E may need to be added to keep the ratio E:PUFA > 0.6 (human milk E:PUFA is 0.9).[82]

Preterm and term milk do not contain sufficient calcium and phosphorus for bone accretion and rickets has developed in LBW infants who are not supplemented. It is because the requirement for bone growth at this point in the growth curve is high. Calcium and phosphorus fetal accretion increases steadily over the last trimester. Magnesium accretion is unchanged in that time period.[73]

Mineral accretion is a complex phenomenon dependent on a number of variables beyond simple levels of calcium, phosphorus, magnesium, and vitamin D.[2] Absorption and retention are altered by the quantities of other minerals as well as other nutrients, including fat, protein, and carbohydrate. Although the CA:Phos ratio in human milk is more physiologic than cow's milk, the low levels of phosphorus lead to loss of calcium in the urine.

Even with optimal vitamin D and magnesium, the amount of calcium absorbed from preterm milk is not enough to meet intrauterine accretion rates without supplementation.[148] Because human milk phosphorus levels are low even in the face of high intestinal absorption and high renal tubular reabsorption compared to the needs of the premature infant, supplementation is necessary to avoid depletion or deficiency.

Vitamin D requirements in this period of high skeletal development depend on maternal vitamin D status, as there is significant correlation between maternal serum and preterm infant cord serum 25-OH D values. LBW infants quickly become dependent on exogenous vitamin D, as fetal storage is minimal. The recommended daily allowance (RDA) of 400 units of vitamin D appears to be appropriate for all LBW infants, regardless of feedings, as well as for term infants. Although there are unresolved questions regarding its absorption and excretion, there is a toxic level of vitamin D, so more may not be better.

Other vitamin needs of LBW infants depend on body stores, intestinal absorption, bioavailability of the vitamin, and rates of utilization and excretion, too. There is little information to suggest that there are major differences in absorption between term and LBW infants, although fat-soluble vitamins depend on bile acids for absorption. Details of vitamin requirements appear in Chapter 9 (Diet and Dietary Supplements). It is recommended that LBW infants receive daily vitamin supplements to especially address the increased need and borderline levels provided in the volume of human milk they can reasonably consume. The necessary supplements are shown below.

Vitamin supplements for LBW infants fed human milk*			
Vitamin B$_{12}$	(only if mother's diet deficient)	Vitamin D	400 IU/d
Folic acid	(HM usually adequate)	Vitamin K	(All infants should receive 0.5
Thiamin B$_1$	Borderline		to 1.0 mg at birth)
Riboflavin B$_2$	Borderline		Recommend 5 µg/kg/d—
B$_6$	(HM usually adequate)		human milk borderline
Niacin	(HM usually adequate)	Vitamin E	25 IU/d for the first month
Vitamin A	1000 to 1500 IU/d		5 IU/d after the first month
Vitamine C	If infant receives supplementary protein up to 60 mg/d		

*Derived from multiple sources.

Table 14-3. Required calcium, phosphorus, and magnesium intake (mg/kg/day) to meet fetal accretion rate of 27 and 30 weeks*

	27 weeks			30 weeks		
	Ca	P	Mg	Ca	P	Mg
Accretion (mg/kg/day)	121	72	3.37	123	72	3.17
Retention (% intake)	50	89	59	50	89	59
Intake (mg/kg/day)	242	81	5.70	246	81	5.37

From Steichen JJ, Krug-Wispe S, and Tsang RC: Clin Perinatol 14:131, 1987.
Assuming a weight of 1000 g and 1250 g, respectively, in an infant fed human milk.

The mineral supplementation required for LBW infants fed human milk is based on intrauterine accretion rates, which may not actually be achieved. The values are provided in Table 14-3. Not all premature infants fed human milk develop rickets. In fact, it is uncommon above 1500 g. The VLBW infant does need supplementation, and cases of rickets are well documented in the literature for this group.[142] Supplements are usually not necessary when the infant reaches 40 weeks post conceptual age. Hypophosphatemia is a sensitive biochemical indicator of low bone mineralization in VLBW infants fed human milk. Weekly measurements of serum phosphorus for the first month and biweekly until 2000 g or 40 weeks' gestation are recommended by Steichen et al.[148] A level below 4 mg/dl should be followed by x-ray of the wrists for osteopenia and rickets. Supplementation should be based on the infant's needs. Calcium levels should also be obtained weekly, as levels above 11 mg/dl should be evaluated for too much calcium or too little phosphorus.[142] Supplements of calcium and phosphorus are incorporated in available human milk supplements and are presented in Tables 14-4 to 14-6.

Trace minerals in general appear in physiologic amounts in human milk and are more bioavailable from human milk than other formulae. The minimum daily requirements for LBW infants are based on daily accretion rates as calculated from third-trimester data and calculated obligatory losses. Zinc is known to be readily available in human milk, although zinc deficiency syndromes from hyperalimentation are well known in the literature and in neonatal intensive care units (NICUs).

Zinc requirements are probably met by mother's own milk, but pooled milk will be lower, as zinc levels drop from term birth levels to 6 months, and this milk will need supplmentation. Copper accretion requires 59 μg/kg/day, and absorption is thought to be 50% to 70%. Copper levels also decline in milk from term to 6 months postpartum. It is recommended that VLBW infants require additional 30 to 40 μg/d of copper for the first 3 months. Manganese represents an apparent deficiency, as the minimum daily requirement is calculated to be 7 μg/kg/day; the provision in human milk is 0.35 ng/ml or 0.5 μg/k/day, but no information is available recommending supplementation. The selenium suggested requirement is 1.5 to 2.5 μg/kg/day (1 μg minimum), and human milk provides 1 to 2 μg/dl and is stable throughout lactation so that no supplementation has been recommended.

Iodine levels in human milk are sufficient to meet daily requirements in the LBW infant. Chromium requirements are calculated to 1.0 to 2.0 μg/kg/day based on an ac-

Table 14-4. Composition of infant feeding using human milk with and without various supplements

	Preterm human milk*		Similac natural care*	50:50 Mix Similac natural care and preterm human milk*		Enfamil human milk fortifier (4 Pkts)	4 Pkts Enfamil human milk fortifier added to preterm human milk*	
Weeks postpartum	1	4		1	4		1	4
Kilocaries	67	70	81	72	76	14	81	84
Protein (g)	2.44	1.81	2.1	2.27	1.96	0.7	3.14	2.5
Carbohydrate (g)	6.05	6.95	8.6	7.3	7.8	2.7	8.75	9.65
Fat (g)	3.81	4.00	3.6	3.7	3.8	0.04	3.85	4.04
Vitamin A, IU†	330	230	550	440	390	780	1110	1010
Vitamin E (mg)†	0.9	0.25	3	2.0	1.61	3.4	4.3	3.65
Vitamin K (g)†	NA	1.5	10	NA	5.8	9.1	NA	10.6
Vitamin D (IU)†	NA	2.5	120	NA	61	260	NA	262
Thiamin (g)	5.4	8.9	200	103	104	187	192	196
Riboflavin (g)	36.0	26.6	500	268	263	250	286	277
Niacin (mg)	0.11	0.21	4.0	2.1	2.1	3.1	3.2	3.3
Pyridoxine (g)	2.6	6.2	200	101	103	193	196	199
Folate (g)	2.1	3.1	30	16.1	16.6	23	25	26
Vitamin B$_{12}$ (g)	0.1	0.1	0.45		0.27	0.21		0.3
Vitamin C (mg)†	7	5	30	19	18	24	31	29
Calcium (mg)	25	22	170	98	96	60	85	82
Phosphorus (mg)	14	14	85	50	50	33	47	47
Magnesium (mg)	3	2.5	10	6.5	6.3	4	7	6.5
Iron (mg)	0.1	0.1	0.3	0.2	0.2	0	0.1	0.1
Sodium (mEq)	2.2	1.3	1.7	2.0	1.5	0.3	2.5	1.6
Potassium (mEq)	1.8	1.7	2.9	2.4	2.3	0.4	2.2	2.1
Chloride (mEq)	2.5	1.6	2.0	2.3	1.8	0.5	3.0	2.1
Zinc (mg)	0.48	0.39	1.2	0.84	0.80	0.31	0.79	0.70
Copper (mg)	0.08	0.06	0.2	0.14	0.13	0.08	0.16	0.14
Manganese (g)†	NA	0.4	NA	NA	NA	9	NA	9.4
Biotin (g)	0.15	0.54	NA	NA	NA	0.8	0.95	1.34
Pantothenic acid (mg)	0.16	0.23	1.5	0.83	0.87	0.79	0.95	1.02
Osmolality†	302	305	300	301	303	+60	362	365

*Volume 100 ml.

†Listed values for 1 and 4 weeks reflect reported values for full-term transitional and mature human milk, respectively.

Table 14-5. Protein, calcium, and sodium requirements by growing premature infants and composiiton of banked human milk

	Protein (g/100 kcal)	Calcium (mg/100 kcal)	Sodium (mEq/100 kcal)
Estimated requirements for hypothetical growing premature infants*	2.54	132†	2.3
Composition of banked human milk	1.50	43	0.8

From Fomon SJ, Ziegler EE and Vazquez HD: Am J Dis Child 131:463. 1977. Copyright 1977, American Medical Association.
*Assumed body weight is 1200 g; weight gain, 20 g/day, energy intake, 120 kcal/kg/day. The basis for estimating requirements is described in the text.
†This estimate does not apply to infants fed formulas from which calcium absorption is less than 65% of intake.

Table 14-6. Weight gain supported by intake of 180 ml human milk/kg at selected body weights

	Weight gain (gm/day)			
	800g	1000 g	1500 g	2000 g
Ca	4	5	6.7	8.4
P	4	5	6.8	8.7
N	10	12	16	21
Na	5	7	11	15
Mg	12	15	22	28
Cl	22	30	48	68
K	21	33	49	66

Based on data compiled by Forbes GB: Nutritional adequacy of human breast milk for premature infants. In Lebenthal E, editor: Textbook of gastroenterology and nutrition, New York, 1981, Raven Press.

cretion rate of 0.1 to 0.2 μg/kg/day and only 10% absorption. Levels in human milk are reported to be 0.03 μg/dl, which with 150 ml/kg/day intake would supply 0.045 μg/kg/day. Supplementation is not usually provided, and absorption in human milk is probably greater than 10%. Molybdenum levels in human milk are believed sufficient to meet LBW accretion rates (1 μg/kg/day).[148]

Iron requirements are a complex issue, and intrauterine accretion rates are not appropriate values on which to base requirements.[88,127] Iron stores partially enlarged by hemoglobin breakdown in early life will eventually be used up if no iron is provided. Providing iron, however, interferes with the immunologic properties of human milk, especially the bacteriostatic properties of lactoferrin in the gut.

The recommendations for iron supplementation for infants receiving human milk (either own mother's or donor milk, which are similar in iron) are based on age and weight of the infant. Supplementation should begin at 2 to 3 months or when birth weight has doubled. For birth weight under 1000 g, the infant should receive 4 mg elemental iron/kg/day; 1000 to 1500 g should receive 3 mg/kg/day.[88,127] It is necessary to also assure adequate vitamin C and vitamin E supplementation (4 to 5 mg/day).

Use of human milk for premature infants

A clear distinction must be made between an infant's own mother's milk and pooled human milk for the feeding of LBW infants. An infant's own mother's milk has some higher level of nutrients but never lower levels than term milk. Mothers who donate to milk banks are also feeding their own infants, who may be any age from birth to 6 months (but no donor should be more than 6 months postpartum). Donor milk must also be prepared by sterilization, and in only a few milk banks is fresh or fresh frozen donor milk available. An infant's own mother's milk may be fed fresh or fresh frozen and is rarely heat treated. Chapter 19 discusses milk storage and milk banking.

When the volume of milk produced by the mother is not sufficient to meet the infant's needs each day, there is a clear need to provide additional nourishment by formula or donor milk.

A 2001 to 2500 g infant without complications may be weaned from the incubator to an open crib within 24 hours. Although his suck reflex may be poor, he can usually be nipple fed. If he is vigorous enough, he can be nursed at the breast. If he can stimulate the breast briefly and obtain the rich, antibody-containing, cell-filled colostrum, it will protect against infection while providing nutrition. If the infant cannot suck and must be tube fed, any colostrum the mother can manually express or pump from the breast can be given by gavage tube along with donor milk or the prescribed formula necessary for nourishment. The value of colostrum to the infant has been thoroughly reviewed in Chapter 5. A study in Guatemala that was repeated in the special care nursery of the Rainbow Children's Hospital in Cleveland showed that the infection rate among sick and premature newborns was greatly diminished by providing 15 ml of human colostrum contributed by random donors daily.[94] These findings were especially dramatic in Guatemala, where the mortality from infection in the nursery is extremely high. It has been suggested that mixed feedings of an infant's own mother's milk and formula to necessary volume be calculated over a 24-hour period so that the infant receives some mother's milk at each feeding and a supplement of formula, in contrast to alternating feedings or using all mother's milk until it runs out and finishing the day with formula. The reasoning is based on the concept of "inoculating" every feeding with human milk to provide the enzymes and immunologic properties with each feeding. Generous levels of active enzymes in the milk will also assist in the digestion and absorption of the formula. The immunologic properties are less measurable, but the only known interference with function is the addition of iron, which blocks the effectiveness of lactoferrin. Therefore the nutritional and infection-protection properties are also spread throughout each feeding around the clock.

Supplementation of mother's own milk or pooled milk

Although some banks can provide single-donor milk for a specific baby and resources are usually more than enough for the newly born recipient, no supplement is needed if the infant is over 1500 g.

The options for supplementing an infant's own mother's milk depend on need for additional volume or for specific nutrients, especially protein, calcium, and phosphorus, based on birth weight and growth rates.

The ideal supplementation is one using human milk nutrients and is referred to as lacto-engineering, where increasing nutrient concentration is done by adding specific nutrients derived from human milk.[67] Techniques involve separating the cream and protein fractions, reducing the lactose content, and heat treating the product by high-temperature short-time (HTST) process of pasteurization. This completely human milk product provides higher protein and energy needs so that weight gains and nitrogen retention are similar to intrauterine rates. Using a feeding prepared from human milk protein and medium-chain triglyceride supplementation of human milk for VLBW infants was reported by Rönnholm et al.[133] Forty-four infants averaging 30 weeks' gestation with birth weights ranging from 710 to 1510 g were nourished by one of four protocols: plain human milk, human milk and protein, human milk and triglycerides, or human milk and protein and triglycerides. The triglycerides did not influence weight and length, but the two groups receiving added protein gained along a curve comparable to the intrauterine growth for their birth weight, gaining faster from 4 to 6 weeks than the unsupplemented. The protein-supplemented groups also grew in length; however, head circumference growth was similar in all groups.

Fortified mother's milk containing an infant's own mother's milk plus skim and cream components derived from mature donor milk was fed *fresh* during the first two postnatal months to 18 VLBW infants (birth weight of 1180 ± 35 g, gestation of 29 ± 0.2 weeks).[34] A comparison group of 16 VLBW infants (birth weight of 1195 g ± 30 g, gestation of 29 ± 0.1 weeks) were fed commercial formula with comparable nitrogen and energy distribution. Balance studies were performed on both groups. Growth measurements were similar in the two groups. Metabolizable energy was 109 kcal/kg/day in both groups, as was fat absorption. The only recorded difference was a high serum calcium but lower serum phosphorus in the mother's milk group.

Schanler and Garza[140] compared plasma amino acid levels in VLBW infants (mean age 16 days, mean birth weight 1180 g, mean gestation 29 weeks) fed either human milk fortified with human milk or whey dominant cow milk–based formula. They received continuous enteral infusions of isonitrogenous, isocaloric preparations. Taurine and cystine were significantly higher in the human milk–fed infants, and threonine, valine, methionine, and lysine were significantly higher in formula-fed infants.

The authors[140] suggest that synthesis of specific functional proteins in the cow protein–based formulae fed to VLBW infants requires further review. Human milk supplements for human milk are not commercially available although ideal from most aspects.[140-142]

Supplementing an infant's own mother's milk with specially prepared formula supplements is an alternative that still provides the riches of human milk. There are available commercial preparations for such supplementation that are intended to complement human milk and not be used an an exclusive formula. They are different and are used differently. They are outlined in Table 14-3. The powdered supplement is intended to add special nutrients to an adequate volume of mother's own milk (Enfamil human milk fortifier), or it can be used to enhance pooled donor human milk. The osmolarity is increased to 60 mOsm/kg H_2O. The liquid supplement (Similac natural care) is intended to provide 50% of the volume of the daily feeding for an infant whose mother's own milk supply has diminished below daily needs. This extends the mother's milk and provides the additional nitrogen, calcium, phosphorus, and vitamins for an LBW infant. If an infant is fed his own mother's milk, pooled donor milk, and a fortifier, the sum total should meet the infant's daily requirements as outlined in Table 14-4.

Studies comparing fortified mother's milk with premature formulas have shown comparable growth in weight, length, and head circumference, making it possible to retain the many advantages of mother's milk while providing the additional nutrients for appropriate accretion rates.[149]

LBW infants averaging 31 weeks' gestation and weighing 1600 g were fed human milk plus banked drip milk to volume or special premature formula by enteral feeds at first and then breast or bottle. The investigators found no differences in the two groups in routine hematologic or biochemical variables or in plasma insulin, blood glucose, lactate, pyruvate, or ketone levels. Plasma amino acids showed higher methionine and threonine levels in the formula group. There was a postnatal surge by day 6 in plasma motilin, neurotensin, enteroglucagon, cholecystokinin, and gastric-inhibiting polypeptide levels. The total nutritional value of the human milk in this study must be questioned, since mother's milk was augmented with bank milk collected by drip method, which is known to be low in protein and fat compared to pumped or suckled milk.

When a preterm infant's own mother's milk was fortified with protein (0.85 g/dl), calcium (90 mg/dl), and phosphorus (45 mg/dl), the rate of weight gain was greater than the unfortified group and comparable to the Similac special care formula group.[71-73] Bone mineralization improved over the 6 weeks of the study but did not reach the intrauterine accretion rate of 150 mg/kg/day. The relative phosphorus deficiency occurred in the human milk groups both with and without supplementation. Greer et al.[71] conclude that fortifying preterm mother's milk permits biochemically adequate growth comparable to that provided by special care formula. Similar results using fortified human milk have been obtained by other investigators.

The effect of calcium supplementation on fatty acid balance studies in LBW infants fed human milk or formula has been shown to be significant by Chappell et al.[34] They showed a decrease in total fatty acid absorption both in LBW infants fed their own mother's milk or the formula-fed (SMA 20) infants when calcium was added. Fecal output of fat and fatty acid excretion were higher in the formula-fed infants. Mother's milk–fed infants' total fat absorption and coefficient of absorption were higher.

Vitamin E

Preterm milk with routine multivitamin supplementation (providing 4.1 mg of to-copherol) uniformly resulted in vitamin sufficiency in VLBW infants when they received iron as well as when they were not iron supplemented in a control study by Gross and Gabriel.[77] VLBW infants were fed preterm milk, bank milk, or formula, utilizing 2 mg/day of iron. Vitamin E content of preterm milk does not differ significantly from that of term human milk from days 3 to 36.[82]

Growth parameters when breastfeeding VLBW infants following discharge. Weight gain, growth in length, and head circumference are similar posthospitalization growth parameters in VLBW infants breastfed or given standard formula. Bone mineral status, however, was followed at 10, 16, and 25 postnatal weeks in those NICU graduates who had formerly received fortified human milk. At 16 and 25 weeks, the breastfed infants had lower bone mineral content and bone mineral content/bone width ratio, and serum phosphorus concentration and higher alkaline phosphatase activity than the formula-fed group. These data suggest a need to monitor this select group of VLBW infants very carefully for suboptimal bone accretion while receiving their mother's milk.

Iron status has also been studied in LBW infants at 6 months chronological age. The incidence of iron deficiency was 86% in the breastfed group of LBW and only 33% in those receiving iron-fortified formula.[2] The breastfed group had significantly lower serum ferritin and hemoglobin values at 4 months of age. The authors recommend that these special breastfed infants should receive iron from 2 months of age, since they have a risk of developing iron deficiency not seen in term infants.

Late hypertriglyceridemia was detected in a group of VLBW infants fully breastfed at home following premature births (30 weeks) and mean birth weight of 1140 g.[72] Blood samples were collected at 31, 33, and 35 days post conceptual age and 6 weeks after hospital discharge. During hospitalization, triclycerides average 153 to 166 mg/dl. The mean fat content of the mother's milk was 3.2 to 3.4 g/dl, and the mean fat intake was 5.0 to 5.5 g/kg/day. At home they received ad lib feedings at the breast and the formula-fed infants received standard 20 cal/oz formula 3.6 g/dl fat. Six of the 13 LBW infants fed human milk had serum triglyceride concentrations >300 mg/dl, none of the formula-fed infants had levels >300, and only three were <200 mg/dl. Only two of 25 term breastfed infants had levels >300. Three LBW infants had levels over 700 mg/dl and demonstrated hyperchlomicronemia. The meaning of these findings is unclear but deserves watching.[72] The role of lipase and postheparin plasma lipolytic activity is undetermined. The recommendations in the boxed material have been modified from the work of Streichen, Krug-Wispe, and Tsang.

Antimicrobial properties of preterm breast milk

The infection-protective properties of human milk have been considered a key reason to provide human milk for high-risk infants who are prone to devastating infections including necrotizing enterocolitis, sepsis, meningitis, and viral infections such as a respiratory syncytial virus (RSV) and rotavirus. The antimicrobial properties of milk produced by mothers who deliver preterm have been studied by several investigators.

The cells of preterm milk were compared to those of term milk and found to be similar in number and in capacity to phagocytose and kill staphylococci.[121] The ability of the preterm cells to produce interferon on stimulation with mitogens was marginally better than that of term cells. The cells survived 24 hours refrigerated at 4° C; at 48 hours there was a reduction in number but not function. Passing the milk through a feeding tube did not diminish the number or function of the cells. The levels of lactoferrin and lysozyme

---

Feeding schedule for human milk in LBW infants

1. Use *refrigerated milk* from the preterm infant's mother when it is available and has been collected within 48 hours of feeding.
2. When fresh milk is not available, use *frozen human milk* from the infant's mother. This milk should be provided in the sequence that it was collected to provide the greatest nutritional benefit.
3. When the preterm infant is tolerating human milk at greater than 100 ml/kg/day, supplementation using a human milk *fortifier* is started.
4. If the mother's milk supply is inadequate to meet her infant's feeding needs, an *infant formula designed* for preterm feeding is used as described.
5. Fortification of human milk is recommended until the infant is taking all feedings from the breast directly or weighs 1800 g to 2000 g, depending on nursery policy on infant discharge weight. During the transition from feeding human milk by gavage or bottle and nipple to feeding at the breast, only those feedings given by gavage or bottle require fortification.
6. *Multivitamin* supplementation is started once feeding tolerance has been established. This supplementation varies depending on the composition of human milk fortifier.
7. *Iron supplementation* providing 2 mg/kg body weight/day is started by the time the infant has doubled birth weight.

were greater in preterm milk than in term milk from the second to the twelfth week postpartum.[68] Secretory IgA (sIgA) was the predominant form of IgA, and values increased from the sixth to the twelfth week in preterm milk. The increase in IgA was not dependent on method of collection, rate of flow, or time of day, but the concentration varied inversely with the milk volume; thus, total production of IgA in 24 hours is thought by some investigators to be comparable for the two groups.[33,75] When preterm (31 to 36 weeks' gestation) infants were fed human milk and compared to a matched group of premature infants fed infant formula, the serum levels of IgA at 9 to 13 weeks were higher in the formula-fed infants.[139] Those infants who received at least 60% of their own mother's milk had higher IgA levels at 3 weeks of age than those receiving less than 30% of the feedings from their mothers' milk. Serum IgG levels were higher in the breast milk group, and serum IgM levels were similar in the two feeding groups. Samples of precolostrum collected from undelivered mothers was assayed and found to contain equal or greater amounts of IgA, IgG, IgM, lactoferrin, and lysoxyme than mature colostrum.[104]

When the impact on actual prevention of infection among premature infants is reviewed, significantly less infection is found in infants receiving human milk as compared with those receiving formula (9 of 32 breast milk; 24 of 38 formula).[122] In a planned prospective evaluation of the anti-infective property of varying quantities of expressed human milk for high-risk LBW infants, infections were found to be significantly less in the groups that received human milk.[152]

The intestinal flora in the second week of life in hospitalized preterm infants who had been treated previously with antibiotics and were fed stored frozen human milk was compared to the flora of those fed formula.[123] The flora were very different from term infants, and both groups contained enterobacteriaceae predominantly. Human milk did not alter the flora in these antibiotic-treated infants. Studies have shown that the acidic pH in the stomach of the human milk–fed LBW infants protects against the bacteria in the unpasteurized milk.[161] Although cultures of the milk (feeding sample) had grown both pathogens and nonpathogens, the two-hour postfeeding cultures of the gastric contents had no growth and a pH of <3.5.

In South Africa, where mothers remain with and help care for their premature babies, a study compared feeding an infant its own mother's milk with pooled pasteurized breast milk. Birth weights were between 1000 and 1500 g. Nonventilator babies were begun on feedings by 96 hours of age. There was significantly greater weight gain using untreated mother's milk, regaining birth weight and reaching 1800 g sooner. The SGA and AGA infants both did better on own mother's milk. This decreased hospital stays and decreased hospital-acquired infection. The authors attribute the advantages to the fact it was fed fresh with early initiation of feeding at the breast compared to pasteurization of the bank milk.[149]

The Committee on Nutrition, American Academy of Pediatrics, has published the "Nutritional Needs of LBW Infants," in which they suggest that mother's own milk and new special formulas for those babies needing breast milk substitutes are promising alternatives.[37] *The Nutrition and Feeding of Preterm Infants* is published as a report of the Committee on Nutrition of the Preterm Infant of the European Society of Paediatric Gastroenterology and Nutrition.[38] The report enthusiastically supports mother's own milk as the preferred nourishment, recognizing the need to supplement certain nutrients for the VLBW infant. They recommend 180 to 200 ml/kg/day as soon as possible, adding sodium, phosphate, and, in some cases, protein and calcium. They recommend heat treatment for donor milk.[38]

Special characteristics of premature infants. The anatomic differentiation of the intestinal tract begins at 20 weeks' gestation, but the functional development is very limited prior to 26 weeks.[101] Different parts of the fetal gut develop at different times so that some nutrients are better tolerated than others (Tables 14-7 and 14-8). The present concentration of digestive enzymes determines the rate of digestion and absorption, along with the maturity of membrane carriers. The impact of human milk on gut maturation has been discussed in Chapter 3. The presence of active enzymes in the gut improves the digestion and absorption of human milk. The gastric emptying time in preterm infants when given human milk is biphasic, with an initial fast phase where 50% has left the stomach in the first 25 mintues.[32] After an hour 25 ml of human milk has left the stomach. The formula feeding, on the other hand, follows a linear pattern with half emptying in 51 minutes and a total of 19 ml in 1 hour.

Milk production by mothers of premature infants. The production of milk by a mother who is not actively nursing her infant, as is frequently the case in LBW infants

Table 14-7. Development of gastrointestinal tract in the human fetus: first appearance of developmental markers

Anatomic part	Developmental marker	Weeks of gestation
Esophagus	Superficial glands develop	20
	Squamous cells appear	28
Stomach	Gastric glands form	14
	Pylorus and fundus defined	14
Pancreas	Differentiation of endocrine and exocrine tissue	14
Liver	Lobules form	11
Small intestine	Crypt and villi develop	14
	Lymph nodes appear	14
Colon	Diameter increases	20
	Villi disappear	20
Functional ability		
Suckling	Mouthing only	28
Swallowing	Immature suck-swallow	33 to 36
Stomach	Gastric motility and secretion	20
Pancreas	Zymogen granules	20
Liver	Bile metabolism	11
	Bile secretion	22
Small intestine	Active transport of amino acids	14
	Glucose transport	18
	Fatty acid absorption	24
Enzymes	Alpha-glucosidases	10
	Dipeptidases	10
	Lactase	10
	Enterokinase	26

From Lebenthal E and Leung Y-K: Pediatr Ann 16:215, 1987.

Table 14-8. Digestion and absorption

Factors	First detectable (week gestation)	Term neonate (% of adult)
Protein		
H+	at birth	<30
Pepsin	16	<10
Trypsinogen	20	10-60
Chymotrypsinogen	20	10-60
Procarboxypeptidase	20	10-60
Enterokinase	26	10
Peptidases (brush border and cytosol)	<15	>100
Amino acid transport	?	>100
Macromolecular absorption	?	>100
Fat		
Lingual lipase	30	>100
Pancreatic lipase	20	5-10
Pancreatic colipase	?	?
Bile acids	22	50
Medium-chain triglyceride uptake	?	100
Long-chain triglyceride uptake	?	10-90
Carbohydrate		
Alpha-amylases		
pancreatic	22	0
salivary	16	10
Lactase	10	>100
Sucrase-isomaltase	10	100
Glucoamylase	10	50-100
Monosaccharide absorption	11-19	>100 (?)

From Lebenthal E and Leung Y-K: Pediatr Ann 16:215, 1987.

and other neonates in ICU, is a challenge indeed to the resources of the NICU and the postpartum staff. Insufficient milk production is a common problem that becomes more critical as time passes, as production continues to drop, and as the infant's needs increase. Evaluation of various protocols has been undertaken by investigators who looked at times of onset of pumping postpartum, frequency of pumping, and duration in total minutes per day and length of time when no pumping occurred.

Thirty-two healthy mothers, 19 of whom had no previous breastfeeding experience, were entered into a study protocol by Hopkinson et al.[87] Their infants were 28 to 30 weeks' gestation. All the mothers initiated pumping between day 2 and 6, and the day of initiation was correlated with the volume of milk at 2 weeks but not at 4 weeks with mothers who had nursed previously and initiated pumping sooner. Parity, gravidity, age, and prior nursing experience were not correlated with volumes at 2 weeks. Parity and prior nursing experience were associated with milk volume at 4 weeks, with multiparas producing 60% greater volumes. These investigators found no significant relationship between 24-hour milk volume and frequency, duration, or maximal night interval. The change in milk volume from 2 weeks to 4 weeks was correlated with frequency and duration of pumping but not to maximal night intervals. The range in number of pumpings per day was 4 to 9. The authors[87] concluded that optimal milk production occurs with at least five expressions per day and pumping durations that exceed 100 minutes/day.

The frequency of milk expression was evaluated by deCarvelho et al.[42] in a cross-over design study of 25 mothers who delivered between 28 and 37 weeks' gestation. Frequent expression of milk was significantly associated with greater milk production (342 ± 229 ml) than infrequent expression (221 ± 141 ml). They compared three or less pumpings a day to four or more times. The mean number was 2.4 vs 5.7, neither number being the frequency with which a mother would usually feed her infant in the first few weeks.

When the physiology of lactation is applied to the practical management of inducing a milk supply without benefit of the infant's participation, it is apparent that mimicking natural breastfeeding is most effective. Although some women succeed with manual expression, it is rare and a good pump should be recommended. None of the hand pumps can truly duplicate the milking action of the infant and are essentially vacuum extractors. They should only be used as a stopgap measure when the electric pump is unavailable. Electric pumps are discussed in Chapter 19. A pump that is provided for pumping both breasts simultaneously saves time but has also been shown to generate higher levels of prolactin and greater total milk volume compared to pumping each breast separately for the same length of time.[124] Pumping should be initiated as soon as the mother's condition permits, and offering this opportunity to the mother should be part of the supportive care offered by the postpartum staff. All the points of preparation for pumping should be included: comfortable position, tranquil atmosphere, preparation of the breast with gentle stroking and warmth, confidence, and reassurance. The obstetrician is in an important position to initiate the offer to pump, as he knows during the mother's prenatal care that she wants to breastfeed. She may not know it is appropriate to ask about it. Providing knowledgeable, accurate, consistent, and sensitive support should be the rule in every perinatal center, especially for mothers of high-risk infants who wish to breastfeed.[124,163] Providing an appropriate room for pumping after the mother has been discharged is critical to individual success and is an expression of commitment to breastfeeding. This room should be clean, bright, and cheery and accommodate more than one mother and companion at a time. It should have a sink for washing hands and storage for equipment and supplies. A nurse call button or other alarm system is also essential. Additional nice features are soft music, a telephone, and reading material. The hospital should have a supply of approved electric pumps and individual disposable attachment packets for each mother. There should be a place to store her properly labeled and dated milk in a freezer or refrigerator. Sterile storage containers should be readily available.

A mother should be encouraged to rent a pump for home use and around-the-clock pumping. These are available from medical supply stores, pharmacies, home care services, and hospitals. Insurance companies reimburse for the cost of rental when the milk is prescribed for a high-risk infant. The neonatologist can provide an appropriate letter of support. The hospital support staff that is coordinating the mother's care or the NICU staff should be sure that mother understands how to use the equipment effectively. Ideally, NICUs have at least one staff member experienced in lactation counseling who will coordinate this effort under the direction of the obstetrician, pediatrician, and neonatologist. Key strategies for successful pumping when the infant is unable to suckle the breast are outlined in the boxed material on p. 336.

Initiating milk supply without infant sucking

A. Begin as soon after delivery as condition permits.

B. Initiate use of electric pump while in hospital.

C. Begin slowly, increasing time over first week.

D. Pump on more regular basis as soon as engorgement is evident.

E. Pump at least five times in 24 hours.

F. Allow a rest period for uninterrupted sleep of at least 6 hours.

G. Pump a total of at least 100 minutes/day.

H. Use "double" pump to pump both breasts simultaneously; can cut total time proportionately.

I. Preparation of breast with warm soaks, gentle stroking, and light massage maximizes pumping.

Mothers of LBW infants who provide milk

Maternal choice to breastfeed or provide milk for a LBW infant is influenced by many factors beyond those which interplay in most feeding decisions of normal full-term infants. Lucas and colleagues[108] sought to answer two major questions in a study of 925 mother/infant pairs in five hospitals from 1982 to 1985: Do health care professionals in neonatal units exert a major influence on a mother's feeding preference and availability of her milk for her infant, and are there population differences between mothers who do and do not provide their milk?

Mothers had delivered at a mean of 31 weeks' gestation infants weighing less than 1850 g with a mean of 1370 g. More educated mothers provided their milk (98%) than uneducated (40%). Higher social economic class, lower parity, or fewer living children, being married, and being over 20 years of age were associated with providing milk. Boys were more apt to receive mother's milk, as shown in other studies. Birth weight and extreme immaturity were not a determinant, nor was transfer of infant to another center. In this study a cesarean section mother was more likely to breastfeed than one who had delivered vaginally.[163] In this study among five centers, the demographic characteristics of the mother were important, not the staff. This study did not look at success rates, however. Another study of breastfeeding LBW infants showed an inverse relationship with maturity and size; the smaller and less mature were not breastfed, nor were those with respiratory distress syndrome (RDS).

Feeding the premature infant at the breast

Large premature infants of 36 weeks of gestation or older may be nursed at the breast if otherwise stable. Particular care should be given to assist the mother in getting the infant to suckle, especially if the breast and/or nipples are large or engorged.[124] Weight should be followed closely to prevent excessive weight loss. In our experience, infants who receive sugar water and formula supplements lose more weight than those who are nursed frequently at the breast without supplementation. If breastfeeding is going well, the infant could be discharged with his mother from the hospital as soon as he begins to gain substantially.

Feeding at the breast when the infant is under 1500 g is considered too strenuous by many neonatologists. When the feeding of infants of less than 1500 g was examined, however, the growth of those fed at the breast was comparable to matched control infants fed expressed human milk by bottle. Breastfeeding was started when sucking movements were observed. Initially they all received supplementary human milk by tube plus 800 units of vitamin D and 60 mg vitamin C daily. Unrestricted visiting of parents to the neonatal unit, an optimistic and knowledgeable attitude of the nursing staff toward breast-feeding, and the avoidance of a bottle for the infants are important to success. They also encouraged the expression of milk by the mothers early in the postpartum period. The main deterrent to successful breastfeeding was lack of maternal interest and commitment.

When infants weighing less than 1500 g are fed by nasogastric tube, it has been shown that offering the infant a pacifier to suck while being tube fed improves gastric emptying and weight gain. Those mothers who wish to breastfeed can put the infant to breast at the time of the tube feeding to avoid introduction of a rubber nipple. If there is concern for swallowing and aspiration of fluid, the mother can pump her breasts first and milk can be given by tube. Infants in our unit have suckled at breast while being tube fed without complications.

Small-for-gestational-age infants

Infants who are below the tenth percentile (or 2 SD) in weight for their gestational age are termed small for gestational age (SGA). These infants may also be shorter in length and have smaller heads, depending on when in the gestational life the insult to their growth occurred. The more general the growth failure, the earlier the intrauterine effect. For example, rubella in the first trimester causes total growth retardation, whereas hypertension in the mother in the third trimester predominantly affects weight. The more profound the growth retardation, the more difficult the nutritional problems.

SGA infants are prone to be hypocalcemic; however, if they can be provided with adequate breast milk early, this complication may be avoided. Other problems, including hypothermia and hypoglycemia, which lead to a vicious circle of acidosis and associated problems, can be triggered by unmonitored exposure of the infant to thermal stress in the first hours of life and failure to identify the hypoglycemia early. Thus the perinatal nursery staff may appear to be obstructive to breastfeeding when they hover over this infant or even insist on his transfer to the nursery. Initially breastfeeding at delivery is permissible if adequate external heat is provided. Testing the blood sugar should be performed in the delivery room recovery area and the infant sent to the nursery if hypoglycemia or hypo-thermia cannot be controlled. Frequent breastfeeding can be initiated unless the blood sugar level is too low (below 30 mg/100 ml or unresponsive to oral treatment). It may not be possible for even an actively lactating multipara to sustain an SGA infant initially, but the infant should be put to breast at least every 3 hours and given IV glucose in addition. SGA infants often have a poor suck and poor coordination with the swallow reflex. There may be considerable mucus with gagging and spitting. A simple lavage of the stomach with a no. 8 feeding tube (or 5, if the infant weighs less than 2600 g) and warmed glucose water usually relieves the gagging. Once this SGA infant begins to eat, he will do well and will require sufficient kilocalories to meet the needs of an infant who is appropriate for gestational age. The mother may need to use a breast pump to stimulate lactation initially.

•   •   •

Infants who are less than 1800 g at birth and have to be gavaged or infants of any weight who are acutely ill present a complex problem. The mother should be instructed to express her milk initially and contribute any colostrum she produces. This can be given

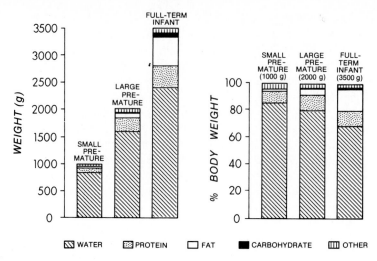

Fig. 14-2. Absolute and relative body composition of infants weighing 1000, 2000, and 3000 g at birth. (Reproduced with permission from Heird WC and Anderson TL: Nutritional requirements and methods of feeding low birth weight infants. In Gluck L et al, editors: Current problems in pediatrics, vol 7, no 8, Chicago, 1977, Year Book Medical Publishers, Inc., Copyright © 1977.)

by gastric or nasojejunal tube. An electric pump is effective in helping a mother increase the volume produced. When the infant is born at 1000 g, requires ventilator support for days, and is not discharged for 8 weeks, it is difficult to maintain a large volume of milk by pumping, but it can be done with supportive counseling by staff. When the infant is strong enough, he may nurse at the breast while still in the hospital (see Fig. 17-3). When the infant is sent home, the breast milk may be limited in volume, or the infant may refuse the breast because he has to suckle properly to obtain the milk after becoming accustomed to soft premature rubber nipples that run automatically. He becomes frustrated and may even turn away screaming.

A mother reported when seen in the follow-up clinic at the University of Rochester that it took her 4 days to break her premature into breastfeeding, and she gave him nothing but the breast during that siege. She thought he might have to starve first! One can see that the reserves of the premature are limited if one studies the absolute and relative body composition of infants at birth (Fig. 14-2). If one considers how long it takes to starve a premature compared to a full-term infant,[83] the risks of starving a premature infant while he adapts to nursing at the breast are real (Fig. 14-3). The solution to the problem is to provide nourishment while the infant stimulates maternal milk production by suckling at the breast. There is equipment called nursing supplementer that will provide this set-up very effectively. It was developed to provide nourishment for the adopted infant that is being nursed by a mother who has not been pregnant or has never lactated and sustains the infant while the mother's milk supply develops (Chapter 17). The same effect can be provided for the premature or sick infant who has not nursed at the breast since birth and needs nourishment while the mother's supply develops. Experience to date at the University of Rochester with mothers who have taken home infants 4 to 12 weeks of age to nurse has been good. The infant can continue to gain weight while stimulating the breast. The volume required from the nursing supplementer dropped continually in all but one case so

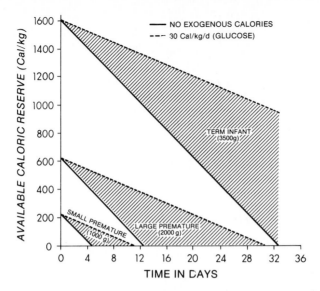

Fig. 14-3. Estimated survival of starved and semistarved infants weighing 1000, 2000, and 3500 g at birth. (Reproduced with permission from Heird WC and Anderson TL: Nutritional requirements and methods of feeding low birth weight infants. In Gluck L et al, editors: Current problems in pediatrics, vol 7, no 8, Chicago, 1977, Year Book Medical Publishers, Inc., Copyright © 1977.)

that the infants were on the breast alone after a week. In one case the infant required the supplementer for a month. Chapter 17 gives details of the equipment. The nursing supplementer provides a simple means of assuring adequate nourishment while adapting to the breast. It is preferable to using supplemental bottles because the infant is not confused by the rubber nipple, which requires a different mechanism of sucking than the human nipple. Furthermore, the suckling breast provides the continued stimulus necessary for milk production.

Hyperbilirubinemia in VLBW infants fed human milk. In a randomized study of 186 premature infants weighing less than 1850 g at birth at a mean 31 weeks' gestation and a mean birth weight of 1385 g, infants were fed their own mother's milk or randomly assigned to receive donor bank milk or formula.[147] These supplements were randomly provided to the own mother's milk group who needed more volume. Those infants receiving human milk had significantly higher peak bilirubin concentration and a more prolonged hyperbilirubinemia than those receiving formula. They had a four times greater chance of having a bilirubin of 11.7 mg% (200 μmol/L).

POSTMATURE INFANTS

Postmature infants are full-grown mature infants who have stayed in utero beyond the full vigor of the placenta and began to lose weight in utero. They are usually "older looking" and look around wide eyed. Their skin is dry and peeling and subcutaneous tissue is diminished; thus the skin appears too big. These infants have lost subcutaneous fat and lack glycogen stores. Initially they may be hypoglycemic and require early feedings to maintain blood glucose levels of 40 mg/100 ml or higher. If breastfed, the infant should go to the breast early, giving care to maintain body temperature, which is quite labile. Blood sugar levels should be followed. These infants may feed poorly initially and require considerable prodding to suckle. If the infant becomes hypoglycemic despite careful management, consideration should be given to a feeding of 10% glucose in water. In extreme cases of hypoglycemia an intravenous infusion may be necessary, and management should follow guidelines for any infant who has hypoglycemia that is resistant to routine early feedings. Calcium problems, on the other hand, although common in these infants, generally are uncommon if the infant is adequately breastfed early. This is due to the physiologic ratio of calcium and phosphorus in breast milk. Once a postmature infant begins to feed well, he is apt to catch up quickly and continue to adapt very well. Problems with hyperbilirubinemia are uncommon.

Fetal distress and hypoxia

Infants who have been compromised in utero or during delivery because of insufficient placental reserve, cord accidents, or other causes of intrauterine hypoxia have had very low Apgar scores at birth and need special treatment. An asphyxiated infant cannot be fed for at least 48 hours, and depending on associated findings it may be 96 hours or more before it is safe to put food in the gastrointestinal tract. He will have to be maintained on intravenous fluids. If the mother is to breastfeed, her colostrum will be valuable to the infant and will be better tolerated by the intestinal tract when he can feed, which has usually suffered hypoxic damage in these circumstances. The mother will need help initiating lactation and understanding the pathophysiology of the infant's disease. These infants often have a poor suck and do not coordinate with the swallow, so that nursing at breast is difficult. The mother may need to hold her breast in place and hold the infant's chin as well. These infants are especially susceptible to nipple confusion, so other means of sustaining nourishment should be sought other than a bottle. Weaning slowly from the intravenous fluids while breastfeeding is introduced is helpful. Using a dropper and using the nursing supplementer are options. These infants may continue to feed poorly for neurologic reasons. They do not do better with a bottle. If the mother is taught to cope with the problem, nursing should progress satisfactorily. There are positions in which the infant can be held that may help an individual baby adapt better. The "football hold" is a popular but poorly named position where the infant is held to the mother's side with the feet to her side. The head and face are squarely in front of the breast and steadied by the arm and hand on that side. Cupping the breast and the jaw in one hand facilitates the infant's seal around the breast with the mouth. This position has been called the "dancer hold" by Sarah Coulter Danner,* who has prepared a pamphlet for mothers feeding the neurologically impaired infant. It is well illustrated and is directed toward the mother and her specific problem. One of the most valuable suggestions is the use of a sling or pleat seat to hold the infant's body in a flexed position, thus giving the mother both hands free to hold the head and the breast in position for feeding. Pacing the feedings and pumping following feedings will increase mother's milk supply when the infant is unable to suck vigorously enough. Giving the pumped milk by lactation supplementer or dropper ensures proper weight gain in the early weeks.[115]

---

*Danner SC and Cerutti ER: Nursing your neurologically impaired baby, Childbirth Graphics, Ltd., 1210 Culver Road, Rochester, NY 14609; (716)482-7940.

In a study of energetics and mechanics of nutritive sucking in preterm and term neonates, Jain et al.[89] compared 38-week infants with 35-week infants and noted that preterm infants use less energy to suck the same volume of milk. The preterm infant took up to 0.5 ml per suck and generated lower pressures and a lower frequency. The development of nonnutritive sucking in a rhythmical manner has been demonstrated as early as 30 weeks' gestation.

The work of feeding, and more importantly "the work" of feeding at the breast, has been the argument against allowing an immature infant in the Western world to breastfeed at under 1800 g. Survival of LBW infants in Third World countries has been dependent on early breastfeeding. Nonnutritive sucking using a pacifier was evaluated measuring transcutaneous oxygen tension, heart rate, and respiratory rate while sleeping. Infants were 32 to 35 weeks post conceptual age.[24] The oxygen tension increased 2.3 mm Hg during suckling the pacifier at 32 to 33 weeks and 4.0 mm Hg at 34 to 35 weeks but not at 36 to 39 weeks. Respiratory rates remained stable, and heart rate rose slightly. Transcutaneous oxygen pressure (to Po_2) and body temperature were monitored during feedings in five VLBW infants during bottle feeding and breastfeeding. Tracings were made from the first oral feeding to time of discharge. Sequential to Po_2 values showed small undulations across baseline (above and below) while breastfeeding, and substantial dips while bottle feeding with recovery, but not above baseline. The quality and quantity of variation was very different in the two modes, with large drops occurring during actual sucking of the bottle but only during burping or repositioning while breastfeeding. The author concludes that the findings do not support the widely held view that breastfeeding is more stressful.[118] The comparative data suggest that both pacifier and bottle feeding are more stressful than suckling at the breast.

It has been suggested that perioral stimualtion enhances an immature or neurologically impaired infant's ability to suck and to coordinate suck and swallow. Perioral stimulation, consisting of stimulating the skin overlying the masseter and buccinator muscles by manually applying a quick-touch pressure stimulus lasting 1 second, was studied. This is accomplished by simultaneously squeezing (the bucal fat) both cheeks. Suck monitoring equipment revealed that perioral stimulation increased the sucking rate, suggesting that this may facilitate sucking.[115] Exercising the mouth of infants who already have excessive mouth movements may not be appropriate.

When the infant is ready for nonnutritive sucking in the NICU, it is possible to allow sucking at the empty breast (prepumped) instead of a pacifier. Considerable literature supports the contention that digestion and gastrointestinal motility are enhanced by sucking.[128] Enteral tube feedings are usually given while using a pacifier in most NICUs. Mothers who have been using an electric pump to produce milk for their VLBW infant find "nonnutritive" suckling by their infant very helpful. Premature infants with a post conceptual age of 35 weeks can discriminate between sweet and not-sweet.[154] They respond with greater sucking when given glucose water rather than plain water, so they may well respond better to the human nipple than the rubber pacifier.

Stimulating milk production in mothers of LBW infants who are pumping to provide milk for their infants has been recommended by several authors as reported by Ehrenkranz and Ackerman.[46a] They used 10 mg Metoclopramide orally every 8 hours for 7 days, tapering over 2 more days. This drug is a substituted benzamide, which has selective dopamine-antagonist activity. Milk production increased within 2 days, but after therapy decreased, milk production decreased. Prolactin levels also increased during the treatment.

MULTIPLE BIRTHS

It is possible to nurse twins and triplets. Many case reports support this fact. That a single mother can provide adequate nourishment for more than one infant has been documented for centuries. In the seventeenth century in France, wet nurses were allowed to nurse up to six infants at one time. Foundling homes provided wet nurses for every three to six infants. The key deterrent to nursing twins is not usually the milk supply but time. If the mother can nurse both infants simultaneously, the time factor is minimized. Many tricks have been suggested to achieve this feat. As the infants become larger and more active, it may be difficult to keep them simultaneously nursing with only two hands to cope. If the mother has help at home to assist with feedings, it can be accomplished. The first year of life for the mother of a set of twins is an extremely busy one and really requires additional help, particularly if the mother is going to breastfeed. She will need time for adequate rest and nourishment. She often benefits from suggestions from other mothers of twins.*

Twins

The challenge of breastfeeding twins was investigated by Addy,[4] who reviewed 173 questionnaires returned by mothers who were members of the Mothers of Twins Clubs of Southern California. This is a national organization that offers help and advice to mothers of twins. No other socioeconomic information was available. Forty-one mothers (23.7%) breastfed from birth, although 30% of the infants were premature. Of those who did not breastfeed, 9% were told not to by their doctor, 11% did not think it was possible, and 11% did not think they would have enough milk for two. Of multiparas who had breastfed their first child, an equal number breastfed and bottle fed. Of those mothers who breastfed, 39 breastfed over 1 month and 12 over 6 months.

Eight healthy women breastfeeding twins and one breastfeeding triplets participated in a study by Saint and colleagues[138] to determine the yield and nutrient content of their milk at 2, 3, 6, 9, and 12 months postpartum. At 6 months, they fed on the average 15 feeds per day. Fully breastfeeding women produced 0.84 to 2.16 kg in 24 hours. Those partially breastfeeding produced 0.42 to 1.392 kg in 24 hours. The mother feeding triplets at 2½ months produced 3.08 kg/day, and they were fed 27 times per day. At 6 months the twins received 64% to 100% of energy and at 12 months received 6% to 13%. This demonstrates that the breast is capable of responding to nutritional demands upon it contrary to previous suggestions that there was a finite limit of production that was well under a liter.

FULL-TERM INFANTS WITH MEDICAL PROBLEMS

Infants who have self-limited acute illnesses, such as fever, upper respiratory infection, colds, diarrhea, or contagious diseases like chickenpox, do best if breastfeeding is maintained. Because of breast milk's low solute load, an infant can be kept well hydrated despite fever or other increased fluid losses. If respiratory symptoms are significant, an infant seems to nurse well at the breast and poorly with a bottle. This observation has

*Make Room for Twins—A Complete Guide to Pregnancy, Delivery and the Childhood Years, 1987, Terry Pink Alexander. Available from Bantam Books, Inc., 666 Fifth Ave., New York, NY 10103.

been documented many times when nursing mothers have "roomed-in" with their sick infants in the hospital. The studies of Johnson and Salisbury[93] on the synchrony of respirations in breastfeeding in contrast to the periodic breathing or gasping apnea pattern of the normal bottle fed infant may well be the underlying explanation for the phenomenon of an acutely ill infant continuing to nurse at the breast.

In addition to the appropriateness of the human milk for a sick infant, there is the added comfort of nursing because of the closeness with the mother. If the infant is suddenly weaned, psychologic trauma is added to the stress of the illness.

It may become difficult to distinguish the effect of the trauma of acute weaning from the symptoms of the primary illness, such as poor feeding or lethargy, if the acutely weaned infant fails to respond to adequate treatment. Going back to breastfeeding may be the answer because the stress of acute weaning will be removed.

It is not appropriate to give the mother medicine intended to treat the infant, especially antibiotics. This has been tried to the detriment of the child, since variable amounts of the drug reach the infant, depending on the dose, dosage schedule, and amount of milk consumed.

Gastrointestinal disease

Bouts of diarrhea and intestinal tract disease are much less common in breastfed infants than in bottle fed infants, but when they occur, the infant should be maintained on the breast if possible. Human milk is a physiologic solution that normally causes neither dehydration nor hypernatremia. Occasionally an infant will have diarrhea or an intestinal upset because of something in the mother's diet. It is usually self-limited, and the best treatment is to continue to nurse at the breast. If the mother has been taking a laxative that is absorbed or has been eating laxative foods such as fruits in excess, she should adjust her diet. Intractable diarrhea should be evaluated as it would be in any infant. Allergy to mother's milk is extremely rare and would require substantial evidence to support the diagnosis.

A rare case of severe colitis in a totally breastfed infant usually with onset in the neonatal period suggests an intrinsic metabolic disorder in the infant or an exquisite intolerance to something in mother's milk such as cow milk protein.[98] Six cases of protein-induced enterocolitis presenting in the first month of life with severe bloody diarrhea are reported to respond to weaning and use of hydrolyzed protein formula. Other cases have been reported requiring long periods of hyperalimentation and utilization of special formulas such as Nutramigen. A case of fucose intolerance is reported in a breastfed infant who was not intolerant of lactose but the by-product of the oligosaccharides in human milk, passing large amounts of fucose in the stool.[20] The infant tolerated Pregestemil and then weaned to SMA.

The management of protracted diarrhea in infants never breastfed is reported by many human milk banks on a case-by-case basis. Eleven of 24 children managed by MacFarlane and Miller[112] in a hyperalimentation referral unit recovered when fed banked human milk orally without protracted IV therapy. All the infants had been tried on all the available special formulas first. A study of oral rehydration in 26 children under the age of 2 years showed that the children who continued to breastfeed while receiving rehydration fluid had fewer stools and recovered more rapidly than those receiving only rehydration fluid.[96] The PIMA Infant Feeding Study clearly showed that in less developed and disadvantaged communities in the United States, exclusive breastfeeding protected against severe diarrhea and other gastrointestinal disorders.[59]

Lactase deficiency may be manifested by chronic diarrhea and failure to thrive of a marked degree. Lactose intolerance is a manifestation of a deficiency of lactase, the enzyme that digests lactose, which is in high concentration in human milk. Prematures and infants recovering from severe diarhhea have transient lactose intolerance, and very rarely it occurs as an autosomal-dominant trait and is more common in males than females. The only treatment is a lactose-free diet, which excludes human milk. Reports of lactose-hydrolyzed human milk are published, suggesting that banked human milk can be treated with lactase (Kerulac), which will hydrolyze the lactose (900 enzyme activity units to 200 ml breast milk degraded 82% of the lactose).[146] In one case the reason for using human milk was that the infant became infection prone when he was weaned from the breast when the initial diagnosis was made. He showed marked improvement with human milk.

Some chronic diseases are better controlled on breast milk, and symptoms become more severe with weaning. Should an infant be weaned and do poorly on formula, relactation of the mother might be considered. With the availability of the nursing supplementer, this possibility is no longer remote (Chapter 17). Childhood celiac disease is disappearing, according to Littlewood and Crollick,[106] a trend they attribute to the increasing incidence of breastfeeding and the decreased use of straight cow's milk. They have seen a reduction in gastroenteritis. The delayed use of gluten in the diet may also be secondarily important. Infants who have been breastfed and had introduction of solids after 4 months have not been seen to have celiac disease.

In a retrospective study of 146 children with celiac disease, Greco et al.[70] initially confirmed that children breastfed 3 months or more showed a marked delay in onset of the disease unrelated to when gluten was introduced. In a case control study of 216 children in Italy with celiac disease and their siblings, Auricchio et al.[18] reported that formula-fed infants from birth or infants breastfed less than 1 month have four times greater risk of celiac disease than infants breastfed over 1 month. The time of introduction of gluten into the diet was not a factor. The incidence in Ireland of celiac disease is also decreasing and was related to the protective effect of breastfeeding by Stevens et al.[150] Of interest is the work of Troncone and colleagues,[158] who measured the passage of gliadin into breast milk following the ingestion of 20 g wheat gluten. Fifty-four of 80 samples showed 5 to 95 ng/ml of gliadin, which peaked in the milk 2 to 4 hours after ingestion but did not appear in serum. The authors[158] suggest that the transfer of gliadin from mother to infant might be critical for the development of an appropriate specific immune response. The epidemiologic data suggest that breastfeeding would be especially appropriate in celiac disease–positive families.

The development of Crohn's disease later in life has increased in recent decades. Since it has been suggested that breast milk is essential for the development of the normal immunological competence of the intestinal mucosa, the association of breastfeeding and later Crohn's disease was studied.[22] Bergstrand and Hellers[22] studied 826 patients who developed Crohn's disease between 1955 and 1974 and their matched controls. Mean length of breastfeeding was 4.59 months among patients and 5.76 among controls (<0.01). Crohn's disease patients were overrepresented among those with no or very short periods of breastfeeding.

Induced colitis in infants is usually due to some dietary insult, such as exposure to cow's milk.[98,145] It has been reported in breastfed infants, most of whom responded to removal of cow's milk from the maternal diet. Several had been given formula at birth. The symptoms included bloody diarrhea, and sigmoidoscopy revealed focal ulcerations, edema, and increased friability of the intestinal mucosa. On relief of symptoms by dietary change, the intestinal tract biopsy returns to normal.

Botulism

Considerable justifiable concern has been expressed because of the reports of sudden infant death from botulism. Infant botulism is distinguished from food-borne botulism from improperly preserved food containing the toxin and from wound botulism from spores entering the wound. Infant botulism occurs when the spores of *Clostridium botulinum* germinate and multiply in the gut and produce the botulinal toxin in the gastrointestinal tract.[12] The toxin binds presynaptically at the neuromuscular junction, preventing acetyl-choline release. The clinical picture is descending, symmetric flaccid paralysis. The gut of only some infants is susceptible, as many infants and adults are exposed. When a previously healthy infant under 6 months of age develops constipation, then weakness, and difficulty sucking, swallowing, crying, or breathing, botulism is a likely diagnosis. The organisms should be looked for in the stools; electromyography may or may not be helpful.

In a group reviewed by Arnon et al.,[13] 33 of 50 patients hospitalized in California were still being nursed at onset of the illness. A beneficial effect of human milk was observed in the difference in the mean age at onset, breastfed infants being twice as old as formula-fed infants with the disease, and the breastfed infants' symptoms were milder. Breastfed infants receiving iron supplements developed disease earlier than those who were beastfed but unsupplemented. Of the cases of sudden infant death from botulism, there were no infants who were breastfed within 10 weeks of death. All were receiving iron-fortified formulas. The only known food exposure that has been implicated is honey, in not more than 35% of the world cases. It has been recommended that honey not be given to infants under 12 months of age as a result. This includes putting honey on a mother's nipples to initiate an infant's interest in suckling.

A review of the first 10 years of infant botulism monitoring worldwide was prepared by Arnon.[11] The disease has been reported from 41 of the 50 states and from eight countries on four continents. The relationship to breastfeeding and human milk is unclear. In general, the acid stools (pH 5.1 to 5.4) of human milk-fed infants encourage *Bifidobacterium* spp, and very few facultatively anaerobic bacteria, and clostridia as spores are virtually absent. In contrast, formula-fed infants have stool pHs ranging from 5.9 to 8.0 containing few *Bifidobacterium,* clostridia, anaerobic streptococci, and facultative anaerobic bacteria. *C. botulinum* and toxin production declines with pH and usually stops below 4.6. Breast milk also contains the protective immunologic components. The relationship between the introduction of solid foods or weaning in both formula and breastfed infants and the onset of botulism remains unclear. It has been suggested that for the breastfed infant, the introduction of solid food causes a major change in the gut with a rapid rise in the growth of enterobacteria and enterococci followed by progressive colonization by *Bacteroides* spp, clostridia, and anaerobic streptococci. Adding solids to formula-fed infants changes nothing. Although more hospitalized infants have been breastfed, sudden death victims are younger and have been formula fed, which supports the concept that there is immunologic protection in the gut of the breastfed infant. The role of honey remains unchallenged. Much work remains to understand the disease. Clinically, constipation, weakness, and hypotonicity in a previously healthy child should be viewed with infant botulism in mind, especially if there have been recent dietary changes.

Respiratory illness

Infants who develop respiratory illnesses should be maintained at the breast. The added advantages of antibodies and anti-infective properties are valuable to the infant. A sick infant can nurse more easily than cope with a bottle. Furthermore, the comfort of having his mother nearby is important whenever the infant has a crisis, but weaning during illness may be devastating.

Otitis media in infants occurs less frequently in breastfed infants. Recurrent otitis media is associated with bottle feeding in a study of 237 children in contrast to prolonged breastfeeding, which had a long-term protective effect up to 3 years of age.[136]

A regional birth cohort of 5,356 children was followed prospectively regarding the occurence of infectious disease in the first year of life.[95] One third developed otitis media. Median age of onset was 8 months, and 10% had had three episodes by 1 year of age. Breastfeeding for 9 months or longer had a significant impact on otitis, as did the number of siblings and day care. Otitis media in Greenland in 3- to 8-year-old children was studied as a national concern for the incidence and associated deafness. Children who were breastfed were spared, especially if nursed a long time.[129]

Young infants who have older siblings may well be exposed to some virulent viruses and bacteria. Developing croup or chickenpox, for instance, may make the infant seriously ill. Hydration can be maintained by frequent, short breastfeedings. Studies have shown that respirations are maintained more easily when feeding on human milk than on cow's milk. Nursing at the breast permits regular respirations, whereas bottle feeding is associated with a more gasping pattern. Thus breastfed infants continue to nurse when they are ill. If the infant is hospitalized, every effort should be made to maintain the breastfeeding if he can be fed at all. One should provide rooming-in for the mother if a care-by-parent ward is not available. Neutralizing inhibitors to respiratory syncytial virus (RSV) have been demonstrated in the whey of most samples of human milk tested.[157]

Colostrum and milk contain large amounts of IgA antibody, some of which is RSV specific. Breastfed but not bottle fed infants have IgA in their nasal secretions.[157] IgG anti-RSV antibodies are present in milk and in reactive T lymphocytes. Breastfeeding-induced resistance to RSV was associated with the presence of interferon as well as virus-specific lymphocyte transformation activity, suggesting that breastfeeding has unique mechanisms for modulating the immune response of infants to RSV infection.[35] Clinical studies indicating a relative protection from RSV in breastfed infants were clouded by other factors.[156] The populations were unequal because of socioeconomic factors and smoking (i.e., bottle feeding mothers were in lower socioeconomic groups and smoked more). In general, if breastfed infants become ill, they have less severe illness.[156,157]

Galactosemia

Galactosemia, which is due to the deficiency of galactose-1-phosphate uridyl transferase, is a rare circumstance in which the infant is unable to metabolize galactose and must be placed on a galactose-free diet. The disease can be rapidly fatal in the severe form. The infant may have severe and/or persistent jaundice, vomiting, diarrhea, electrolyte imbalances, cerebral signs, and weight loss. This does necessitate weaning from the breast to a special formula because human milk contains high levels of lactose, which is a disaccharide that splits into glucose and galactose. The diagnosis is suspected when reducing substances are found in the urine and confirmed by measuring the enzyme uridyl transferase in the red and white blood cells.

Inborn errors of metabolism

Other metabolic deficiency syndromes are usually only apparent as mild failure to thrive syndrome until the infant is weaned from the breast and the symptoms become severe. This particularly applies to inborn errors of metabolism due to an inability to handle one or more of the essential amino acids. Infection is often a complication early in the lives of these infants with inborn errors. In the process of treating the acute infection the infant may be weaned, and the metabolic disorder then becomes apparent precipitously.

An infant in a coma was transferred to the intensive care unit of the University of Rochester Medical Center from another hospital where he had been admitted at 7 weeks of age. He had been entirely well until 3 weeks of age, when he was abruptly weaned from the breast because he developed sepsis and possible meningitis. He became acutely acidotic, then comatose with shock symptoms. On transfer he had a blood ammonia level of 1600 μmol/L. He was ultimately diagnosed postmortem, after heroic efforts to bring the ammonia to normal levels. The disease, propionic acidemia, was incompatible with life, but the parents were able to console themselves in their loss because the child had had a few apparently "healthy, happy weeks" while being breastfed.

If one refers to Table 4-9, it will be observed that there is significantly less of certain amino acids in human milk than in cow's milk, such as phenylalanine, methionine, leucine, isoleucine, and others associated with metabolic disorders. Management of an amino acid metabolic disorder while breastfeeding would depend on careful monitoring of blood and urine levels of the specific amino acids involved. Since these are essential amino acids, a certain amount is necessary in the diet of all infants, including those with the disease. An appropriate combination of breastfeeding and a milk free of the offending amino acid could be developed. The care of such infants should be in consultation with a pediatric endocrinologist. Transient neonatal tyrosinemia, which has been reported to occur in a high percentage (up to 80%) of neonates fed cow's milk, is associated with blood tyrosine levels 10 times those of adults. Wong et al.[166] have associated severe cases with learning disabilities in later years.

The most common of the amino acid metabolic disorders is phenylketonuria (PKU), in which the amino acid accumulates for lack of an enzyme. The treatment has been phenylalanine-free formula, Lofenalac (Mead Johnson, Evansville, Indiana) with added formula to provide a little phenylalanine because every infant needs a small amount. If the infant is breastfed, the mother is usually reluctant to stop. It has been demonstrated in our own hospital and elsewhere that an infant may supplement the Lofenalac with breast milk. With careful monitoring of the blood levels and control of the amount of breastfeeding, a balance can be struck that permits optimal phenylalanine levels and some breastfeeding. The infant will require some Lofenalac to provide enough calories and nutrients. There is a detailed outline of management available called *Guide to Breastfeeding the Infant with PKU* prepared by Ernest, McCabe, Neifert and O'Flynn. It is available from the Superintendent of Documents, U.S. Government Printing Office, Washington, DC 20402.[49]

Literature values for phenylalanine range from 29 to 64 mg/100 ml in human milk.

The amount for Lofenalac and human milk for a given baby are calculated by weight, age, blood levels, and needs for growth. As an example, a 3-week-old weighing 3.7 kg whose blood level was 52.5 mg/100 ml when he was getting an estimated 570 ml of breast milk would receive 240 ml Lofenalac and 360 ml breast milk (four breastfeedings a day with before and after weighing). The details of every step of management are available in the *Guide* to assist the physician in planning treatment. Since infants with PKU are more prone to thrush infection, the mother should be alerted to watch for symptoms in the infant and the onset of sore nipples that could be due to *Candida albicans*. Treatment is nystatin for mother and baby. The other benefits of human milk make the effort to breastfeed valuable for the infant and for the mother who usually wishes to continue to contribute to her infant's nourishment. The prognosis for intellectual development is excellent if treatment is initiated early and the blood levels maintained at less than 10 mg/100 ml.

α_1 Antitrypsin deficiency

α_1Antitrypsin (α_1AT) is a serum protease inhibitor that inactivates a number of proteases. There are more than 24 genetic varients of this disease designated B through Z, with the M-variant being most common. Children with α_1AT deficiency are at increased risk for liver disease, occurring most often during infancy and often progressing to cirrhosis and death. Udall and colleagues[160] investigated the relationship between early feedings and the onset of liver disease. Severe liver disease was present in eight (40%) of the bottle-fed and one (8%) of the breastfed infants (breastfed for only 5 weeks). Of the 32 infants, 24 were still alive at the end of the study; 12 had been breastfed and 12 bottle fed during their first month of life. All eight of the deceased children had been bottle fed; SGA and preterm infants had been exluded from the study so that all infants were equally stable at birth and capable of breastfeeding. A bottle fed infant was seven times more likely to develop liver disease.

With the increasing early diagnosis of α_1 antitrypsin deficiency disease, it would appear that encouraging a mother to breastfeed if her infant is affected would have a significant impact on long-range liver disease in her infant.

Acrodermatitis enteropathica (Danbolt-Closs syndrome)

Acrodermatitis enteropathica is a rare but unique disease in that feeding with human milk may be lifesaving. It is inherited as an autosomal recessive trait. It is characterized by a symmetric rash around the mouth, genitalia, and periphery of the extremities. The rash is an acute vesicobullous and eczematous eruption often secondarily infected with *C. albicans*. It may be seen by the third week of life or not until late in infancy and has been associated with weaning from the breast. Failure to thrive, hair loss, irritability, and chronic severe intractable diarrhea are often life-threatening. The disease has been associated with extremely low plasma zinc levels. Oral zinc sulfate has produced remission of the disease.

Human milk contains less zinc than does bovine milk, with zinc concentrations of both decreasing throughout lactation. Eckert et al.[46] studied the zinc binding in human and cow's milk and noted that the low-molecular-weight binding ligand isolated from human milk may enhance absorption of zinc in these patients. Gel chromatography indicated that most of the zinc in cow's milk was associated with high-molecular-weight fractions, whereas zinc in human milk was associated with low-molecular-weight fractions. The copper/zinc ratio may also be of significance, since the ratio is lower in cow's milk.

The zinc binding ligand from human milk was further identified as prostaglandin E by chromatography, ultrafiltration, and infrared spectroscopy by Evans and Johnson.[50] These patients also have low arachidonic acid levels. Arachidonic acid is a precursor of prostaglandin. The efficacy of human milk in the treatment of acrodermatitis enteropathica results from the presence of the zinc-prostaglandin complex.

The clinical significance of the relationship of human milk to onset of the disease and its treatment is in developing lactation in the mother of such an infant, rare as the disease may be. Delayed lactation or relactation is possible and should be offered as an option to the mother of such an infant (Chapter 17).

Several reports of isolated cases of zinc deficiency during breastfeeding have appeared in the literature.[5,6,14,120] In some cases, zinc levels in the milk were low; in others, they were not measured.[168] One child had a classic "zinc-deficient" rash that responded to oral zinc therapy. It is advisable to keep in mind that any deficiency is possible and consider intake deficiency when symptoms occur in the breastfed infant.

Down's syndrome

Infants with Down's syndrome or other trisomies may be difficult to feed. When they are breastfed, it takes patience on the part of the mother to teach the infant to suck with sufficient vigor to initiate the let-down reflex and to stimulate adequate production of milk. Using manual expression to start flow and holding the breast firmly for the infant so that the nipple does not drop out of the mouth when the infant stops suckling will assist the process.

Initially, an infant with Down's may have surprisingly good tone and may even suck well at the breast only to develop problems once the mother and infant have been discharged home. Providing support for the head, the jaw, and the general body hypotonia will require considerable coordination on the part of the mother. Propping the baby firmly with a pillow in mother's lap or supporting the infant in a sling as recommended by McBride and Danner[115] frees up a much-needed hand for steadying the jaw and breast. It is clearly a time for a nurse-clinician knowledgeable and experienced in dealing with neurologically impaired infants to be available. The initial goals for the mother-infant pair are developing confidence in handling the infant, adjusting to the infant's problem, and dealing with the parental grief and sense of loss. If the mother has breastfed other children, the emphasis on breastfeeding modifications are more successful, and milk supply usually responds to manual expression and pumping. Initiating sufficient stimulus to the breast to increase milk production is critical in the first few days to induce good prolactin response, especially in a primipara. Renting an electric breast pump is a good investment justifiable for reimbursement from health insurance by physician prescription.

The pediatrician in developing a discharge plan for this infant will need to coordinate the team to avoid the fragmented care that develops with a multiproblem situation, which may have required the consultation of a geneticist, a genetic counselor, a cardiologist, and other medical experts to deal with the problems. Ideally, the pediatrician and the office nurse-practitioner can provide the additional support and counsel necessary. Many families prefer to leave the hospital early to retreat to the comfort and privacy of their home and the health care provider they selected. Home visits by the pediatrician's staff can provide the necessary monitoring of weight gain and nutrition, as well as counseling by someone capable of handling all the problems that arise including the breastfeeding. No referrals should be made without the pediatrician's knowledge and agreement. The pediatrician has the advantage of knowing both the family and the child.

In a study of 59 breastfed infants with Down's syndrome, Aumonier and Cunningham[17] reported that 31 of the 59 infants had no sucking difficulty, 12 infants were successfully nursing within a week, and 16 required tube feeding initially, but this was associated with other medical problems including LBW, cardiac lesions, and jaundice. Hyperbilirubinemia is common in trisomy and was seen in 49% of these study infants. Eighteen babies had multiple medical conditions, and 11 of them sucked poorly. The authors[17] point out that the initial sucking ability of the infants did not appear to be a major cause for nonmaintenance of breastfeeding. Ten of the 13 mothers who discontinued breastfeeding cited insufficient milk as a contributing cause, which might have been prevented by early pumping.

The birth of an infant with a major genetic abnormality is a shock, even to the strongest parents. If the mother wants to breastfeed, she should be offered all the encouragement and support necessary. Usually she needs to talk with someone just to express her anguish about the infant, not the feeding per se. A sympathetic nurse-practitioner can be invaluable in providing the support as well as the expertise necessary to help with the various management problems.

It is especially important that these infants be breastfed if possible because they are particularly prone to infection. Before the advent of antibiotics, they often died of overwhelming infection and rarely survived past 20 years of age. These infants and most other infants with developmental disorders do better with stimulation and affection, so the body contact and communication while at the breast are especially important. Those who have associated cardiac lesions not only can suckle, swallow, and breathe with less effort at the breast but also receive a fluid more physiologic to their needs. Breastfed or bottle fed, these infants gain poorly; thus, switching to a bottle does not solve the problem. The recommendation that the Down's child receive extra vitamins was tested in a controlled study in children 5 to 13 years of age, and there was no sustained improvement in the children's appearance, growth, behavior, or development.[21]

Hypothyroidism

It has been reported by Bode et al.[27] that an infant with congenital cretinism was spared the severe effects of the disease because he was breastfed. This was attributed to significant quantities of thyroid hormone in the milk. In a prospective study of 12 cases of hypothyroidism in breastfed infants, Letarte et al.[103] found no protective effect on the disease, nor was the onset of the disease delayed. Anthropometric measurements, biochemical values, and psychologic testing at 1 year of age did not differ from those in the 33 bottle fed hypothyroid infants. Successful diagnosis of congenital hypothyroidism in four breastfed neonates was also reported by Abbassi and Steinour.[1] Sack et al.[137] measured thyroxine (T_4) concentrations in human milk and found it to be present in significant amounts. Varma et al.[162] have reported the study of thyroxine (T_4), triiodothyronine (T_3), and reverse triiodothyroxine (rT_3) concentrations in human milk in 77 healthy euthyroid mothers from the day of delivery to 148 days postpartum. They calculated from their data that if an infant received 900 to 1200 ml of milk/day, he would receive 2.1 to 2.6 μg of T_4/day, based on 238.1 ng/100 ml of milk after the first week. This amount of T_4 is much less than the recommended dose for the treatment of hypothyroidism (18.8 to 25 μg/day of levo-triiodothyronine). T_4 was essentially unmeasurable in the milk sampled. In another study, however, comparing 22 breastfed and 25 formula-fed infants who were 2 to 3 weeks old, the levels of T_3 and T_4 were significantly higher in the breastfed infants.[80] No definite relationship between the levels of T_3 and rT_3 could be found.

A 6-week-old female was diagnosed to have congenital hypothyrodism by routine neonatal screening when the thyroxine was reported at 3 mg/dl (normal >7 mg/dl).[41] The mother gave a history of multiple applications of povidone iodine during pregnancy and continuing during lactation. Further testing revealed TSH of 0.9 μU/ml (normal 0.8-5 μU/ml). Iodine treatment was stopped and breastfeeding continued while treatment of thyroid replacement was begun. At 1 year, growth and development were normal. It is therefore suggested that neonatal screening for thyroid disease may be even more urgent if the clinical symptoms are apt to be masked in a breastfed infant. There is no contraindication to breastfeeding when the infant is hypothyroid, and it may well be beneficial. Appropriate therapy should also be instituted promptly.

Adrenal hyperplasia

In an analysis of 32 infants presenting with salt-losing congenital adrenal hyperplasia in adrenal crisis, 8 had been breastfed, 5 had been breastfed with formula supplements, and 19 had been formula-fed.[39] Infants who were breastfed were admitted to the hospital later than the formula-fed infants, although the breastfed infants had lower serum sodium levels on admission. The breastfed infants did not vomit and remained stable longer, although they all had severe failure to thrive. Weaning initiated vomiting and precipitated crises in the breastfed infants. The authors[39] suggest that congenital adrenal hyperplasia should be considered in failure to thrive in a breastfed infant. Electrolytes should be obtained before weaning to make the diagnosis and avoid precipitating a crisis.

Neonatal breasts and nipple discharge

It is not uncommon for the newborn to have swelling of the breasts for the first few days of life, whether male or female; this is unrelated to being breastfed. If the breast is squeezed, milk can be obtained. This has been called witch's milk. The constituents of neonatal milk were studied by McKiernan and Hull,[116] who measured electrolyte, lactose, total protein, and lipid concentrations in the milks of 18 normal newborns and infants with sepsis, adrenal hyperplasia, cystic fibrosis, and meconium ileus. Electrolyte values were similar to those in adult women in all the infants except one with a mastitis, in which the sodium was elevated and the potassium decreased. Total protein and lactose were also similar to those in adult women. The fat was different, increasing with postnatal age and being higher in short-chain fatty acids. It was indeed true milk.

Two infants, one female and one male, were reported to have bilateral bloody discharge from the nipples at 6 weeks of age. Cultures and smears were unrevealing.[23] No biopsy was done. The female infant's swelling and discharge cleared after 5 months; the male's was still present at 10 weeks, when he was lost to follow-up. Galactorrhea or persistent neonatal milk has been reported in association with neonatal hyperthyroidism. In another report, a 21-day-old infant female was seen because of a goiter and galactorrhea. The infant had 50% 24-hour ^{131}I uptake and elevated prolactin levels, which slowly responded to Lugol's solution treatment for hyperthyroidism.[111]

Hyperbilirubinemia and jaundice

Jaundice in the newborn has become a source of considerable misinformation, confusion, and anxiety in recent years. There is a higher incidence of jaundice in full-term infants than a decade ago. More physicians are paying attention to the development of hyperbilirubinemia in newborns. These two factors serve to increase the frequency of the question of the role of breastfeeding in the development of hyperbilirubinemia. Some of the confusion and inconsistencies associated with the management can be attributed to the indecisive terminology. An attempt will be made to clarify the issues and outline the causes and effects of hyperbilirubinemia.

Why the concern about jaundice

Bilirubin is a cell toxin, as can be demonstrated dramatically by adding a little bilirubin to a tissue culture, which will be quickly destroyed. Excessive bilirubin causes concern because when there is free, unbound, unconjugated bilirubin in the system it can be deposited in various tissues, ultimately causing necrosis of the cells. The brain and brain cells, if destroyed by bilirubin deposits, do not regenerate.[81] The full-blown end result is bilirubin encephalopathy or kernicterus, which is essentially a pathologic diagnosis that depends on identifying the yellow pigmentation and necrosis in the brain, especially the basal ganglion, hippocampal cortex, and subthalamic nuclei. About 50% of the infants with kernicterus at autopsy also have other lesions due to bilirubin toxicity. There may be necrosis of the renal tubular cells, intestinal mucosa, or pancreatic cells or associated gastrointestinal hemorrhage. The classic clinical manifestations of bilirubin encephalopathy are characterized by progressive lethargy, rigidity, opisthotonos, high-pitched cry, fever, and convulsions. The mortality rate is 50%. Survivors usually have choreoathetoid cerebral palsy, asymmetric spasticity, paresis of upward gaze, high-frequency deafness, and mental retardation.[45] Premature infants are particularly susceptible to bilirubin-related brain damage and may have kernicterus at autopsy without the typical clinical syndrome. There is a significant correlation between level of bilirubin and hearing impairment in newborns. Classic full-blown kernicterus rarely occurs today, but what may well develop are mild effects on the brain that will be manifested clinically in later life as incoordination, hypertonicity, and mental retardation or perhaps learning disabilities, symptoms sometimes collectively called minimal brain damage.[81] Bilirubin encephalopathy is the appropriate term for conditions in which bilirubin is thought to be the cause of brain toxicity.

Mechanism of bilirubin production in the neonate

The normal full-term infant has a hematocrit in utero of 50% to 65%. Because of the low oxygen tension delivered to the fetus via the placenta, the fetus requires more hemoglobin to carry the oxygen. As soon as the infant is born and begins to breathe room air, the need is gone. The infant bone marrow does not make more cells, and excess cells are destroyed and not replaced. The life span of a fetal red blood cell is 70 to 90 days instead of the adult's 120 days. Normally when red cells are destroyed, the released hemoglobin is broken down to heme in the reticuloendothelial system (RES). The reticuloendothelial cells contain a microsomal enzyme, heme oxygenase, which is capable of oxidizing the alpha-methene bridge carbon of the heme molecule after the loss of the iron and the globin to form biliverdin, a green pigment, according to Gartner and Lee.[66] Biliverdin is water soluble and is rapidly degraded to bilirubin. A gram of hemoglobulin will produce 34 mg of bilirubin.

The reticuloendothelial cell releases the bilirubin into the circulation, where it is rapidly bound to albumin. Bilirubin is essentially insoluble (less than 0.01 mg/100 ml soluble). Adult albumin can bind two molecules of bilirubin, the first more tightly than the second. Newborn albumin has reduced molar binding capacities that vary with maturity and other factors.[132]

Unconjugated bilirubin is removed from the circulation by the hepatocyte, which converts it by conjugation of each molecule of bilirubin with two molecules of glucuronic acid into direct bilirubin. Direct bilirubin is water soluble and is excreted via the bile to the stools. The balance between hepatic cell uptake of bilirubin and the rate of bilirubin production determines the serum unconjugated bilirubin concentration.

Evaluation and management

Normal full-term newborns have serial bilirubin tests to determine the range of values. Many have observed that the cord bilirubin level may be as high as 2.0 mg/100 ml and rise over the first 72 hours to 5 to 6 mg/100 ml, which is barely in the visible range, and gradually taper off, assuming adult levels of 1.0 mg/100 ml after 10 days. Fewer than 50% of normal infants are visibly jaundiced in the first week of life. Why any normal infant is visibly jaundiced is not known, although it has been suggested by Gartner and Lee[64] that it is due to insufficient enzyme synthesis, inhibition of enzymatic activity by naturally occurring substances, deficient synthesis of the glucuronide donor UDPGA, or a combination of factors. This would suggest the jaundice is idiopathic, not physiologic. The acceptable level of bilirubin depends on a number of factors. In some premature infants, even bilirubin levels under 10 mg/100 ml may be of concern.

Factors that influence significance. For a given level of bilirubin, several associated factors may need to be considered. If there has been acidosis, anoxia, asphyxia, hypothermia, hypoglycemia, or infection, even lower levels of bilirubin may have a significant risk of causing deposition of bilirubin in the brain cells. These factors increase the susceptibility of the brain to bilirubin deposition: prematurity, asphyxia, hypoxia, hypoglycemia, hypothermia, acidosis, and infection. The most important of these is prematurity, which affects both liver and brain metabolism. There is an increased incidence of elevated bilirubin levels in certain races and populations. Asian populations—including Chinese, Japanese, and Korean—and American Indians may have bilirubin levels averaging between 10 and 14 mg/100 ml. There is also a higher incidence of autopsy-identified kernicterus in these populations. It does not seem to be related to G_6PD deficiency, however, which is also common in these groups.

Determination of cause of jaundice. If one follows the chain of events from the red cell and its destruction in the newborn through to the final excretion of conjugated bilirubin in the stools, it simplifies understanding the cause of a specific case of jaundice. Causes include (1) increased destruction of red cells, (2) decreased conjugation in the glucuronidase system, (3) decreased albumin binding, and (4) increased reabsorption from the gastrointestinal tract.

When albumin binding is altered, the visibility of the jaundice is not affected. The bilirubin level may not be very high, but the substance is not bound to albumin and is available at lower levels to pass into the brain cells. Premature infants have much lower albumin levels and thus have fewer binding sites. Drugs that also bind to albumin compete for binding sites. These drugs include aspirin and sulfadiazine, for instance. A lower level of bilirubin puts the infant who has these medications in his system at risk because the bilirubin is unbound and available to enter tissue cells, including brain cells.

Reabsorption of bilirubin from stool in the gastrointestinal tract can increase the bilirubin level. This occurs when the conjugated bilirubin that was excreted into the colon is unconjugated by the action of intestinal bacteria and reabsorbed, which happens when stools are decreased or slowed in passage. Poor feedings, pyloric stenosis, and other forms of intestinal obstruction are common causes of this type of jaundice. Some bacteria are more apt than others to unconjugate conjugated bilirubin.

Safe levels of bilirubin. Safe levels of bilirubin depend on a number of factors noted previously, including acidosis, hypoxia or anoxia, and sepsis. A handy rule of thumb is the correlation of birthweight in the premature infant and the indirect bilirubin level, using a value 2 to 3 mg lower when the infant has multiple problems.

In a well infant weighing under 2000 g, the peak tolerated bilirubin corresponds roughly: 1800 g/18 mg%, 1500 g/15 mg%, 1200 g/12 mg%, and 1000 g/10 mg%. Because of stripping of the bilirubin from the binding sites in the capillaries of the brain in some situations such as prematurity or presence of a competing drug in the serum, more bilirubin is available to be deposited than is measured to be "free" in the plasma.[132]

Any value of 20 mg/100 ml or over warrants treatment. Phototherapy is generally begun when the bilirubin is roughly 5 mg/ml below the exchange level. Jaundice visible under 24 hours of age is of special concern because it is usually associated with an incompatibility or infection. Rapidly rising bilirubin levels are also of concern, and a 0.5 mg/100 ml rise/hour is also an indication for treatment.

Treatment. Treatment depends on identifying the cause. Blood incompatibilities may be treated by exchange transfusion if severe enough (i.e., bilirubin 20 mg/100 ml or rising at 0.5 mg/100 ml/hour or dropping hematocrit). The exchange transfusion removes affected red blood cells (RBC) and antibodies and improves excessive bilirubin levels. If the cause is sepsis, the infection should be treated immediately as well as the bilirubin problem. About half the cases of jaundice will not have an identified cause and are classified as idiopathic (rather than physiologic jaundice). Refer to standard texts of pediatrics and neonatology for more extnesive discussions of neonatal hyperbilirubinemia.

Hyperbilirubinemia and breastfeeding. Two major clinical conditions exist that associate the breastfed infant with hyperbilirubinemia, one very common, one rare. The major clinical features of these two conditions are outlined in Table 14-9. They will be discussed separately. The more common condition has been called *early breast milk jaundice* by Gartner and others[60,61] but might be called *jaundice while breastfeeding,* as probably not the breastfeeding but the failure to stool and the decreased calories are at fault. Since some bottle fed infants also are jaundiced, the appropriate term would be bottle feeding jaundice for this latter group.

Early jaundice while breastfeeding. Many studies of bilirubin levels in normal newborn nurseries have been conducted looking at method of feeding. Unfortunately, very few have detailed frequency of feeds, supplementation, and stool pattern.[43,113,147] A review of multiple published studies summarizing results in 13 studies covering over 20,000 infants was reported by Schneider[143] to show a relationship between breastfeeding and jaundice. A pooled analysis of 12 studies showed 514 of 3,997 breastfed infants to have a bilirubin $\geq$12 mg/dl versus 172 of 4,255 bottle fed infants. In a smaller group of studies, 54 of 2,655 breastfed infants had bilirubins $\geq$15 mg/dl versus 10 of 3,002 bottle fed infants. Eleven of 13 studies reported that breastfed infants had higher mean bilirubins. In a series of over 12,000 infants, the risk of a breastfed infant's becoming jaundiced had an odds

Table 14-9. Hyperbilirubinemia while breastfeeding

Early jaundice	Late jaundice
Occurs 2-5 days of age	Occurs 5-10 days of age
Transient—10 days	Persists >1 month
More common in primipara	All children of a given mother
Infrequent feeds	Milk volume not a problem
	May have abundant milk
Stools delayed/infrequent	Normal stooling
Receiving H_2O or D_5W	No supplements
Bilirubin peaks ≤15 mg/dl	Bilirubin may >20 mg/dl
Treatment none or phototherapy	Treatment: phototherapy
	Disc. breastfeeding
	Rarely exchange transfusion
Associations low Apgars, H_2O, or D_5W supplement, prematurity	None identified

ratio of 1.8. The risk of becoming jaundiced for a premature was 3.6; for an Asian race, 3.56; and with prolonged rupture of membranes, 1.91. No doubt jaundice is more common in normal newborns as compared to the 1950s, when bilirubin was rarely measured in normal babies, although hospital stays averaged 5 to 7 days. It is clear from many studies that more breastfed infants are jaundiced than bottle fed, and the cause of this needs attention.

Relationship of bilirubin level to passage of stools. There are 450 mg of bilirubin in the meconium in the intestinal tract of the average newborn infant. Passing this meconium is critical to avoid the deconjugation and reabsorption of this bilirubin from the gut into the serum. Failure to pass meconium is correlated with elevated serum bilirubin. Time of first stool is also correlated with level of serum bilirubin. Bottle fed infants were reported by DeCarvalho et al.[44] to excrete more stool (82 g) and more bilirubin (23.8 mg) in the first 3 days than breastfed infants, who excreted 58 g of stool and 15.7 mg bilirubin. The serum bilirubin levels were 6.8 mg/dl in bottle fed and 9.5 mg/dl in breastfed infants. Furthermore, when the breastfed infants excreted more stools and more bilirubin, they had lower bilirubins.

Feeding practices and early hyperbilirubinemia. A retrospective study of over 200 infants in our nursery looked at weight loss, number of feeding, amount of supplementation with water or dextrose water, body temperature, number of stools, and third-day serum bilirubin. The infants who received water or dextrose water passed fewer stools, had higher bilirubins, and had more problems nursing beyond 4 days of life. Full-term breastfed infants who were receiving water or dextrose supplements had higher serum bilirubin levels on the sixth day of life than bottle babies in a study by Nicoll et al.[125] Supplementation with water or dextrose did not reduce hyperbilirubinemia that had already developed. This is not surprising, since bilirubin is excreted in the stool rather than the urine, and these jaundiced infants usually show no signs of dehydration. When the number of feedings at the breast in the first 3 days of life was related to bilirubin levels, DeCarvalho et al.[44] were able to display a significant relationship. The greater the number of breastfeedings, the lower the bilirubin. Those infants with more than eight feedings per day were not significantly jaundiced. These authors also found that water and dextrose supplements were associated with higher bilirubin levels. When the feeding practices were studied in breastfed infants, Kuhr and Paneth[97] noted that sugar-water intake in the first 3 days negatively affected the volume of breast milk available on the fourth day. The infants with high glucose intake had higher bilirubins. There does not appear to be a correlation with weight loss and bilirubin level in these studies, although breastfed infants may lose more weight than bottle fed infants.

When production of bilirubin was measured by Stevenson et al.[151] by measuring pulmonary carbon monoxide excretion in both breastfed and bottle fed infants, there was no difference in the amount of bilirubin produced in the two groups.

Sucking behavior of jaundiced newborns. Nutritive sucking was assessed by measurement of rate, duration, and pressure of sucking and by clinical observation in a study by Alexander and Roberts.[7] Milk consumption and duration and pressure of sucking increased over the period from the second to the sixth day, but rate was unaffected by age. Serum bilirubin levels showed no correlation with milk consumption or with sucking. Elevated bilirubin did not impede sucking ability.

Caloric deprivation and starvation. Reduced caloric intake or starvation has been associated with hyperbilirubinemia in adult humans and in many animals. The association with starvation and early neonatal jaundice has been described by Gartner.[60] Gartner and Lee[66] have postulated that starvation may increase bilirubin production, shift bilirubin pools, reduce hepatic bilirubin uptake, diminish hepatic bilirubin conjugation, or increase enteric bilirubin reabsorption. Adequate caloric intake may simply diminish intestinal bilirubin absorption. Infants with intestinal obstruction at birth or in the early weeks of life (pyloric stenosis) are often jaundiced.

Treatment of early hyperbilirubinemia. When 50 jaundiced infants were randomly assigned to phototherapy or discontinuing breastfeeding in a study by Amato et al.,[8] they found both treatments equally successful. The infants under phototherapy were breastfed and given 10% dextrose. Both treatments required approximately 51 hours. Three breast-feeding-treated infants and ten phototherapy infants had rebound of the bilirubin. The authors suggest that discontinuing breastfeeding is better than phototherapy. The amount of stress generated by separation from her infant for phototherapy was measured by urine cortisol levels and compared to levels in mothers who roomed-in with their infants.[48] The separated mothers were more stressed and were more likely to discontinue breastfeeding than those who remained with their infant.[48]

When Maisels and Gifford[113] measured serum bilirubin levels in the newborn and the relationship to breastfeeding, they reported 8 of 10 infants with serum bilirubin >12.9 mg/dl were breastfed. They suggested that rather than use phototherapy to treat the jaundice, the cause, namely, breastfeeding, be treated by temporary cessation of breastfeeding. This approach implies a substance in the milk causing the problem, whereas it is the process of altered nourishment. To truly treat the cause, i.e., failed breastfeeding or inadequate stooling or underfeeding, quite the opposite is recommended. The breastfeeding should be reviewed for frequency, length of suckling, and apparent supply of milk, adjusting the breastfeeding to improve any deficits. If stooling is the problem, the infant should be stimulated to stool. If starvation is the problem, the infant should receive additional calories (formula) while the milk supply is being increased by better breastfeeding techniques. The same would apply to bottle feeding jaundice (i.e., any infant with *idiopathic* jaundice who is being bottle fed and has a bilirubin over 12.9 mg/dl). Stooling, frequency of feeds, and kilocalories would be improved. A management schema for preventing or treating jaundice

---

Management outline for early jaundice while breastfeeding

1. Monitor all infants for initial stooling. Stimulate stool if no stool in 24 hours.
2. Initiate breastfeeding early and frequently. Frequent short feeding more effective than infrequent prolonged, although total time may be the same.
3. Discourage water, dextrose water, or formula supplements.
4. Monitor weight, voidings, stooling in association with breastfeeding pattern.
5. When bilirubin level approaches 15 mg/dl, stimulate stooling, augment feeds, stimulate breast milk production with pumping, and use phototherapy if this aggressive tack fails.
6. There is no evidence that early jaundice is associated with "an abnormality" of the breast milk, so that withdrawing breast milk as a trial is only indicated if jaundice persists >6 days or rises about 15 mg/dl or the mother has a history of previously affected infant.

---

in the breastfed infant is provided in the boxed material. All infants must have the appropriate laboratory studies performed.

Breastmilk jaundice—late-onset breastmilk jaundice or breastmilk jaundice syndrome. Apart from the frequent but low level (usually under 12 mg/dl) hyperbilirubinemia, there is a rare association of breastfeeding with delayed but prolonged hyperbilirubinemia, which, if unchecked, may exceed 20 mg/dl. This has been called variously *breastmilk jaundice, late-onset jaundice,* or *breastmilk jaundice syndrome.*[66] It occurs in 1 in 200 births or less; the numbers are imprecise because not all mothers breastfeed. This is a syndrome associated with the milk of a particular mother and will occur with each pregnancy in varying degrees, depending on each infant's ability to conjugate bilirubin (i.e., a premature sibling might be more severely affected). (Early-onset jaundice is related to the process of breastfeeding, not the milk itself.) It is essential to rule out other causes of prolonged or excessive jaundice, especially hemolytic disease, hypothyroidism, G_6PD deficiency, inherited hepatic glucuronyl transferase deficiency (Gilbert syndrome, etc.), and intestinal obstruction.

The pattern of this jaundice is distinctly different. Normally idiopathic jaundice peaks on the third day and then begins to drop. Breastmilk jaundice, however, becomes apparent or continues to rise after the third day, and bilirubin levels may peak any time from the seventh to the tenth day, with untreated cases being reported to peak as late as the fifteenth day. Values have ranged from 10 to 27 mg/100 ml during this time. There is no correlation with weight loss or gain, and stools are normal.

The syndrome of breastmilk jaundice had been attributed by Arias et al.[10] to a substance in the milk of some mothers that inhibits the hepatic enzyme glucuronyltransferase, preventing the conjugation of bilirubin. The substance has been identified as 5β-pregnane-3α,20β-diol, a breakdown product of progesterone and an isomer of pregnanediol that is not usually found in milk but occurs normally in about 10% of the lactating population. Although this material had also been isolated from the milk and serum of mothers whose infants were jaundiced, this work has not been duplicated. Foliot et al.,[53] on the other hand, showed that pathologic breastmilk from mothers of jaundiced infants will inhibit bromsulphalein (BSP)-Z protein binding only when stored under conditions that also cause the appearance of the capacity to inhibit bilirubin comjugation in vitro, as well as cause the liberation of nonesterified fatty acids. They conclude that the appearance of this inhibitory capacity in vitro seems linked to the lipolytic activity peculiar to pathologic milks.

It has been reported by Luzeau et al.[109,110] that milks with inhibitory activity contain increased concentrations of free fatty acids. These simple forms of fat are presumed to be derived by the enzymatic breakdown of the triglycerides normally present in milk, suggesting a greater lipase activity. Some type of synergistic effect between pregnanediol and free fatty acids may be responsible for the clinical syndrome of breastmilk jaundice.

The role of lipoprotein lipase and bile salt-stimulated lipase in breastmilk jaundice continues under investigation. The role of free fatty acids and the possibility of abnormal lipases is unresolved. The undisputed cause of breastmilk jaundice continues to elude investigators.

As in early jaundice associated with breastfeeding, jaundiced infants at 3 weeks do not produce more bilirubin than their unjaundiced breastfed peers or bottle fed infants.

Gardner and others[64] have suggested that bilirubin reabsorption from the gut may be enhanced by the milk of mothers whose infants are jaundiced. The studies relate 60% reabsorption of bilirubin in the presence of this milk when reabsorption is usually close to zero. This abnormal milk also inhibited hepatic glucuronyl transferase and contained free fatty acids tenfold greater than normal milks. Gardner speculates that these three abnormal properties may enhance enterohepatic circulation of bilirubin with this increased load of bilirubin exceeding the capacity of the liver.

Diagnosis depends on circumstantial evidence, since there is no easy, rapid laboratory test. All other causes, including infection, should be ruled out in the usual manner and a thorough history taken, including medications and family history. If the mother has nursed other infants, were they jaundiced? Usually 70% of the previous children of a given mother whose infant has breastmilk jaundice have been jaundiced. The difference may be related to the greater maturity of the liver of a given infant who then is able to handle the increased demands on the glucuronyltransferase system. To establish the diagnosis firmly, and this is necessary when the bilirubin level is above 15 mg/100 ml for more than 24 hours, a bilirubin reading should be obtained 2 hours after a breastfeeding and then breastfeeding discontinued for at least 12 hours.[63] The infant must be fed fluids and calories. In some cases, a mother of a nonjaundiced infant is available to nurse the child or provide breastmilk. The infant's mother should be assisted in pumping her breasts to maintain her supply. Even more urgent is providing the mother with a sympathetic explanation of the problem and the process. After at least 12 hours without mother's milk, the bilirubin level should be measured. If there is a significant drop of more than 2 mg/100 ml it is diagnostic. When the level is below 15 mg/dl the infant can be put to the breast. Bilirubin levels should be obtained to determine if the bilirubin rises again and, if so, how much. In most cases, in the time not breastfeeding the infant's body equilibrates the levels sufficiently, so there is only a slight increase in bilirubin on return to breastfeeding followed by a slow but steady drop. If that is the case, breastfeeding can continue. The bilirubin level should be checked at 10 days and 14 days to be certain the bilirubin is truly clearing.

If the bilirubin has not dropped significantly after 12 hours off the breast, the time off the breast should be extended to 18 to 24 hours, measuring bilirubin levels every 4 to 6 hours. If the bilirubin rises while the infant is off the breast, the cause of jaundice is clearly not the breastmilk; breastfeeding should be resumed and other causes for the jaundice reevaluated.

Phototherapy and breastmilk jaundice. Phototherapy is the use of light energy from a fluorescent light source, which provides light in the white to blue range of the photo spectrum. Fluorescent lamps (20W)—daylight, cool white, or blue—are usually used and provide 420 to 500 nm. A fluorescent bulb provides this light energy for only about 400 hours of its usual 14,000-hour life. Standard lamps are available for use with Plexiglas screens to filter out the small amount of ultraviolet light and protect the infant should the bulb break. They should be at least 16 inches (40 cm) from the unclothed infant. Phototherapy can destroy the retina in 12 hours; thus, protecting the eyes with opaque eye covers is mandatory. Lights should be turned off to collect blood samples. The infant should be fed with the lights and eye covers off to provide a cycle of light and dark for the establishment of normal circadian rhythms. For discussion of the "bronze baby" syndrome, congenital erythropoietic porphyria, and other complications of phototherapy, refer to standard neonatology texts.

If the bilirubin is over 20 mg/dl in a full-term infant (or proportionately lower in a preterm infant), it is a medical emergency to lower the bilirubin promptly; thus the phototherapy should be initiated as soon as the bloodwork is drawn. The relationship to breastfeeding can be established later. Often intravenous fluids are also necessary.

If one is attempting to establish the diagnosis of breastmilk jaundice, phototherapy should not be used while breast milk is being discontinued. If establishing the diagnosis is not necessary (perhaps because of the same diagnosis in older siblings), phototherapy can be used to bring the values to a more acceptable range, that is, under 12 mg/100 ml. When phototherapy is discontinued, it is most important to establish that there is no rebound hyperbilirubinemia. In addition, it will be important to follow the infant at home after discharge through at least 14 days of life or longer if the values are not below 12 mg/100 ml. It should not be assumed that the diagnosis is breastmilk jaundice when breastfeeding has been stopped and phototherapy initiated simultaneously.

Late diagnosis of breastmilk jaundice. With the frequency of early discharge from the hospital, especially for families enjoying the birthing center concept, breastfed infants are often discharged before jaundice for any reason has developed. Since breastmilk jaundice is apt to be delayed to the fourth or fifth day, peaking at 10 to 14 days of age, most normal infants are already home. Occasionally an infant is observed in the pediatrician's office at 10 days of age or older with a bilirubin level over 20 mg/100 ml, often 23 to 25 mg/100 ml. This is a medical emergency. It necessitates the admission of this infant to the hospital for a complete bilirubin workup. It is important to recognize that other causes of hyperbilirubinemia must be ruled out, including blood-type incompatibilities. At this age it is also necessary to rule out biliary obstruction and hepatitis, which might have a high direct or conjugated bilirubin level. An immediate exchange transfusion may be considered or breast milk discontinued and phototherapy used for 4 to 6 hours to establish whether this therapy will be effective in dropping the level sufficiently. It has been our approach to stop breastfeeding and start phototherapy immediately on admission while the diagnostic workup is being performed. (The bilirubin level should be obtained first, but the result need not be reported before initiating therapy if the infant is 7 days or older as long as an exchange transfusion for a blood type incompatibility is not omitted because of the temporary effect of phototherapy.) It usually takes about 4 hours to do the diagnostic workup and prepare compatible blood for an exchange transfusion; thus no time is actually lost. In only one family have we had to do an exchange transfusion in what appeared to be a "breastmilk jaundice" infant; all three siblings required treatment, although the mother was fully lactating and producing abundant milk.

Persistent jaundice in the breastfed infant. It has been acknowledged that breastmilk jaundice is extremely rare, but in that rare case, the infant will be observed to maintain a bilirubin level over 12 mg/100 ml if breastfed. Pediatricians in Rochester have reported that this persists beyond 6 weeks of age and is altered only by giving one or two feedings of formula a day to dilute the effect of the breastmilk or by discontinuing breastfeeding altogether. There are no prospective studies of a 7-year long-range nature to confirm that this is a benign condition. It has been the policy to give enough formula feeding to keep the bilirubin level under 12 mg/100 ml (preferably 10 mg/100 ml), which is actually arbitrarily selected. Occasionally levels will hover at 15 mg/100 ml or higher with some formula feeding, at which point breastfeeding is discontinued (two cases in 5 years). An exchange transfusion might be an alternative to drop the bilirubin significantly and continue breastfeeding. The physician needs to weigh the advantages and risks with the family and document the final care plan. Rechecking the direct bilirubin level and the color of the urine and stools to rule out hepatitis and biliary obstruction is also appropriate. Phenobarbital has not been effective in the postnatal period.

INFANTS WITH PROBLEMS REQUIRING SURGERY
Immediate neonatal period
First arch disorders

Feeding of any sort may be greatly hindered by abnormalities of the jaw, nose, and mouth. A receding chin may be a minor problem and require only positioning the jaw forward. A mother can hook the angle of the jaw with her finger and draw it forward. If the tongue is too large for the jaw, the infant will actually nurse better at the breast than at the bottle because the human nipple fits into the mouth with less bulk. Infants with first arch abnormalities usually require considerable help in feeding. A cleft palate may also be present. It may be necessary to insert semipermanent nasal tubes so that the infant can be fed orally until he is older; definitive surgery may be necessary later. Once the nasal tubes are in place, the infant can manage at the breast. Feeding by any technique, however, is never easy.

Cleft lip

A solitary cleft lip is usually repaired in the first few weeks of life. Prior to surgery the infant will need some help, but he can nurse at the breast if a seal around the areola can be developed. Actually the breast may fill the defect, and suckling will go well. Mother may be able to put her thumb in the cleft to create a seal as she holds the breast to the infant's mouth. It is important to encourage the infant to suck to strengthen the tongue and jaw muscles. If all else fails, a breast shield can be tried, affixing a special cleft lip nipple to the shield.

The mother may have to express or pump milk and offer it by dropper or other means if sucking is ineffective. The pediatrician, plastic surgeon, and parents should work together as a team from the time of birth to determine a coordinated plan of treatment. Some surgeons have special protocols before and after surgery to assure optimal healing. It is important to make all plans for feeding around the surgical plan. There are reports in the literature of individual mothers' experiences nursing infants with lip defects. The major caution in sharing these experiences is to consider that the supportive surgical approach may differ from those reported in the cases in the literature.[84]

Cleft palate

The prognosis for successful feeding of an infant with a cleft palate depends on the size and position of the defect (soft palate, hard palate) as well as the associated lesions. Lubit[107] recommends the application of an orthopedic appliance to the neonatal maxilla to close the gap, thus aiding nursing, stimulating orofacial development, developing the palatal shelves, preventing tongue distortions, preventing nasal septum irritation, and decreasing the number of ear infections. This will aid the plastic surgeon and help the mother psychologically as well. Lubit further relates that a cleft involving the secondary palate can interfere with normal nursing. For the infant to suckle, the nose must be sealed off from the mouth, creating a negative pressure in the oral cavity. The milk may also run out the nose. The absence of the palatal tissue can prevent expulsion of milk from the nipple. The orthopedic appliance prosthetically restores the anatomy of the palate, permitting normal suckling.

Since the purpose of the negative pressure in the mouth is to hold the nipple and areola in place and not to extract milk from the breast, a seal is needed to keep the pressure. One mother was able to perform the positioning task by holding the breast to her infant's mouth firmly between two fingers, as in Fig. 8-10. The infant was then able to milk the areola and nipple with the tongue pressing it against the roof of the mouth, even with the cleft. The breast had to be held in position much as a bottle would be held throughout the feeding.[69]

In assessing 143 infants with cleft lip and palate over a five-year period, Clarren and colleagues[36] found that by assessing the infant's ability to generate negative intraoral pressure and to move the tongue against the nipple, they could identify effective feeding techniques. They summarized these findings in relation to the possibility of breastfeeding (Table 14-10). They point out that normal children with a cleft can swallow normally. A defect in the bony structure of the palate, however, creates a hole that is difficult to plug; thus these children are harder to feed. The authors point out that problems with intraoral muscular movements are associated with bilateral cleft lip, which causes severe anterior projection of the premaxilla that precludes stabilizing the nipple; and with wide palatal clefts that offer no back guard for tongue movements and retroplaced tongues that cannot compress the nipple effectively. When there are neurologic problems causing dysrhythmic tongue movements or a weak tongue or grinding of the gum on the nipple, it is more than a simple anatomic problem and is usually part of a syndrome such as first arch syndrome. These children usually have swallowing problems as well (such as Pierre Robin syndrome).

Feeding procedures for each infant vary. Early assessment of the infant and the mother can usually lead to successful feeding within 1 to 2 days. The infant should not go hungry, nor should mother spend hours struggling with a system that is not successful for this child. The lactation supplementer can be very helpful, since mother can control the flow by squeezing the reservoir, and the infant can have some suckling experience, which will strengthen the oral structure and avoid the trauma of invasive devices. Mother may need to pump to increase her milk supply.

A program of early repair in breastfeeding infants with cleft lip is reported by Weatherley-White and colleagues.[164] Repair has been initiated earlier and earlier, but these authors present 100 consecutive repairs: 51 were older than 3 weeks, and 49 were younger, of whom 26 were operated on at a week or less of age. There was no increase in complication rate and no increase in need for revision of repair. Sixty mothers were offered the opportunity

Table 14-10. Assessment of sucking and feeding techniques for infants with clefts of lip and palate

	Assessment*		
Condition	**Generation of negative pressure**	**Ability to make mechanical movements**	**Feeding techniques**
Cleft lip and palate	−	+ / −	Breast feeding unlikely Deliver milk into the mouth
Cleft palate only	+ / −	+	Breast feeding sometimes succeeds Soft artificial nipples with large openings effective May need delivery of milk into the mouth
Cleft of soft palate	+ / −	+	Breast feeding or normal bottle feeding usually works well Nipple shape may make functional difference
Robin malformation sequence	+ / −	−	Breast feeding unlikely Nipple position critical Many need delivery of milk into the mouth
Cleft lip only	+ / −	+	Breast feeding works well Artificial nipple with large base works well

From Clarren SK, Anderson B, and Wolf LS: Cleft Palate J 24:244, 1987.
*+ = present; − = absent; + / − = partial.

to breastfeed immediately postoperatively; 38 began within hours. Of these, 16 breastfed over 6 weeks, 22 converted by 6 weeks, and 22 were fed by cup or syringe. Breastfed infants gained more weight, and hospital stay was a day shorter.

Similar experience with early surgery and breastfeeding is confirmed by Fisher,[52] who reports performing reconstructive surgery in the Third World, where breastfeeding is undisputed and is very successful. He also reports greater success rate with breastfeeding but notes it requires the conviction not only of the surgeon and pediatrician but also of the nurse, nutritionist, mother, and grandmother. It takes all these for success, but it takes only one for failure.

It has been noted in this chapter that breastfed infants have fewer bouts with otitis media, which has been attributed to the position of the infant while feeding at the breast as well as the anti-infective properties of the milk. It is certainly an important consideration in infants with cleft palates, who have been identified as having more ear infections in general than other infants.

Children with cleft palates may also fail to thrive, not only as a function of their feeding difficulty but also because there may be an underlying increased metabolic need. In a study of 37 children with cleft palates and no other anomalies it was seen that the median birthweight was at the thirtieth percentile.[19] By 1 to 2 months, weights had dropped to the twentieth percentile and did not recover to the thirtieth until 6 months.

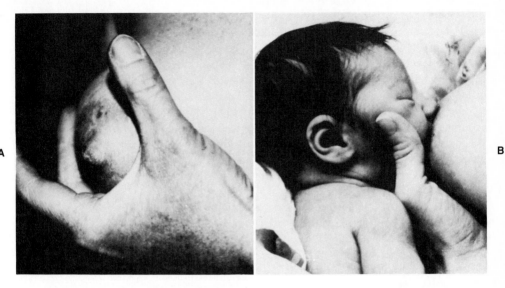

A   B

Fig. 14-4.   Dancer hold. **A,** Illustrates hand position of Mother. **B,** Infant in position
at the breast with support. (From McBride MC and Danner SC: Clin Perinatol 14:109,
1987.)

Feeding infants with oral defects requires extra effort. Each infant is slightly different.
Usually mothers learn to feed their own infants more effectively, even when bottle feeding,
than the skilled professional can. This amplifies the fact that it requires a special patience
and knack. Breastfeeding can be successful. Infants with cleft lip or palate should be
managed as normal infants. Cupping of the infant's jaw and filling the defect with the
mother's thumb while supporting the breast in place for suckling will allow effective
breastfeeding in the infant with cleft lip. This has been referred to as the "dancer hold"[115]
(Fig. 14-4). The infant should be brought to the mother to feed and for rooming-in, as
with any infant. Reinforcing the fact that the infant is normal and merely needs some
reconstructive surgery is important in helping the parents adjust. Here parent-to-parent
programs are most helpful.

Intestinal tract disorders

Infants with anomalies of the gastrointestinal tract that cause obstruction develop
symptoms that depend on the location of the problem in the intestinal tract.

Tracheoesophageal fistula. Tracheoesophageal (T-E) fistula is apparent early and,
depending on the exact anatomy of the lesions, shows respiratory symptoms and signs of
obstruction. This is a surgical emergency. If no feedings have been given or no milk has
been aspirated, surgery can be done as soon as possible. If pneumonia develops, the course
is protracted and the infant may have to be maintained on peripheral venous alimentation
until surgery can be done and healing takes place.

A mother who wishes to breastfeed an infant with a T-E fistula can manually express
milk or pump, saving all samples in the freezer until the infant can take oral milk feedings.
If the infant has a gastrostomy tube in place, small feedings may be started fairly early
postoperatively, and human milk is ideal if available because of its easy digestibility and

anti-infective properties. If there is initially a need to partially supplement the milk with intravenous fluids, the fluids can be calculated to make up the difference between needs and nutrients supplied by breast milk taken by tube. As nutrition progresses, if supply does not keep up with requirements, feedings can be supplemented with other nutrients. When ready for oral feedings, a full-term or large premature infant can nurse at the breast. Unless the mother is able to spend most of the day and night at the hospital, the infant will have to receive bottle feedings as well. If the mother has been able to store up enough milk, the infant may be able to fulfill his needs from breast milk. Once the infant is discharged and begins to nurse at the breast every feeding for a few days, the supply will increase immediately. If there is concern for nutritional lag between needs and production, the lactation supplementer device can be used briefly to stimulate the breast without starving and exhausting the infant (Chapter 17).

Pyloric stenosis. Pyloric stenosis occurs in about 2 to 5/1000 live births. There is a family tendency, but the disease is more common in first-born males. Usually it occurs between the second and sixth weeks of life, although it can occur anytime after birth. Vomiting is characteristic. It is intermittent at first and progresses to include every feeding and is often projectile. These infants are eager feeders and go back for more milk until the weight loss and dehydration make them anxious and irritable.

Large epidemiologic studies published in recent years have failed to show a relationship between pyloric stenosis and breastfeeding. Although pyloric stenosis and breastfeeding have both increased in the last decades, there does not appear to be a relationship. The study in western Australia links LBW, short gestational age, and paternal family history.[86] In Atlanta, the rates were unchanged, but the victims are white male, larger birthweight, upper class, and the infants are most likely to be breastfed in this generation but not in 1970.[99]

In the investigation of vomiting, it is important to keep in mind that overfeeding can cause spitting and vomiting, even projectile vomiting, but it is not associated with weight loss, decreased urine and stools, and dehydration. Therapy consists of pyloromyotomy following correction of the dehydration and associated electrolyte abnormalities. If the procedure is uncomplicated, the infant can go back to the breast in 6 to 8 hours after a trial of water at 4 hours shows the infant is alert and sucking well. The breastfed infant may be discharged in 24 hours if nursing has gone well. If the duodenum is entered at the time of surgery, gastric decompression and intravenous fluids will be necessary and oral feeding delayed several days until signs of healing occur. A breastfed infant may resume nursing earlier than a bottle fed infant returns to formula because of the rapid emptying time of the stomach and the zero curd tension of the milk.

Disorders of the small intestine. Disorders of the small intestine, including duodenal obstruction, malrotation, jejunal obstruction, and duplications, require surgery. Depending on the extent of the lesion, whether the bowel wall is opened, whether bowel segments are removed, and whether there are associated lesions such as annular pancreas, the infant will need postoperative maintenance on intravenous fluids and possibly alimentation. The mother who wishes to breastfeed may or may not have ever nursed the infant, depending on the time of onset of symptoms and their severity. The mother should be counseled about the prognosis and encouraged to manually express and pump if it appears feasible for her to breastfeed eventually. The decision should be made among the parents, surgeon, neonatologist, and pediatrician. Frequently infants with atresias are also small or premature.

Disorders of the colon. Disorders of the colon occur more commonly in full-term infants. Hirschsprung's disease or congenital aganglionic megacolon is the most common lesion. There is usually delayed passage of meconium; however, only 10% to 15% of all children with delayed passage of meconium have Hirschsprung's disease. Constipation and abdominal distention are the most frequent initial symptoms. They may begin during the first few days of life and gradually progress to include bilious vomiting. The clinical picture may be indistinguishable from meconium ileus, ileal atresia, or large bowel obstruction. In any infant with perforation of the colon, ileum, or appendix, Hirschsprung's disease should be considered. The breastfed infant may have milder symptoms and delayed onset of real stress because the breast milk stools are normally loose and seedy and easily passed. The pH and flora of the intestinal tract are also different, leading to less distention. Enterocolitis may occur at any age and is the major cause of death. No data have been located to distinguish the incidence of this complication in breastfed and bottle fed infants, although an argument could be mounted regarding the projected value of sIgA and intestinal flora of the breastfed infant. The treatment depends on the symptoms, x-ray findings, and results of biopsy for the identification of the aganglionic segment. Usually colostomy is done at the time of diagnosis and definitive surgery is done later in the first year of life. Feedings can be resumed as soon as the infant is stable, after the colostomy has healed sufficiently to permit bowel activity. Human milk has the same advantages for early postoperative feeding in this disease as well because of its anti-infective properties and easy digestibility.

Meconium plug syndrome and meconium ileus. Meconium plug syndrome and meconium ileus are less common and less severe in breastfed infants who have received a full measure of colostrum. Colostrum has a cathartic effect and stimulates the passage of meconium. Should either disorder be diagnosed, the infant should continue to nurse in addition to any other treatment.

Necrotizing enterocolitis. Although necrotizing enterocolitis (NEC) has been known for 100 years, only since 1960 has it been identified with any frequency, which suggests an iatrogenic component. It is most common in premature infants and infants compromised by asphyxia. It has been associated with umbilical catheters, exchange transfusions, polycythemia, hyperosmolar feedings, and infection. Its cause is not clear. Work with animals has suggested that human breast milk, specifically colostrum, provides protection against the disease. A good control study to evaluate this in human infants has not been reported. A "dose or two" of human milk may not be enough. Reported cases of NEC have occurred so early in life that no feedings were given. Present regimens of treatment call for cessation of all oral feedings and use of oral and systemic antibiotics, gastric decompression, plasma or blood transfusions, and rigorous monitoring for progression or perforation with serial x-ray studies as well as a septic workup. Further study is necessary to determine cause and possible prevention and the role colostrum or breast milk might play.

The organisms generally associated with NEC are gram-negative organisms such as *Bacteroides, E. coli,* and especially *Klebsiella.* Brown et al.[29] reported that 89% of the infants with NEC had received cow's milk formulas and that gram-negative bacteria and endotoxins were present in the stool. Colonization of breastfed infants with *Klebsiella* does not occur, and *Lactobacillus bifidus* predominates, according to Mata and Urrutia.[114] The uncommon occurrence of NEC in Helsinki, at the University of Helsinki Children's Hospital intensive care nursery, is remarkable. Jelliffe and Jelliffe[92] report that all the premature infants are routinely fed with colostrum and breast milk in Helsinki.

Imperforate anus. Defects in the rectum and anal sphincter are usually diagnosed in the first few hours on physical examination or because a rectal thermometer cannot be passed. When the blind pouch is more generous, diagnosis may depend on the evaluation of failure to stool. Depending on associated lesions and fistulas to bladder or vagina, the surgical decompression can be performed. Until this time, oral feedings are withheld. High lesions require an immediate colostomy with later final repair, whereas low lesions may be repaired at the primary procedure through a perineal approach. Infants may be breastfed as soon as any bowel activity can be permitted, often 2 to 3 days postoperatively.

Gastrointestinal bleeding. The most common cause of vomiting blood or passing blood via the rectum in a breastfed infant is a bleeding nipple in the mother, which may or may not be painful. Any time fresh blood is found in the vomitus or stool of any newborn, the blood should be tested for adult or fetal hemoglobin. If it is adult hemoglobin, it indicates the source is maternal. This is done by a qualitative test, the Apt test. (Mix blood with 2 to 3 ml normal saline solution, add 2 to 3 ml of 10% NaOH [0.25M]. Mix gently. Observe for color change. Fetal hemoglobin is stable in alkali and will remain pink, whereas adult hemoglobin turns brown. Use a known adult sample as a color control.) If the blood is adult hemoglobin in a breastfed infant, the possibility of a cracked and bleeding nipple should be ruled out by inspection of the maternal breast (see Chapter 8).

If the blood is fetal hemoglobin, the differential diagnosis for bleeding in any neonate should be followed. Breastfeeding can be maintained meanwhile, unless a lesion requiring surgery is identified. More than 50% of the cases of gastrointestinal bleeding in the neonate go undiagnosed. Anorectal fissure is uncommon as a cause in breastfed infants. Allergy to human milk is unreported as a cause of intestinal bleeding. The distribution of causes of intestinal bleeding in the neonate, without selection for type of feeding is: idiopathic, 50%; hemorrhagic disorders, 20%; swallowed maternal blood, 10%; anorectal fissures, 10%; intestinal ischemia, 5%; and colitis, 5%.

Congenital dislocation of the hip

When procedures or treatments need to be initiated for an infant previously thought to be normal, breastfeeding may not go smoothly. Using congenital dislocation of the hip as a prototype, Elander[47] looked at overall breastfeeding success. Compared to a randomly chosen control group of 113 infants, the 30 study infants who required the von Rosen splint were less successfully fed. There was, however, a higher incidence of cesarean section in the study group (30% vs 4%). There were equal numbers of primiparas (50% vs 48%). Once breastfeeding was established, the long-range success rate was no different. Mothers were pleased to be able to do something special for their splinted children (i.e., breastfeed). This would suggest that special support and guidance around breastfeeding issues may be needed along with details on how to apply the splint.

Malformations of the central nervous system

Malformations of the central nervous system (CNS) diagnosed at birth include the clinical spectrum from anencephaly and complete craniorachischisis to dermal sinuses. Defects of the spinal column run from complete spinal rachischisis to spina bifida occulta. Those that are incompatible with life or are inoperable present the additional problem to the mother who had planned to breastfeed of coping with her desire to nurse her infant. If the infant is to be given normal newborn care and the mother desires to nurse this infant, breastfeeding should be discussed by the pediatrician and parents together. It has been well demonstrated that parents grieve more physiologically if they have contact with their abnormal infants, but their imaginations are more vicious than some abnormalities of development. The professional's personal bias as to how to deal with this infant should not overshadow the discussion with the parents. If the mother chooses to nurse the infant who has no life expectancy and the infant is to be fed at all by mouth, she should have that choice.

Infants with CNS abnormalities requiring surgery can be breastfed until the operation and postoperatively as soon as oral intake is permitted. In these cases in which the gastrointestinal tract is not involved, breastfeeding can be initiated 6 to 8 hours postoperatively, at the surgeon's discretion. The risk of lung irritation from breast milk is minimal. The rapid emptying time of the stomach and other anti-infective factors serve as advantages in the postoperative course.

Fifth-day fits

Fifth-day fits is a syndrome described in the literature affecting neonates on the fifth day of life and variously associated with toxic, viral, or deficiency states. In a comprehensive study of thousands of births since 1984, a sudden stop to new cases was noted that correlated precisely with the cessation of the habit of giving all infants 10% glucose and then formula to supplement breastfeeding until the seventh day, when they were put completely on the breast.[51] It is not seen in fully breastfed infants.

Surgery or rehospitalization beyond the neonatal period

The infant who requires surgery or rehospitalization can and should be breastfed postoperatively in most cases. The gravity of the surgery and the length of the recovery phase will determine the time necessary for the mother to pump and manually express her milk to keep her supply available. The infant who is hospitalized is already traumatized by the separation, the strange surroundings and people, and the underlying discomfort of the disease process itself. If he is to be fed orally, it should be at the breast as much as possible. If the mother can room-in or the hospital has a care-by-parent ward, this works out well. If obligations to other family members make it impossible for mother to stay around the clock, she can pump her milk and bring it in fresh day by day or frozen if the time interval between visits is longer than a day. Freezing will destroy the cellular content, but that is not a major problem beyond the immediate neonatal period. The infant should not be subjected to the added trauma of being weaned from the breast when he needs the security and intimacy of nursing most unless it is absolutely unavoidable.

The medical profession needs to be aware of this infant and mother and their special needs for support. An opportunity to discuss the breastfeeding aspect of the infant's management should be offered by the physician. The parents should not have to fight for the right to maintain breastfeeding. Plans for pumping and saving milk should be discussed and provided for. If the infant is housed in an open ward or even a room with other infants and their parents without adequate privacy, a separate room should be provided for the mother to nurse or pump her milk. This room should be clean, neat, adequately illuminated, and equipped with a sink for washing hands. Storerooms, broom closets, and staff dressing rooms are inappropriate. If a mechanical pump is to be used, it should be kept clean, sterile, and operable with disposable tubing and attachments that come in contact with the milk.

Arrangements for providing sterile containers for collecting milk and storing it should be discussed (Chapter 19). Occasionally a mother may become so concerned about the adequacy of her milk for her infant that she may nurse far too frequently. Actually her child will need much more nonnutritive cuddling and holding than usual. The physician may need to reassure the mother when pointing this out. The father should also be encouraged to understand all the tubes, bandages, and appliances the infant may have attached. He is an important member of the parenting team and should provide some of the cuddling and soothing as well.

Nursing bottle caries in breastfed infants

The development of rampant dental caries can occur in breastfed infants and is reported in the literature.[28] Usually the children have been nursed for 2 to 3 years, spending long stretches at the breast. One infant had early signs at 9 months, and by 18 months she required full mouth reconstruction.

The physician should be alert to the potential for dental decay when infants nurse frequently, especially through the night. Family history of dental enamel problems is worth investigating. Certainly these children were candidates for fluoride treatment.

REFERENCES

1. Abbassi V and Steinour TA: Successful diagnosis of congenital hypothyroidism in four breast-fed neonates, J Pediatr 97:259, 1980.
2. Abrams SA, Schanler RJ, and Garza C: Bone mineralization in former very low birth weight infants fed either human milk or commercial formula, J Pediatr 112:956, 1988.
3. Adams JA, Hey DJ, and Hall RT: Incidence of hyperbilirubinemia in breast vs formula-fed infants, Clin Pediatr 24:69, 1985.
4. Addy HA: The breast feeding of twins, Environ Child Health 21:231, 1975.
5. Aggett PJ et al: Symptomatic zinc deficiency in a breast-fed preterm infant, Arch Dis Child 55:547, 1980.
6. Ahmed S and Blair AW: Symptomatic zinc deficiency in a breast-fed infant, Arch Dis Child 56:315, 1981.
7. Alexander GS and Roberts SA: Sucking behavior and milk intake in jaundiced neonates, Early Hum Dev 16:73, 1988.
8. Amato M, Howald H, and von Murah G: Interruption of breastfeeding versus photo therapy as treatment of hyperbilirubinemia in full term infants, Helv Paediatr Acta 40:127, 1985.
9. Anderson DM et al: Length of gestation and nutritional composition of human milk, Am J Clin Nutr 37:810, 1983.
10. Arias IM et al: Prolonged neonatal unconjugated hyperbilirubinemia associated with breast feeding and steroid pregnane-3α,20β-diol in maternal milk that inhibits glucuronide formation in vitro, J Clin Invest 43:2037, 1964.
11. Arnon SS: Infant botulism: anticipating the second decade, J Infect Dis 154:201, 1986.
12. Arnon SS: Infant botulism, Ann Rev Med 31:541, 1980.
13. Arnon SS et al: Protective role of human milk against sudden death from infant botulism, J Pediatr 100:568, 1982.
14. Atinmo T and Omololu A: Trace element content of breast milk from mothers of preterm infants in Nigeria, Early Hum Dev 6:309, 1982.
15. Atkinson SA, Anderson GH, and Bryan MH: Human milk: comparison of the nitrogen composition in milk from mothers of premature and full-term infants, Am J Clin Nutr 33:811, 1980.
16. Atkinson SA et al: Macro-mineral content of milk obtained during early lactation from mothers of premature infants, Early Hum Dev 4:5, 1980.
17. Aumonier ME and Cunningham CC: Breast-feeding in infants with Down's syndrome, Child-care Health Dev 9:247, 1983.
18. Auricchio S, Follo D, de Ritis G et al: Does breast feeding protect against the development of clinical symptoms of celiac disease in children? J Pediatr Gastr Nutr 2:428, 1983.
19. Avedian LV and Ruberg RI: Impaired weight gain in cleft palate infants, Cleft Palate J 17:24, 1980.
20. Barfoot RA, McEnery G, Ersser RS et al: Diarrhea due to breast milk: a case of fucose intolerance? Arch Dis Child 63:311, 1988.
21. Bennett FC et al: Vitamin and mineral supplementation in Down's syndrome, Pediatrics 72:707, 1983.
22. Bergstrand O and Hellers G: Breastfeeding during infancy in patients who later develop Crohn's disease, Scand J Gastroenterol 18:903, 1983.

23. Berkowitz CD and Inkelis SH: Bloody nipple discharge in infancy, J Pediatr 103:755, 1983.
24. Bernbaum JC, Pereira GR, Watkins JB et al: Non-nutritive sucking during gavage feeding enhances growth and maturation in premature infants, Pediatrics 71:41, 1983.
25. Billeaud C, Senterre J, and Rigo J: Osmolality of the gastric and duodenal contents in low birth weight infants fed human milk or various formulae, Acta Paediatr Scand 71:799, 1982.
26. Bitman J et al: Comparison of the lipid composition of breast milk from mothers of term and preterm infants, Am J Clin Nutr 38:300, 1983.
27. Bode HH, Vanjonack WJ, and Crawford JD: Mitigation of cretinism by breast feeding, Pediatr Res 11:423, 1977.
28. Brams M and Maloney J: "Nursing bottle caries" in breast-fed children, J Pediatr 103:415, 1983.
29. Brown EG, Ainbender E, and Sweet AY: Effect of feeding stool endotoxins: possible relationship to necrotizing enterocolitis, Pediatr Res 10:352, 1976.
30. Calvert SA, Soltesz G, Jenkins PA et al: Feeding premature infants with human milk or preterm milk formula, Biol Neonate 47:189, 1985.
31. Carey DE, Rowe JC, Goetz CA et al: Growth and phosphorus metabolism in premature infants fed human milk, fortified human milk, or special premature formula, Am J Dis Child 141:511, 1987.
32. Cavell B: Gastric emptying in preterm infants, Acta Paediatr Scand 68:725, 1979.
33. Chandra RK: Immunoglobulin and protein levels in breast milk produced by mothers of preterm infants, Nutr Res 2:27, 1982.
34. Chappell JE, Clandinin MT, Kerney-Volpe C et al: Fatty acid balance studies in premature infants fed human milk or formula: effect of calcium supplementation, J Pediatr 108:439, 1986.
35. Chiba Y, Minagawa T, Mito K et al: Effect of breastfeeding on responses of systemic interferon and virus-specific lymphocyte transformation in infants with respiratory syncytial virus infection, J Med Virol 21:7, 1987.
36. Clarren SK, Anderson B, and Wolf LS: Feeding infants with cleft lip, cleft palate, or cleft lip and palate, Cleft Palate 24:244, 1987.
37. Committee on Nutrition, Academy of Pediatrics: Nutritional needs of low birth weight infants, Pediatrics 75:976, 1985.
38. Committee on Nutrition of the Preterm Infant, European Society of Paediatric Gastroenterology and Nutrition: Nutrition and feeding of preterm infants, Acta Paediatr Scand 76(Suppl):336, 1987.
39. Curtis JA and Bailey JD: Influence of breastfeeding on the clinical features of salt-losing congenital adrenal hyperplasia, Arch Dis Child 58:71, 1983.
40. Dahms BB et al: Breast feeding and serum bilirubin values during the first 4 days of life, J Pediatr 83:1049, 1973.
41. Danziger Y, Pertzelin A, and Mimount M: Transient congenital hypothyroidism after topical iodine in pregnancy and lactation, Arch Dis Child 62:295, 1987.
42. De Carvalho M, Anderson DM, Giangreco A et al: Frequency of milk expression and milk production by mothers of non-nursing premature neonates, Am J Dis Child 139:483, 1985.
43. DeCarvalho M, Klaus M, and Merkatz RB: Frequency of breast-feeding and serum bilirubin concentration, Am J Dis Child 136:737, 1982.
44. De Carvalho M, Robertson S, and Klaus M: Fecal bilirubin excretion and serum bilirubin concentrations in breastfed and bottle fed infants, J Pediatr 107:786, 1985.
45. DeVries LS, Lary S, Whitelaw AG et al: Relationship of serum bilirubin levels and hearing impairment in newborn infants, Early Hum Dev 15:269, 1987.
46. Eckhert CD et al: Zinc binding: a difference between human and bovine milk, Science 195:789, 1977.
46a. Ehrenkranz RA and Ackerman BA: Metoclopramide effect on faltering milk production by mothers of premature infants, Pediatrics 78:614, 1986.
47. Elander G: Breastfeeding of infants diagnosed as having congenital hip joint dislocation and treated in the von Rosen splint, Midwifery 2:147, 1986.
48. Elander G and Lindberg T: Hospital routines in infants with hyperbilirubinemia influence the duration of breastfeeding, Acta Paediatr Scand 75:708, 1986.
49. Ernest AE et al: Guide to breast feeding the infant with PKU, Washington DC, 1980, US Government Printing Office.
50. Evans GW and Johnson PE: Defective prostaglandin synthesis is acrodermatitis enteropathica, Lancet 1:52, 1977.
51. Fabris C, Licata D, Stasiowska B et al: Is type of feeding related to fifth day fits of the newborn? Acta Paediatr Scand 77:162, 1988.
52. Fisher JC: Early repair and breastfeeding for infants with cleft lip, Plastic Reconstruct Surg 79:886, 1987.
53. Foliot A et al: Breast milk jaundice: in vitro inhibition of rat liver bilirubin-uridine diphosphate glucuronyltransferase activity and Z protein-bromosulfophthalein binding by human breast milk, Pediatr Res 10:594, 1976.
54. Fomon SJ, Ziegler EE, and Vazquez HD: Human

milk and the small premature infant, Am J Dis Child 131:463, 1977.

55. Forbes GB: Nutritional adequacy of human breast milk for premature infants. In Lebenthal E, editor: Textbook of gastroenterology and nutrition, New York, 1981, Raven Press.

56. Forbes GB: Human milk and the small baby, Am J Dis Child 136:577, 1982.

57. Forbes GB: Fetal growth and body composition: implications for the premature infant, J Pediatr Gastroenterol Nutr 2(suppl):552, 1983.

58. Ford JE et al: Comparison of the B vitamin composition of milk from mothers of preterm and term babies, Arch Dis Child 58:367, 1983.

59. Forman MR, Graubard BI, Hoffman HJ et al: The PIMA infant study: breastfeeding and gastroenteritis in the first year of life, Am J Epidemiol 119:335, 1984.

60. Gartner LM: Breast milk jaundice. In Maisels MJ, editor: Hyperbilirubinemia in the newborn, Report of the 85th Ross Conference on Pediatric Research, Columbus, Ohio, 1983, Ross Laboratories.

61. Gartner LM: Disorders of bilirubin metabolism. In Oski FA and Naiman JL, editors: Hematologic disorders of the fetus and newborn, Philadelphia, 1972, WB Saunders Co.

62. Gartner LM: Disorders of bilirubin metabolism. In Nathan DG and Oski FA, editors: Hematology of infancy and childhood, ed 3, Philadelphia, 1987, WB Saunders Co.

63. Gartner LM and Arias IM: Temporary discontinuation of breast feeding in infants with jaundice, JAMA 225:532, 1973.

64. Gartner LM and Auerbach KG: Breast milk and breastfeeding jaundice, Acta Pediatr 34:249, 1987.

65. Gartner LM and Lee KS: Effect of starvation and milk feeding on intestinal bilirubin absorption, Pediatr Res 14:498, 1980.

66. Gartner LM and Lee KS: Jaundice and liver disease. In Behrman RE, Driscoll JM Jr, and Seeds AE, editors: Neonatal-perinatal medicine diseases of the fetus and infant, ed 2, St Louis, 1977, The CV Mosby Co.

67. Garza C, Hopkinson J, and Schanler RJ: Human milk banking. In Howell RR, Morriss FH, and Pickering LK, editors: Human milk in infant nutrition and health, Springfield Ill, 1986, Charles C Thomas, Publishers.

68. Goldman AS et al: Effects of prematurity on the immunologic system in human milk, J Pediatr 101:901, 1982.

69. Grady E: Breastfeeding the baby with a cleft of the soft palate: success and its benefits, Clin Pediatr 16:978, 1977.

70. Greco L, Mayer M, Grimaldi M et al: The effect of early feeding on the onset of symptoms in celiac disease, J Pediatr Gastroenterol Nutr 4:52, 1985.

71. Greer FR and McCormick A: Improved bone mineralization and growth in premature infants fed fortified own mother's milk, J Pediatr 112:961, 1988.

72. Greer FR, McCormick A, Kashyap ML et al: Late hypertriglyceridemia in very low birth weight infants fed human milk exclusively, J Pediatr 111:466, 1987.

73. Greer FR and Tsang RC: Calcium, phosphorus, magnesium, and vitamin D requirements for preterm infants. In Tsang RC, editor: Vitamin and mineral requirements for preterm infants, New York, 1985, Marcel Dekker.

74. Gross SJ: Growth and biochemical response of protein infants fed human milk or modified infant formula, N Engl J Med 308:237, 1983.

75. Gross SJ et al: Elevated IgA concentration in milk produced by mothers delivered of preterm infants, J Pediatr 99:389, 1981.

76. Gross SJ et al: Nutritional composition of milk produced by mothers delivering preterm, J Pediatr 96:641, 1980.

77. Gross SJ and Gabriel E: Vitamin E status in preterm infants fed human milk or infant formula, J Pediatr 106:635, 1985.

78. Guerrini P et al: Human milk: relationship of fat content with gestational age, Early Hum Dev 5:187, 1981.

79. Hagelberg S et al: The protein tolerance of very low birth weight infants fed human milk protein enriched mother's milk, Acta Paediatr Scand 71:597, 1982.

80. Hahn HB et al: Thyroid function tests in neonates fed human milk, Am J Dis Child 137:220, 1983.

81. Hansen TWR and Bratlid D: Bilirubin and brain toxicity, Acta Paediatr Scand 75:513, 1986.

82. Haug M, Laubach C, Burke M, and Harzer G: Vitamin E in human milk from mothers of preterm and term infants, J Pediatr Gastroenterol Nutr 6:605, 1987.

83. Heird WC and Anderson TL: Nutritional requirements and methods of feeding low birth weight infants. In Gluck L, editor: Current problems in pediatrics, vol VII, no 8, Chicago, 1977, Year Book Medical Publishers, Inc.

84. Hemmingway L: Breastfeeding a cleft-palate baby, Med J Aust 2:626, 1972.

85. Hibberd CM et al: Variations in the composition of breast milk during the first 5 weeks of lactation: implications for the feeding of preterm infants, Arch Dis Child 57:658, 1982.

86. Hitchcock NE, Gilmour AI, Gracey M et al: Pyloric stenosis in western Australia, 1971-1984, Arch Dis Child 62:512, 1987.

87. Hopkinson JM, Schanler RJ, and Garza C: Milk production by mothers of premature infants, Pediatrics 81:815, 1988.
88. Iwai Y, Takanashi T, Nakao Y et al: Iron status in low birth weight infants on breast and formula feeding, Eur J Pediatr 145:63, 1986.
89. Jain L, Sivieri E, Abbasi S et al: Energetics and mechanics of nutritive sucking in the preterm and term neonate, J Pediatr 111:894, 1987.
90. Järvendää AL: Feeding the low-birth-weight infant. IV. Fat absorption as a function of diet and duodenal bile acids, Pediatrics 72:684, 1983.
91. Järvendää AL et al: preterm infants fed human milk attain intrauterine weight gain, Acta Paediatr Scand 72:239, 1983.
92. Jelliffe DB and Jelliffe EFP: Human milk in the modern world, Oxford, 1976, Oxford University Press.
93. Johnson P and Salisbury DM: Breathing and sucking during feeding in the newborn. In Hofer MA, editor: Ciba Foundation Symposium no 33, Parent-infant interaction, Amsterdam, 1975, Elsevier Scientific Pub. Co.
94. Kennell JH et al: Early neonatal contact: effect on growth, breast feeding and infection in the first year of life, Pediatr Res 10:426, 1976.
95. Kero P and Piekkala P: Factors affecting the occurrence of acute otitis media, Acta Paediatr Scand 76:618, 1987.
96. Khin-Maung-U, Nyunt-Nyunt-Wai, Myo-Khin et al: Effect on clinical outcome of breastfeeding during acute diarrhea, Br Med J 290:587, 1985.
97. Kuhr M and Paneth N: Feeding practices and early neonatal jaundice, J Pediatr Gastroenterol Nutr 1:485, 1982.
98. Lake AM, Whitington PF, and Hamilton SR: Dietary protein-induced colitis in breast-fed infants, J Pediatr 101:906, 1982.
99. Lammer EJ and Edmonds LD: Trends in pyloric stenosis incidence, Atlanta, 1968 to 1982, J Med Genet 24:482, 1987.
100. Lawrence RA: Infant nutrition, Pediatr Rev 5:133, 1983.
101. Lebenthal E and Leung Y-K: The impact of development of the gut on infant nutrition, Pediatr Ann 16:211, 1987.
102. Leonard EL, Trykowski LE, and Kirkpatrick BV: Nutritive sucking in high-risk neonates after perioral stimulation, Phys Ther 60:299, 1980.
103. Letarte J et al: Lack of protective effect of breastfeeding in congenital hypothyroidism: report of 12 cases, Pediatrics 65:703, 1980.
104. Lewis-Jones DI and Reynolds GJ: A suggested role for precolostrum in preterm and sick newborn infants, Acta Paediatr Scand 72:13, 1983.
105. Linn S, Schoenbaum SC, Monson RP et al: Epidemiology of neonatal hyperbilirubinemia, pediatrics 75:770, 1985.
106. Littlewood JM and Crollick AJ: Childhood coeliac disease is disappearing, Lancet 2:1359, 1980.
107. Lubit EC: Cleft palate orthodontics: why, when, how, Am J Orthod 69:562, 1976.
108. Lucas A, Cole TJ, Morley R et al: Factors associated with maternal choice to provide breast milk for low birth weight infants, Arch Dis Child 63:48, 1988.
109. Luzeau R et al: Demonstration of a lipolytic activity in human milk that inhibits the glucuronoconjugation of bilirubin, Biomedicine 21:258, 1974.
110. Luzeau R et al: Activity of lipoprotein lipase in human milk: inhibition of glucuroconjugation of bilirubin, Clin Chim Acta 59:133, 1975.
111. Macaron C: Galactorrhea and neonatal hyperthyroidism, J Pediatr 101:576, 1982.
112. MacFarlane PI and Miller V: Human milk in the management of protracted diarrhea of infancy, Arch Dis Child 59:260, 1984.
113. Maisels MJ and Gifford K: Normal serum bilirubin levels in the newborn and the effect of breastfeeding, Pediatrics 78:837, 1986.
114. Mata LJ and Urrutia JJ: Intestinal colonization of breast fed children in a rural area of low socioeconomic level, Ann NY Acad Sci 93:1976, 1971.
115. McBride MC and Danner SC: Suckling disorders in neurologically impaired infants: assessment and facilitation of breastfeeding, Clin Perinatol 14:109, 1987.
116. McKiernan J and Hull D: The constituents of neonatal milk, Pediatr Res 16:60, 1982.
117. Meberg A, Willgraff S, and Sande HA: High potential for breast feeding among mothers giving birth to pre-term infants, Acta Paediatr Scand 71:661, 1982.
118. Meier P: Bottle- and breast-feeding: effects on transcutaneous oxygen pressure and temperature in preterm infants, Nurs Res 37:36, 1988.
119. Meier P and Anderson GC: Responses of small preterm infants to bottle- and breast-feeding, Maternal Child Nurs 12:97, 1987.
120. Mendelson RA, Anderson GH, and Bryan MH: Zinc, copper and iron content of milk from mothers of preterm and fullterm infants, Early Hum Dev 6:145, 1982.
121. Murphy JF, Neale ML, and Mathews N: Antimicrobial properties of preterm breast milk cells, Arch Dis Child 58:198, 1983.
122. Narayanan I et al: Partial supplementation with expressed breast-milk for prevention of infection in low-birth-weight infants, Lancet 2:561, 1980.

123. Narayanan I, Prakash K, Prabhakar AK et al: A planned prospective evaluation of the anti-infective property of varying quantities of expressed human milk, Acta Paediatr Scand 71:441, 1982.

124. Neifert M and Seacat J: Practical aspects of breastfeeding the premature infant, Perinatol Neonatol 12:24, 1988.

125. Nicoll A, Ginsburg R, and Tripp JH: Supplementary feeding and jaundice newborns, Acta Paediatr Scand 71:759, 1982.

126. Oberkotter LV, Pereira GR, Paul MH et al: Effect of breastfeeding vs formula feeding on circulating thyroxine levels in premature infants, J Pediatr 106:822, 1985.

127. Oski FA: Iron requirements of the premature infant. In Tsang RC, editor: Vitamin and mineral requirements in preterm infants, New York, 1985, Marcel Dekker.

128. Paludetto R, Robertson SS, Hack M et al: Transcutaneous oxygen tension during non-nutritive sucking in preterm infants, Pediatrics 74:539, 1984.

129. Pedersen CB and Zachau-Christiansen B: Otitis media in Greenland children: acute, chronic and secretory otitis media in three to eight year olds, J Otolaryngol 15:332, 1986.

130. Putet G, Rigo J, Salle B et al: Supplementation of pooled human milk with casein hydrolysate: energy and nitrogen balance and weight gain composition in very low birth weight infants, Pediatr Res 21:458, 1987.

131. Reichman B et al: Dietary composition and macronutrient storage in preterm infants, Pediatrics 72:322, 1983.

132. Robinson RJ and Rapoport SI: Binding effect of albumin on uptake of bilirubin by brain, Pediatrics 79:553, 1987.

133. Rönnholm KAR, Perheentupa J, and Siimes MA: Supplementation with human milk protein improves growth of small premature infants fed human milk, Pediatrics 77:649, 1986.

134. Rönnholm KAR, Sipilä I, and Siimes MA: Human milk protein supplementation for the prevention of hypoproteinemia without metabolic imbalance in breast milk-fed, very low-birth-weight infants, J Pediatr 101:243, 1982.

135. Rowe JC et al: Nutritional hypophosphatemic rickets in a premature infant fed breast milk, N Engl J Med 300:293, 1979.

136. Saarinen UM: Prolonged breast feeding as prophylaxis for recurrent otitis media, Acta Paediatr Scand 71:567, 1982.

137. Sack J, Amado O, and Lunenfeld B: Thyroxine concentration in human milk, J Clin Endocrinol Metab 45:171, 1977.

138. Saint L, Maggiore P, and Hartman PE: Yield and nutrient content of milk in eight women breastfeeding twins and one woman breastfeeding triplets, Br J Nutr 56:49, 1986.

139. Savilahti E, Järvenpää AL, and Räihä NCR: Serum immunoglobulins in preterm infants: comparison of human milk and formula feeding, Pediatrics 72:312, 1983.

140. Schanler RJ and Garza C: Plasma amino acid differences in very low birth weight infants fed either human milk or whey-dominant cow milk formula, Pediatr Res 21:301, 1987.

141. Schanler RJ, Garza C, and Nichols BL: Fortified mother's milk for very low birth weight infants: results of growth and nutrient balance studies, J Pediatr 107:437, 1985.

142. Schanler RJ, Garza C, and Smith EO: Fortified mother's milk for very low birth weight infants: results of macro mineral balance studies, J Pediatr 107:767, 1985.

143. Schneider AP: Breast milk jaundice in the newborn, JAMA 255:3270, 1986.

144. Senterre J et al: Effects of vitamin D and phosphorus supplementation on calcium retention in preterm infants fed banked human milk, J Pediatr 103:305, 1983.

145. Shmerling DH: Dietary protein-induced colitis in breast-fed infants, J Pediatr 103:500, 1983.

146. Similä S, Kokkonen J, and Kouvalainen K: Use of lactose-hydrolyzed human milk in congenital lactase deficiency, J Pediatr 101:584, 1982.

147. Sirota L, Nussinovirtch M, Landman J et al. Breast milk jaundice in preterm infants, Clin Pediatr 27:195, 1988.

148. Steichen JJ, Krug-Wispe SK, and Tsang RC: Breastfeeding the low birth weight preterm infant, Clin Perinatol 14:131, 1987.

149. Stein H, Cohen D, Herman AAB et al: Pooled pasteurized breast milk and untreated own mother's milk in the feeding of very low birth weight babies: a randomized controlled trial, J Pediatr Gastroenterol Nutr 5:242, 1986.

150. Stevens FM, Egan-Mitchell B, Cryan E et al: Decreasing incidence of coeliac disease, Arch Dis Child 62:465, 1987.

151. Stevenson DK: Pulmonary excretion of carbon monoxide in human infants as an index of bilirubin production. In Maisels MJ, editor: Hyperbilirubinemia in the newborn, Report of the 85th Ross Conference on Pediatric Research, Columbus Ohio, 1983, Ross Laboratories.

152. Stevenson DK, Yang C, Kerner JA et al: Intestinal flora in the second week of life in hospitalized preterm infants fed stored frozen breast milk or a proprietary formula, Clin Pediatr 24:338, 1985.

153. Sturman JA, Rassin DK, and Gaull GE: A mini review: taurine in development, Life Sci 21:1, 1977.

154. Tatzer E, Schubert MT, Timischi W et al: Discrimination of taste and preference for sweet in premature babies, Early Hum Dev 12:23, 1985.
155. Tikanoja T et al: Plasma amino acids in preterm infants after a feed of human milk or formula, J Pediatr 101:248, 1982.
156. Toms GL et al: Secretion of respiratory syncytial virus inhibitors and antibody in human milk through lactation, J Med Virol 5:351, 1980.
157. Toms GL and Scott R: Respiratory syncytial virus and the infant immune response, Arch Dis Child 62:544, 1987.
158. Troncone R, Scarcella A, Donatiello A et al: Passage of gliadin into human breast milk, Acta Paediatr Scand 76:453, 1987.
159. Tyson JE et al: Growth, metabolic response, and development in very low birth weight infants fed banked human milk or enriched formula. I. Neonatal findings, J Pediatr 103:95, 1983.
160. Udall JN, Dixon M, Newman AP et al: Liver disease in α-antitrypsin deficiency, JAMA 253:2679, 1985.
161. Usowicz AG, Dab SB, Emery JR et al: Does gastric acid protect the preterm infant from bacteria in unheated human milk? Early Hum Dev 16:27, 1988.
162. Varma SK et al: Thyroxine, tri-iodothyronine, and reverse tri-iodothyronine concentrations in human milk, J Pediatr 93:803, 1978.
163. Verronen P: Breastfeeding of low birth weight infants, Acta Paediatr Scand 74:495, 1985.
164. Weatherly-White RCA, Kuehn DP, Mirreh P et al: Early repair and breastfeeding for infants with cleft lip, Plast Reconstruct Surg 79:886, 1987.
165. Whyte RK et al: Energy balance and nitrogen balance in growing low birth weight infants fed human milk or formula, Pediatr Res 17:891, 1983.
166. Wong PWK, Lambert AM, and Komrowe GM: Tyrosinaemia and tyrosinuria in infancy, Dev Med Child Neurol 9:551, 1967.
167. Wong YK and Wood BSB: Breast milk jaundice and oral contraceptives, Br Med J 4:403, 1971.
168. Zimmerman AW et al: Acrodermatitis in breast-fed premature infants: evidence for a defect of mammary gland zinc secretion, Pediatrics 69:176, 1982.

Medical complications of the mother

15

OBSTETRIC COMPLICATIONS
Cesarean section

When delivery takes place by cesarean section, the mother becomes a surgical patient with all the inherent risks and problems. If the section is anticipated because of a previous section, cephalopelvic disproportion, or some other identifiable reason, a mother can prepare herself psychologically for the event and usually tolerates the process better. When the section is unplanned and done during the process of labor, it is psychologically more traumatic, and the mother tends to feel as if she has failed in her female role. In addition to this unexpected disappointment, there may be medical emergencies that also have an impact on the mother's well-being, such as a long hard labor, abruptio placentae, blood loss, toxemia, or infection.

The mother who plans to breastfeed following a cesarean section should be able to do so provided the infant is well enough. The method of delivery makes no significant difference to the timing of the milk coming in or the changes in the concentration of the major milk constituents in the first 7 days postpartum.[60] Depending on the type of anesthesia and the associated circumstances, the mother may feel alert enough to put the infant to breast within the first 12 hours. Mothers frequently nurse in the first hour after the surgery is over.

Bupivacaine is being used for epidural block for cesarean section or for vaginal delivery because it does not show the decrease in muscle tone and strength reported in neonates whose mothers have received lidocaine or mepivacaine.[68,86] There is a rapid distribution of the drug, and elimination appears to be well developed at birth.

Regional anesthesia permits the mother to remain awake, and she may be ready to nurse as soon as the intravenous lines and urinary catheter are all stabilized. The mother will need considerable help from the nursing staff. She should remain flat if she has had a spinal anesthetic to prevent developing a spinal headache. She can turn to one side and offer the nipple by placing the infant on his side and stroking the infant's perioral area with the nipple. If he is a normal full-term infant and has not been depressed by maternal medication, he should do well. If the mother can be turned to the other side, the infant should nurse on both sides. The bedside rails will help the mother turn as well as provide safety for her.

Fluids and medications in the first 48 hours postoperatively should not affect the infant adversely. Pain medication is required usually for 72 hours or so. It is best given immediately after breastfeeding to permit the level to peak before the next feeding. The medication used should be limited to short-acting drugs that the adult eliminates quickly (i.e., within 4 hours) and that the newborn is able to excrete also. Aspirin and acetaminophen are in that category because they are readily excreted by both adult and infant. Codeine is also acceptable (Chapter 11). Low-grade fever is not uncommon and should not interrupt lactation.

There are some very positive factors associated with breastfeeding for the mother who has had a cesarean section. Lactation is advantageous to the postoperative uterus in that the oxytocin production stimulated by suckling will assist in the involution of the uterus. In addition, the traumatized psyche of a mother whose delivery did not occur naturally as planned is more quickly healed when she can demonstrate her maternal capabilities by breastfeeding.

Whether breastfeeding can be introduced early or must await stabilization of medical problems in the mother or infant, it is a reasonable goal for the mother to seek, in most cases. Supportive nursing care will be critical to establishing successful lactation. But none of this can take place unless the physician has carefully assessed the condition of the mother and the infant in light of the advantages and disadvantages of breastfeeding to both.

The management should include the following:

1. A postoperative care plan must include sufficient rest. Most postpartum wards are not scheduled to include adequate rest for postoperative patients.
2. The family must be instructed on the needs for rest at home and assistance with the household chores.
3. The infant should be considered, when possible, in writing medication orders.
4. If the infant cannot be put to breast, arrangements should be made to pump the mother's breast on a regular basis with a quality electric pump at least every 3 hours during waking hours.

Toxemia

Toxemia presents a problem in management anytime it occurs. The clinical onset is insidious and may be accompanied by a variety of subtle symptoms but the diagnosis depends on the presence of hypertension and proteinuria.[15] It usually begins after the thirty-second week of gestation and has been observed to occur 24 to 48 hours or later postpartum. Convulsions, renal disease, and cerebral hemorrhage in the mother are all complications to be prevented by careful management. Because serious toxicity in the mother may necessitate delivery of a premature infant or an infant compromised by a poorly profused placenta or maternal medications, there are a number of contraindications to breastfeeding in the immediate postpartum period. Initial treatment of the preeclamptic patient includes bed rest, preferably lying on her side in a room that is darkened to prevent photic stimuli. Blood pressure and proteinuria are to be carefully watched. Sedation with phenobarbital or diazepam (Valium), salt restriction, and possibly diuretics such as thiazide or furosemide are used. Hydralazine (Apresoline) and methyldopa (Aldomet) may be indicated as well, to bring down the blood pressure. Magnesium sulfate may also be used and is safest for the breastfeeding infant. Many patients recover quickly once the infant and placenta are delivered, requiring only 24 to 48 hours of postpartum sedation. Often the infant is small for gestational age or premature and may require special or intensive care; therefore the decision when to initiate to breastfeeding depends on the infant's condition. If the infant is full term and well, then the breastfeeding is initiated when toxemia precautions are discontinued and when the mother's phenobarbital intake has been tapered off to about 180 mg/day or less, calculating that initially the amount of milk obtained is not so great as to provide a large dose of drug to the infant. Careful observation should be made to be sure the infant is not depressed by the accumulation of phenobarbital, however. Phenobarbital is a drug that can be and is given to newborns for several indications and therefore is of low risk. It is preferable to wait until the other medications can be discontinued, especially the diuretics, hydralazine, and methyldopa.

Once the risk of convulsions is past, some attention can be given to manual expression or pumping even if the infant cannot be nursed yet. If medications are a problem temporarily, the milk will have to be discarded, but the expression of milk will serve to stimulate the breast and initiate lactation. Diminution of stress is a critical factor in toxemia therapy so that anxiety of the mother about being able to nurse must be managed with open discussion of the overall plan and where nursing fits in. On the other hand, the stress of early feedings that do not go well because the infant has been confused by initial bottle feedings may also present a hazard in the course of management of toxemia. The single most important element in every case is communication with the patient about her expectations or needs regarding breastfeeding. The physician's therapeutic management design can put this in appropriate perspective.

Retention of the placenta and lactation failure

Three cases of failure of the onset of lactation were reported by Neifert et al.[75] Although the original references to the association of the placenta with delayed lactation were made at the turn of the century, most reports of retained placenta merely discuss persistent hemorrhage as a recognized symptom. In each of these cases the failure of breast engorgement and leakage of milk was evident from the time of delivery, but the hemorrhage and emergency curettage occurred at 1 week, 3 weeks, and 4 weeks postpartum, respectively. In each case spontaneous milk began immediately postoperatively, after the removal of placental fragments. The authors suggest that failure of lactogenesis may be an early sign of retained placenta that should not be ignored.[75]

Venous thrombosis and pulmonary embolism

Venous thrombosis and pulmonary embolism are the most common serious vascular diseases associated with pregnancy and the postpartum period.[15] Pulmonary embolism has assumed relatively greater importance because of the decline in morbidity and mortality from sepsis and eclampsia. Varicose veins also present more problems during pregnancy than at any other time. These diseases all represent common features in vein physiology as associated with the perinatal period.

The major concerns during lactation, in addition to the well-being of the mother, include the diagnostic procedures that might be necessary to establish the diagnosis and the systemic medications necessary for treatment that could have an impact on the nursing infant via the milk. Accurate diagnosis is urgent and is far more complex than therapy. Besides the health of the mother in this life-threatening state, any program of contraception after childbirth is fundamentally affected by the established diagnosis of thromboembolism. Thus the diagnosis must be accurate.

Diagnosis

Laboratory procedures such as evaluation of arterial blood gases, liver function studies, and fibrin/fibrinogen derivatives are not a problem to nursing. It might be noted that the absence of fibrin split products in plasma and serum virtually excludes the diagnosis of embolism, although their presence does not confirm it. The most definitive diagnosis is made with radioactive scanning procedures and angiography. At present, computed tomography and ultrasound are effective in major arterial aneurysms only. Radioactive materials vary in their half-lives and disappearance time from breast milk. They all appear in breast milk (Chapter 11).

Treatment

Anticoagulant therapy is the treatment of choice for established venous thrombosis with or without embolism. Heparin can be given parenterally, since this large molecule does not cross the placenta or appear in breast milk. This therapy is adequate for the hospitalized patient, in whom constant monitoring of coagulation is possible. Warfarin has been considered the best replacement for heparin, but it is secreted in the breast milk (Chapter 11 and Appendix E). The amount transmitted is miniscule, and it is considered safe to breastfeed while taking warfarin. The prothrombin time should be monitored in the infant and vitamin K given if necessary.

MATERNAL INFECTIONS
Bacterial infections

Bacterial infections due to streptococci, staphylococci, or other transmissible organisms may cause skin lesions, pharyngitis, pneumonia, or endometritis. These should be treated promptly with antibiotics and the infant permitted to breastfeed as soon as a therapeutic level of medications has been established for at least 12 hours. Usually infants who are bottle fed are separated from their mothers longer, since they do not receive the valuable anti-infective properties of human milk. Often the question of isolation from the mother and interruption of feeding at the breast comes when symptoms of fever, pain, or malaise first develop in the mother and the diagnosis is still in question. A clinical judgment must be made as to the organ infected, whether bacteria are being actively extruded from the infected source, and the estimated virulence of the organism. A draining incision that appears to show that the infection is streptococcal in origin suggests early isolation and a conservative approach, whereas a low-grade fever within 24 hours of delivery with no localizing signs might warrant continuing active breastfeeding.*

Staphylococcal infections may be passed back and forth between the mother and infant. Identification of the infection and the etiologic agent is important so that appropriate treatment may be initiated. Not all staphylococci are pathologic, and removing this flora

---

*It should be pointed out that engorgement may be associated with a low-grade fever. The patient should be evaluated as to other possible causes, but if none is identified the probable diagnosis is engorgement. The best treatment is to nurse the infant as often as possible and see that the breasts are gently expressed to assure proper drainage of all alveoli.

may permit growth of real pathogens. A mother and nursing infant with nonepidemic staphylococcal disease under medication need not be separated from each other. They should be isolated from other mothers and infants. Sometimes the best plan when the symptoms are mild is to discharge the nursing couple to prevent spread in the hospital and permit freedom of contact at home, with reasonable precautions (Table 15-1).

Urinary tract infection

Urinary tract infections are the most common of the postpartum bacterial infections. Any apparent infection is of concern because of the risk to the infant. Urinary tract infections, however, are "closed infections" and do not constitute a hazard except when

Table 15-1. Management of infectious disease

Organism	Condition	Isolate from mother
Bacteria	Premature rupture of membranes; longer than 24 hr without fever	
	Full-term infant	No
	Premature infant	No
	Maternal fever greater than 38° C twice, 4 hr apart, 24 hr before to 24 after delivery, or endometriosis; full-term or premature infant	Yes, until mother afebrile 24 hr if not breastfeeding
Salmonella, Shigella		No
Staphylococcus		No
Group B β-streptococcus	Mother with possible cervical culture but otherwise negative obstetrical history	No
	Mother with possible cervical possible cervical culture and obstetrical history of fever, premature rupture of membranes >24 hr, fetal distress, meconium, low Apgar score, any symptoms of prematurity	No
	Infant with surface colonizing	

the infection is due to β-hemolytic streptococci. The mother should be reminded to wash her hands thoroughly before handling the infant. The choice of medication is important when the mother is breastfeeding, since the majority of antibiotics reach the milk in some concentration. The medication should be one that could also be given to the infant, such as penicillin, ampicillin, and gentamicin. Under 1 month postpartum, sulfadiazine and sulfa-containing medications should not be given, since the hazard of interfering with bilirubin binding to albumin is significant. Beyond 1 month of age sulfa drugs are actually given to infants directly. Tetracycline and chloramphenicol should not be used unless the mother's survival is in jeopardy. Forcing fluids and acidifying the urine via the diet are always helpful.

Mother can visit nursery	Mother can breastfeed	Immediate treatment	Contact with pregnant women allowed
Yes	Yes	Observe	Yes
Yes	Yes	Treat with antibiotics	Yes
No, until mother afebrile 24 hr	Yes	Treat with antibiotics	Yes
Yes, if culture negative	Yes, if culture negative	In most cases	Yes
Yes	Yes	Yes	Yes
Yes	Yes		Yes
Yes	Yes, after treatment	Treat with antibiotics	Yes

Continued.

Table 15-1. Management of infectious disease—cont'd

Organism	Condition	Isolate from mother
	Negative history and physical examination	No
	With premature rupture of membrane or maternal infection	No
Group A streptococcus	Mother with infection	Yes
Gonorrhea	Mother with positive smear or culture; infant well	No
	Infant with conjunctivitis	No
Syphilis	Mother with positive VDRL test or clinical disease not treated	Only if mother with second-stage disease or with skin lesions
	Mother treated	No
Tuberculosis	Mother with inactive disease	No
Hepatitis	Mother had in first trimester, well at delivery	No
	Mother with active hepatitis at delivery or in third trimester	No, may room-in after good handwash technique followed
	Mother is chronic carrier	No
Protozoa		
Toxoplasma	Toxoplasmosis	No

Toxic shock syndrome

A postpartum woman developed toxic shock syndrome 22 hours after delivery, and coagulase-positive staphylococcus was recovered from the vagina. Breast milk specimens collected on days 5, 8, and 11 contained staphylococcal enterotoxin. The mother and infant lacked significant antibody in their sera. This case, reported by Vergeront et al.,[98] represents the first isolation of staphylococcal enterotoxin from a body fluid from a patient with toxic shock syndrome.

Mother can visit nursery	Mother can breastfeed	Immediate treatment	Contact with pregnant women allowed
Yes	Yes	Observe	Yes
Yes	Yes	Treat with penicillin	Yes
Not in acute stage	Not in acute stage; after 24 hr treatment	Prophylactic penicillin for 10 days	Yes
Yes, after treatment	Yes, after treatment	Antibiotic to the eyes, once in delivery room and once in nursery	Yes
Yes, after treatment	Yes, after treatment	Penicillin IM or IV, plus chloramphenicol drops topically	Yes
No, if skin lesions; yes, otherwise	Yes	Penicillin IM or IV after workup done; follow-up after discharge	Yes
Yes	Yes		Yes
Yes	Yes	Consider BCG if follow-up in doubt	Yes
Yes	Yes		Yes
No	Yes, after HBIG and Heptavax	HBIG and immunization with Heptavax	Yes
Yes, not kiss other infants	Ask for infectious disease opinion	Immunization	Yes
Yes	Yes		No

Group B β-hemolytic streptococcal infection

Streptococci (GBS) are a significant cause of perinatal infections including maternal endometritis, amnionitis, and urinary tract infections and focal infections in the infant. The neonate is subject to early-onset GBS, which is associated with respiratory distress, apnea, shock, and pneumonia. Late-onset GBS is usually manifest as meningitis or osteomyelitis. All five serotypes are associated with neonatal disease. The colonization rate in postpartum women and newborns varies from 5% to 35%. Transmission in early-onset disease in the neonate occurs in utero. Late onset, after the fourth day of life, is due to person-to-person contact. Penicillin is treatment of choice and may need to be given for 3 weeks depending on manifestations of late-onset disease in the neonate. The mother may be without symptoms. Two cases associated with group B β-hemolytic streptococci in the maternal milk were reported by Schreiner et al.[87] and one by Kenny.[56] It is not clear yet whether the transmission is mother to baby or the reverse. When a breastfed infant becomes infected, it is appropriate to culture the milk, and consider treating the mother as well.

Tuberculous mastitis

Mastitis due to the tuberculous tubercle has occurred in Third World countries; it is usually found in association with tuberculosis of the tonsils in the neonate. With the migration to industrial communities, this should always be kept in mind when mastitis progresses to abscess despite antibiotic therapy.

Gonorrhea

When gonorrhea is specifically diagnosed by identification of bacteria in the cervical smear or culture prior to delivery, antibiotics should be started immediately; the mother may handle and/or feed her infant 24 hours after the initiation of therapy. Because of the occasional occurrence of established infection in the neonate despite use of silver nitrate in the eyes at birth, it is appropriate to isolate the infant from the rest of the nursery population, although the infant need not be isolated from his mother once her treatment has been established. The Credé method of eye prophylaxis may fail because it is improperly done or the infection was established prior to birth because of prolonged ruptured membranes or the development of inclusion conjunctivitis.

Syphilis

Syphilis has increased in incidence in many urban areas and must be considered when a newborn has multisystem disease. In addition to transplacental infection, an infant can contract the disease from lesions on the nipple or breast. Open moist lesions of primary or secondary stages teem with spirochetes. A mother with positive syphilis serum reaction, which indicates a primary infection, should be treated immediately. If there are primary or secondary lesions that could contain the treponeme, the infant should be isolated from the mother as well as from other infants. The infant should have a diagnostic workup for congenital syphilis and treatment instituted when appropriate. If there are lesions around the breast and nipple, nursing is contraindicated until treatment is complete and the lesions are clear. The neonate should be treated with the standard neonatal protocol pending the classic nontreponemal Venereal Disease Research Laboratory (VDRL) slide test.[20]

Chlamydial infections

One of the most frequently sexually transmitted pathogens is *Chlamydia trachomatis,* which causes urethritis and epididymitis in men and cervicitis and salpingitis in women. Infants may be infected during delivery and develop conjunctivitis and pneumonitis. Diagnosis is made by culture and serology. Specific *Chlamydia* colostral IgA was present in the milk of a group of postpartum women who were seropositive.[89] Chlamydial-specific IgA was also found in the milk of five out of six women who had positive vaginal cultures. No data are available on the role milk antibodies play in protection against infection in the infant.

Tuberculosis

Controversy exists around the management of tuberculosis during pregnancy and lactation. All mothers with positive tuberculin test reaction but no radiologic evidence of tuberculosis are considered by Huber[45] to be infected but not diseased. Recent tuberculin conversion, which represents a state of undetermined activity, should be distinguished from well-contained tuberculosis. Dates and results of previous skin tests and recent exposure to active cases are important parts of the history. Because of the hazard that tuberculosis presents to the newborn, careful family studies, including tuberculin skin testing and chest x-ray examinations, should be performed on contacts of both the mother and the infant. Huber[45] states that all mothers with a newly positive skin test and negative chest film should be started on a course of isoniazid at the beginning of the third trimester of pregnancy. Therapy is continued for a year postpartum. If no active cases are identified in the household, no special precautions are indicated to protect the newborn. At one time, however, approximately half the neonates born to tuberculin-positive but bacteriological-negative mothers later became infected with tuberculosis. Since the advent of antituberculous drugs in recent years, however, breastfeeding has been permitted without difficulty in these cases.

When the mother has a positive tuberculin test and a positive chest film, considerable effort should be made to identify the organism in the sputum or gastric washings. If the mother is bacteriologically positive, she should receive therapy of isoniazid (INH), and ethambutol for 18 months or INH and rifampin for 9 months. INH is secreted into breast milk, but no adverse affects are reported. There are no data for rifampin in breast milk, but since it appears in tears, saliva, and urine, which turn red-orange, a change in color of the milk to red-orange would demonstrate its presence. The benefit of ethambutol and rifampin for the therapy of active disease in the mother outweighs the risk to the infant according to the Committee on Infectious Disease of the Academy of Pediatrics.[20] Streptomycin and pyrazinamide should not be used unless they are essential to controlling the disease. If the mother is bacteriologically negative, she should receive isoniazid in the third trimester. Minimum active tuberculosis is defined as parenchymal involvement without cavities. The pregnant woman with minimum active tuberculosis should be hospitalized for evaluation. Sputum sampling and gastric washings should be done and triple treatment begun immediately. It has been shown these patients are no longer infective to others as soon as therapy is initiated. Therapy should continue for 2 years. It is important to reassure the mother that if she is given triple treatment, there is no reason to believe the newborn will have the disease at birth. The controversy arises on postpartum management and separation of mother and infant.

When maternal pulmonary tuberculosis has been treated for at least a week, and if compliance with regard to maternal therapy is assured, infant and maternal contact can be permitted, provided the infant is receiving INH prophylaxis. The INH prophylaxis (30 mg/kg/day in two doses) is always indicated when the mother has any disease requiring triple therapy, even without any contact. If the mother has been treated during pregnancy and cultures are negative, 10 mg of INH/kg/day is indicated for the infant and no period of separation is necessary.

If it is safe for the mother to be in contact with her infant, then it is safe to breastfeed except for consideration regarding the medications. Since both mother and infant will be taking INH, it would be a matter of assuring that the accumulation in the infant is not excessive because INH does pass into the breast milk. Dosages for infants range from 10 to 20 mg/kg/day. Hepatotoxicity is possible in either the mother or infant, which can be monitored with serial serum glutamic-oxaloacetic transaminase (SGOT) tests. INH is relatively safe for children. Jelliffe and Jelliffe[49] point out that in technically undeveloped countries, maternal pulmonary tuberculosis is not a contraindication to breastfeeding. Active treatment is given the mother, while the infant receives INH or BCG vaccine with an INH-resistant strain. In these countries the risk to the infant of not being breastfed far outweighs any risk of drug-related toxicity. The isolated populations of the American Indian as well as recently landed Southeast Asians and Caribbeans are the chief victims of tuberculosis. In these populations that would greatly benefit from breastfeeding meticulous care must be given to assure that both mother and infant receive proper medication and vaccination against tuberculosis. Newborns and young infants are the most vulnerable group with the highest rate of complication.

Leprosy

Leprosy is not a contraindication to breastfeeding, according to Jelliffe and Jelliffe.[49] The urgency of breastfeeding is recognized in leprosariums, where the infant and mother are treated with diaminodiphenylsulfone by mouth. No mother-infant contact is permitted except to breastfeed.

Listeriosis

Listeriosis has been identified as the infecting organism in neonatal sepsis and meningitis in recent years and can result in neonatal death. *Listeria*, causing abortion, stillbirth, prematurity, and neonatal death, was described in the 1930s under various titles, including argyrophilic septicemia and pseudotuberculosis of the newborn. The early infection frequently is not recognized and is confused with aspiration pneumonia because of the respiratory symptoms. Examination of the meconium, placenta, and maternal lochia may locate the chief sources of the bacteria, since the symptom complex is not pathognomonic. Symptoms in the mother may be flulike or similar to those of infectious mononucleosis. The manifestations in the adult are protean and in the pregnant woman may lead to an early delivery of an infected infant. Otherwise the infection in adults may be mild and unrecognized, except in retrospect.

The outcome of listeriosis in the neonate depends on early and effective antibiotic therapy, since untreated infants usually do not survive over 4 days. Both mother and infant should be treated. At present, ampicillin plus an aminoglycoside is the treatment of choice and should be maintained pending culture sensitivities in the newborn through the fourth week of life. Treatment in the mother should be maintained 6 to 8 days after symptoms have cleared or cultures are negative. If the mother's symptoms were mild and/or brief and she is well postpartum, she can breastfeed as soon as the infant is well enough to be fed. Usually such infants require intravenous fluids and nutrition, at least briefly. Once the mother has had adequate medication to show negative cultures, her colostrum or milk can be expressed and given to the infant. The management of lactation and feeding in listeriosis is conducted supportively as it is in any situation in which the infant is extremely ill. Hospitalization is usually required for 4 weeks.

Bacterial diarrhea

Neonatal diarrhea due to various bacteria, but especially *Escherichia coli*, is best managed by breastfeeding. Diarrhea in the mother due to infection is not a contraindication. Although infections of the gastrointestinal tract are among the principal causes of illness and death in infants in much of the world, death usually does not occur until after 4 months of age because of the incidence of early breastfeeding in other countries. Even when a diagnosis of infectious diarrhea is made in the mother, it is appropriate to treat her with antibiotics that are also safe for the neonate and to start or continue breastfeeding. One should also obtain a culture from the infant although asymptomatic and treat accordingly. If this is a hospital-acquired disease, then the rigors of establishing the source of the outbreak are to be instituted. Epidemiologic investigation and management of cases and contacts should be initiated. A surveillance system should be established for those in the cohort who are already discharged home.

In developing countries where diarrheal disease has significant morbidity and mortality, many mothers have demonstrable breast milk antibodies against *E. coli* and *Vibrio cholerae*. A prospective study to measure the protective value of these antibodies against disease was done by Glass et al.[40] There were no differences in antibody levels in the milk received by infants who became colonized in an epidemic and those who did not. Among those who were colonized, however, the children who developed symptoms had received milk with lower levels of antibodies than the asymptomatic infants. Apparently the antibodies do not prevent colonization but do protect against disease.

Antibodies against *Shigella, Salmonella,* and enteropathogenic *E. coli* have all been found in breast milk. Parenteral vaccination of lactating women in epidemic areas with killed cholera vaccine or with cholera toxoid vaccine have produced a booster effect on specific milk antibody levels.[70]

Viral infections
Rubella

Rubella can produce a variety of effects on the newborn in intrauterine infections from a classic constellation of defects to no apparent effect. Silent infections in the young infant are much more common than symptomatic ones. Prospectively, over 4,000 infants were examined after the 1964 rubella epidemic using virologic and serologic techniques for the detection of infections in the newborn. The overall rate of congenital rubella was in excess of 2% during the epidemic, whereas it is usually 0.1% in endemic years. During the neonatal period 68% of the infected newborns in that study had subclinical infection; 71% of this group of neonates developed evidence of disease in the first 5 years of life. The infant who is shedding virus is contagious; he should be isolated until the presence or absence of infection can be established. The mother's virus is not considered contagious once the placenta is delivered. The infant can be breastfed. Isolation of the infant should not interfere with breastfeeding except for its inherent inconveniences. If the infant is clinically well, the mother and infant can be discharged, even without all the laboratory results reported. At home they can nurse without restriction. Regardless of method of feeding, the family should protect pregnant women from contact with the infant until the rubella status is determined.

Rubella infection in the mother postpartum will be spread to the neonate long before it is identified. If there is breastfeeding, it should be continued. A sick breastfed infant does better when breastfeeding is maintained.

Herpesvirus

Cytomegalovirus. Cytomegalovirus (CMV) is one of four known herpesviruses in the human. In addition to *Herpesvirus hominis* (herpes simplex), *Herpesvirus varicellae* (varicella-zoster, V-Z), and Epstein-Barr virus (EBV), CMV has also been found to have

Table 15-2. Incidence of CMV in human milk of seropositive women

Postpartum day	Number tested	Number positive	Percent positive
1-6 days	37	4	10.8
1-13 weeks	26	13	50.0

From Hayes K: N Engl J Med 287:177, 1972. Reprinted by permission from the *New England Journal of Medicine.*

ultrastructure and physiochemical properties of a herpesvirus. CMV, EBV, and V-Z are believed to be antigenically related on the basis of cross-reactions observed in indirect fluorescent antibody tests. Herpes simplex and V-Z have antigenic similarities in cross-neutralization tests. Two or more subgroups are believed to exist in the CMV group. About 1% of all infants are excreting CMV at birth; however, those infants who are born to mothers having their first infection are at greatest risk for serious congenital infection. Maternal cervical infection is very common. In daycare centers, the prevalence of CMV in urine and saliva of apparently healthy children is high. Seroepidemiologic studies suggest the infection is acquired in early infancy.[20]

Various studies[30,91] have detected that 3% to 28% of pregnant women have CMV in cervical cultures; 4% to 5% have CMV in their urine. CMV is found in the milk of seropositive women. The data on these women with CMV-complement fixing (CF) antibody are shown in Table 15-2.

The time at which the virus gains access to the fetus may be an important determinant in the prognosis. Women who seroconvert early in pregnancy are more apt to have symptomatic infants, whereas infants born to mothers who seroconvert late in pregnancy are born with silent infections. The newborn infant may be exposed to the virus at a time when he has received the passive transfer of antibodies from this mother. The lack of infection in the neonatal period may well be due to this passive and active transfer protection. These data provide evidence that infected mothers who are seropositive can breastfeed their infants safely.

In random study of postpartum women, 39% had CMV in their milk, vaginal secretions, urine, and saliva.[30] Of the infants receiving this milk, 69% developed infections; although there were specific antibodies in the milk, they prevented neither shedding nor transmission. There were, however, no sequelae in any of these infants, although they continued to shed virus. Two preterm infants, however, developed meningitis. The risk to milk-bank recipients is major, since they would not have immunity and are already at high risk for serious disease.[91] It has been observed that many infants are exposed to CMV during the descent through the birth canal because infections of the cervix at birth are not uncommon. This type of exposure is not associated with disease. The presence of CMV in donor milk from milk banks has led most banks to pasteurized milk, although the virus reportedly is destroyed by freezing. The major cause of serious CMV infections is in compromised neonates who receive infected blood or milk.

Herpes simplex. Herpes simplex virus (HSV) infection in the neonatal period is often fatal or severely debilitating. Reviews spanning a 39-year period, including 276 patients, have been reported by Nahmias et al.[74] The mode of transmission has been a critical question in management. Transplacental infections have been diagnosed because of the presence of HSV lesions at birth, recovery of the virus from the placenta or cord blood, demonstration of histologic changes or the virus itself in the placenta, detection of elevated IgM levels in the cord blood, presence of typical congenital malformations, or presence of HSV viremia. Because the risk of exposure of the newborn to individuals has not been fully determined, the question of removing personnel with herpetic lesions or subclinical infections from the nursery is still unsettled.

A report of the combined deliberations of the Committee on the Fetus and Newborn and the Committee on Infectious Disease[19] regarding perinatal HSV infections has recommended that with careful attention to hygiene measures a mother and infant need not be separated when the mother has genital lesions. Breastfeeding is acceptable if there are no herpetic lesions on the breast and the lesions that are present are adequately covered. This precaution of handwashing, clean covering, and no fondling or kissing of the infant pertains at home too until all the lesions are dried.[83]

A case of disseminated herpes simplex type 1 (HSV-1) was reported to have been acquired postnatally in an infant, and the only source of the virus was the mother's milk.[29] The infant survived with significant residual CNS symptoms. Two separate cases of fatal herpes infection has been reported. In one case the infant developed oral lesions and then fulminating disease, and he died on the eighth day.[93] The mother developed lesions of both breasts, which were positive for herpes simplex type 2 (HSV-2), as were the vulva and the cervix cultures and all the infant tissue cultures including the oral lesions. Another fatal case was reported in an infant breastfed from birth.[83] The mother developed a skin sore on the areola of the left breast on the third day. On the fourth day the infant developed lesions in the corner of the mouth and on the chin. The mother had no other lesions. All infant and maternal breast lesions grew HSV-1 with the same profile. Antibody titers in mother and infant were 1:4 and, later, 1:16. A history was obtained of oral breast contact 3 weeks prior to the birth from the father who had a history of recurrent oral-labial herpes.

Two cases of areola lesions diagnosed as being due to herpes, although cultures are not reported, are discussed by Riordan.[85] Both women had extreme pain on nursing. One infant was 5 months old and continued to nurse uneventfully. The second infant was 17 months old and was weaned but remained well. No antibody titers were obtained on either mothers or babies, but it is possible that there was sufficient antibody protection by 5 months of age. It would also be important to know the mother's history of oral and genital lesions. From these cases it cannot be assumed it is safe to breastfeed with active breast lesions.

It is significant that infants with fatal generalized herpes reported in the literature were 3 weeks old or less at the time of onset.[103] It is equally interesting that the presence or absence of antibodies did not correlate with the outcome. Mouth lesions were the most common site, second to skin lesions. In an extensive review of adults, no mention is made of lesions on the breast.[22]

Herpesvirus cultures are easily obtained and the virus grows in a few days; smears of secretions and the cervix are also readily available, as are serum antibody titers. Thus the clinician can obtain a definitive diagnosis when there are suspicious lesions.

Chickenpox. Chickenpox ranks as one of the most communicable diseases, in a class with measles and smallpox. The vaccine is not available for everyone. The incidence is reported at 5 cases/10,000 pregnancies.[105] There is no known reservoir of V-Z. Transfer is believed to be by respiratory droplet; contact infection from the lesions is also possible. In pregnancy, V-Z may be transmitted across the placenta, resulting in congenital or neonatal chickenpox. Most mothers and hospital personnel have had the disease and are not at risk. When chickenpox occurs in pregnancy, it is a highly lethal disease for the mother with death, when it occurs, usually resulting from varicella pneumonia, although there may be a bias of selective reporting.

Perinatal chickenpox

Postnatally acquired chickenpox usually begins at 10 to 28 days of age and is more common than the congenitally acquired form but generally mild. Transmission in neonates is of a low order. Congenital chickenpox by definition occurs in infants less than 10 days of age. The attack rate is about 24% when the mother has the disease within 17 days of delivery. V-Z does not readily cross the placenta. Congenital chickenpox is associated with significant mortality. The case/fatality ratio is only 5%; that is, 95% will either not get the disease or will not die. When the disease occurs more than a week before delivery, antibody titers in maternal and cord blood are the same. When the disease occurs within 4 days of delivery, maternal titers are positive and cord blood tests are negative. The greatest risk of nosocomial chickenpox exists when the mother develops lesions within 6 days of delivery. If the infant has lesions, he should be isolated with his mother and discharged as soon as his condition permits. This infant should be allowed to breastfeed if the mother is well enough (Table 15-3).

When maternal chickenpox occurs within 6 days of delivery or immediately postpartum and no lesions are present in the neonate, mother and infant should be isolated separately. Only half the infants born to mothers who developed the disease 7 to 15 days before delivery will develop the disease. They should receive zoster immune globulin (ZIG) if available.[20] If no lesions develop by the time the mother is noninfectious, they may be sent home together. When the mother and infant can be together, the child can be breastfed (Table 15-1). Antibodies appear in the milk within 48 hours of the disease onset, so that the infant can be breastfed as soon as it is appropriate for the mother and infant to be together.

Measles

Measles is a highly communicable childhood disease that is more severe in adult life or in the neonatal period. Measles is also a disease that can be prevented by immunization. The disease is contagious from the onset of the rash. Incidence of the disease in pregnancy prior to immunization is low, 0.4/10,000 pregnancies, because most adults are immune.[105] Perinatal measles include transplacental infection as well as disease acquired postnatally by the respiratory route. Measles acquired in the first 10 days of life may be considered transplacental. When measles occur after 14 days, it is due to extrauterine exposure. The course of extrauterine exposure is mild. A case is described in which an infant developed the disease on the fourteenth day of age, and it had a very benign course. The infant had been nursed at the breast by his mother in whom the prodromata of measles occurred on the first day of postpartum. Since secretory antibodies occur within 48 hours of onset, it is possible that the disease was mitigated by the presence of measles-specific IgA in the mother's milk.[58]

As with chickenpox, the incidence of disease postpartum is minimal. The same precautions noted in the discussion of varicella are appropriate. If the mother is exposed just before delivery, mother and infant should be isolated separately, since only half the infants will acquire the disease. If the mother and infant can be isolated together because the infant has the disease, he can be breastfed. Since specific antibodies are present in the milk in 48 hours, the value of the antibodies after that time would outweigh any theoretic risk (Table 15-1). The incidence of measles in the generation just reaching the childbearing years should diminish, since they should have been immunized during childhood. Epidemics still occur where there are pockets of unimmunized individuals.

Table 15-3. Guidelines for preventive measures after exposure to chickenpox in the nursery or maternity ward

Types of exposure or disease	Locale of chickenpox lesions		Disposition
	Mother	Neonate	
A. Siblings at home have chickenpox when neonate and mother are ready for discharge from hospital	No	No	1. Neonate: protective isolation indicated. 2. Mother: with history of previous chickenpox, she may either remain with neonate or return to older children. Without previous history, she should remain with neonate until older siblings are no longer infectious. She may breastfeed.
B. Mother with no history of chickenpox exposed during period 6-20 days antepartum*	No	No	1. Exposed mother and infant: send home at earliest date unless siblings at home have communicable chickenpox. 2. Other mothers and infants: no special managment indicated. 3. Physicians and nurses in delivery room and nursery: no precautions indicated if there is a history of previous chickenpox or zoster. In absence of history, immediate serologic testing† is indicated to determine immune status. Nonimmune personnel should be excluded from patient contact for 20 days.
C. Onset of maternal chickenpox antepartum‡ or postpartum	Yes	Yes	1. Infected mother and infant: isolate together until clinically stable, then send home. May breastfeed. 2. Other mothers and infants: send home at earlier date. ZIG§ or immune serum globulin may be given to exposed neonates. 3. Hospital personnel: same as B-3.
D. Onset of maternal chickenpox antepartum‡ or postpartum	Yes	No	1. Infected mother: isolate until no longer infectious.‡ 2. Infected mother's infant: administer ZIG and isolate separately from mother. Send home with mother if no lesions develop by the time mother is noninfectious. 3. Other mothers and infants: same as C-2. 4. Hospital personnel: same as B-3.
E. Congenital chickenpox	No	Yes	1. Infected infant and its mother: same as C-1. 2. Other mothers and infants: same as C-2. 3. Hospital personnel: same as B-3.

From Young NA: Chickenpox, measles, and mumps. In Remington JS and Klein JO, editors: Infectious disease of fetus and newborn infant, Philadelphia, 1976, WB Saunders Co.

*If exposure occurred less than 6 days antepartum, mother would not be potentially infectious until at least 72 hours postpartum.

†Send serum to virus diagnostic laboratory for determination of complement-fixing (CF) antibodies or, preferably, indirect fluorescent antibodies. Personnel may continue to work for period of 9 days after exposure pending serologic results, since they are not potentially infectious during this period. CF antibodies to V-Z virus >1:2 probably are indicative of immunity in the absence of recent infection caused by herpes simplex virus.

‡Considered noninfectious when no new vesicles have appeared for 72 hours and all lesions have progressed to the stage of crusts.

§ZIG (zoster immune globulin) is available from Center for Disease Control, Atlanta, Georgia, or from regional consultants.

Mumps

Mumps is also an acute generalized communicable disease. It is characterized by parotid gland swelling and involvement of other glands. It is also preventable by immunization. It is less contagious, thus more adults are still susceptible. Incidence in pregnancy is from 0.8 to 10 cases/10,000 pregnancies.[105] Mumps in pregnancy, however, is generally benign. Mumps virus has been isolated on the third postpartum day from the milk of a woman who developed parotitis 2 days antepartum.[57] She did not breastfeed, and her infant did not develop clinical mumps.

Mumps is not a major hazard in newborn nurseries. A mother with the disease should be isolated from the other patients but need not be separated from her infant. Clinically apparent mumps with parotitis during the first year of life tends to be very mild. Although mastitis is a rare complication of mumps in any mature female, no data are available to suggest that the incidence is greater in lactating women. Should mumps occur, breastfeeding should continue because the exposure has already occurred during the prodromata and the IgA in the breast milk may help to mitigate the symptoms in the infants.

Hepatitis

The two major types of hepatitis are hepatitis A virus (HAV) and hepatitis B virus (HBV). HAV is defined as the virus that causes the short incubation form of viral hepatitis; it has also been referred to as infectious hepatitis. Its virus has not yet been isolated, although electron microscopy has identified probable virus particles.

There is no indication for use of immunoglobulin or for withholding breastfeeding in HAV. In the rare circumstance in which the mother is in an active phase of the disease with jaundice, breastfeeding might be postponed temporarily.

HBV is the virus that causes the long-incubation form of viral hepatitis. This form has also been called serum hepatitis and Australian antigen hepatitis. Most of the information available on epidemiology, immunology, mode of transmission, pathogenesis, and clinical disease is about HBV, mainly because its virus has been isolated. HAV and the immune reactions to it are considered distinct from those of HBV.[26]

Transmission

Carrier state in mothers. The chief concern here is the mode of transmission of the virus from mother to infant. The transmission of HBV from mothers whose blood contains hepatitis B surface antigen HBsAg to their infants has been described. This is called vertical transmission. It may occur transplacentally in utero, at the time of delivery, or shortly after delivery. The transmission between any two individuals who may be close contacts is termed horizontal transmission. Work in Taiwan, where hepatitis occurs in 5% to 20% of the people (one of the highest rates in the world), showed that 51 infants of 158 carrier mothers developed antigenemia within 6 months of life. This high frequency has not been observed in other populations. When the mother had a prenatal CF titer in her serum of 1:64 for HBsAg, over 90% of the infants were positive. This appears to be vertical transmission. The high incidence of transmission of HBV in Taiwan and Japan from carrier mothers to infants suggests that the virus passes the placental barrier easily. In other countries, there has been almost no evidence (0% to 8.3%) of transplacental transmission as infants of carrier mothers remain negative.

Care of infants whose mothers are HBsAg positive. The management of newborns whose mothers have active hepatitis B has changed since the availability of human vaccine.[20] At birth in the delivery room, the newborn is given hepatitis B immune globulin (HBIG)

(0.5 ml). Screening during pregnancy all women at risk for hepatitis is therefore imperative. Newborn infants should also receive three doses of 10 μg (0.5 ml, i.e., half the adult dose) of hepatitis vaccine (Heptavax). The first dose is given immediately after delivery with the HBIG in separate syringes in two sites. The second and third doses are given 1 and 6 months later.

The virus has been isolated from breast milk. With the immediate administration of protection, however, the infant may be breastfed in this country and worldwide.[88] Infants breastfed in Taiwan and in England by mothers who are HBsAg positive have had no increased risk of the disease.

There is a high incidence of prematurity (35%) in infants born to mothers with hepatitis. Most infected infants acquire the infection in the birth canal. The long-term effects of perinatal hepatitis are unknown, but in the Third World, the risk of dying from diarrhea before the age of 1 year is so great that breastfeeding is imperative even when the HBIG and Heptavax cannot be given immediately.

Toxoplasmosis

Toxoplasmosis is one of the most common infections of humans throughout the world.[84] The protozoan organism is ubiquitous and is the cause of a variety of illnesses that were previously thought to be due to other agents or unknown causes. The normal host is the cat. The pregnant or lactating woman should not handle kitty litter. It should, however, be disposed of daily, as the oocysts are not infective for the first 48 hours after passage. In humans, prevalence of positive serologic test titers increases with age, indicating past exposure, and there is equal distribution in males and females in the United States, but not in Norway, El Salvador, or Poland. The risk to the fetus is related to the time when the maternal infection occurs. In the last months of pregnancy, the protozoa are most frequently transmitted to the fetus, but the infection is subclinical in the newborn. Early in pregnancy, the transmission to the fetus occurs less often but does result in severe disease. Once the placenta has been infected, it remains so throughout pregnancy. *Toxoplasma gondii* have been isolated from the milk, menstrual fluid, placenta, lochia, amniotic fluid, embryo, and fetal brain in 33% of the subjects in one series.

In various animal models, the toxoplasmas have been transmitted via the milk to the suckling young. They have been isolated from colostrum as well. The newborn animals became asymptomatically infected when nursed by an infected mother when her colostrum contained *T. gondii*.

Transmission during breastfeeding in humans has not been demonstrated. It is possible that unpasteurized cow's milk could be a vehicle of transmission. The human mother, however, would provide appropriate antibodies via her milk. From this information it appears there is no evidence to support depriving the neonate of his mother's milk when the mother is known to be infected with *T. gondii*[84] (Table 15-1).

Vulvovaginitis

Normally during pregnancy there is an increase in cervical and vaginal secretions. Only about 1% of women have symptomatic vulvovaginitis.[20] The normal flora of the vagina at a pH of 4.5 includes predominantly Döderlein's bacilli with some bacteroides, enterococci, group B β-hemolytic streptococci, diphtheroid organisms, or coliform bacteria. Vaginitis is identified when there is inflammation and discharge associated with an alkaline pH and absence of Döderlein's bacilli. The usual pathogens are *Trichomonas vaginalis* and *Candida albicans*.

Monilial vulvovaginitis

Monilial vulvovaginitis is usually bothersome but benign, except during pregnancy and lactation, when it is difficult to treat. The infant may become infected coming through the birth canal. The infection is manifested in the newborn as an oral infection, or thrush. The breastfed infant may transmit the oral infection to the breast and then the infection is passed back and forth unless both mother and infant are adequately treated. *C. albicans,* the causative organism, is a fungus, which thrives on milk in the breast or in the mouth. Early lesions in a newborn who is bottle fed can be treated by rinsing the mouth with water after each feeding so there are no curds on which the fungi can thrive. Water treatment is effective in early mild cases. Sodium bicarbonate should not be recommended because of the risk of hypernatremia. Sodium bicarbonate is not more effective than plain water. Furthermore, solutions mixed at home tend to be supersaturated, which further predisposes the infant to increased sodium intake. When the infant is breastfed, however, it is important to be vigorous with treatment immediately in an effort to avoid a chronic *Candida* infection of the breast. When an infant is harboring *Candida,* the mouth may not show the typical plaques of caseous material, but the infant has a perianal diaper rash instead. *Candida* infection of the breast, because it is bilateral, may be hard to identify. The nipple and aerola may be slightly swollen and violetious in color. The hallmark symptom, however, is exquisite pain, due probably to inflammation of the ducts. In cases resistant to therapy or recurrent, ketoconazole has been recommended as a 2% cream applied to the nipple and areola after each nursing.[46]

The recommended treatment for the infant is rinsing his mouth with water after each feeding and giving 1 ml of nystatin (Mycostatin) suspension carefully by dropper onto the oral lesions. This treatment should be used for 2 weeks, even if the mouth appears to have cleared before the fourteenth day. The major reason for apparent relapse is that therapy is terminated as soon as the caseous plaques seem to disappear. Simultaneous treatment of the mother should include the use of nystatin ointment to both nipple and areola areas after each feeding and appropriate washing each day. The absorbent pads the mother uses in her nursing brassiere should be changed with each feeding and be of the disposable variety. Nystatin plus cortisone in an ointment is often more effective for the breast, not the infant.

If this infant also is given a rubber nipple or uses a pacifier, these should be boiled daily for 20 minutes and discarded after a week of therapy and new ones used. Reseeding can occur from other articles that are placed in the mouth. Properly treated, thrush should not be a cause for weaning from the breast.

Trichomonas vaginalis infection

A common cause of vaginitis is the parasite *T. vaginalis,* which usually causes an asymptomatic infection in both male and female. The parasite is found in 10% to 25% of women in the childbearing years. It is transmitted predominantly by sexual intercourse. Symptoms are common in pregnancy when the infection is more difficult to cure. There is some evidence that growth of the parasite is enhanced by estrogens. It is more difficult to treat in women taking oral contraceptives. The difficulty encountered in lactation stems from the fact that the drugs of choice are contraindicated for the infant during lactation. The organism has not been identified as a particular threat to the neonate who is otherwise healthy. The treatment of choice is metronidazole (Flagyl). Metronidazole, however, does appear in the breast milk with milk levels paralleling serum levels. Severe systemic reactions occur, including headache, nausea, vomiting, and diarrhea, when metronidazole is taken in conjunction with alcohol. Leukopenia and neurologic symptoms have been described in adults who take metronidazole. Concern has been expressed because of the tumorgenicity in laboratory animals. On the other hand, metronidazole is given to children beyond the neonatal period with serious infections with sensitive parasites such as amebiasis. It is recommended, therefore, that the use of metronidazole be limited to those patients in whom local palliative treatment has been inadequate. The peak serum levels occur about 1 hour after oral ingestion. A single 2 g dose, discarding milk for 24 hours, is the recommended treatment. Most of the drug clears in 24 hours. It should be pointed out again that the infant who is solely breastfed is at greater risk than the older infant who is getting other nourishment (Chapter 11). Thus the older infant (over 6 months of age) may not get much drug when doses are carefully timed to avoid peak serum time.

Parasites

Information is emerging on the protective qualities of human milk in the face of parasitic infections in the mother. Parasites have been a serious problem in underdeveloped countries because they cause debilitation in any victim and growth failure in the young. Actually parasitic disease is increasing in industrial countries. *Giardia lamblia* is one of the more frequent infestations and is the cause of some diarrheas and malabsorption syndromes. It has been shown by Gillin[39] that human milk from uninfected donors has antiparasitic activity, and this activity is not from specific antibodies but from lipase enzymatic activity, which acts in the presence of bile salts to destroy the trophozoites as they emerge from their cysts in the intestinal tract.

Giardia have also been reported to appear in mother's milk, and the parasite has been transmitted to newborns via that route. The interrelationships of the parasite and the breastfed host continue to be studied.[39]

MATERNAL PROBLEMS
Pituitary disorders
Persistent lactation due to hyperpituitary activity

After an infant stops breastfeeding it is not unusual for the mother to be able to express milk from the breasts for many weeks, although spontaneous flow ceases in 14 to 21 days. Postlactation milk is partially a function of the length of established lactation. When spontaneous lactation persists for more than 3 months after the infant has stopped nursing, some thought should be given to the cause. The physician should evaluate the mother to make a specific diagnosis. Galactorrhea is characterized by spontaneous milky, multiple-duct, bilateral nipple discharge. It is thought to be due to increased prolactin production, either by the pituitary or be removal of hypothalamic inhibition.[99] Pituitary adenomas are not an uncommon cause. Galactorrhea can occur with normal ovulatory function for 1 or more years postpartum if everything else appears normal. Galactorrhea has been reported to occur in thyrotoxicosis with such frequency (80%) that it should be part of the differential for galactorrhea. Amenorrhea and galactorrhea are also associated with hypothyroidism which is not surprising, since thyrotropin releasing hormone (TRH) is known to be a prolactin-stimulating hormone. More complex disorders are rare and are usually named for the physician who first described them. During pregnancy there is a risk of pituitary tumor expansion, especially with large tumors. In a series of cases of micro-prolactinomas, Ikegami et al.[47] noted no symptom of tumor enlargement in pregnancy. The serum prolactin levels were at or below pregnancy levels postpartum. They felt breastfeeding in these patients diagnosed as having Chiari-Frommel syndrome may actually have occult microadenomas that may become radiologically evident later.[35] Prolactin levels are elevated in about half the patients with galactorrhea, and the prolactin levels show little correlation with the copiousness of milk flow in the patients. Prolactin levels in milk and plasma in women with inappropriate lactation were compared to those of normally lactating women by Adamopoulos and Kapolla.[1] Women with galactorrhea had milk prolactin concentrations similar to nursing mothers, but plasma levels were significantly lower than in lactating women except for pituitary adenoma–related galactorrheas. Levels in milk remain relatively constant, whereas plasma levels vary by time of day and various stimuli.

Some drugs can cause galactorrhea. These include phenothiazines, tricyclic antide-pressants, rauwolfia alkaloids, theophylline, amphetamines, methyldopa, and even some contraceptives. A copper intrauterine (IUD) device was associated with normoprolactinemic galactorrhea in a fertile woman. When the IUD was removed, the secretion stopped, and when it was reinserted, the flow began again.[37]

Chiari-Frommel syndrome

Patients with persistent postpartum or postlactation lactation extending over months or years should be evaluated for Chiari-Frommel syndrome, especially if there are abnormal menses.[35] Often there will have been irregular menses before the pregnancy as well. The galactorrhea will occur whether the mother breastfeeds or does not breastfeed. The clinical manifestations of Chiari-Frommel syndrome are not only persistent lactation with possible breast engorgement, but also oligomenorrhea or amenorrhea, obesity, uterine and ovarian failure, and in some cases hypothyroidism. Spontaneous remission within 5 years occurs in 40% of cases.

Other possible causes of galactorrhea include other hypothalamoadenohypophyseal disorders including infection and trauma, ectopic production of lactogenic hormone as in hypernephroma, or end-organ hypersensitivity to prolactin.

Hyperprolactinemic women do not respond to breast stimulation with a rise in pro-lactin as breastfeeding women do. The hyperprolactinemic patient has no acute response to suckling in her growth hormone levels either, indicating that the central dopaminergic tonus was not altered but shows regulatory dysfunction.[35]

Sheehan's syndrome/hypopituitarism

Sheehan's syndrome is due to postpartum hemorrhage of such severe degree that it leads to pituitary thrombotic infarction and necrosis or other vascular injury to the pituitary including hypoperfusion. It is the only commonly recognized endocrine disorder associated with lactation failure.[1] It occurs in 0.01% to 0.02% of postpartum women. Secretion of pituitary hormones including prolactin is usually deficient, and thus the patient may fail to lactate postpartum; this is considered a key clinical sign of the syndrome. There have been reports of women with Sheehan's syndrome who do lactate, but the diagnosis had to be established by other means. This is believed to be due to the pituitary lactotropes, which have compensatory activity of hypothalamoadenohypophyseal function.[99] Usually cases manifest hyposecretion of all pituitary hormones, with decreased thyroid and adrenal function. They may experience oligomenorrhea or amenorrhea and utero-ovarian atrophy. Often the obstetric crisis that caused the hemorrhage has also required hysterectomy, however, and these findings are obscured.

Prolactin-stimulating drugs such as sulpiride to augment milk yields require investigation, although they have been successful in women delivering prematurely and unable to breastfeed immediately.[6] In a case of presumed Sheehan's syndrome in our service, use of nasal syntocin spray (see Management, Chapter 8) with each feeding for about 2 weeks resulted in a gradual increase in milk production. The mother weaned herself from the drug and the infant from the lactation supplementer over the next 2 weeks, achieving full lactation for 6 months.

Maternal diabetes

While interest in lactation among diabetics increases, clinical research on the topic is lean.[7,13] The laboratory has been the site of considerable study of the disease in the animal model and of the role of insulin.[11,78] The breast is known to be a target organ for insulin, and there are insulin receptors in the mammary gland acini.[64] The mammary gland is an insulin-sensitive tissue where acute changes in insulin concentration result in a rapid alteration in the rate of lipogenesis and the utilization of glucose. Cultures of mammalian breast tissue serve as ideal models for the exploration of insulin activity.[64]

Pregnancy has become a more common event in the well-controlled diabetic, and fertility rates compare with those of nondiabetics. Much has been said about labor and delivery in the diabetic and almost nothing about lactation in these mothers. Textbooks on diabetes often do not mention lactation except those written prior to 1960, perhaps reflecting the national trends away from breastfeeding. A mother, although diabetic, should be offered the same opportunity to breastfeed that is offered to all patients unless her disease has so incapacitated her that any stress is out of the question. When the diabetic infant's progress is uneventful and he can be treated normally, there is no contraindication to breastfeeding. Lactation may be more difficult in diabetic mothers, perhaps as a result of operative delivery or the need to keep the infant in a special care unit for the first few days of life.

During the last stages of pregnancy in normal women, there is a more or less constant excretion of lactose in the urine, with the height reached on the day of delivery. Following delivery, the lactose excretion immediately drops to a low level where it remains for from 2 to 5 days, followed by a sudden large excretion of lactose in the normal woman. Lactosuria in the diabetic may lead to diagnostic confusion. It occurs normally late in pregnancy and in the postpartum period before the infant takes much milk, if the mother does not nurse, or if the supply of milk exceeds the requirement of the infant. Lactose reabsorbed from the breasts is excreted in the urine.

The sparing effect of lactation on the insulin requirement has been observed by many, beginning with Joselin et al.[50] The depression of the level of the blood sugar in normal nursing diabetic women may lead to hypoglycemic symptoms. The simultaneous lactosuria may be misdiagnosed as glucosuria and excessive insulin be taken. The improved tolerance has been explained by the transference of sugar from the blood to the breast for conversion to galactose and lactose. Joselin and colleagues[50] report that the majority of patients at the Joselin Clinic, as well as those at Johns Hopkins Hospital, breastfeed in whole or in part. They recommend the increased administration of the B vitamins for the diabetic during lactation.

Milk composition in diabetes has been studied by Butte et al.[16] in a group of moderately well-controlled insulin-dependent women (Class B, C, and D) at 3 months postpartum. Diabetic women in pregnancy and postpartum have been observed to have low levels of prolactin, placental lactogen, and parathyroid hormone. Whether the observed decreased placental blood flow is associated with diminished mammary blood flow in lactation has not been established.

In this small sample size, there was not significant difference in the values for total nitrogen, lactose, fat, and calories given the normally wide variations found among controls as well. Mineral content was not different except for sodium, which averaged 140 $\mu g/g$ compared with reference milk's 100 $\mu g/g$. The glucose concentrations were significantly higher in the milk of diabetics, and this varied markedly without any pattern throughout the 24-hour collections, although lactose fluctuated little. The mean glucose value was 0.70 ± 0.11 mg/g in diabetics and 0.32 ± 0.08 mg/g in the reference women. During the collections, the diabetics were noted to have periods of hyperglycemia. Milk glucose concentrations have been shown by Neville et al.[76] to increase with blood glucose in lactating women. Total milk volumes were not measured in Butte's study, but the infants were noted to gain weight appropriately.[16] Measurements of glycosylated hemoglobin within a month of the milk collections were noted to be $8.1\% \pm 0.6\%$, i.e., above the normal range of 4.0% to 7.6%. It is appropriate for the clinician to be aware of the slightly elevated sodium levels, especially if mastitis develops. The glucose elevations probably have little clinical significance to the infant because glucose makes up about 0.4% of the total energy content.

Diet for the lactating diabetic

Although it is clearly demonstrated that all lactating mothers have an increased energy requirement, it is critical to the diabetic to identify this need and provide for it in dietary adjustments (Fig. 15-1). The 300 kcal required by the infant initially means at least 500 to 800 additional kcal in the mother's diet. Since the milk is synthesized from maternal stores and substrates, the plasma glucose levels in the lactating diabetic will be lower. The daily maternal insulin requirement is usually much less. The balance is a significant one between the needs of the infant and the energy and nutrition production in the mother. Most postpartum women, including the diabetic, have fat stores developed during pregnancy in preparation by the body for lactation. The diabetic, when balancing diet and insulin, needs to consider that the course of lactation mobilizes these fat stores as substrate for the mammary gland. It has been recommended that the diet include no less than 100 g of carbohydrate and 20 g of protein. This will permit the continued mobilization of fat stores to produce the glucose needed for mother and milk. When a diabetic increases fat metabolism, there is always the risk of ketonemia and ketonuria. This indicates a need for increased kilocalories in both the diabetic and the nondiabetic. With some careful observations of blood and urine sugar levels and anticipatory guidance, lactation can be managed without hypoglycemia or hyperglycemia.

A critical analysis of dietary intake and outcome of lactation in a group of insulin-dependent diabetic women (IDDM) was undertaken by Ferris et al.[32] in three major obstetrical services in Connecticut. Sixteen of the 30 IDDM women chose to breastfeed and 14 to bottle feed (53%), compared with the 57% of the general maternity population at that time. The authors found that the IDDM women who sustained lactation received average diet prescriptions of 31 kcal/kg/day (based on maternal weight at 3 days postpartum) or 35 kcal/kg/day (based on preconceptual weight). The mothers who stopped nursing had received only 25 kcal/kg/day (based on maternal weight at 3 days postpartum)

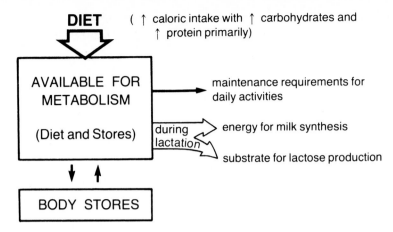

Fig. 15-1. Glucose utilization in lactation. (From Asselin BL and Lawrence RA: Clin Perinatol 14:71, 1987.)

or 31 kcal/kg/day (based on preconceptual weight), which was the same as that for bottle-feeding diabetics. When compared to general recommendations, RDA for lactation is 2000 kcal + 500 kcal extra. Only one mother who continued to nurse and none who had stopped nursing met this. Mothers who lactated successfully actually consumed more than they thought, and those who "failed" consumed less than they thought when it was calculated, which supports the recommendation that IDDM breastfeeding mothers need a knowledgeable dietary counselor as well as other support systems. The weight-loss patterns of these women reinforced this observation. Those women who stopped lactating lost considerably more weight than the successful breastfeeders, the bottle feeders, or the normal controls. Fasting blood sugars were lower (60 mg/dl) in the successful lactators without an increased insulin dosage.

Adjustments to lactation for the diabetic

The mild, or class A, diabetic whose condition can be controlled by diet alone will have to modify her diet to include the increased caloric needs, taking adequate protein in particular. Class A diabetics who have been taught to control the problem in pregnancy by diet often continue this dietary awareness postdelivery so that appropriate counseling for lactation should continue. The mother with insulin-dependent diabetes will usually be able to increase her diet and maintain her insulin level, although some may find insulin requirements will be reduced also. Monitoring blood sugars and acetone will be necessary at first to achieve the correct balance.

Although hypoglycemia does not cause a reduction in lactose in the milk, the phenomenon of hypoglycemia itself will cause increased secretion of epinephrine in insulin shock. The epinephrine will inhibit milk production and the ejection reflex. Acetone signals a need for increased calories and carbohydrate. In addition, elevated acetone can cause increased acetone in the milk itself, which is a stress to the newborn liver. If one merely increases insulin to clear the acetone, it may predispose the patient to hypoglycemia. Each mother will identify the point below which she cannot reduce her insulin dosage without producing acetonuria. While the infant is nursing exclusively at the breast, adjustment is usually smooth. Weaning may present some need for day-to-day adjustment, since the amount of milk taken by the infant varies. Many infants take more one day and less the next, and it is less predictable. If blood sugars cannot be controlled by diet during this time, then insulin will have to be decreased. If the weaning is gradual and continuous, the adjustment will be similar.

Problems among IDDM mothers in the first days after delivery

Fewer infants of mothers with diabetes are put to the breast in the first few days, as noted by Ferris.[32] Most infants of diabetics are admitted to the NICU for 8 hours or more of observation. Not only does this delay breastfeeding, but it also increases the amount of formula and number of rubber nipples taken. The breastfeeding IDDMs breastfed for the first time at 35 + 5 hours, whereas the bottle feeding mothers did so for the first time at 43 + 24 hours! In this study, only two diabetics and no controls were offered a pump. All the mothers who stopped breastfeeding had infants who received a total of 9 oz or more of formula.

Weaning was precipitated in these IDDMs by problems they saw with the baby such as crying, fussing, and problems sucking—not that there was insufficient milk. No IDDM was told by her physician to stop. Control mothers all cited insufficient milk as the cause of weaning. Severity of the disease influenced the decision to bottle feed and to wean early.

Hospital management is critical to successful lactation in diabetics as well.[7] When 42 IDDM mothers who breastfed were followed by Whichelow and Doddridge,[101] they found the most important factor in success was the lapsed time to the first breastfeeding. This, of course, is usually a function of the medical stability of the infant. They were able to initiate a change in hospital policy that minimized separation of infant and mother. Duration of lactation was inversely related to the delay in first suckling.[7]

The insulin requirement at 3 months in Whichelow's study[101] was 43 U daily average compared with 50 U prepregnancy in bottle feeders and 40 U at 3 months compared with 45 U prepregnancy in the breastfeeders. Ferris et al.[32] reported that insulin dosages were not different among breast and bottle feeders, but they were not reported. The subjects in Butte et al.[16] received less insulin while lactating (35 ± 10 U/day compared with 63 ± 14 U/day during pregnancy).

Special features of lactation for the diabetic

Some diabetics enjoy a postpartum remission of their diabetes that may be minimal or complete. The remission may last through lactation; it may last several years. This remission has been attributed to the hormone interactions that affect the hypothalamus and pituitary gland during pregnancy, labor, delivery, and lactation. Many diabetics report a feeling of well-being during lactation.

Diabetics are prone to infection,[13] and therefore mastitis presents a particular problem. With careful anticipatory care, avoidance of fatigue, and antibiotics for at least 10 days when indicated, mastitis should not pose a threat. Monilial infections are more common because of the glucose-rich vaginal secretions, and most diabetic women are alert to the early signs of a fungal vaginitis. Infection of the nipples can also occur due to *C. albicans,* even though the infant does not have obvious thrush. Early specific treatment with nystatin ointment to the breast and nystatin suspension for the infant whenever sore nipples do not respond to the usual nonspecific treatment is recommended. Treatment of both mother and infant simultaneously is necessary or they will reseed each other.

Infants of diabetics present a special problem in breastfeeding, as noted by Lubchenco,[65] because they are often premature, frequently have respiratory distress syndrome and hyperbilirubinemia, and may be poor feeders at first. Hypoglycemia is the immediate problem, and its management may initially preclude dependency on breast milk as the sole source of nourishment. Since less than half do develop problems, many need not be separated from their mothers. For those requiring special or intensive care, lactation may have to be postponed briefly, depending on the infant's status.

Providing an electric breast pump and assistance in pumping is essential if the infant is too ill to be fed. Attention to this detail is important regardless of the reason for separation of the mother and infant.[7]

The hypoglycemia of the infant of a diabetic occurs early and is proportional to the level of hyperglycemia in the mother at the time of delivery. Cord blood sugar and micro sugars at ½ and 1 hour of age will give the curve of glucose disappearance and potential for hypoglycemia. If lactation can be established, the glucose can be managed by breast-feeding, but it must be closely monitored so that intervention can be initiated when necessary. There is also a high incidence of hypocalcemia in infants of diabetic mothers, which is believed to be due to functional hypoparathyroidism since phosphorus and calcitonin levels are normal.[77] The role of magnesium in this balance has not been clearly defined.

Breastfeeding and the onset of diabetes

Several epidemiologic reports[9,34,38] have appeared suggesting that breastfeeding has a protective effect on the onset of diabetes in childhood. Children to the age of 14 years who were studied in western Australia had an incidence of 0.59 diabetics per 1000.[41] No significant trends or associations with illness were made except that breastfeeding beyond 1 week of age was less frequent in diabetics than nondiabetic cohorts. In a study of 95 IDDM children and their nondiabetic siblings and peers, the incidence of breastfeeding was only 18% but comparable in all three groups. Twice as many diabetic children had received soy formula as the other children. In a study of IDDMs in Scandinavian populations, fewer children were breastfed, and those who were breastfed were breastfed for shorter periods of time.[9] The authors suggest that insufficient breastfeeding of genetically susceptible newborn infants may lead to β-cell infection and IDDM in later life. The prevalence of diabetes in black populations throughout Africa is usually considerably lower than in Western countries inversely proportional to the rate of breastfeeding, according to Gill.[38] These interesting observations need the careful scrutiny of the strict epidemiologic protocol before conclusions can be drawn.

Thyroid disease

The thyroid gland is intimately involved with hormone activity of pregnancy. The metabolic and hormonal demands of pregnancy alter the thyroid gland. Conversely, the outcome of pregnancy may be altered by changes in the thyroid gland. The thyroxine-binding globulin increases secondary to the increased estrogens. The normal pregnant woman may be euthyroid, yet there are changes in the basal metabolic rate, radioactive iodine uptake, and thyroid size.

Thyroid disease is four times more common in women than men, and thyroid abnormality is common in pregnancy. The diagnosis is more difficult to make during pregnancy because of problems with the interpretation of thyroid function tests. Treatment must take into account the presence of the fetus once the management decision is made.

Maternal hypothyroidism

It has long been held that hypothyroidism is associated with infertility. There is a low incidence of hypothyroidism during pregnancy. Because of the difficulty in maintaining pregnancy in hypothyroid individuals, the number of women who are truly hypothyroid at delivery is also low. There are women who are maintained on thyroid treatment for one reason or another who do have children. If hypothyroidism is diagnosed, it should be treated with full replacement therapy equivalent to 3 grains of desiccated thyroid daily. The medication should be continued after delivery. The mother should be permitted to breastfeed without question. Previous reports have indicated that thyroid does not appear in human milk. Data from Bode et al.[8] indicate there is measurable thyroid in the milk of normal women. In any event, breastfeeding is not contraindicated. If the mother is truly hypothyroid, particular care should be used to rule out hypothyroidism in the infant, using neonatal screening with thyroxine (T_4) and thyroid-stimulating hormone (TSH) if necessary. Diagnosis can be performed by evaluating blood values and is not a hazard to the nursling.[97]

Hyperthyroidism

The diagnostic procedures and therapeutic management of the mother with possible hyperthyroidism presents some hazards to the breastfed infant. The diagnosis can be made without radioactive material. The combination of an elevated serum T_4 and a normal resin triiodothyronine (T_3) uptake is helpful. These two determinations can be combined to obtain a free T_4 index, which reflects these determinations in a single value. Whether the patient is operated on eventually or not, her thyrotoxicosis must first be medically stabilized.

The treatment includes antithyroid medication with thiourea compounds, which inhibit the synthesis of thyroid hormone by blocking iodination of the tyrosine molecule. Propylthiouracil (PTU) and methimazole (Tapazole) are the treatments of choice for the mother. The major difficulty in their use in pregnancy is that PTU may cause fetal goiter and possibly hypothyroidism. The goiter is thought to be the result of inhibition of fetal thyroid hormone production by PTU with resulting increase in fetal TSH and thyroid gland enlargement. In 41 pregnancies in 30 patients receiving antithyroid medication, five infants developed goiters. Goiter development was not dose related. It has been recommended that the maternal therapy also include desiccated thyroid on the basis that the various components of thyroid metabolism cross the placenta at different rates.[15]

The lactating mother presents a somewhat similar problem. Thiouracil appears in the milk in significant levels and is contraindicated. Methimazone appears in the milk with a milk/plasma (M/P) level of 1. A 40 mg dose of methimazole would yield 70 µg for the infant. Lamberg et al.[61] treated 12 lactating women with methimazole derivative, carbimazole, in doses ranging from 5 to 15 mg daily, which is comparable to 3.3 to 10 mg methimazole. All the infants maintained normal thyroid function studies at 4, 14, and 21 days. Two infants were followed to 3 and 4 months and remained normal. Levels of PTU in milk were reported by Kampmann et al.,[52] who calculated that minimal amounts reach the milk, since the drug is ionized and protein bound. They found no evidence of effect in the infants with careful follow-up with T_4 and TSH measurements. It has been suggested that the infant can be breastfed and monitored biochemically. Microtechniques are available for determining T_3, T_4, and TSH levels, and monitoring should not be a technical problem.[97] Physical examination would reveal bradycardia or other signs of hypothyroidism and goiter. It has also been suggested that the infant may be given 0.125 and 0.25 grain of thyroid daily. Certainly this situation should be under close medical surveillance and continually monitored by microanalysis. The clinical judgment rests with the physician as to whether sufficient medication is reaching the infant. The older infant (over 6 months of age) who is getting other diet such as solids would be at less risk than the newborn, who depends solely on breast milk. Lamberg et al. recommend doses of ≤ 150 mg/day PTU.[61]

When PTU is not an effective drug for the mother, Cooper[21] suggests methimazole or carbimazole in doses ≦10 mg with close monitoring of the infant who is breastfeeding with thyroid function tests biweekly. (Lamberg et al. recommended ≤15 mg/day.)

Cystic fibrosis

Patients with cystic fibrosis are living longer and enjoying more stable lives as diagnostic and therapeutic advances in the disease continue. Reports have appeared indicating that a number of women with cystic fibrosis have become pregnant and have delivered normal infants. A case was reported of such a mother who had high sodium levels (132 and 280 mEq/L) in her milk. It happens that this mother had not been breastfeeding and expressed her milk for the studies only. As pointed out by Alpert and Cormier,[2] milk from involuting breasts is different, and sodium may be closer to serum levels. Since that time, Welch et al.[100] reported one case and Alpert and Cormier[2] reported two cases of successful breastfeeding with maternal cystic fibrosis. Sodium and chloride levels in the milks were normal. These studies demonstrate that mothers with pulmonary and pancreatic disease of cystic fibrosis can breastfeed and their infants do well. It is appropriate, however, to test milk samples occasionally for sodium and chloride.

Hyperlipoproteinemia

The study of a mother with type I hyperlipoproteinemia nursing her second child is reported by Steiner et al.[92] The milk and plasma were carefully analyzed, and it appeared that the deficit of lipoprotein lipase extended to the mammary gland. The milk had low total lipids and bizarre composition of fatty acids. Her milk differed greatly from her plasma triglycerides in comparison to normal mothers, where fatty acid profile in the milk matches the plasma. Low concentrations of essential linoleic (C 18:2) and arachidonic (C 20:4) acids in her milk made it inadequate for her infant.

Galactosemia

The case of a 25-year-old woman who had been diagnosed herself at the age of 3 weeks to have galactosemia is reported by Forbes et al.[33] at the time of her first baby whom she breastfed. The woman had blood transferase activity that hovered from zero to 1.9 units (normal is 18 to 25 U/g hemoglobin). Despite irregular menses, she conceived and delivered a normal female who thrived on breastfeeding exclusively. Solid foods were added at 5 months. The analysis of her milk by Forbes et al.[33] at 4½ weeks postpartum revealed protein 1.42 g/dl, lactose 7.5 g/dl, fat 4.25 g/dl, and calculated energy content 74 kcal/dl. Fatty acid profile was normal except for 18:3, which was low. Macro minerals were all within normal range. Glucose was 26 mg/dl and galactose was <15 mg/dl. The authors point out that since "lactose can be found from uridine diphosphogalactose (by means of epimerase) and glucose (a reaction stimulated by lactalbumin) in the absence of transferase enzyme, one could have predicted that lactose would be present in her milk."

Malignancy and other situations requiring radioactive exposure

The treatment of a lactating women with malignancy may well necessitate the use of radioactive compounds for diagnosis and treatment or the use of antimetabolites. Since the breast is a minor route of excretion for most of these compounds, it is probably inappropriate to continue nursing during such exposure. Although the dose of the material in a single aliquot of milk may be small, the effects are cumulative (Appendix E). There are no long-range studies to indicate the outcome of offspring exposed in utero. In addition, a mother with malignancy should be encouraged to spare all her resources to overcome the disease. Lactation is as draining in such a situation as pregnancy.

Diagnostic or therapeutic measures using radioactive materials are contraindicated in pregnancy and lactation, since they tend to accumulate in the fetoneonatal thyroid and the maternal breast. If radioactive testing is deemed essential before treatment can be carried out, a test dose of ^{131}I can be given and breastfeeding discontinued for 48 hours. The validity of the test during lactation has been questioned because the mammary gland may divert a disproportionate amount of ^{131}I to the milk. The milk should be expressed during the 48-hour period and discarded.[12]

An additional question about the young cancer patient is what additional risk lactation adds to long-range prognosis of the mother. The automatic response tends to be not to become pregnant and, in any event, not to breastfeed. This question was examined by Hornstein et al.,[44] who indicate that "the current data suggest that pregnant women with early breast carcinoma may be treated in the same way as nonpregnant women without affecting the pregnancy." The disease that is detected toward the end of pregnancy may be treated with surgery immediately and then the patient may receive adjuvant therapy if indicated after delivery. Advanced disease should be treated aggressively and the infant delivered and not breastfed. During lactation, the diagnosis of breast carcinoma requires the immediate suppression of lactation by medications other than estrogens. The carcinoma is then treated by standard methods. When a woman has already had a radical mastectomy for breast cancer, she can have subsequent pregnancies, but they should be delayed until the period of greatest risk is over (i.e., at least 3 to 5 years). She may also breastfeed.

The authors report that 7% of fertile women have one or more pregnancies after mastectomy.[51] Seventy percent of these pregnancies have occurred within 5 years after treatment. Women who have pregnancies after potentially curative mastectomy have survival rates of 5 to 10 years—as good or better than those who do not become pregnant. The patients with the best prognosis, however, may be a function of selection because they are healthier and thus able to become pregnant. Uneventful pregnancy does not guarantee cure, although the highest rate of recurrence is in the first 3 years and gradually declines. It is never zero. Metastases to the axilla increase the risk. Recurrence in the chest wall during pregnancy can be treated with local shielded radiation, but anything more extensive requires aggressive intervention. The importance of careful monitoring during pregnancy is obvious. One of the major contributors to a more grave prognosis of the original disease that appears during pregnancy and lactation is not the underlying disease, but the difficulty detecting the lesion during pregnancy and lactation and the reluctance of patient and doctor to make a diagnosis and initiate treatment. The greatest risk of neoplastic growth occurs in the first 20 weeks of pregnancy, when the immune system is suppressed and growth of the mammary tissues is at its peak under the stimulus from estrogen, progesterone, and prolactin levels.[63] The authors give no data on the influence of postmastectomy lactation on long-range survival. There are women who have wished to nurse on the remaining breast. The decision would necessitate consideration of the individual situation. It represents a different risk/benefit ratio than pregnancy itself. Extensive epidemiologic studies of large populations of women do not show any evidence that breastfeeding has any relationship to the overall risk of breast cancer. Epidemiologic data about breastfeeding on the remaining breast are not available.[63] The incidence of cancer in the remaining breast has fueled the question of prophylactic contralateral mastectomy. The women who are at greatest risk for cancer in the second breast are those who have a family history of breast cancer in their mother or sister, who have had onset in childbearing years, or whose original cancer involved multiple lesions in the primary breast. In their discussion of the other breast, Leis and Urban[63] state that if a postmastectomy patient were to become pregnant and deliver, "it would be rare indeed that the patient would allow or the attending physician would condone the use of the remaining breast for nursing." Although some women cherish the remaining breast, most in the experience of Leis and Urban are ashamed of it and keep it hidden.[63]

Lactation following primary radiation therapy for carcinoma of the breast was reported in a major literature search by Burns[14] to have occurred successfully in one patient whose primary lesion was in the tail of Spence. One year after radiation she became pregnant and successfully breastfed. She had less milk on the treated side. Her malignancy had not recurred. Another patient received radiotherapy following biopsy for an invasive duct carcinoma known to be present for a year. She had a week of boost therapy 8 weeks later. She became pregnant a year later, delivering a full-term infant 22 months after the original radiation. She successfully established lactation on the uninvolved side but was unable to obtain any response from the irradiated breast. No comment was made about the radiated breast's response to pregnancy. She weaned her infant at 6 weeks.[27] Two years posttreatment she remains well without evidence of recurrence.

Adult T-cell leukemia

The transmission of adult T-cell leukemia retrovirus (HTLV-1) from mother to child has been demonstrated by Ando et al.[5] in a study of breastfed and bottle fed infants. In 11 of 24 breastfed infants born to HTLV-1 seropositive women, antigen-positive cells were detected in their peripheral blood at 12 months of age. In sharp contrast, only 1 of the 11 bottle fed infants had positive cells, suggesting some other transmission route. The authors concluded that HTLV-1 infections from mother to infant occur mainly via the breast milk and not the placenta or during birth.

Autoimmune thrombocytopenic purpura

Reports are conflicting regarding the passage of antibodies to platelets via the breast milk in mothers with autoimmune thrombocytopenic purpura.[43,71] Laboratory efforts to demonstrate absorption of these antibodies from the breast milk failed. There is a case report of the successful breastfeeding of a severely affected premature infant who had required exchange transfusion and multiple platelet transfusions at birth.[69] There were no relapses on the introduction of maternal milk at 5 days of age. Steroids were discontinued at 2 weeks, and the infant thrived at the breast.

Hypertension

The published literature on the excretion of antihypertensive agents into human milk has been reviewed by White[102] as successful management of hypertension is pharmacologic. Before one considers the drugs involved, it is appropriate to consider that lactation may present some therapeutic advantages. The high levels of prolactin may be physiologically soothing to the mother, and it has been shown in animals that females given high levels of prolactin respond with nesting and mothering behavior. The breast is also an organ of secretion, and a liter or so of fluid is produced a day. In dehydrated women, lactation continues while urine production diminishes. The appropriate use of low-dose diuretics may control the disease whereas high-dose thiazides can cause suppression of lactation. Chlorothiazide, hydrochlorothiazides, and chlorthalidone are minimally excreted in milk (see Chapter 11, Drugs and Appendix E) as is spironolactone and its metabolite canrenone, according to single-dose kinetics.

Propranolol has been widely studied and is probably the safest of the beta blockers during lactation because of its low level in milk compared to other beta blockers, which are weak bases with an average pKa of 9.2 to 9.5, predisposing them to appear in slightly acidic human milk. Methyldopa appears in low amounts in milk, but its direct action on the pituitary to suppress prolactin release presents a theoretical risk of suppressing milk production. The obstetrician should be aware of the potential if lactation is going poorly. Reserpine is a recognized risk to the infant during delivery and postpartum. Other drugs appropriate to hypertension management are discussed in Chapter 11, Drugs.

Renal transplantation

Pregnancy following renal transplant is relatively safe when renal function is adequate before conception and when maintenance immunosuppressive therapy is instituted. Most patients receive azathioprine and prednisone or methylprednisolone. Breastfeeding has been discouraged because of the effect of these medications on the infant especially from the major metabolite of azathioprine, 6-mercaptopurine. The actual levels of these compounds were studied in two patients, one of whom breastfed her infant.[23] Measurements of IgA were also done because of the concept that immunosuppressed women might produce immunoincompetent milk.

The levels of 6-mercaptopurine averaged 3.4 ng/ml in one patient and 18 ng/ml in the other. The therapeutic level is 50 ng/ml with the use of the normal daily dose. The levels of methylprednisolone in the milk (daily dose 6 mg) were at or below the levels measured in normal drug-free controls. The IgA determination in the milk was similar in both transplant and control mothers. The breastfed infant whose mother had a transplant had normal blood cell counts, no increase in infections, and an above-average growth rate.

Glomerular disease and lactation

A high percentage of patients show their first evidence of renal disease probably not because pregnancy precipitates the disease but because it is the first time these young women have had urinalysis and blood pressure studies. In the series of glomerular disease in pregnancy published by Surian et al.,[94] they reported that in most cases the disease is not made worse by pregnancy. A disease with a bad prognosis such as membranoproliferative glomerulonephritis is not worse nor is it made better by pregnancy. When the nonpregnant serum creatine and urea nitrogen levels exceed 3 mg/100 ml and 300 mg/100 ml, respectively, normal pregnancy is uncommon. Lupus nephropathy, however, has a very poor prognosis in pregnancy with considerable fetal loss and morbidity.[28]

Hypertension as a complication influences the obstetric complication rate and the fetal outcome. The infant may be premature, small for gestational age, or both. The option to breastfeed is a matter of the risk-benefit ratio.[7] It involves not only the medical status of the mother but also of the infant and the drugs that must be utilized to keep the mother stable. The obstetrician, nephrologist, and neonatologist will have to determine the appropriateness of breastfeeding on a case-by-case basis.

Breastfeeding and maternal donor renal allografts

With the advent of renal transplants, a whole new mode of investigation with the role of human milk in the host-graft relationship has developed.[7] Large numbers of living maternal lymphocytes are present in human milk. Campbell and colleagues[17] investigated the question of whether exposure of an infant to maternal lymphocytes during breastfeeding would affect the subsequent reactivity of a patient to a maternal donor-related renal transplant. They studied the posttransplant course of 55 patients with a primary maternal donor transplant, 27 of whom were breastfed and 28 of whom were not. The 1-year graft function rate was 82% for those breastfed and 57% for the bottle fed ($p \leq 0.05$) infants. Five-year follow-up did not sustain the statistically significant difference. Paternal donor relationship in a small group of patients did not reveal significant difference. The same group of investigators (Kois et al.[59]) reported the relationship of a history of breastfeeding was associated with improved results in a different patient population (HLA-semi-identical sibling donors). Breastfed patients in whom both donor and recipient were breastfed by the same mother showed dramatic improvements in graft-function rates compared with nonbreastfed counterparts at all intervals studied up to 9 years ($p \leq 0.001$). The authors concluded that the breastfeeding effect is not entirely specific for maternal antigens, since both sibling donor and maternal donor transplantation was improved. They consider a history of being breastfed an important variable in clinically related renal transplantation. Because they were retrospective questionnaires these studies did not take into account the length of time breastfeeding took place, which included all cases "ever breastfed." Although this is potentially important, studies of graft recipients' donors are another means of understanding more about the role of human milk for the human species.

Osteoporosis

Tremendous attention has been focused on osteoporosis in women, particularly following childbirth and lactation. Clearly the demands for calcium and phosphorus during the perinatal period are great, but they can be met by diet with any degree of attention. In addition to dairy products, there are other sources of calcium (Table 15-4). Modern advertising in the wave of the calcium hysteria has suggested women take various medicinal forms of calcium. The incidence of calcium-containing renal calculi has increased as a result.

There is a syndrome of severe osteoporosis associated with pregnancy and lactation. Three cases are reported by Gruber et al.[42] These young women had vertebral fractures and skeletal complications, but most of their studies were normal except for their bony structure. There was no osteomalacia, however. They apparently recovered after lactation ceased and had no residual high-turnover osteoporosis. The author suggests an association with low calcium in the diet.[42]

Crohn's disease and ulcerative colitis

Ulcerative colitis and Crohn's disease (and, recently, rheumatoid arthritis) are treated with salicylazosulphapyridine (SASP). Because of the concern about exposing the fetus

Table 15-4. Calcium content of foods (mg per serving)

100 +	150 +	200 +	250 +
10 Brazil nuts	1 cup ice cream	1 cup beet greens	1 cup almonds
1 med. stalk broccoli	1 cup oysters	1 oz chedder cheese	1 oz cheese (swiss or
1 cup instant Farina	1 cup cooked	1 cup cottage cheese	Parmesan)
3 oz canned herring	rhubarb		1 cup cooked collards
1 cup cooked kale	3 oz canned salmon		1 cup cooked dande-
1 tbsp blackstrap	with bones		lion greens
molasses	1 cup cooked spinach		4 oz self-rising flour
3 tbsp light (regular)			1 cup milk
molasses			3 oz sardines
1 cup cooked navy beans			1 cup cooked turnip
1 cup cooked soybeans			greens
3½ oz soybean curd			
(tofu)			
3½ oz sunflower seeds			
5 tbsp maple syrup			

From Committee on Nutrition: Forbes GB, editor: American Academy of Pediatrics Pediatric nutrition handbook, ed 2, Elk Grove Village Ill, 1985, The Academy.

to sulphisoxazole at the end of pregnancy or during lactation because of the suggestion that sulfas—even at low levels—predispose to kernicterus, this therapy has been discontinued in the third trimester. Recently, it was noted that sulphapyridine (SP), the main split product of SASP, has a low affinity for albumin-binding sites. Esbjorner et al.[31] studied the binding capacities in both mothers and babies and found them low. They measured cord blood levels in the mothers of 11.5 μmol/L and in the infants 20 μmol/L. Follow-up infant blood levels showed a clearance in 70 to 90 hours. Infants who were being breastfed did not increase their levels of SASP or SP. The milk/serum levels for SP were 0.4 to 0.6, and those for SASP were undetectable. Infant serum samples were 10% of maternal SP levels, and only one infant had detectable SASP. No children had complications of hyperbilirubinemia or kernicterus. All the infants were term infants without major complications. The authors[31] conclude it is safe to continue the SASP throughout pregnancy and lactation in full-term infants. The affect on prematures is under study.

Epilepsy

A history of epilepsy in a mother is of concern for the obstetrician in pregnancy, and much has been written on the topic. It is clear that seizures in pregnancy are more dangerous to the fetus than the medication. Antiepileptic drugs (AEDs) include phenobarbital, primidone, phenytoin, carbamazepine, ethosuximide, valproic acid, and diazepam. The concern regarding lactation includes the affect of the disease on the fetus in terms of major and minor malformations, the level of drugs in the infant's serum at birth, and the state of the mother postpartum. Breastfeeding may provide a means of gradually withdrawing the infant from maternal medication and avoiding the syndrome of withdrawal[10] (i.e., hyperirritability, tremor, vomiting, poor sucking, hyperventilation, and sleep disturbances).

Table 15-5. Pharmacokinetic data in newborns

	Free fraction (% unbound)	Volume distribution (1/kg)	Half-life (hours)
Phenobarbital	57–72	0.6–1.5	40–500
Primidone	?	?	7–60
Phenytoin	15–30	0.7–2.0	15–105
Carbamazepine	?	1.1–2.6	8–28
Ethosuximide	?	?	40
Valproic acid	~15	0.2–0.4	14–88
Diazepam	~14	1.8–2.1	40–400

The half-life of various AEDs are listed in Table 15-5. These compounds have a sedating effect and may prevent the infant from suckling adequately in the first few days. Attention must be paid to the infant's behavior to avoid not only undernutrition but also failure to provide sufficient stimulus to the breast. The infant may need some supplementation and the mother some stimulus with an electric pump, carefully coordinated with support.

Whether the infant is breastfed or bottle fed, it is necessary to establish that the mother will remain seizure-free and able to care for the infant.[53] Forty-two infants of 32 epileptic mothers were studied by Kaneko et al.[53] for harmful side affects of AED while breastfeeding. The duration of poor sucking was correlated with the drug and the levels. The poor weight gain of the mixed-fed infants (breast/bottle) was associated with infant drowsiness during feeding and vomiting. These authors recommend mixing feedings (breastfeeding and formula) early postpartum to reduce the medication to the infant until levels in infant serum taper a little and the infant metabolism increases to promote drug clearance. Full breastfeeding can then proceed if care has been taken to establish a good milk supply with supplementary pumping.

Neuropathies associated with breastfeeding

A number of neurologic systems have been described in association with lactation.

During periods of engorgement, pressure on nerves in the axilla, especially from an engorged tail of Spence (see Chapter 2), has caused numbness and tingling down the arms on the flexor surface to the ulnar distribution of the hands similar to crutch palsy. The numbness and tingling usually abate as soon as the infant nurses and then gradually return as the breast fills again. Symptoms gradually disappear after several weeks as engorgement disappears.

Symptoms similar to that associated with tennis elbow—pain and tingling with flexion of the forearm—have developed in nursing women who are pumping milk with a Kaneson-style hand pump. Similar symptoms have been experienced by mothers just holding a newborn over periods of time, especially primiparas.

Carpal tunnel syndrome has been described in pregnancy, causing paresthesia of the hands. Two cases are reported by Yagnik[104] in which symptoms developed 1 month postpartum while breastfeeding. The diagnosis was confirmed by EMG and nerve-conduction studies. The second case was bilateral. Symptoms disappeared after the infants were weaned. Five other cases are described in the literature; all were breastfeeding, all showed improvement with temporary suspension of breastfeeding, and all recovered completely within a month of complete weaning.[90] Treatment recommended is conservative with rest, diuretics, hand splint, and local corticosteroid injection, since it is usually reversible. No cases had residual signs or symptoms, so that perseverance with lactation and symptomatic treatment is appropriate.

Smoking

Mothers who smoke choose bottle feeding more frequently than women who do not smoke. Of those smokers who are breastfeeding on discharge from the hospital, more have discontinued breastfeeding by 6 weeks than those who do not smoke.[67]

The pharmacologic effects of nicotine have been studied in the fetuses of experimental animals. The active components of cigarette smoke, nicotine and carbon monoxide, have been implicated in the birth-weight reduction seen in infants of mothers who are heavy smokers. Nicotine has acetylcholine-like actions on the CNS, skeletal muscle, and upper sympathetic and parasympathetic ganglia. Nicotine initially stimulates and then depresses. Nicotine has been shown to interfere with the let-down reflex, but it does not appear to disrupt lactation once it has been initiated. Smoking has been associated with a poor milk supply. It has been reported that women who smoke 10 to 20 cigarettes a day have 0.4 to 0.5 mg of nicotine/L in their milk. Calculations indicate this is equivalent to a dose of 6 to 7.5 mg of nicotine in an adult. In an adult, 4 mg of nicotine has produced symptoms, and the lethal dosage is in the range of 40 to 60 mg for adults. On the basis of gradual intake over a day's time the neonate would metabolize it in the liver and excrete the chemical through the kidney. Low-grade responses to nicotine would be subtle in the neonate and require specific monitoring to detect.

When a group of lactating women who smoked more than 15 cigarettes a day were compared with lactating women who did not smoke at all, the basal prolactin levels were significantly lower in smokers, but suckling induced acute increments in serum prolactin and oxytocin-linked neurophysin were not influenced.[3] These experiments showed no influence on oxytocin when two cigarettes were smoked before a feeding. Serum nicotine and plasma epinephrine but not dopamine or norepinephrine were significantly increased in the mothers during smoking. The smokers weaned their babies more quickly than nonsmokers.[67] The heavy smokers had the lowest prolactin levels and weaned earliest.

Newborn infants nursed by smoking mothers and kept in the newborn nursery to avoid passive smoke showed serum concentration of nicotine 0.2 ng/ml and cotinine, the main metabolite, 5 to 30 ng/ml.[24] They excrete measurable amounts in their urine also. Infants exposed to passive smoking but not breastfed also had nicotine in their urine. Thus, breastfeeding by smoking women contributes to the nicotine in infants.

In counseling the nursing mother who smokes, consideration should be given to the data. The data suggest that mothers should not smoke while nursing, or in the infant's presence. If it is not possible to stop, they should cut down and also consider low-nicotine cigarettes.

If the mother smokes marijuana, an entirely different risk is created. Animal studies have shown that structural changes occur in the brain cells of newborn animals nursed by mothers whose milk contained cannabis. Nahas et al.[72,73] describe impairment of DNA and RNA formation and of proteins essential for proper growth and development. Results seen in some humans suggest that serious and long-lasting effects can occur. Impairment of judgment and behavioral changes may actually interfere with an individual's ability to care for the infant or adequately breastfeed. If the mother smokes while nursing, there is not only the drug in her milk but also the effect of the smoke that the infant inhales from the environment. Since brain cell development is still taking place in the first months of life, any remote chance that DNA and RNA metabolism is altered should be viewed with concern.

The mother who requires hospitalization
Emergency admission

The mother who suddenly develops an emergency condition that requires hospitalization presents a unique problem in management. It is patently obvious that the emergency condition must be dealt with appropriately, medically, surgically, or psychiatrically. It is equally important in all three situations to deal with the patient as a lactating mother, since failure to do so may have an impact on the successful outcome of the primary condition.

Medical admission. Medical problems such as acute infection or metabolic disturbances should be analyzed in relationship to lactation and to the infant and, in addition, to any other children at home. Is it contagious? In the case of lactation, will the drugs pass into the breast milk? If so, are there alternative treatments? What is the prognosis for recovery? Is the recovery phase more or less than 2 weeks and is maintaining lactation realistic? This decision should not be made in the abstract without an understanding of the mother's commitment to further breastfeeding. If the prognosis is poor for recovery or the drugs involved are contraindicated for the infant but necessary for the mother, provision should be made for the mother's adjusting. It should be kept in mind that abrupt cessation of lactation can cause a flulike syndrome, which will confuse the management picture. It may be advisable to include the mother's obstetrician or pediatrician in the discussion to provide the mother with the necessary support to accept alternatives (Chapter 11).

Surgical admission. Surgical emergencies such as trauma, appendicitis, or chylocystitis will require immediate attention, including anesthesia and surgery. If it is a self-limited disease with a short postoperative course, as in appendicitis, the mother can go back to breastfeeding on her return home. If the hospitalization will be more prolonged, as in trauma with immobilizing fractures, different considerations are important. It is possible to have the infant brought to the hospital several times a day for nursing. Unless the mother is mobile enough to provide some of the infant's bedside care, rooming-in is too taxing to the recovering patient. It is also stressful to other patients and staff who are not equipped for neonates. The mother would require a single room. If she has provision for her own nursing care or if the nursing staff is agreeable, an arrangement could be worked out. The only contraindication would be whether it would interfere with recovery. When bone healing is important, attention should be given to the dietary demands of bone healing and lactation, especially in calcium, phosphorus, and vitamin intakes. If the mother is to be cared for but immobilized at home, nursing is easier, but provision for ample assistance would be mandatory. The need for assistance would not differ for the breastfed or bottle fed infant of the same age. Home care services are available in most communities.

Psychiatric admission. The onset of a psychiatric crisis in a lactating mother rarely occurs unless the mother has already been identified as having a psychiatric problem. Childbirth has an established etiologic role in postpartum psychosis. There is a report in the literature, however, of a case of mania precipitated in a mother each time she weaned her children from the breast but at no other time. We had treated a patient with a known psychiatric disorder who decompensated during pregnancy, did well during lactation, and had difficulty after weaning. With her fourth child, she weaned abruptly at 3 months and committed suicide 2 weeks later.

Breastfeeding of itself does not cause psychosis, although women with a postpartum psychosis have acutely decompensated when they wean abruptly. The management of weaning is a very important part of the mother's treatment, and the process should be orchestrated by the psychiatrist and not the pediatrician or the obstetrician.

As the number of women who breastfeed increases, there will be increased understanding of the relationship of these physiologic events to psychiatric disease. The role of the mother in lactation will be a part of her psychiatric care, and the decision to breastfeed or not should be worked out with her psychiatrist. Most psychiatric wards can accommodate young infants whether they are breastfed or bottle fed, so it is less of a novelty than on the medical and surgical wards. The management of postpartum psychosis includes the concerns of the mother caring for the infant as part of recovery. The drugs used when the mother is nursing should be appropriate for both mother and nursing infant.

Elective maternal admission to the hospital

There are occasions when a lactating mother may have to plan for hospitalization. The urgency will be determined by the underlying disease. If the admission date can be made for over a month away, there is time for gradual weaning of the infant if this is necessary. If weaning is appropriate and/or necessary, the impact will largely be determined by the age of the infant. A very young infant who would profit greatly by continued breastfeeding is one type of problem. If the child is a year old, it may be less traumatic for him to be weaned when the separation time is going to be greater than 48 to 72 hours. A child who is also receiving solids and some other liquids from a cup can sustain himself during the separation without much more than sadness. If the caretaker and the surroundings are familiar, the support of this infant is easier. For the mother of the older child the impact of forced separation during hospitalization is also easier and less likely to produce "milk fever."

The young infant can be sustained by bottle feedings or "cross-nursing" by another lactating mother until he can be breastfed by his own mother again. The mother in the first few months of lactation will have more problems with engorgement, discomfort, and even malaise. Provision should be made to express or pump milk to maintain the supply if the mother will be nursing again or pumping minimally for comfort if lactation is to be discontinued. Milk can be collected in sterile bottles and sent home for the infant. When the admission is elective, plans can be made in advance to have a pump available, renting one if the hospital is not equipped. Methods for collecting, refrigerating, and getting milk home to the infant can be planned along with her other needs, such as a baby-sitter.

During an elective admission for a self-limited disease, rooming-in for the infant may be possible if the circumstances of the illness permit. It should be pointed out that the prime purpose of the hospitalization is to treat an illness. If surgery is involved, rooming-in should not be a stress to the mother when she is in the operating room, in the recovery room, or heavily medicated. Day-of-surgery, same-day surgery, and ambulatory surgery units have minimized hospital stays and the need for alternative nourishment for the infant.

The purpose of this section is to point out that it is possible to maintain lactation when hospitalization is necessary for the mother. It is possible to have the infant accompany the mother or vice versa in a rooming-in arrangement. The theoretic threat of infection in the hospital setting is outweighed by the advantages of human milk in most cases. On the other hand, the decision rests with the physician in charge of the case, who will have the responsibility of looking at the total picture including the medical problem in question, the necessary treatment, and the short-range prognosis for resuming normal breastfeeding. Here again the expertise of the mother's obstetrician and the infant's pediatrician may be invaluable. They can also assist in coping with family and friends who have confused the mother with their experiences or opinions.

The evaluation of nipple discharge

Most nipple discharges are due to benign lesions, and many do not require surgical intervention. They could, however, represent a malignant condition and deserve careful investigation. Nipple discharges associated with lactation have a different etiologic incidence profile, but they are no less significant. In general, discharge is more common in older women. Most texts discussing discharge from the nipple are written by surgeons, and the distinction regarding the relationship to breastfeeding is not made.

Milky discharge

Persistent bilateral lactation is the presentation following breastfeeding and, as noted, may represent pituitary disease. If there is no surgical disease such as an adenoma, medical treatment to suppress prolactin such as estrogens or bromocriptine are usually employed. In the nonlactating woman this finding is called galactorrhea and is a spontaneous, milky, multiduct, bilateral discharge.[82] Galactorrhea has been discussed on pp. 394-395.

Multicolored and sticky discharge

Duct ectasia, so-called *comedomastitis,* is the most common cause of multicolored sticky discharge.[82] It begins as a dilation of the terminal ducts and may occur during pregnancy, although it is most common between the ages of 35 and 40. It is rare in virgins and most common in women who have lactated. An irritating lipid forms in the ducts producing an inflammatory reaction and nipple discharge. Cytology shows debris and epithelial cells. Duct ectasia may be associated with burning pain, itching, and swelling of the nipple and aerola. Palpation reveals a wormlike tubular feeling once called *varicocele tumor of the breast.* As the disease progresses, a mass may develop that mimics cancer, and chronic inflammation leads to fibrosis. Surgery is not indicated unless the discharge becomes bloody. The disease is usually treated with thorough cleansing with pHisoHex or povidone-iodine (Betadine) daily and avoidance of nipple manipulation. Lactation would aggravate preexisting diseases but would not be an absolute contraindication.

Purulent discharge

Purulent discharge is due to acute puerperal mastitis, chronic lactation mastitis, central breast abscess, or plasma cell mastitis. It is usually unilateral, involving one or two ducts. Once it is diagnosed, the treatment is with antibodies. When an abscess does not clear after cessation of lactation and adequate treatment, a biopsy should be done to rule out secondary necrosis and infection of an underlying lesion.

Watery, serous, serosanguineous, and bloody discharges

Nipple discharges are primarily of surgical significance. They are the second most common indication for breast surgery. Watery or colorless, serous or yellow, serosanguineous or pink and sanguineous discharges are more common over the age of 50, but younger women do not escape them.[82] Bloody discharge in pregnancy and lactation is most commonly due to vascular engorgement or trauma of the breast. The next most common causes in pregnancy and lactation are intraductal papilloma (50%) and fibrocystic disease (31%). Because the type of discharge does not identify the malignant or nonmalignant nature of the problem, all patients with unusual discharge should be seen by an appropriate surgeon for diagnosis.

In intraductal papilloma, the discharge is usually spontaneous, unilateral, and from a single duct. It is occasionally associated with a nontender lump in the subareolar area. Symptoms may include bleeding, which is usually painless during pregnancy. It is possible to excise the involved duct and wedge of tissue, leaving the rest intact to preserve mammary function, when surgery is required for intraductal papilloma. Painless bleeding during pregnancy may be bilateral or unilateral and may cease after delivery. After serious disease has been ruled out, lactation is possible.

To be significant a discharge should be true, persistent, spontaneous, and nonlactational. Single-duct unilateral discharges are more apt to be surgically significant. A true discharge comes from a duct to the surface of the nipple. Pseudodischarges occur on the surface and may be associated with inverted nipples, eczematoid lesions, trauma, herpes simplex, infections of the Montgomery glands, and mammary duct fistulas. Discharges are more common in women taking oral contraceptives, tranquilizers, or rauwolfia and in those who are postmenopausal and menopausal. Cytologic examination should be part of any examination for an abnormal discharge from the breast, although there is a high percentage of false negatives and there are some false positives. Absence of a mass is reassuring but should not dissuade one from further diagnostic studies.

Lumps in the breast

The lactating breast is lumpy to palpation, and the lumps shift day by day. The most common cause of a persistent lump is a plugged duct (see Chapter 8); the second most common cause is a mass associated with mastitis. Lumps that persist beyond a few days and do not respond to palliative treatment deserve review.

Adenomas of the breast and ectopic breast under lactational influences were reviewed by O'Hara and Page.[79] They reported five ectopic lactating ademonas located in the axilla, chest wall, and vulva. Tubular adenomas have been associated with lactation and described to show lactational changes in a fibroadenoma, thus making diagnosis difficult by fine-needle aspiration. Fine-needle aspiration of the breast has been recommended as a safe, easy diagnostic tool to use in an ambulatory setting without interrupting lactation.

Fibrocystic disease

Fibrocystic disease is a diffuse parenchymal process in the breasts that has many synonyms, none of which is satisfactory. The process involves hormonally produced benign proliferations of the alveolar system of varying degrees that occur in response to the normal menstrual cycle. In a full-blown case there are pain, tenderness, palpable thickenings, and nodules of varying sizes that are most symptomatic with menses. The disease is prominent in the childbearing years and regresses during pregnancy. It is not a contraindication to breastfeeding. Some women have achieved relief by totally eliminating caffeine and related products from their diet.

Breast cysts

Benign cysts of the breast are being identified in younger and younger women, probably because of the more careful self-examination of the breast now recommended. They should be removed and biopsied but do not interfere with lactation. Fibroadenomas that are due to disturbance in the normal menstrual cycle usually proliferate and regress before the age of 30. Pregnancy and lactation stimulate their growth. They are firm, smooth, lobulated masses and are freely movable without fixation. They can be diagnosed radiologically and do not interfere with lactation. They can be removed under local anesthesia if necessary without stopping breastfeeding.

Lipomas

Lipomas are very common in the breast, which has considerable fat in its stroma. They are usually solitary, asymptomatic, slowly growing, freely movable, soft, and well delineated. They can be easily identified radiologically or with ultra sound imagery in the lactating breast, which has less fat present.

Fat necrosis

Fat necrosis is usually associated with trauma and is caused by local destruction of fat cells with release of free lipid and variable hemorrhage. Organization with fibrosis may lead to fixation. Fat necrosis can be identified radiologically and looks like a fat density or oil cyst with a capsule.

Hematomas

Hematomas of the lactating breast may occur from trauma or in women on anticoagulant therapy. They generally regress without treatment. When they occur with minimal trauma, the presence of a tumor should be considered.

Plastic surgery of the breast
Augmentation mammoplasty

Augmentation mammoplasty has become a more acceptable procedure and techniques have improved tremendously.[95] The implantation of inert material is the approach. Young women may request it and then wish to lactate. There should be no destruction of breast tissue or interruption of ducts, nerve supply, or blood supply to the gland or nipple, so that breastfeeding is possible and successful (Fig. 15-2). Injections of silicone are no longer used. The silicone did cause fibrosis and duct destruction.

Breasts requiring augmentation mammoplasty may in some cases lack adequate functional breast tissue. A woman may wish to have this evaluated by real-time ultrasound prior to the insertion of an implant if she wishes to breastfeed later.

Anytime there is surgical manipulation of the breast, there may be residual loss of sensation for several months and only rarely permanently. The nerve involved is the anterior cutaneous branch of the fourth lateral cutaneous nerve, which passes deep into the breast tissue unaccompanied by arteries. Preoperative and postoperative evaluation of breast sensation was reported by Courtiss and Goldwyn.[25] Preoperatively they found the areola to be the most sensitive. For 2 weeks following augmentation mammoplasty, sensation was decreased to the areola and nipple. Erectility did return in all cases. The return of significant

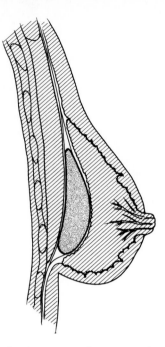

Fig. 15-2. Placement of implant in augmentation mammoplasty. There is no interruption of vital ducts, nerve supply, or blood supply.

sensitivity, however, usually took 6 months or longer, even 2 years, with the larger implants being associated with the greatest loss. Hyperesthesia and paraesthesia were also reported. Immediately following reduction mammoplasty, breasts were insensitive to testing, and it took about 6 months for sensation to return. The greater the resection, the greater the loss of sensation. Nipple erectility returned before complete sensation in the skin in about 2 months, but complete recovery took about 1 year. Mastopexy for sagging breasts had normal sensation in the skin in about 2 months, but complete recovery could take up to a year.

Postlactation involution of a severe degree occasionally occurs. Some women note considerable regression and seeming atrophy after weaning, which alarms them. The fat deposition has not recurred when the ducts regress. In most of these women the breasts return to their normal contour in about 3 years if there has been no further pregnancy or lactation. Loss of tissue turgor and fat padding occurs without pregnancy or lactation as well (Fig. 15-3). Certainly augmentation is possible if desired once the childbearing is completed. If subsequent pregnancy occurs, the breast regenerates and lactates well.

Reduction mammoplasty

There are women with breasts so large they cause shoulder and back pain, deep grooves in the shoulders from brassiere straps, and negative self-image. These women sometimes want surgical correction. Reduction mammoplasty is more destructive than augmentation because of the necessity of replacing the nipple symmetrically, which requires

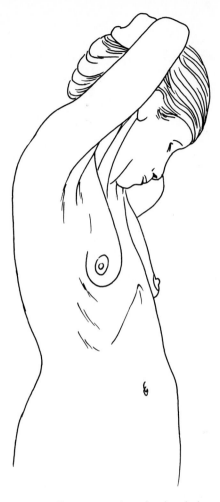

Fig. 15-3. Extreme postlactation involution.

interrupting the ducts.[95,96] Although plastic surgeons report that these women do not wish to breastfeed, it is our experience that many of them do wish to breastfeed later when they bear a child and are suddenly aware of their maternal role. At the time of surgery they are consumed with their perceived affliction. The surgeon should clearly discuss the options with the patient or provide a procedure that leaves the ducts intact. If the ducts are intact, breastfeeding can be successful postoperatively. The nerve must also be intact for tactile sensations to trigger let-down.

In general, surgery of the breast for nonmalignant lesions does not preclude breast-feeding unless the ductal structure has been interrupted. Surgeons need to consider mammary function in counseling young women about breast surgery.

REFERENCES

1. Adamopoulos DA and Kapolla N: Prolactin concentration in milk and plasma of puerperal women and patients with galactorrhea, J Endocrinol Invest 7:273, 1984.
2. Alpert SE and Cormier AD: Normal electrolyte and protein content in milk from mothers with cystic fibrosis: an explanation for the initial report of elevated milk sodium concentration, J Pediatr 102:77, 1983.
3. Andersen AN et al: Suppressed prolactin but normal neurophysin levels in cigarette smoking breast-feeding women. Clin Endocrinol 17:363, 1982.
4. Andersen AN and Tabor A: PRL, TSH and LH responses to metoclopramide and breast feeding in normal and hyperprolactinaemic women, Acta Endocrinol 100:177, 1982.
5. Ando Y, Nakano S, Saito K et al: Transmission of adult T-cell leukemia retrovirus (HTLV-1) from mother to child: comparison of bottle with breastfed babies, Jpn J Cancer Res 78:322, 1987.
6. Aono T et al: Effect of sulpiride on poor puerperal lactation, Am J Obstet Gynecol 143:927, 1982.
7. Asselin BL and Lawrence RA: Maternal disease as a consideration in lactation management, Clin Perinatol 14:71, 1987.
8. Bode HH, Vonjonack K, and Crawford JT: Mitigation of cretinism by breast feeding, Pediatr Res 11:423, 1977.
9. Borch-Johnsen K, Mandrup-Poulsen T, Zachau-Christiansen B et al: Relation between breastfeeding and incidence rates of insulin-dependent diabetes mellitus, Lancet 2:1083, 1984.
10. Bossi L: Neonatal period including drug disposition in newborns: review of the literature. In Janz D et al, editors: Epilepsy, pregnancy and the child, New York, 1982, Raven Press.
11. Botta RM, Donatelli M, Bucalo ML et al: Placental lactogen, progesterone, total estriol and prolactin plasma levels in pregnant women with insulin-dependent diabetes mellitus, Eur J Obstet Gynecol Reprod Biol 16:393, 1984.
12. Briggs GG, Freeman RK, and Yaffe S: Drugs in pregnancy and lactation, ed 2, Baltimore, 1986, Williams & Wilkins.
13. Buchanon TA, Unterman TG, and Metzger BE: Medical management of diabetes in pregnancy, Clin Perinatol 12:625, 1985.
14. Burns PE: Absence of lactation in a previously radiated breast (letter), Int J Radiation Oncol Biol Phys 13:1603, 1987.
15. Burrow GN and Ferris TF: Medical complications during pregnancy, Philadelphia, 1975, WB Saunders Co.
16. Butte NF, Garza C, Burr R et al: Milk composition of insulin-dependent diabetic women, J Pediatr Gastroenterol Nutr 6:936, 1987.
17. Campbell DA, Lorber MI, Sweeton JC et al: Breastfeeding and maternal-donor renal allografts, Transplantation 37:340, 1984.
18. Check JH and Adelson HG: Amenorrhea-galactorrhea associated with hypothalamic hypothyroidism, Am J Obstet Gynecol 139:736, 1981.
19. Committee on Fetus and Newborn/Committee on Infectious Disease, Academy of Pediatrics: Perinatal herpes simplex virus infections, Pediatrics 66:147, 1980.
20. Committee on Infectious Disease: Report of the Committee, Red Book, ed 21, Elk Grove Village Ill, 1988, Academy of Pediatrics.
21. Cooper DS: Antithyroid drugs: to breastfeed or not to breastfeed, Am J Obstet Gynecol 157:234, 1987.
22. Corey L et al: Genital herpes simplex virus infections: clinical manifestations, course, and complications, Ann Intern Med 98:958, 1983.
23. Coulam CB et al: Breastfeeding after renal transplantation, Transplant Proc 14:605, 1982.
24. Counsilman JJ and McKay EV: Cigarette smoking by pregnant women with particular reference to their past and subsequent breastfeeding behavior, Aust NZ Obstet Gynecol 25:101, 1985.
25. Courtiss EH and Goldwyn RM: Breast sensation before and after plastic surgery, Plastic Reconstruct Surg 58:1, 1976.
26. Crumpacker CS: Hepatitis. In Remington JS and Klein JO, editors: Infectious disease of fetus and newborn infant, ed 2, Philadelphia, 1976, WB Saunders Co.
27. David FC: Lactation following primary radiation therapy for carcinoma of the breast, Int J Radiation Oncol Biol Phys 11:1425, 1985.
28. Davidson JM, Katz AI, and Lindheimer MD: Kidney disease and pregnancy: obstetric outcome and long term renal prognosis, Clin Perinatol 12:497, 1985.
29. Dunkle L, Schmidt RR, and O'Connor DM: Neonatal herpes simplex infection possibly acquired via maternal breast milk, Pediatrics 63:250, 1979.
30. Dworsky M et al: Cytomegalovirus infection of breast milk and transmission in infancy, Pediatrics 72:295, 1983.
31. Esbjorner E, Jarnerot G, and Wranne L: Sulphasalazine and sulphapyridine serum levels in children of mothers treated with sulphasalazine

during pregnancy and lactation, Acta Paediatr Scand 76:137, 1987.

32. Ferris AM, Dalidowitz CK, Ingardia CM et al: Lactation outcome in insulin-dependent diabetic women, J Am Dietetic Assoc 88:317, 1988.

33. Forbes GB, Barton LD, Nicholas DL et al: Composition of milk produced by a mother with galactosemia, J Pediatr 113:90, 1988.

34. Fort P, Lanes R, Dahlem S et al: Breastfeeding and insulin-dependent diabetes mellitus in children, J Am College Nutr 5:439, 1986.

35. Frantz AG and Wilson JD: Endocrine disorders of the breast. In Wilson JD and Foster DW, editors: Textbook of endocrinology, Philadelphia, 1985, WB Saunders Co.

36. Frinkel N, Dooley SL, and Metzger BE: Care of the pregnant woman with IDDM, N Engl J Med 313:96, 1985.

37. Giampietro O, Ramacciotti C, and Moggi G: Normoprolactinemic galactorrhea in a fertile woman with a copper intra-uterine device (copper IUD), Acta Obstet Gynecol Scand 63:23, 1984.

38. Gill G: Breastfeeding and diabetes (letter), Lancet 2:1283, 1984.

39. Gillin FD, Reiner DS, and Gault MJ: Cholate-dependent killing of Giardia lamblia by human milk, Inf Immun 47:614, 1985.

40. Glass RK et al: Protection against cholera in breast-fed children by antibodies in breast milk, N Engl J Med 308:1389, 1983.

41. Glatthaar D, Whittall DE, Welborn TA et al: Diabetes in western Australian children: descriptive epidemiology, Med J Aust 148:117, 1988.

42. Gruber HE, Butteridge T, and Baylink DS: Osteoporosis associated with pregnancy and lactation: bone biopsy and skeletal features in three patients, Metab Bone Dis Rel Res 5:159, 1984.

43. Hanson LA: The mammary glands as an immunological organ, Immunol Today 3:168, 1982.

44. Hornstein E, Skornick Y, and Rozin R: The management of breast carcinoma in pregnancy and lactation, J Surg Oncol 21:179, 1982.

45. Huber GL: Tuberculosis. In Remington JS and Klein JO, editors: Infectious disease of fetus and newborn infant, ed 2, Philadelphia, 1976, WB Sauders Co.

46. Hughes WT, Bartley DL, Patterson GG et al: Ketoconazole and candidiasis, J Infect Dis 147:1060, 1983.

47. Ikegami H, Aono T, Koizumi K et al: Relationship between the methods of treatment for prolactinomas and the puerperal lactation, Fertil Steril 47:867, 1987.

48. Jarrett RJ: Breastfeeding and diabetes (letter), Lancet 2:1283, 1984.

49. Jelliffe DB and Jelliffe EFP: Human milk in the modern world, Oxford, 1978, Oxford University Press.

50. Joselin EP et al: The treatment of diabetes mellitus, Philadelphia, 1959, Lea & Febiger.

51. Kalache A, Vessey MP, and McPherson K: Lactation and breast cancer, Br Med J 1:223, 1980.

52. Kampmann J et al: Propylthiouracil in human milk, Lancet 1:736, 1980.

53. Kaneko S, Suzuki K, Sato T et al: The problems of antiepileptic medication in the neonatal period: is breastfeeding advisable? In Janz D et al, editors: Epilepsy, pregnancy, and the child, New York, 1982, Raven Press.

54. Kapcala LP: Galactorrhea and thyrotoxicosis, Arch Intern Med 144:2349, 1984.

55. Kelemen E, Szalay F, and Peterfy M: Autoimmune (idiopathic) thrombocytopenic purpura in pregnancy and the newborn (letter), Br J Obstet Gynecol 85:239, 1978.

56. Kenny JF: Recurrent group B streptococcal disease in an infant associated with the ingestion of infected mother's milk, J Pediatr 91:158, 1977.

57. Kilham L: Mumps virus in human milk and in milk of infected monkey, JAMA 146:1231, 1951.

58. Kohn JL: Measles in newborn infants (maternal infection), J Pediatr 3:176, 1933.

59. Kois WE, Campbell DA, Lorber MI et al: Influence of breastfeeding on subsequent reactivity to a related renal allograft, J Surg Res 37:89, 1984.

60. Kulski JK, Smith M, and Hartmann PE: Normal and caesarean section delivery and the initiation of lactation in women, Aust J Exp Biol Med Sci 59:405, 1981.

61. Lamberg BA, Ikonen E, Osterlund K et al: Antithyroid treatment of maternal hyperthyroidism during lactation, Clin Endocrinol 21:81, 1984.

62. Lee GL: Fine-needle aspiration of the breast: the outpatient management of breast lesions, Am J Obstet Gynecol 156:1532, 1987.

63. Leis HP and Urban JA: The other breast. In Gallager HS et al, editors: The breast, St. Louis, 1978, The CV Mosby Co.

64. Lobato MF, Careche M, Ros M et al: Effect of prolactin and glucocorticoids on P-enolpyruvate carboxykinase activity in liver and mammary gland from diabetic and lactating rats, Molecular Cell Biochem 67:19, 1985.

65. Lubchenco, CO: Infants of diabetic mothers, an editorial, Keeping Abreast J 1:107, 1976.

66. Luck W and Nau H: Nicotine and cotinine concentrations in serum and urine of infants exposed via passive smoking or milk from smoking mothers, J Pediatr 107:816, 1985.

67. Lyon AJ: Effects of smoking on breast feeding, Arch Dis Child 58:378, 1983.

68. Magno R et al: Anesthesia for caesarian section. IV. Placental transfer and neonatal elimination of bupivacaine following epidural anlages for elective cesarean section, Acta Anaesthesiol Scand 20:141, 1976.

69. Martin JN, Morrison JC, and Files YC: Autoimmune thrombocytopenic purpura: current concepts and recommended practices, Am J Obstet Gynecol 150:86, 1984.

70. Merson MH et al: Maternal cholera immunization and secretory IgA in breast milk, Lancet 1:931, 1980.

71. Meschengieser S and Lazzari MA: Breastfeeding in thrombocytopenic neonates secondary to maternal autoimmune thrombocytopenic purpura, Am J Obstet Gynecol 154:1166, 1986.

72. Nahas GG: Marijuana, JAMA 233:79, 1975.

73. Nahas GG et al: Inhibition of cellular mediated immunity in marijuana smokers, Science 183:419, 1974.

74. Nahmias AJ and Visintine AM: Herpes simplex. In Remington JS and Klein JO, editors: Infectious disease of fetus and newborn infant, ed 2, Philadelphia, 1976, WB Saunders Co.

75. Neifert MR, McDonough SL, and Neville MC: Failure of lactogenesis associated with placental retention, Am J Obstet Gynecol 140:477, 1981.

76. Neville MC, Hay WW, Lutes V et al: Glucose clamp studies in lactating women: effects of glucose and insulin on milk glucose and lactose secretion, Fed Proc 95:901, 1986.

77. Noguchi A, Eren M, and Tsang RC: Parathyroid hormone in hypocalcemic and normocalcemic infants of diabetic mothers, J Pediatr 97:112, 1980.

78. Nylund L, Lunell NO, Lewander R et al: Uteroplacental blood flow in diabetic pregnancy: measurements with indium 133^m and a computer-linked gamma camera, Am J Obstet Gynecol 144:298, 1982.

79. O'Hara MF and Page DL: Adenomas of the breast and ectopic breast under lactational influences, Hum Pathol 16:707, 1985.

80. Osborne MP: Breast development and anatomy. In Harris JR, Hellman S, Henderson IC, and Kinne DW, editors: Breast diseases, Philadelphia, 1987, JB Lippincott.

81. Paulus DD: Benign diseases of the breast, Radiol Clin North Am 21:27, 1983.

82. Pilnik S and Leis HP: Nipple discharge. In Gallager HS et al, editors: The breast, St. Louis, 1978, The CV Mosby Co.

83. Quinn PT and Lofbera JV: Maternal herpetic breast infection: another hazard of neonatal herpes simplex, Med J Aust 2:411, 1978.

84. Remington JS and Desmonts G: Toxoplasmosis. In Remington JS and Klein JO, editors: Infectious disease of fetus and newborn infant, ed 2, Philadelphia, 1976, WB Saunders Co.

85. Riordan J: A practical guide to breastfeeding, St. Louis, 1983, The CV Mosby Co.

86. Scalon JW et al: Neurobehavioral responses and drug concentrations in newborns after maternal epidural anesthesia with bupivacaine, Anesthesiology 45:400, 1976.

87. Schreiner RL et al: Possible breast milk transmission of group B streptococcal infection, J Pediatr 91:159, 1977.

88. Sinata FR et al: Perinatal transmitted acute icteric hepatitis B in infants born to hepatitis B surface antigen-positive and anti-hepatitis B$_e$-positive carrier mothers, Pediatrics 70:557, 1982.

89. Skaug K et al: Chlamydial secretory IgA antibodies in human milk, Acta Pathol Microbiol Immunol Scand 90:21, 1982.

90. Snell NJC, Coysh HL, and Snell BJ: Carpal tunnel syndrome presenting in the puerperium, Practitioner 224:191, 1980.

91. Stagno S et al: Breast milk and the risk of cytomegalovirus infection, N Engl J Med 302:1073, 1980.

92. Steiner G, Myher JJ, and Kuksis A: Milk and plasma lipid composition in a lactating patient with type 1 hyperlipo-proteinemia, Am J Clin Nutr 41:121, 1985.

93. Sullivan-Bolyai JZ et al: Disseminated neonatal herpes simplex virus type I from a maternal breast lesion, Pediatrics 71:455, 1983.

94. Surian M, Imbasciati E, Cosci P et al: Glomerular disease and pregnancy, Nephron 36:497, 1985.

95. Synderman RK: Augmentation mammoplasty. In Gallager HS et al, editor: The breast, St. Louis, 1978, The CV Mosby Co.

96. Synderman RK: Reduction mammoplasty. In Gallager HS et al, editors: The breast, St. Louis, 1978, The CV Mosby Co.

97. Varma SK et al: Thyroxine, tri-iodothyronine, and reverse tri-iodothyronine concentrations in human milk, J Pediatr 93:803, 1978.

98. Vergeront JM et al: Recovery of staphylococcal enterotoxin F from the breast milk of a woman with toxic-shock syndrome, J Infect Dis 146:456, 1982.

99. Vorherr H: The breast, morphology, physiology, and lactation, New York, 1974, Academic Press, Inc.

100. Welch MJ, Phelps DL, and Osher AB: Breastfeeding by a mother with cystic fibrosis, Pediatrics 67:664, 1981.

101. Whichelow MJ and Doddridge MC: Lactation in diabetic women, Br Med J 287:649, 1983.

102. White WB: Management of hypertension during lactation, Hypertension 6:297, 1984.

103. Whitley RJ et al: The natural history of herpes simplex virus infection of mother and newborn, Pediatrics 66:489, 1980.

104. Yagnik PM: Carpal tunnel syndrome in nursing mothers, South Med J 80:1468, 1987.

105. Young NA: Chickenpox, measles, and mumps. In Remington JS and Klein JO, editors: Infectious disease of fetus and newborn infant, ed 2, Philadelphia, 1976, WB Saunders Co.

Human milk as a prophylaxis in allergy

16

THE NATURAL HISTORY OF ATOPIC DISEASE

The association of allergy with cow's milk has been documented in the literature for decades.[9,34] The incidence of this allergy in the general population has been noted to increase progressively since the original comments on the subject by Rowe[47] in 1931. The incidence has been said to have increased ten times in 20 years and has been attributed to increased recognition, increased incidence of exposure to known allergens, and a gradual decrease in infection as a source of morbidity due to the use of antibiotics and immunization revealing an underlying allergic component to chronic symptoms. Glaser[12] attributed this rapid increase in the development of allergic diseases to the abandonment of breastfeeding when safe pasteurized milk became available. It was noted that 20% of all children were allergic by 20 years of age. Studies of office pediatrics[54] have shown that one third of the visits are due to allergy. One third of all chronic conditions under age 17 are due to allergy, and one third of the days lost from school are due to asthma. In the evaluation of 2,000 consecutive unselected newborns in pediatric practice, it was found that 50% had allergic family histories. Grulee et al.[17] observed as early as 1934 that eczema was seven times more common in infants fed cow's milk than in those who were breastfed. McCombs et al.[43] reported in 1979 that asthma caused more than 2,000 deaths and the loss of 94 million days of activity and initiated 183,000 hospital admissions and more than 1 million hospital days in 1 year in the United States alone. The disease costs the American public over a billion dollars annually.

The question of heredity

There is no question that heredity plays a part in the development of allergic disease, an observation first recorded by Maimonides in his *Treatise on Asthma* in the twelfth century. Most studies in the past 60 years have concurred with the concept of a recessive mode of inheritance.[25]

Kern[33] has noted that the outstanding etiologic factor in human hypersensitivity is heredity. He states that there are few diseases in which heredity is so clearly identified and so common.

Hamburger[21] reported that children with both parents atopic had 47% chance of developing atopic disease. When only one parent was atopic, there was a 29% chance of developing atopy; when neither parent was allergic, there was only a 13% risk of the disease. Falliers et al.,[7] in a study of asthmatic monozygotic twins, observed similar serum IgE, blood eosinophil counts, and positive skin tests to allergens in both twins but dissimilar responses to infection and methacholine. This finding suggests there is also an acquired component to bronchial hyperactivity. Apparently several mechanisms are involved in antigen processing. To identify infants at high risk for developing atopy, several approaches have been suggested. Cord serum total IgE levels of greater than 100 U/ml are associated with five to ten times greater risk than lower levels. Eosinophilia and lymphocytes may prove to be markers, but at present only the family allergic history and the cord blood IgE have been significantly reliable predictors according to Bousquet et al.[1]

Glaser speculated in the 1930s that if a child was at high risk for developing allergy, prophylaxis should be able to change the outcome. The original work on prophylaxis was done by Glaser and Johnstone[15] and reported in 1953. Only 15% of a group of children whose mothers controlled their own diet in pregnancy and controlled the infant's diet and environment at birth did develop eczema, whereas 65% of the sibling controls and 52% of nonrelated controls receiving cow's milk developed similar allergic illnesses. Although as a retrospective study it was open to some criticism, it did begin to look at a very significant issue, that is, reducing the incidence of allergic manifestations in high-risk individuals by a new type of preventive measure.

A second study was designed in 1953 and carried out prospectively by Johnstone and Dutton[26] to investigate dietary prophylaxis of allergic disease. They observed a difference over 10 years in the incidence of asthma and perennial allergic rhinitis in those fed soybean milk (18%) and those fed evaporated milk (50%). No infant in this study of 283 children was breastfed, however. Halpern[19] reported the study of 1753 children fed breast milk, soy milk, and cow's milk from birth to 6 months of age who were followed until they were 7 years or older. The children included those with high-risk, low-risk, and no-risk family histories for allergy. They reported in 1973 no difference in outcome related to early diet. There was a relationship to the family history, however.

In a prospective study to identify the development of reaginic allergy, infants of allergic parents were placed in a study or control group. The study group followed an allergen-avoidance regimen, including breastfeeding. At 6 months and 1 year there was less eczema than the controls had had at 6 months. Lower serum total IgE levels were also reported.[41]

PROPHYLAXIS OF ATOPIC DISEASE

Efforts to alter the incidence of atopic illness have continued to challenge investigators who now have access to increased methodologic sophistication. Prevention of IgE-mediated disorders could be directed at interfering with any of the major forces responsible for the phenotypic expression of atopy. Practically, however, it is not yet possible to mask IgE genes or manipulate cellular components of the response organ. Clinicians are limited to manipulating the effect of the environment by reducing the allergenic load.

Review of the plethora of studies directed at measuring the impact of dietary manipulations on the incidence of atopic disease demonstrates that retrospective studies show little or no difference in the incidence of asthma and eczema, whereas prospective studies

Table 16-1. Prevention of atopy: prospective studies

Authors	Year	Number years followed	Number subjects*	Type feeding	Impact on atopy†
Johnstone & Dutton[26]	1953	10 yr	235	Soy-cow's milk	↓ asthma and rhinitis
Mathew et al[41]	1977	1 yr	53 (26)	Breast and soy milk	↓ eczema
Chandra[3]	1979	>24 mo	134	Breast milk	↓ eczema and asthma
Saarinen et al[48]	1979	3 yr	(256)	Breast milk	↓ eczema, food allergy, and asthma
Hamburger[22]	1981	1 yr	(300)	Breast milk	↓ eczema and asthma
Kaufman et al[31,32]	1981	2 yr	(94)	Breast milk	↓ asthma
Hide & Guyer[23]	1981	1 yr	843 (266)	Breast <6 mo, soy milk, cow's milk (maternal diet not controlled)	↓ eczema slight and rhinitis
Gruskay[18]	1982	15 yr	908 (328)	Breast milk 4 mo, soy milk, cow's milk	breast ↓ symptoms; soy no effect
May et al[42]	1982	6 mo	67 normal	Soy/cow's/modern formula	↑ antibodies no disease symptoms
Businco et al[2]	1983	2 yr	(101)	Breast milk <6 mo, soy/cow's milk	↓ asthma and eczema
Kajosaari & Saarinen[30]	1983	1 yr	(135)	All breast milk <6 mo, ½ solid foods early	↑ eczema and food intolerance in those fed solids
Moore et al[44]	1985	1 yr	525	Exper–breastfed 3 mo; control–SMA	not clear as 74% failed to breastfeed or gave cow's milk in experimental group

Modified from Busino L et al: Ann Allergy 51:206, 1983.
*Number in study; parentheses indicate number at risk for atopy.
†Arrows indicate decrease or increase compared with the control group.

tended to demonstrate a significant reduction in atopic disease in the treated group. These are summarized in Table 16-1. In looking at these data, it is important to recognize that in some studies the risk of the population developing atopic disease on a hereditary basis was not considered. In other studies, breastfeeding may have been carried out for only a few weeks or months. The evidence is clear that 6 months or longer of exclusive breastfeeding makes a difference. In addition, some studies did not control the breastfeeding mother's diet.

Hamburger et al.[22] carried out prospective prophylactic studies to include measuring IgE and skin radioallergosorbent test (RAST) on mother, father, and infant. They found a significant correlation between maternal IgE and infant IgE and potential allergy in the infant (Tables 16-2 and 16-3). This study had been done by controlling the environment and the diet. The process had been initiated in pregnancy to protect the fetus and continued at birth. Considerable attention, therefore, has been directed toward breastfeeding in this and other studies.

Table 16-2. Relationship of maternal total serum IgE level to cord and 4-month serum IgE level in prophylaxis group infants

Maternal IgE U/ml	Cord IgE <0.5 Number (%)	(U/ml) ≥0.5 Number (%)	4-month IgE <5.0 Number (%)	(U/ml) ≥5.0 Number (%)
≥100	35 (71)	14 (29)	41 (87)	6 (13)
>100	14 (42)	19 (58)	24 (73)	9 (27)
Total	49	33	65	15

From Hamburger RN et al: Ann Allergy 51:281, 1983.
P < 0.01 by chi square for maternal IgE <100 vs >100 for cord IgE with a trend (p < 0.08) at 4 month IgE.

Table 16-3. Relationship of paternal total serum IgE level to cord and 4-month serum IgE level in prophylaxis group infants

Paternal IgE U/ml	Cord IgE <0.5 Number (%)	(U/ml) ≥0.5 Number (%)	4-month IgE <5.0 Number (%)	(U/ml) ≥5.0 Number (%)
≥100	29 (63)	17 (37)	40 (83)	8 (17)
>100	10 (56)	8 (44)	14 (82)	3 (18)
Total	39	25	54	11

From Hamburger RN et al: Ann Allergy 51:281, 1983.

The effect of breastfeeding on allergic sensitization is both direct through the elimination of nonhuman milk protein as an exposure to antigen and indirect by affecting the absorption of antigen through the intestinal tract.[34] Maternal antibody is transferred to the breastfed infant as part of what has been called the enteromammary immune system[35] (Fig. 16-1). The secretory IgA antibody present in the milk is the result of enteric immune response of the mother to antigens in her gut. This IgA in her milk provides protection against bacterial, viral, and toxic exposures. Prospective studies in infants have shown that infants at high risk for atopic illness from a hereditary standpoint had significantly less disease when breastfed and also reared in a protected environment with delayed use of solid foods, compared with children of similar risk fed cow's milk and regular solid foods. Serum IGE concentrations were also markedly reduced under 6 months and 12 months of age in the breastfed group. Infants with a low incidence of T-lymphocytes were at greater risk to develop allergies if fed cow's milk rather than breast milk, according to work of Juto.[27,28] Infants with reduced T cells fed cow's milk also demonstrated higher serum IgE levels and peripheral eosinophil counts.[27,29] Juto also reported that with careful prophylaxis, greater than 50% of infants in whom both parents have serum IgE levels above 100 μg/ml evidenced both elevated cord and 4-month IgE levels. More than 80% of those infants whose parents had IgE levels below 100 μg/ml, however, had both low cord blood and low 4-month IgE levels. Such data confirm the genetic effect of both maternal and paternal genes.

The predictive value of cord blood IgE in the development of atopic disease was tested by Chandra and colleagues[5] in a study of 226 infants, 120 of whom had a positive family history of atopic disease in first-degree relatives (parents and siblings) and 106

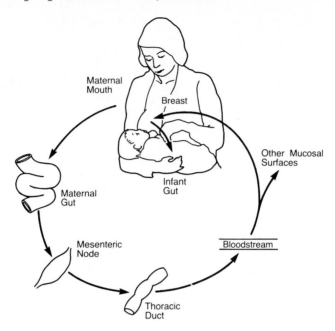

Fig. 16-1. Maternal serum antibodies affect the passage of foreign antigens into the milk, affecting the processing of antigen in the infant's intestine. (Redrawn from Kleinman RJ: Ann Allergy 51:222, 1983.)

whose family history was negative for atopy. Using ≥ 0.7 U/ml IgE, these authors found the level of cord blood IgE correlated significantly with the subsequent development of atopic disease. These investigators further tested the effect of feeding.[6] In the group with IgE <0.7 mg/100 ml who were breastfed, none developed atopy, and only one on formula did by 2 years of age. Of the 39 infants breastfed with elevated IgE, 12 developed atopy (30.7%), while in the 31 with elevated IgE who were formula fed, 26 (83.3%) developed eczema and/or wheezing in the first 2 years, a highly significant finding (p = 0.001). Of the entire study group, 12% of breastfed and 32% of formula fed infants developed atopy. The authors[6] consider cord blood IgE antibody levels a significant marker for development of atopy when the level ≥ 0.7 µg/ml is used. The history of family atopy was a significant indicator of high IgE levels.

Investigating the influence of maternal food antigen avoidance during pregnancy and lactation on the incidence of atopic eczema in infants, Chandra et al.[6] reported the outcome of a randomly assigned prospective study of 120 women with a history of a previous child with atopic disease. The study group avoided all milk, dairy products, egg, fish, beef, and peanuts throughout pregnancy and lactation. The control group had no restrictions. Maternal antigen avoidance was associated with less and milder eczema, particularly in those who were breastfed. Of 55 women who completed the avoidance regimen, 17 infants developed atopy; 5 of 35 were breastfed and 12 of 20 were formula fed. Of the 54 unrestricted mothers, 11 of 36 breastfed infants developed atopy and 13 of 18 fed formula developed atopy. The researchers thus concluded that "avoidance of common dietary allergens during pregnancy and lactation enhanced the preventive beneficial effect of exclusive breastfeeding on the incidence of atopic eczema among infants at high risk."[6]

IMMUNOLOGIC ASPECTS OF ALLERGY

Interest in identifying the immunologic aspects of clinical allergy led to a number of additional studies.[20,21] Kletter et al.[36] reported that hemagglutinating antibodies to cow's milk were present in the sera of some newborns but usually at levels lower than those of the mother. The earliest rise in titer was detected at 1 month, and a peak was seen at 3 months in infants given cow's milk from birth. Antibodies belonged mainly to the IgG group with their rise and fall parelleling hemagglutinating antibodies. IgA antibodies were in low titer and IgM rarely detected. The delayed exposure to cow's milk in breastfed infants resulted in lower mean values of milk antibodies, and peak values were attained more slowly. An inverse relationship exists between duration of breastfeeding and levels of titers of humoral antibodies.

Antibody-facilitated digestion and its implications for infant nutrition have been presented by Freed and Green.[8] They suggest a model of digestion in which oligopeptides in the small bowel are bound to secretory antibodies, which hold them in contact with proteases. This facilitates the breakdown and utilization of the oligopeptides. They consider immunity and digestion to be closely related. Breastfeeding, they point out, with colostrum and then mature human milk provides the immature gut of the infant with both immunity and "digestivity."

Eighteen patients with documented malabsorption of cow's milk, which improved by feeding them human milk, were studied by Savilahti[49] after challenge with powdered milk. Eight patients had clinical reactions; the number of IgA- and IgM-containing cells increased by almost two and a half times in the intestinal mucosa. When breast milk resumed, the findings returned to normal. There was a rise in serum antibodies of both hemagglutination and IgA. There was no change in IgE antibodies or serum complement. Multiple other findings, including villous atrophy and round cell infiltration, were noted. After the age of 2, all the infants became tolerant of milk, which the researches suggest indicates immunologic immaturity is part of the pathogenesis. Walker presented similar arguments and conclusions in a symposium discussion.[59]

The role of heredity in allergy was studied by Kaufman and Frick.[31] They described unilateral family history as allergy in one parent, bilateral as involving both parents. They followed 94 infants from birth for 24 months. Significantly more infants developed allergy if they were from a bilaterally allergic family. In the first 3 months there was less atopic dermatitis in the breastfed infants with unilateral history than with bilateral history. Businco et al.[2] present similar relationships to family history in a study of breastfed infants.

These data are augmented by findings by Murray[45] examining nasal-secretion eosinophilia in relationship to respiratory allergy, associated with a screening procedure for hearing loss. In a group of children with a history of allergy in the immediate family, an association between early introduction of solid food and the presence of a nasal-secretion eosinophilia was significantly positive.

Further follow-up on the Isle of Wight Infant Feeding Survey was conducted by Hide and Guyer[23,24] when the children were 2 and 4 years old, producing data on 486 of the original 843 children. The authors report not only on eczema and asthma but also on recurrent croup. Both asthma and recurrent croup showed strong predictability with a positive family history. More atopy was seen in the breastfed group; however, more mothers with a family history of eczema choose to breastfeed. Breastfeeding had a protective effect against asthma at 1 year but not at 4 years. Recurrent croup did not have a clear relationship to feeding method, but any breastfeeding at all was considered breastfeeding. They found

Table 16-4. Some diseases possibly preventable by protecting relatively
immunodeficient infants from adverse antigen experience

Disease	Status
Eczema	Established
Asthma	Probable
Hay fever	Probable
Infantile gut and respiratory infection	Probable
Intestinal allergy	Probable
Septicemia and renal *E. coli* infection	Probable
Sudden death	Probable
Ulcerative colitis	Possible

From Soothill JT: Proc R Soc Med 69:439, 1976.

a male preponderance and a close association with other signs of allergy in children with
recurrent croup.

Although modern processing of cow's milk has diminished the problem, it has not
eliminated it, and it would appear that given high-risk factors or strong family history of
allergy, an effort to avoid unnecessary exposure to known allergens is an easy way to
avoid some medical problems (Table 16-4).

ACUTE REACTIONS TO COW'S MILK IN BREASTFED INFANTS

External reaction to cow's milk was first described in the literature by Schloss[51] in
1920 and Tisdall and Erb[57] in 1924. At that time the reaction was noted to occur at the
first feeding of cow's milk provided in an effort to wean from the breast at several months
of age. The event included sudden crying as if in pain; swelling of the lips, tongue, and
throat; stridor; even generalized urticaria and wheezing lasting for up to an hour. This type
of cow's milk allergy is the first of two types described by Gerrard and Shenassa[11] and
others. The second type is the well-known reaction to large amounts of cow's milk in a
cow's milk–fed infant and is manifested by vomiting, diarrhea, or colic and is not associated
with cow's milk–specific IgE antibodies. It usually subsides over time. The acute anaphylactic reactions, however, are associated with α-lactalbumin, β-lactoglobulin, and casein
immunity.

Schwartz et al.[50] studied 29 breastfed or soy formula fed infants, who had had acute
urticarial reactions while being fed cow's milk for the first time. One infant had the reaction
in the newborn nursery, suggesting in utero sensitization. Sixteen were identified as having
been given formula, often without an order in the newborn nursery when charts were
carefully reviewed. Twelve could have been sensitized in utero or via the breast milk. The
authors identified elevated serum IgE levels, positive radioallergosorbent tests (RASTs) to
α-lactalbumin, β-lactoglobulin, and casein and recurrent wheezing in 55% (16/29) of the
infants. The study confirms the importance of heredity in this acute reaction by its occurrence
in twins and human leukocyte antigen (HLA) identical siblings as well as children of 28
(89%) positive parent pairs and 56 (70%) parents. Genetic homogeneity could not be
demonstrated by HLA typing.

A case of anaphylactic shock due to cow's milk hypersensitivity in a breastfed infant has been reported by Lifschitz et al.[38] They describe three episodes of shock from two separate feedings of formula and one while breastfeeding. After a prolonged course and the diagnosis of colitis, associated with numerous eosinophils, the infant, at 21 days of age, was able to breastfeed without difficulty after his mother had been placed on a cow's milk–free diet. When challenged, however, with breast milk that had been pumped and stored while the mother was still consuming dairy products, the infant went into profound shock. The child was finally stabilized on breast milk and meat-base formula. At 6 months cereal was added to the diet. At 12 months soy and cow's milk were well tolerated.

Recommendations for management

Intrauterine sensitization and allergy in the newborn breastfed infant were described by Matsumura[40] and his colleagues in Japan. Glaser[13] also identified the fact that under certain conditions an infant with a predisposition for allergy may become actively sensitized in utero because of the mother's overindulgence in certain foods in pregnancy. Shannon[53] demonstrated in 1922 the presence of egg antigen in human breast milk, for instance. The infant will then respond to reexposure with allergic symptoms on first contact with that same food.[10,37] Infant colic associated with maternal ingestion of cow's milk is discussed in Chapter 14. Kuroume et al.[37] showed in intrauterine sensitization that hemagglutinating antibody titers against lactalbumin and soybean in the amniotic fluid were high. They suggest this measurement of amniotic fluid as an instrument to predict future allergy.

The allergens of specific foods ingested by the mother have now been identified in the milk. β-Lactoglobulin was studied by Machtinger and Moss[39] and identified in milk. These same investigators measured IgA in milk and attempted to correlate these levels with symptoms in the infants. High IgA levels were seen in asymptomatic infants. Cant et al.[4] found 49 eczematous infants who were solely breastfed to be sensitized to cow's milk and egg protein; these researchers also concluded it was possible to be sensitized by foods eaten by the mother. They were able to demonstrate ovalbumin in the breast milk of 14 of 19 mothers tested 2 to 4 hours after eating raw egg, whether or not their infants had tested positive to egg albumin. Samples of breast milk collected at various times after the mothers were fed 20 g of gluten, after a period of deliberate avoidance of it, were found by Trocone et al.[58] to contain gliadin in 54 of 80 samples. Levels peaked at 2 to 4 hours. Gliadin could not be detected in maternal serum. The transfer of gliadin to the infant via the milk could be one of the factors producing a protective effect, since breastfeeding is known to decrease the risk of celiac disease according to Greco and co-workers.[16]

It has been suggested that for the first 6 weeks or so of life, the intestinal tract is immature anatomically and immunologically. The early absorption of protein macromolecules in young animals is well recognized.[52] The subepithelial plasma cells of the lamina propria mucosae and lymph nodes do not make IgA initially. Gradually the levels increase until they reach adult values at 2 years of age. Children with a strong family history of allergy have a more prolonged deficiency of IgA, lasting 3 months or longer. The early introduction of foods other than human milk has been associated with a rise in antibodies in the blood and eosinophilia, as noted earlier. Providing the infant with breast milk to which he will not become sensitized is the most direct way of dealing with the problem.[14]

The total approach to the potentially allergic individual should include diet in pregnancy to exclude known common food allergens plus any known to cause problems in the members of that family[55] (Table 16-5). From birth until 6 months the infant should receive

Table 16-5. Idealized strategy and mechanisms for the prevention of allergic diseases in humans

Strategy	Mechanisms
Identify at-risk families	Document IgE reactivity in parents with history of allergic disorders or with existing atopic child
Prevent intrauterine sensitization	Reduce maternal dietary allergenic load during last trimester
Prevent postnatal sensitization to	
1. Food allergens	
a. Transmitted through breast milk	Continue maternal avoidance diet during lactation
b. Ingested by infant	Withhold *all* nonbreast milk foods except Nutramigen for at least 6 months
2. Environmental allergens	Encourage, instruct, and document avoidance of animals, mite, dust and molds as well as unnecessary medications
Maximize immunologic competence	Encourage, instruct, and support breastfeeding for at least 6 months
Minimize nonspecific enhancing factors	Discourage parental smoking; avoid viral illnesses (?), delay pertussis immunization (?)

From Hamburger RN et al: Ann Allergy 51:281, 1983.

no cow's milk formula. In addition, the diet of the mother should be restricted as in pregnancy and the environment made as allergen free as possible. If the infant is not breastfed, he should receive cow's milk–free formula. Even though this regimen will not totally prevent all the potentials for allergy, it will help to minimize the insults by foreign protein (Appendix K).

Walker[59] summarizes by saying that it has been shown that antigens cross the intestinal barrier in physiologic and pathologic states. He states it is most important to prevent excessive penetration of antigens in patients that are susceptible to the disease via the following steps:

1. Identify the population at risk
2. Encourage breastfeeding in infancy
3. Decrease antigen load with elemental formulas
4. Continue to conduct direct research at identification and prevention

REFERENCES

1. Bousquet J et al: Predictive value of cord serum IgE determination in the development of "early-onset" atopy, Ann Allergy 51:291, 1983.
2. Businco L et al: Prevention of atopic disease in "at-risk newborns" by prolonged breastfeeding, Ann Allergy 51:296,1983.
3. Chandra RK: Prospective studies on the effect of breast feeding on incidence of infection and allergy, Acta Paediatr Scand 68:691, 1979.
4. Cant A, Marsden RA, and Kilshaw PJ: Egg and cow's milk hypersensitivity in exclusively breastfed infants with eczema, and detection of egg protein in breast milk, Br Med J 291:932, 1985.
5. Chandra RK, Puri S, and Cheema PS: Predictive value of cord blood IgE in the development of atopic disease and role of breastfeeding in its prevention, Clin Allergy 15:517, 1985.
6. Chandra RK, Puri S, Suraiya C, and Cheema PS: Influence of maternal food antigen avoidance dur-

ing pregnancy and lactation on incidence of atopic eczema in infants, Clin Allergy 16:563, 1986.

7. Falliers C et al: Discordant allergic manifestations in monozygotic twins: genetic identity vs. clinical, physiologic, and biochemical differences, J Allergy 47:207, 1971.

8. Freed DLJ and Green FHY: Hypothesis antibody-facilitated digestion and its implications for infant nutrition, Early Hum Dev 1:107, 1977.

9. Gerard JW: Allergy in infancy, Pediatr Ann 3:9, Oct, 1974.

10. Gerrard JW and Shenassa M: Sensitization to substances in breast milk: recognition, management and significance, Ann Allergy 51:300, 1983.

11. Gerrard JW and Shenessa M: Food allergy: two common types as seen in breast and formula fed babies, Ann Allergy 50:375, 1983.

12. Glaser J: Prophylaxis of allergic disease in infancy and childhood. In Speer F and Dockhorn RJ, editors: Allergy and immunology in children, Springfield Ill, 1973, Charles C Thomas, Publisher.

13. Glaser J: Intrauterine sensitization and allergy in the newborn breast fed infant (editorial), Ann Allergy 35:256, 1975.

14. Glaser J, Daeyfuss EM, and Logan J: Dietary prophylaxis of atopic disease. In Kelley VC, editor: Brennemann's practice of pediatrics, vol 2, Hagerstown Md, 1976, Harper & Row, Publishers, Inc.

15. Glaser J and Johnstone DE: Prophylaxis of allergic disease in newborn, JAMA 153:620, 1953.

16. Greco L, Mayer M, Grimaldi M et al: The effect of early feeding on the onset of symptoms in celiac disease, J Pediatr Gastroenterol Nutr 4:52, 1985.

17. Grulee GG, Sanford HN, and Herron PH: Breast and artificial feeding, JAMA 103:735, 1934.

18. Gruskay FL: Comparison of breast, cow, and soy feedings in the prevention of onset of allergic disease, Clin Pediatr 21:486, 1982.

19. Halpern SR et al: Development of childhood allergy in infants fed breast, soy, or cow milk, J Allergy Clin Immunol 51:139, 1973.

20. Hambuger RN: Allergy and the immune system, Am Sci 64:157, 1976.

21. Hamburger RN: Development of atopic allergy in children. In Johansson SGO, editor: International symposium on diagnosis and treatment of IgE-mediated diseases, Amsterdam, 1981, Excerpta Medica.

22. Hamburger RN et al: Current status of the clinical and immunologic consequences of a phototype allergic disease prevention program, Ann Allergy 51:281, 1983.

23. Hide DW and Guyer BM: Clinical manifestations of allergy related to breast and cows' milk feeding, Arch Dis Child 56:172, 1981.

24. Hide DW and Guyer BM: Clinical manifestations of allergy related to breastfeeding and cow's milk–feeding, Pediatrics 76:973, 1985.

25. Johnstone DE: The natural history of allergic disease in children. Advances in Pediatric Allergy workshop proceedings, Rome, 1982.

26. Johnstone DE and Dutton AM: Dietary prophylaxis of allergic disease in children, N Engl J Med 274:715, 1966.

27. Juto P: Elevated serum immunoglobulin E in T-cell-deficient infants fed cow's milk, J Allergy Clin Immunol 66:402, 1980.

28. Juto P and Bjorksten B: Serum IgE in infants and influence of type of feeding, Clin Allergy 10:593, 1980.

29. Juto P and Strannegard O: T lymphocytes and blood eosinophils in early infancy in relation to heredity for allergy and type of feeding, J Allergy Clin Immunol 64:38, 1979.

30. Kajosaari M and Saarinen VM: Prophylaxis of atopic disease by six months' total solid food elimination. Acta Paediatr Scand 72:411, 1983.

31. Kaufman HS and Frick OL: The development of allergy in infants of allergic parents: a prospective study concerning the role of heredity, Ann Allergy 37:410, 1976.

32. Kaufman HS and Frick OL: Prevention of asthma, Clin Allergy 11:549, 1981.

33. Kern RA: Prophylaxis in allergy, Ann Intern Med 12:1175, 1939.

34. Kleinman RE: The role of developmental immune mechanisms in intestinal allergy, Ann Allergy 51:222, 1983.

35. Kleinman RE and Walker WA: The enteromammary immune system: an important new concept in breast milk host defense, Dig Dis Sci 24:876, 1979.

36. Kletter B et al: Immune response of normal infants to cow milk. I. Antibody type and kinetics of production, Int Arch Allergy 40:656, 1971.

37. Kuroume T et al: Milk sensitivity and soybean sensitivity in the production of eczematous manifestations in breast-fed infants with particular reference to intrauterine sensitization, Ann Allergy 37:41, 1976.

38. Lifschitz CH, Hawkins HK, Guerra C, and Byrd N: Anaphylactic shock due to cow's milk protein hypersensitivity in a breastfed infant, J Pediatr Gastroenterol Nutr 7:141, 1988.

39. Machtinger S and Moss R: Cow's milk allergy in breastfed infants: the role of allergen and maternal secretory IgA antibody, J Allergy Clin Immunol 77:341, 1986.

40. Matsumura T et al: Congenital sensitization to food in humans, Jpn J Allergy 16:858, 1967.

41. Matthew DJ et al: Prevention of eczema, Lancet 1:321, 1977.

42. May CD, Fomon SJ, and Remigio L: Immunologic consequences of feeding infants with cow milk and soy products, Acta Paediatr Scand 71:43, 1982.

43. McCombs R, Lowell F, and Ohman J: Myths, morbidity, and mortality in asthma, JAMA 242:1521, 1979.

44. Moore WJ, Midwinter RE, Morris AF et al: Infant feeding and subsequent risk of atopic eczema, Arch Dis Child 60:722, 1985.

45. Murray AB: Infant feeding and respiratory allergy, Lancet 1:497, 1971.

46. Ratner B: A possible causal factor of food allergy in certain infants, Am J Dis Child 36:277, 1928.

47. Rowe AH: Food allergy, Philadelphia, 1931, Lea & Febiger.

48. Saarinen VM et al: Prolonged breast-feeding as prophylaxis for atopic disease, Lancet 2:163, 1979.

49. Savilahti E: Intestinal immunoglobulins in children with coeliac disease, Gut 13:958, 1972.

50. Schwartz RH, Kubicka M, Dreyfuss EM, and Nikaein A: Acute urticarial reactions to cow's milk in infants previously fed breast milk or soy milk, Pediatr Asthma, Asthma Immunol 1:81, 1987.

51. Schloss OM: Allergy in infants and children, Am J Dis Child 19:433, 1920.

52. Shannon WR: Demonstration of food proteins in human breast milk by anaphylactic experiments in guinea pigs, Am J Dis Child 22:223, 1921.

53. Shannon WR: Eczema in breast-fed infants as a result of sensitization to foods in the mother's diet, Am J Dis Child 23:392, 1922.

54. Soothill JT: Some intrinsic and extrinsic factors predisposing to allergy, Proc R Soc Med 69:439, 1976.

55. Soothill JF: Prevention of atopic allergic disease, Ann Allergy 51:229, 1983.

56. Stevenson DD et al: Development of IgE in newborn human infants, J Allergy Clin Immunol 48:61, 1971.

57. Tisdale FF and Erb IH: Extreme sensitization in infants to cow's milk protein, J Can Med Assoc 15:497, 1925.

58. Troncone R, Scarcella A, Donatiello A et al: Passage of gliadin into human breast milk, Acta Paediatr Scand 76:453, 1987.

59. Walker WA: Antigen absorption from the small intestine and gastrointestinal disease, symposium on gastrointestinal and liver disease, Pediatr Clin North Am 22:731, 1975.

Induced lactation and relactation (including nursing the adopted baby)

17

Induced lactation is the process by which a nonpuerperal woman is stimulated to lactate, in other words, breastfeeding without pregnancy. Relactation is the process by which a woman who has given birth but did not initially breastfeed is stimulated to lactate. This may also apply to the situation in which a mother may have initially breastfed her infant, weaned him, and then wishes to reinstitute lactation. Induced lactation and relactation are not new concepts but rather are well known to history and to other cultures. The motivation historically has been to provide nourishment for an infant whose mother has died in childbirth or is unable to nurse him for some reason. A friend or relative would take on the care of the child and with it the responsibility to nourish the infant at the breast, since there were no other alternatives. Relactation has been used in times of disaster or epidemics to provide safe nutrition to weaned or motherless infants. Numerous accounts of induced lactation are recorded in medical literature and reviewed in the writings of Brown.[5] Mead[19] recorded the phenomenon in her writings about New Guinea in 1935. Other anthropologists have made similar observations in other preindustrialized societies of women who have not borne children who, after a few weeks of placing the suckling infant to the breast, produce milk adequate to nourish the infant. Until recently, Western world literature reported the phenomenon as an anecdotal report as part of the discussion of aberrant lactation. Cohen[9] reported in 1971 a patient who had been nursing an adopted child very successfully for weeks when first seen in his pediatric office.

Today the interest in induced lactation in the industrialized world stems from a desire on the part of some adopting mothers to nurture the adopted child at the breast even if she was unable to carry the infant in utero. The interest in relactation comes from mothers of sick or premature infants who wish to breastfeed their infants after the days and weeks of neonatal intensive care are over. These mothers, although postpartum, have not been lactating.

The process of induced lactation is separate from galactorrhea, or inappropriate lactation, which has been described in the medical literature for over 100 years.[27] Abnormal lactation has been observed in a number of circumstances in nulliparous and parous women and even in males. There are many eponyms for these conditions, usually based on the name of the physician who first described the syndrome, such as Chiari-Frommel and Ahumada-del Castillo-Argonz. Normally in the absence of suckling, lactation ceases 14 to 21 days after delivery. Milk flow that continues beyond 3 to 6 months after abortion or any termination of pregnancy is termed abnormal or inappropriate lactation, or galactorrhea. Also included in this group of galactorrhea is lactation in a woman 3 months after weaning or the secretion of milk in a nulliparous woman in association with hyperprolactinemia and amenorrhea. Although these cases are pathologic in nature and therefore different from the groups under discussion, it is noteworthy that some knowledge of the initiation and maintenance of lactation has been gained from the study of these syndromes.

Lactation has been induced for scientific and commercial purposes in nonpregnant and nonparturient animals by the continual systematic application of a mechanical milking apparatus to the mammary gland of the animal.[16] The response is effected through the release of mammotrophic hormone from the anterior pituitary gland. This effect is abolished if the pituitary stalk is transected. Ruminants respond to the addition of estrogen or estrogen-progesterone combinations, which facilitate mammary growth. Experiments in goats involved applying ointment containing estradiol benzoate to the udders of virgins, which resulted in development of the udder and milk yield almost comparable to normal postpartum animals.[10] It was subsequently shown, however, that a combination of estrogen-progesterone not only had a better milk yield but histologically the lobuloalveolar growth was normal, whereas with estrogen alone growth was cystic and irregular. It was also demonstrated that ovariectomized goats could be stimulated to lactation with these two hormones, with resultant normal histology of the udder and good milk production. Initiation of regular milkings had a significant impact on production of milk. The fact that lactation can be stimulated when the ovaries have been removed but not when the pituitary stalk has been severed has significance for understanding some of the postpartum lactation failures in women. Again in ruminants, growth hormone and thyroid hormone have been shown to increase milk yield, although prolactin does not. This suggests that prolactin is not deficient in ruminants. Selye and McKeown[22] showed in 1934 that suckling stimulus inhibits sexual cyclicity in rats. They further showed that when the main milk ducts to all the nipples are cut and the escape of milk has been rendered impossible, the mechanical stimulation of the nipples by nursing would also inhibit the sexual cyclicity of the normal estric, non-lactating adult rat. These studies demonstrate the significance of suckling in triggering the lactation cycle and suppressing ovulation.

Because the motivation, goals, and physiologic problems may be slightly different, induced lactation and relactation shall be considered separately.

INDUCED LACTATION

When a mother wishes to nurse her adopted infant, the goal is usually to achieve a mother-infant relationship that may also have the benefit of some nutrition. Put in that perspective then, success can be evaluated on the basis of whether or not the infant will suckle the breast and achieve some comfort and security from this opportunity and close relationship with his new mother. As has been well described by Avery,[3] this is nurturing with the emphasis on nursing, not on "breastfeeding" or nutrition. A mother who is interested in inducing lactation to nurse an adopted infant may need to understand that she may never be able to completely sustain the infant by her milk alone without supplementation. Neither the physician nor the mother should be disappointed. The nurturing goal is still achieved.

Preparation for induced lactation

Normally the breast is prepared by the proliferation of the ductal and alveolar system through pregnancy in anticipation of the time when lactation will begin.[19] Thus it is appropriate to assume that a period of similar preparation should take place in induced lactation. It has been suggested that the woman should begin systematically to express the breasts manually and stimulate the nipples for up to 2 months prior to the arrival of the infant, if time permits. A hand pump or other pumping devices can be used, but manual expression may work as well or better. Sometimes some secretion can be produced in this manner if it is carried out systemically on a uniform schedule throughout the day. The schedule should be practical, that is, include times when a mother could take a moment for this activity, such as morning and night plus any times she uses the bathroom or can conveniently handle her breasts.

In other cultures in which lactation is induced as a survival tactic for the infant, no period of preparation is available. The infant is put to the adoptive mother's breast and allowed to suckle. Emphasis has been placed on herbal teas as galactogues and good nourishment for the mother, while the infant is also given prechewed food, gruel, or animal milk. Mead attributes much of the success of induced lactation in New Guinea to the ingestion of ample supplies of coconut milk by the new mother.

Adoption is not an easy process, and in fact, it can be quite stressful to become an instant parent. In assisting such a mother, consideration should be given to the infant's age, previous feeding experience, and any medical problems that may exist. Provision for additional nourishment during the process of establishing some milk secretion is most important. Onset of lactation varies from 1 to 6 weeks, averaging about 4 weeks after initiation of stimulation with the appearance of the first drops of milk. When the infant is actually nursing at the breast and being nourished by supplements, milk may appear as early as 1 to 2 weeks.

Some infants are easily confused by switching back and forth between breast and bottle because the sucking technique is slightly different. Other nourishment can be offered by dropper or as solid foods. There is, however, a unique system for providing nourishment for the infant while suckling at the breast. It involves the use of a device to provide a source of nourishment while the infant suckles at the breast, thus stimulating production. It is further described on p. 441 and in Appendix F and is called Supplemental Nursing System (Medela's SNS) or Lact-Aid Nursing Trainer System.

Drugs to induce lactation

As described in Chapter 2, estrogen and progesterone stimulate the proliferation of the alveolar and ductal systems. These hormones work in association with an increase in prolactin production. Although the prolactin level is high during pregnancy, milk secretion is inhibited by the presence of the estrogen, progesterone and prolactin-inhibiting hormone. After delivery has occurred and the placenta is removed, there is a marked fall in these hormones, and prolactin initiates milk production.[25] Efforts to stimulate this hormonal response have had variable success and are not usually recommended because of the possible effect on the infant via the milk. Women taking birth control pills have been noted in some cases to have breast enlargement. In addition, although estrogen and progesterone may enhance proliferation, they may inhibit lactation per se. The dosage recommended by Waletzky and Herman[29] of conjugated estrogens is 2.5 mg twice a day for 14 days beginning on the fourth day of a regular menstrual cycle. Giving 0.35 mg norethindrone once daily with the morning dose of estrogen prevents breakthrough bleeding. Medication is given for 2 weeks and is comparable in dosage to 2 weeks of birth control pills. This may be accompanied by some side effects. The regimen should include direct efforts to stimulate lactation.

Oxytocin, on the other hand, is a critical component in the milk ejection reflex and may be helpful in the early initiation of ejection. Physiologically stimulation of the nipple in the lactating woman results in the release of oxytocin by the hypothalamus, which then triggers the release of milk by stimulating the contraction of the myoepithelial cells and the ejection of milk (see Chapter 8). The effect of intranasal administration of oxytocin on the let-down reflex in lactating women was well described by Newton and Egli.[20] (Oral administration by tablet has not been as effective, since oxytocin is destroyed in the stomach.) Oxytocin nasal spray has been utilized in nonpuerperal lactation with some success in enhancing let-down but not necessarily altering the volume produced. Continued use of oxytocin over weeks has been associated with diminished effect or even suppression of lactation. The chief benefit of oxytocin is often to break the cycle of failure and instill a feeling of confidence once it has been demonstrated that some secretion can be produced.

Chlorpromazine has been observed to act as a galactagogue as well as a tranquilizer when given to patients in large doses (up to 1000 mg or more). The effect has been observed in both male and female patients in mental institutions. The drug has been reported to increase pituitary prolactin secretion severalfold. It acts via the hypothalamus, probably by reducing levels of prolactin-inhibitory factor (PIF). Using this information, women well motivated to lactate who have attempted induced lactation by suckling a normal infant have had the process enhanced by small doses of chlorpromazine, according to Brown.[7] In a program to induce lactation in refugee camps in India and in Vietnam, nonlactating women were given 25 to 100 mg of chlorpromazine three times a day for a week to 10 days while infants were initially put to breast. Brown reports apparent enhancement of lactation with this treatment.[6] Chlorpromazine has the added pharmacological effect of acting as a tranquilizer. The program of management in these women was supportive in other ways and also included the usual herbal medicines associated with lactation in these Eastern cultures. There was no control group. It is possible that the drug contributed to both the physiologic and psychologic well-being of the women wishing to lactate. It has been suggested that the wish to lactate is a strong component of success, since women whose breasts are frequently stimulated sexually do not begin to lactate. Theophylline can also increase pituitary prolactin secretions, according to Vorherr[28]; therefore both tea and coffee should enhance prolactin secretion and thus lactation. Excessive amounts may inhibit let-down, however.

Since the role of prolactin is the initiation and maintenance of lactation, whereas oxytocin regulates the glandular emptying via the milk-ejection reflex, it is reasonable to speculate that enhancing prolactin release would be productive in inducing lactation. The exact activating mechanism of the neuronal reflex arc from breast to brain has not been deciphered. Secretion of prolactin appears to be influenced, if not controlled, by changes in hypothalamic dopamine turnover. Correspondingly, suckling has been observed to deplete dopamine stores.

Investigation of other drugs that are known to stimulate prolactin release has identified some possible therapeutic materials. McNeilly et al.[18] have reported metoclopramide in-

Table 17-1. Influence of drugs on prolactin secretion

Phamacologic agents	Plasma prolactin concentration	Mechanism of drug action
L-Dopa	Decrease	Increase in hypothalamic dopamine-catecholamine levels, leading to enhanced activity of prolactin-inhibiting factor (PIF)
Ergot alkaloids (ergocornine, ergocryptine)	Decrease	Direct inhibition of adenohypophyseal prolactin secretion; possible increase of hypothalamic PIF activity (continued PIF function)
Thyrotropin-releasing hormone (TRH; pyroglutamyl-histidyl-prolinamide) Theophylline	Increase	Direct stimulation of adenohypophyseal lactotrophs for increased prolactin secretion
Phenothiazines (chlorpromazine) Amphetamine α-Methyldopa	Increase	Decreases in hypothalamic dopamine-catecholamine levels, leading to diminution of PIF activity
Metoclopramide	Increase	Inhibition of hypothalamic PIF secretion through dopamine antagonism
Sulpiride	Increase	Increase in hypothalamic prolactin-releasing hormone

From Vorherr H: Human lactation and breast feeding. In Larson BL, editor: Lactation, New York, 1978, Academic Press, Inc, p 182.

duces prolactin release regardless of the route of administration. Prolactin levels are increased three to eight times normal levels within 5 minutes when a 10 mg dose is given either intravenously or intramuscularly. The effect is achieved within an hour when metoclopramide is given orally. The effect persists for 8 hours. No reports are available for its use in nonpuerperal women at this time, although metoclopramide has been used to enhance lactation and for relactation (p. 441) (see Table 17-5).

The regulation of prolactin secretion in humans has been studied to further the understanding of abnormal lactation as well as provide information on the regulation of pituitary function of the brain. It has been shown experimentally that the hypothalamus secretes PIF, which acts on the mammotropin-releasing cells of the pituitary to inhibit release of the hormone prolactin. The hypothalamus can also regulate prolactin secretion by a stimulatory mechanism, the secretion of thyrotropin-releasing hormone (TRH). When human volunteers (nonpregnant, nonlactating) are given infusions of TRH, increases in thyrotropin and prolactin are observed within minutes of injection with values peaking in 20 minutes. The level of thyroid hormone in the volunteers initially influences the results. Hypothyroid patients have been observed to secrete excessive amounts of prolactin, whereas hyperthyroid patients are relatively insensitive to TRH. This may explain some of the variable results obtained with prolactin-stimulating drugs used to enhance lactation. Studies of relactation have been done using TRH but not of de novo induced lactation.

Table 17-1 summarizes the influence of drugs on prolactin secretion.

Jelliffe[13] points out that the most important factor for continued production of milk is not drugs or hormones but "mulging." He explains that *mulging* (stimulation) is a word

Table 17-2. Composition of normal breast milk and "galactorrhea milk"

Milk components and properties	Normal breast milk	"Galactorrhea milk"	Induced lactation
Components			
Fat (g/100 ml)	3.7	3-8	
Lactose (g/100 ml)	7.0	3-5	5.4
Total protein (g/100 ml)	1.2	2-7	1.6
Sodium (mg/100 ml)	15	70	22.0
Potassium (mg/100 ml)	50	5	19.8
Calcium (mg/100 ml)	35	38	
Chlorine (mg/100 ml)	45	50	18.4
Phosphorous (mg/100 ml)	15	2	
Ash (mg/100 ml)	20	40-70	
Properties			
Specific gravity	1030-1033	1031	
Milk pH	6.8-7.3	7.3	
Daily volume	400-800 ml	1-120 ml	

From Vorherr H: The breast: morphology, physiology and lactation, New York, 1974. Academic Press, Inc; and Kulski J K, et al: Obstet Gynecol 139:597, 1981. Reprinted with permission from the American College of Obstetricians and Gynecologists.

created in 1975 by N.W. Pirie to mitigate the confusion between the words *sucking* and *suckling*. The word comes from the Latin *mulgere,* to milk.

Composition of milk in induced lactation

Concern has been expressed that the composition of the milk produced by stimulation of suckling rather than as a result of pregnancy might indeed differ from "normal human milk."[24] Such induced milk is not different in other species that have been studied extensively, including bovine and rat. In developing countries the fact that the infants showed normal growth and weight gain was taken as evidence that the milk is adequate. Vorherr[27,28] reported the analysis of the galactorrheal secretion produced by the breast following hyperstimulation. The comparative analysis is shown in Table 17-2. The induced lactational milk did not differ from puerperal milk. Brown[5] reported higher values of fat, protein, and lactose in galactorrheal milk, but the volume of secretion was small in these subjects.

The composition of the breast secretion produced by two women who induced lactation artificially by breast hyperstimulation was close to the composition obtained for women with normal lactation, according to Kulski et al.[15] (Table 17-2). These investigators also examined the milk of a woman in whom lactation had occurred when medicated with a psychotropic drug (haloperidol). She had had a pregnancy 4 years previously. Her galactorrhea lasted 38 months. Her milk had composition like that of colostrum for a week but resembled mature milk at 1 month. A woman with hypothyroidism and elevated prolactin and TSH had colostrum-like milk for 53 days of sampling. Two women with galactorrhea and amenorrhea associated with pituitary tumor and hyperprolactinemia had transient colostrum-like secretion, which changed to mature milk. Protein values of milk samples from five mothers without biologic pregnancies were measured by Kleinman et al.[14] Two of the mothers had nursed previous babies and three had never been pregnant and had never breastfed. These authors did not distinguish between them. The mean total protein con-

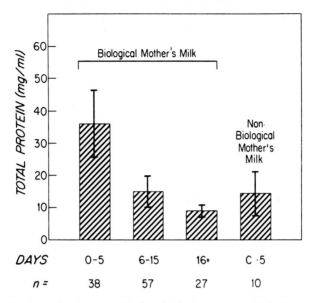

Fig. 17-1. Total protein changes with time: biologic versus nonbiologic mother's milk, protein value ± SD. (From Kleinman R, Jacobson L, Hormann E, and Walker WA: J Pediatr 97:613, 1980.)

centration of milk samples from the "nonbiologic" mothers differs from the "biologic" mothers (Figs. 17-1 and 17-2). If the goal of induced lactation is nurturing, these differences are clinically less important. However, the clinician needs to keep these values in mind when counseling a mother-infant dyad about induced lactation nutrition, especially if the infant was premature or small for gestational age. A creamatocrit test for fat and energy content is an appropriate first step. (See Chapter 19, p. 476.) In tandem nursing, when a mother continues to nurse an older child and puts an adopted newborn on the breast simultaneously, the composition of milk will not return to colostrum as it does with a biologic pregnancy.

Management of the mother and infant when lactation is induced

In the collected experiences of counseling women in the Western world who wish to induce lactation there are several thousand women reported. The request for information and advice is increasing and becoming widespread throughout the United States and other Western countries.[24]

Because there are simple means of supplementing the nutritional needs of the infant, the counseling should center on the relationship and the nurturing aspects. When the process is undertaken in preindustrialized nations, the anti-infective properties become important even though total nourishment may not be possible. Success is measured by having the infant content to nurse at the breast.

The woman should be encouraged to come to the physician's office for a counseling visit prior to the arrival of the adoptive infant to discuss the process of induced lactation. Actually, parents who are planning to adopt an infant should have at least one visit with

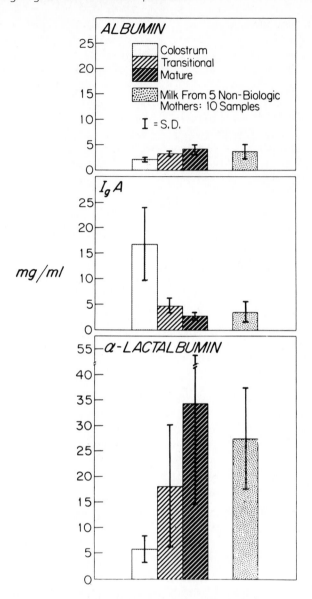

Fig. 17-2. Protein changes with time: biologic versus nonbiologic mother's milk. (From Kleinman R, Jacobson L, Hormann E, and Walker WA: J Pediatr 97:614, 1980.)

their pediatrician so that some understanding of parenting can be discussed, just as any couple should do prior to the birth of their first child. At this visit while discussing lactation with the couple, it is helpful to explore their motives and general concepts of what is involved. It has been pointed out by all authors on the subject that the husband's interest in and support of lactation is critical to success. His participation in the preparation of the breasts may be a means by which the father can share intimately and constructively in the process. Instruction of the mother in preparation of the breast for suckling is also critical in induced lactation, whereas with puerperal lactation it may not be necessary at all.

Exercises to stimulate the nipple should be undertaken several times a day and will be most successful if they are scheduled for times when and situations in which it is easy, feasible, and readily remembered. A few minutes multiple times a day is more successful and less likely to *overemphasize* milk versus mothering than rigid excessive exercises one or twice a day. Manual manipulation with gentle traction or horizontal and vertical stretching can be suggested. Avery[3] suggests that the father be encouraged to assist in breast massage and other techniques. She notes that "many adoptive parents felt that this technique (fondling and suckling of the breasts by the husband) added to the mutual sharing in preparation for adoptive nursing similar to the closeness many couples experience in preparing for natural childbirth." Raphael[21] reports that among 40 adoptive nursing mothers there were dozens of variations on the theme of preparation. A positive attitude seemed to be the only consistent factor.

The need for dietary counseling is obvious. Lip service in behalf of well-balanced nutritious meals is not enough. Discussion should center around the absolute needs in kilocalories, fluids, and nutrients to produce milk (Chapter 9).

The physician should point out that stimulation of the nipples may well cause amenorrhea. Although the variation in menses is not uniform, decreased flow, irregular cycles, or total cessation of menstrual flow is possible. On the other hand, the menstrual cycle may be maintained and the flow of milk may seem to vary during menses. Changes in breast size, heaviness, and feeling of fullness may accompany the induced lactation. There may be an associated weight gain of 10 to 12 pounds, on the average, according to Avery,[3] attributed to the response of the body to developing stores for lactation, just as in pregnancy (i.e., increased fluid retention and appetite increase). The weight gain may be a simple phenomenon of excessive intake. There is no need to gain excessive weight, however, during this experience. Mothers (who may be nutritionally depleted) in non-Western countries who induce lactation are given added diet, nourishment, and herbal teas but do not usually gain weight. Failure to experience change in breast size, menstrual regularity, or weight should not be construed as a failed response.

Auerbach and Avery[2] reported a retrospective questionnaire study of 240 women, 83 of whom had never been pregnant or lactated before, 55 of whom had been pregnant but never lactated, and 102 of whom had breastfed one or more biologic children prior to the adoptive nursing (lactation). Most respondents used more than one technique to stimulate their nipples. The most effective method of nipple stimulation, these mothers felt, was nipple exercises combined with infant suckling. Hand-operated pumps caused soreness and irritation. The nipple exercises included nipple stroking, massaging the breast, and rolling the nipple between thumb and finger. In this study, the infant's willingness to suckle improved over time and was related to the age at which he was first put to breast. Infants who were under 8 weeks of age had over a 75% success rate; those over 8 weeks of age had only 50% success. No infants failed to thrive, but nearly all needed some type of supplementation. Mothers who had nursed a biologic baby before were able to wean from supplementation partially or completely. This group was also more disappointed if they had to supplement.

These few simple guidelines, developed as a result of experiences reported by several authors and many mothers, may be helpful to the physician in counseling the mother to induce lactation:

1. Before arrival of the baby, initiate frequent brief manual stimulation of nipples and breasts, increasing time gradually to about 10 minutes per session. Initiate mechanical pumping stimulus after 2 weeks or so of manual stimulus. Hand pumps

usually cause more soreness. Modern electric pumps with milking action and pressure cycling are most effective.

2. Upon arrival of the baby, depending on age of the infant, provide all sucking of the breast using lactation supplementer if necessary.
3. Breastfeed before any other nourishment is provided for a given feeding.
4. Avoid stressing baby with hunger.
5. When supplementing, use donor human milk or prepared formula, not cow's milk with its long stomach-emptying time.
6. Avoid rubber nipples and pacifiers to encourage appropriate suckling at breast.
7. Provide other supplements by dropper, spoon, cup, or supplementer.
8. Create positive atmosphere—mother the mother.

Rigid conformity to a system of feeding may be a symptom of a more serious problem. Women who are rigid and compulsive may have trouble lactating because of the inability to have a good ejection reflex, which can be inhibited by stress and emotional conflict. Mothers who demonstrate an inordinate attention to volume of production of milk over and above the value of the relationship may feel as if they have failed.

Nutritional supplementation

The need to supplement the infant's intake while the milk supply is being developed should be discussed. The older infant who has already been receiving solid foods can be continued on solids by spoon with careful attention to nutritional content so that the diet includes a balance of protein and other nutrients. Supplements with milk or formula should be appropriate to the age of the infant. The infant under 6 months should receive infant formula rather than whole milk if donor breast milk is not available. The milk supplements should be full strength, 20 kcal/oz and provided during the feeding by dropper or supplementer or after the nursing by dropper, spoon, or cup in preference to rubber nipple, which may confuse the infant in his adaptation to nursing at the breast.

The process of induced lactation requires considerable commitment and determination. It is far more arduous a task than initiating postpartum lactation, but it is possible and worth the effort, according to the many mothers who have attempted it. The situation is better managed if a doula is available. It is appropriate for the physician to suggest that in addition to medical support the mother seek counseling from a lactation counselor experienced in induced lactation. Day-by-day contact for verbal support may be helpful, and these needs may be beyond the scope of a busy office practice. The nurse practitioner may be invaluable in this situation, particularly if home visits are made.

Assuring that the child grows appropriately is the responsibility of the pediatrician; however, this task is best carried out in a nonthreatening way so the mother can concentrate on nurturing and nourishing the infant. Monitoring the usual growth parameters of weight and height as well as the patterns of voiding and stooling is essential.

RELACTATION

The need to relactate exists in a number of circumstances, including the following:

1. A sick or premature infant cannot be fed initially or even until he is several weeks or months old (Fig. 17-3).
2. An infant is weaned prematurely because of illness in the infant or in the mother.
3. An infant who was not previously breastfed develops an allergy or food intolerance.
4. A mother who has lactated weeks, months, or years before and wishes to nurse an adopted infant.

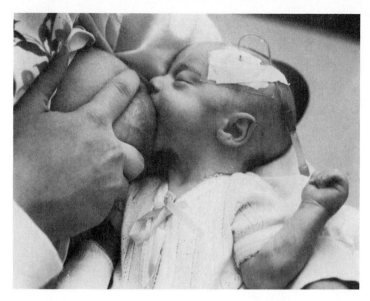

Fig. 17-3. Premature infant (1300 g) at time of photograph at breast.

  5. A mother who is nursing a biologic child begins nursing an adopted child (without
     benefit of pregnancy).

Historical reviews provide many examples of infants suckled in times of crisis by
women who have not lactated for years. The process of reestablishing lactation under these
circumstances is generally easier than that of nonpuerperal lactation. Investigations have
shown that a breast that has been previously primed by pregnancy to respond to prolactin
will produce milk more readily.

Although the general process of nipple stimulation, having the infant suckle the
breast, and setting the stage for lactation is similar, the woman who has experienced
successful lactation previously may have not only the physiologic but also the psychologic
edge.

A prospective study of mothers whose infants were in the neonatal intensive care
unit in Durham, North Carolina, was reported by Bose et al.[4] The profile of the mothers
is listed in Table 17-3. Mother and baby were admitted to the Clinical Research Unit,
where they were assisted with relactating including help using the Lact-Aid. The infant's
nutritional intake was recorded. Mother and infant were discharged when the mother was
comfortable with the Lact-Aid and feeding was established (about 3 days). Follow-up
occurred every week or two. All but one infant were initially reluctant to suckle, but all
received their entire nutritional intake at the breast, with or without Lact-Aid, within the
first week of the study. Most of the mothers had trouble initiating suckling, with the most
significant factor being the length of separation from their infant and not degree of prematurity, postnatal age, weight, or feeding regimen. Nipple tenderness occurred in all
mothers transiently. All the mothers (except number seven, who was an adoptive mother)
produced milk in 1 week, with maximum milk production occurring from 8 to 58 days,
proportional to the time since delivery. Although it was done with a small population, this
study established some important information. Given appropriate techniques and support,
many women appear to be able to relactate, and premature infants can learn to breastfeed
after initial bottle feeding.

Table 17-3. Historical and clinical data of mothers in relactation study

Case number	Gestational age	Time from delivery to entry into study (days)	Time from last lactation to entry into study (days)	Postpartum breast involution*	Time to first breast milk (days)	Time to half breast milk supply† (days)	Time to complete relactation (days)
1	Term	10	10	None	1	4	8
2	Term	120	120	Incomplete	4	20	28
3‡	Twins, 31 wk	49	49	Complete	7	28	Never
4	32 wk	70	42	Complete	7	39	Never
5	28 wk	150	135	Complete	9	Never	Never
6	32 wk	30	16	None	4	17	58
7	Term (adopted)	5 yr	5 yr	Complete	21	Never	Never

From Bose CL et al: Pediatrics 67:565, 1981. Copyright American Academy of Pediatrics 1980.
*Mothers were asked if their brassiere size was different from that before this pregnancy.
†Estimated on the basis of a decrease in formula intake.
‡Ceased to suckle her infant after 28 days in the study to return to full-time employment.

A retrospective study of relactation was reported by Auerbach and Avery[1] in which 366 women responded with a completed questionnaire out of over 500 contacted from a list of names obtained from manufacturer's lists, magazine ads, and requests to breast-feeding support groups. The bias was in favor of well-educated, affluent women who had probably obtained their lactation goals. The population included those who had untimely weaning ($N = 174$), following delivery of low birthweight infants ($N = 117$), and following hospitalization of mother or baby or both ($N = 75$).

Willingness to nurse on the part of the infant was related to his previous suckling experience, but responses in the first week of effort were not directly correlated with ultimate successful suckling. Fifty percent of mothers were able to discontinue supplementing in 1 month, and 24% were never able to eliminate supplements completely. Once established, the nursing patterns were similar to those of ordinary breastfeeding. The authors point out that keeping the baby hungry in the mistaken notion that he will nurse more often and for longer periods does not help and may negatively influence outcome. For the professional it is of interest that fewer than 10% of respondents received helpful advice from health-care professionals.

Tandem nursing

Tandem nursing an adoptive child is a phenomenon in which the adoptive mother is still nursing a biologic child and puts an adopted infant to the breast and intends to nourish the newcomer totally. Usually the older child is a toddler and feeding only a few times a day or for comfort and receiving the major nourishment from other food and drink. In biologic tandem nursing, the milk returns to colostrum-like constituency with the birth of the new baby; however, in the absence of a pregnancy the milk volume may increase with increased nipple stimulus while the constituents do not change. Data of milk constituents beyond a year postpartum or in the case of relactation have been noted (see p. 436). In most cases reported anecdotally the adopted infant is several weeks or months old, so the absence of colostrum is less of a problem. On the other hand, the active state of lactation in terms of immediate availability of milk is actually an advantage. An additional concern, as in any situation of tandem nursing, is the development of the younger child. The physician will need to be alert to these issues in counseling the family and assuring adequate total nutrition for the adopted child. Eighteen respondents to the survey on adoptive nursing by Auerbach and Avery[2] reported tandem-nursing experiences. Eleven of these mothers were able to discontinue supplements totally (two within the first month). Most of the infants were started on solids by 4½ months, which may be the most effective method of supplementing if nutritional value is maintained. For the physician it is important to be knowledgeable about tandem adoptive nursing and to support the family accordingly.

Drugs to induce relactation

Some medications that have been tried in relactation seem only to work when the breast has been primed by mammogenesis, that is, by pregnancy.

Thyrotropin-releasing hormone (TRH, pyroglutamyl-histidyl-prolinamide) (Thyroliberin), has been used by Tyson[26] and others to induce lactation. Each woman in their study was primed with estrogens beforehand. TRH stimulates the pituitary to release both TSH and prolactin. Drugs that produce a decrease in hypothalamic catecholamines, such as phenothiazines, reserpine, meprobamate, amphetamines, and α-methyldopa, cause an increase in prolactin secretion by blocking hypothalamic PIF.

Table 17-4. Basal and stimulated serum prolactin concentrations (ng/ml)

Case number	TRH stimulation		Suckling stimulation: presuckling/postsuckling					
	Basal	15 min/30 min	1st wk*	2nd wk	3rd wk	4th-5th wk	6th-7th wk	8th-9th wk
1	179.2	611.1/423.5	136.9/155.4	72.3/123.8	...	...	...	...
2	38.7	80.9/70.3	17.2/119.3	38.6/214.3	16.6/180.6	186.2/244.5	...	...
3	19.9	89.6/77.3	17.9/23.5	...	...	...	...	...
4	9.5	89.9/63.4	12.5/12.7	...	7.0/437.6	5.5/47.3	...	...
5	13.9	40.6/36.3	21.1/58.2	37.8/82.0	38.3/57.7	77.2/98.5	24.6/54.2	...
6	31.7	335.6/274.7	9.5/11.4	...	16.5/18.4	11.8/16.3	7.8/13.3	...
7	43.6†	78.8/69.9	8.8/59.6	17.0/77.7	...	...	34.4/147.1	19.2/60.5

From Bose CL et al: Pediatrics 67:565, 1981. Copyright American Academy of Pediatrics 1980.

*Suckling test performed on day 1 or 2 of study.

†In this mother, suckling test was done first, followed 1 hour later by thyrotropin-releasing hormone (TRH) infusion; thus, 8.8 is the true basal concentration.

The feasibility of pharmacologically manipulating puerperal lactation was demonstrated by Canales et al.[8] using bromocriptine and TRH sequentially. They suppressed lactation using bromocriptine orally for 8 days in four mothers whose infants were premature and/or ill and could not be nursed. These mothers did not lactate during this time. On the eighth day they were given TRH intravenously and then daily orally for 4 days (eighth to twelfth postpartum day). On the fourteenth day they initiated breastfeeding by putting the infant to the breast. Prolactin levels were measured from the day of birth. Levels were depressed by bromocriptine and noted to rise when the TRH was given. The mothers subsequently nursed successfully.

Bose et al.[4] also studied TRH and the basal and stimulated serum prolactin concentrations. Prolactin concentrations were measured followed by levels of 15 and 30 minutes after intravenous infusion of 200 µg of thyrotropin-releasing hormone (TRH). Prolactin levels are also measured before and after suckling at weekly intervals. Serum prolactin levels rose 15 minutes after infusion of TRH (Table 17-4). The absolute rise in prolactin concentrations did not appear to be related to establishment of milk production. The change over time in the basal prolactin levels was not predictably related to lactation progress.

Lactation can be reestablished with metoclopramide, according to Sousa et al.[23] Metoclopramide is a derivative of procainamide, as is sulpiride. Studies done by McNeilly et al.[18] showed that metoclopramide and sulpiride are potent stimulators of prolactin release. These authors demonstrated marked increase in prolactin when metoclopramide is given, as noted earlier in this chapter. Sousa et al.[23] used metoclopramide to reestablish lactation in women who had experienced diminished milk supply. All five mothers experienced increased production of milk when 10 mg was given orally every 8 hours for 7 to 10 days. No side effects were noted, although this drug is known to cause cardiac arrhythmias and extrapyramidal signs in some adults. No side effects were noted in the infants either, but the level of drug was not measured in the milk. The results were encouraging, but further study is needed to determine the minimum dosage necessary to produce the effect and the amount passed into the milk. The summation of the data on patients treated by Sousa et al.[25] is recorded in Table 17-5.

In a controlled double-blind study with a placebo, Lewis et al.[17] found no difference in the success rate of induced lactation in 10 patients medicated with 10 mg metoclopramide orally three times daily for 7 days compared to 10 matched patients medicated with lactose capsules. Successful lactation was attributed to the special advice and support provided

Table 17-5. Data regarding mothers taking metoclopramide

Number	Age of mother (yr)	Age of infant (mo)	Daily dose (mg)	Length of treatment (days)	Side effects	Result	Education level of mother
1	27	2	30	6	None	Increase in milk volume; infant not weaned	University
2	25	10	30	10	None	Same as above	University
3	29	1	20	7	None	Same as above	High school
4	35	3	30	7	None	Same as above	University
5	20	2	20	7	None	Same as above	High school

From Sousa PLR et al: J Trop Pediatr 21:214, 1975.

equally for these women by the nursery staff. Before conducting the study, these authors measured the amount of drug that appeared in the milk of 10 women after a single 10 mg dose of metoclopramide orally given at 7 to 10 days postpartum. The mean 2-hour postdose plasma level was 68.5 ± 29.6 ng/ml. The simultaneous mean concentration in the breast milk was 125.7 ± 41.7 ng/ml. Consuming a liter of milk a day, the dose to the infant would be calculated at 130 mg or 45 mg/kg, a subtherapeutic dose. These data do not address possible accumulation in the infant, however, when multiple doses are given to the mother.

SPECIAL DEVICES

Although many mechanical devices have been developed since Roman times to augment lactation and give other feeding opportunities, lactation supplementing devices provide a unique ability to nourish an infant adequately while he suckles at the inadequately lactating breast (Fig. 17-4). The suckling stimulates the mother's own supply. On the other hand, the infant continues to suckle the breast because there is milk available. The devices have been carefully engineered to provide a source of milk that is obtained by suckling, not by gravity. The capillary tube through which the milk flows can be placed along the human nipple without interfering with suckling. The plastic containers that serve as reservoirs for the supplemental milk are sterilizable or disposable. The milk is naturally warmed by hanging the bag beside the mother's breast, as shown in Fig. 17-4. See Appendix F for a full description.

Gradual weaning from the supplementer can be provided by putting less and less in the container each day so that the infant can obtain milk from the breast in increasing amounts as the nipple stimulation affects milk production.

An increasing number of mothers wish to nurse their sick premature infants; however, it is often not possible to put the infant to breast for weeks. Meanwhile the mother may pump but only obtain minimal volume. When the infant is finally ready for discharge from the hospital, it is mandatory that he continue to receive reliable nourishment every day. Starving the infant into submission is inappropriate and dangerous. A lactation supplementer is an excellent alternative.

For years mothers of premature and sick infants have been assisted in breastfeeding their infants in preparation for discharge from the hospital and during early weeks at home by using dropper feeding, complementary feeds by bottle after each breastfeeding, or solids. The success rate was low and the aggravation for the mother often insurmountable.

Weaning from the device is usually not a problem for most of the infants. It was a problem, however, for an occasional mother who could not nurse without the supplementer even though it contained less than an ounce of formula per feeding and the breast was supplying the rest. Mother may use it as a "crutch." Careful anticipatory counseling should avoid this.

Special equipment should be started with a full understanding of its role in nourishment of the infant as well as with a plan for weaning from it that begins the first day. Weaning should be appropriate to the age of the infant and his nutritional needs. The nourishment provided should be donor human milk or regular-strength formula, 20 kcal/oz and not just water, sugar water, or diluted formula. Starvation, even for a day or so, in a premature infant compromises the growth, especially of the brain. An infant who has been in the intensive care nursery is in special jeopardy (Fig. 14-13). Several alternative devices have been suggested by professionals interested in the transient supplementation

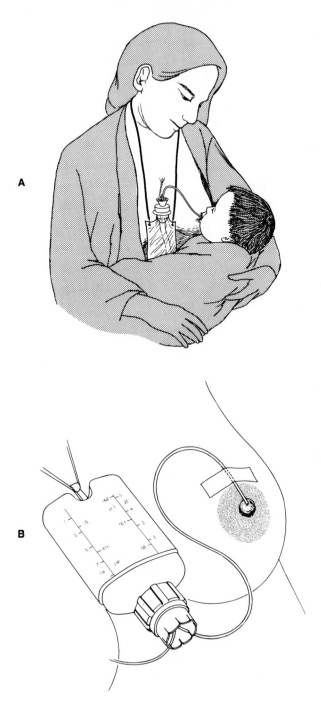

Fig. 17-4.   A, Lact-Aid Nursing Trainer System (Lact-Aid International, Inc.). **B,** Lactation Supplementer by Medela, which provides additional nourishment to the infant while suckling at the underproducing breast.

of lactation while a mother increased her milk supply for her full-term baby. Usually these are situations where lactation failure has been the result of inadequate initial advice. The devices are rigged from readily available feeding tubes and syringes but lack the special engineering and safety features of the supplementer. Special precautions are advised when employing such hand-made equipment to avoid milk aspiration by the infant, which is the chief hazard. Because they will allow milk to flow without sucking, they do not stimulate the infant to suck. Other devices, such as hand pumps, the electric pumps, and the Whittlestone physiologic breast milker, which are useful in initiating relactation or induced lactation as well as puerperal nursing, are illustrated in Chapter 19.

SUMMARY

Careful medical management of the adopted infant who is breastfed is important. Many times the prenatal care of this infant as a fetus in utero has not been optimal. Any failure in growth should be identified quickly so that appropriate supplementation can be provided. In cases of relactation to provide for sick or premature infants, close follow-up is mandatory. A child who does not have a powerful suck may well appear to be very content yet be underfed. This situation was clearly described by Gilmore and Rowland[12] who reported three cases of malnutrition while breastfeeding, attributed to the failure of the mother to recognize signs of growth failure and dehydration.

Relactation and induced lactation are special events requiring the positive support of medical personnel. The physician can serve as a well-informed stable resource in a process that will require considerable effort and commitment by the participants.

Mother-initiated preparation for induced lactation or relactation

1. Nipple stimulation: hand massage and nipple exercises, hand pump, electric "milkers"
2. Diet supplementation: fluids and calories, especially protein
3. Reading, learning, and communication with others with similar experience

Physician-initiated preparation for induced lactation or relactation

1. Knowledgeable, sympathetic support
2. Preparatory hormones and lactagogues to promote mammogenesis may be considered
3. Induction of let-down: oxytocin nasal spray to initiate or enhance let-down
4. Counseling about breast preparation and diet supplementation in the context of total care of the mother and the infant
5. Use of lactation supplementing devices

REFERENCES

1. Auerbach KG and Avery JL: Relactation: a study of 366 cases, Pediatrics 65:236, 1980.
2. Auerbach KG and Avery JL: Induced lactation: a study of adoptive nursing by 240 women, Am J Dis Child 135:340, 1981.
3. Avery JL: Induced lactation: a guide for counseling and management, Denver, 1979, Resources in Human Nurturing, International.
4. Bose, CL et al: Relactation by mothers of sick and premature infants, Pediatrics 67:565, 1981.
5. Brown RE: Some nutritional considerations in times of major catastrophe, Clin Pediatr 11:334, 1972.
6. Brown RE: Breast-feeding in modern times, Am J Clin Nutr 26:556, 1973.
7. Brown RE: Relactation: an overview, Pediatrics 60:116, 1977.
8. Canales ES et al: Feasibility of suppressing and reinitiating lactation in women with premature infants, Am J Obstet Gynecol 128:695, 1977.
9. Cohen R: Breast-feeding without pregnancy: letter to the editor, Pediatrics 48:996, 1971.
10. Cowie AT, Forsyth IA, and Hart IC: Hormonal control of lactation, Monographs on Endocrinology, vol 15, New York, 1980, Springer-Verlag.
11. Evans TJ and Davies DP: Failure to thrive at the breast: an old problem revisited, Arch Dis Child 52:974, 1977.
12. Gilmore HE and Rowland TW: Critical malnutrition in breast fed infants, Am J Dis Child 132:885, 1978.
13. Jelliffe DB: Hormonal control of lactation. In Schams D, editor: Ciba Foundation Symposium no 45, breast feeding and the mother, Amsterdam, 1976, Elsevier Scientific Publ Co.
14. Kleinman R et al: Protein values of milk samples from mothers without biologic pregnancies, J Pediatr 97:612, 1980.
15. Kulski JK et al: Changes in the milk composition of nonpuerperal women, Obstet Gynecol 139:597, 1981.
16. Larson BL: Lactation: a comprehensive treatise. IV. The mammary gland/human lactation/milk synthesis, New York, 1978, Academic Press, Inc.
17. Lewis PJ, Devenish C, and Kahn C: Controlled trial of metoclopramide in the initiation of breast-feeding, Br J Clin Pharmacol 9:217, 1980.
18. McNeilly AS et al: Metoclopramide prolactin, Br Med J 2:729, 1974.
19. Mead M: Sex and temperament in three primitive societies, New York, 1963, Dell Publishing Co, Inc.
20. Newton M and Egli GE: The effect of intra-nasal administration of oxytocin on the let-down of milk in lactating women, Am J Obstet Gynecol 76:103, 1958.
21. Raphael D: Breast feeding the adopted baby. In Raphael D: The tender gift: breast feeding, New York, 1976, Schocken Books.
22. Selye H and McKeon T: The effect of mechanical stimulation of the nipples on the ovary and the sexual cycle, Surg Gynecol Obstet 59:886, 1934.
23. Sousa PLR et al: Re-establishment of lactation with metoclopramide, J Trop Pediatr 21:214, 1975.
24. Thearle JJ and Weissenberger R: Induced lactation in adoptive mothers, Aust NZ J Obstet Gynecol AEC 24:283, 1984.
25. Turkington RW: Human prolactin, Am J Med 53:389, 1972.
26. Tyson JE: Mechanisms of puerperal lactation. In Tyson JE, editor: Symposium on pregnancy, Med Clin North Am 61:153, 1977.
27. Vorherr H: The breast: morphology, physiology and lactation, New York, 1974, Academic Press, Inc.
28. Vorherr H: Human lactation and breast feeding. In Larson BL, editor: Lactation, New York, 1978, Academic Press, Inc.
29. Waletzky LR and Herman EC: Relactation, Am Fam Pract 14:69, 1976.

18

Reproductive function during lactation

FERTILITY

Although gonadotropic and ovarian function during lactation have been investigated, the major body of knowledge has been collected about the postpartum return of the menstrual cycle and ovulation in the woman who is lactating as compared to the nonlactating woman.

The amenorrhea of lactation has been attributed to an imperfect balance of hypo-thalamoanteropituitary function and gonadotropin secretion, although the complex process by which lactation inhibits ovulation and the menstrual cycle is incompletely understood. It is clear that frequent suckling, which results in high prolactin levels, is closely associated with altered luteinizing hormone (LH) secretion and amenorrhea.[32]

Secretion of follicle-stimulating hormone (FSH) and LH is generally diminished whenever prolactin is released from the acidophilic cells of the hypothalamoanteropituitary axis. Although the inhibition of FSH and LH has been reported by some, other investigators found no difference between lactating and nonlactating postpartum women (see Fig. 18-1). It has been suggested[8] that the ovaries are refractory to gonadotropic stimulation during the early postpartum period and lactation. This has been attributed to the conditions in pregnancy in which high sex steroid plasma levels and large amounts of human chorionic gonadotropin (HCG) led to ovarian inactivity. The ovarian quiescence has been observed in the early postpartum period as well (Figs. 18-2 to 18-4). The antigonadotropic activity of prolactin present during the early months of nursing augments this effect on the ovary. The levels of gonadotropin in all postpartum women for the first weeks of the postpartum period are decreased, which substantiates the theory that there is postpartum ovarian re-fractoriness. In the first 2 weeks postpartum low levels of FSH are found in urine and plasma. Beling et al.[4] report estrogen excretion to be low with a linear increase during the first 5 to 8 weeks. When lactating postpartum women are given intramuscular gonadotro-pins, there is no increase in urinary steroids, according to studies by Zarate et al.[52] The prolactin cell predominance may be responsible for the decreased activity of the pituitary-ovarian axis postpartum. Myometrial and endometrial involution are also considered to reduce fertility. Animal studies have shown that the release of FSH and LH is inhibited by intense suckling. In addition, animals in which the nipple is stimulated while the milk ducts have been tied off still show a suppression of estrous and menstrual cycles. Selye and McKeown[44] concluded that interruption of sexual cyclicity during lactation is a result

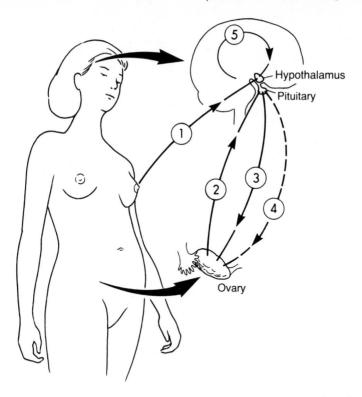

Fig. 18-1. Possible mechanisms of lactational amenorrhea: (1) Nervous impulse from nipple produces not only a rise in prolactin but also (2) changed hypothalamic sensitivity to ovarian steroid feedback and (3) altered gonadotrophin secretion. It is not established if (4) prolactin itself contributes directly to changes in hypothalamic sensitivity or blocks gonadotrophin activity at ovarian level. (5) Suckling may also stimulate release of beta endorphin, thus suppressing gonadotrophin releasing hormone from hypothalamus. (Redrawn from Winikoff B, Semeraro P, and Zimmerman M: Contraception during breastfeeding: a clinician's source book, New York, 1988, The Population Council.)

of the suckling and not due to the secretory activity of the mammary gland. The more the sucking stimulus in frequency and duration, the more consistent the suppression of ovulation.[31]

The inhibition of secretion of dopamine from the hypothalamus has been associated with the neural impulses from stimulation of the nipple during lactation. Normally dopamine inhibits the secretion of prolactin, and conversely when dopamine is inhibited, prolactin rises. Two pathways of ovulation inhibition are possible as a result of the rise in prolactin. One is a lack of responsiveness to ovarian steroids of the hypothalamic pituitary axis of the lactating woman, leading to diminished (rather than inefficient or inappropriate) release of pituitary gonadotropins, FSH and LH, which in turn results in absent or reduced ovarian activity. The second possible pathway is that the ovarian response to gonadotropins is impaired. It is possible that both pathways function as a result of prolactin. The possible mechanisms are illustrated in Fig. 18-1.

Clinically, the perceptible measurement of the return of fertility is the onset of menstruation. Return of reproductive function varies, depending on the length and degree

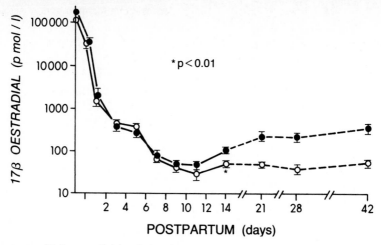

Fig. 18-2. 17 β-oestradial levels in postpartum period in lactating (circles) and non-lactating (dots) women. (From Neville MC: Regulation of mammary development and lactation. In Neville MC and Neifert MR, editors: Lactation: physiology, nutrition, and breastfeeding, New York, 1983, Plenum Press.)

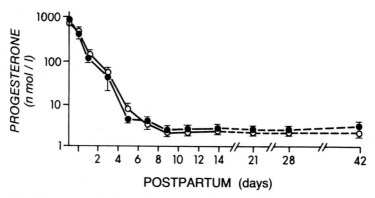

Fig. 18-3. Progesterone levels in postpartum period in lactating (circles) and nonlactating (dots) women. (From Neville MC: Regulation of mammary development and lactation. In Neville MC and Neifert MR, editors: Lactation: physiology, nutrition, and breastfeeding, New York, 1983. Plenum Press.)

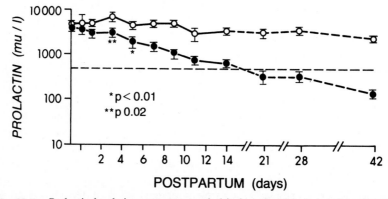

Fig. 18-4. Prolactin levels in postpartum period in lactating (circles) and nonlactating (dots) women. (From Neville MC: Regulation of mammary development and lactation. In Neville MC and Neifert MR, editors: Lactation: physiology, nutrition, and breastfeeding, New York, 1983, Plenum Press.)

Table 18-1. Percentage of ovulatory first cycles by duration from birth and nursing status at time of first bleeding day postpartum*

Ovulatory first cycles	Day of first bleeding			Total
	0-29	30-59	60 or more	
Fully nursing				
No. of patients	—	8	19	27
Ovulatory (%)	—	0	58	41
Partial nursing				
No. of patients	—	7	38	45
Ovulatory (%)	—	29	79	75
Nursing suspended				
No. of patients	—	18	80	98
Ovulatory (%)	—	83	93	91

From Perez A et al: Am J Obstet Gynecol 114:1041, 1967.
*In the 12 patients who became pregnant during amenorrhea, first bleeding day is defined as ovulation day plus 9.

of lactation. Most studies do not, in fact, report the completeness of lactation, that is, whether the infant is totally breastfed or is also receiving solid foods or supplemental bottles.[23] By the end of the third month only 33% of lactating women have had a menstrual period, whereas 91% of nonlactating women have had at least one period. At 9 months, 65% of those women who are still lactating have had the return of menstruation. Vorherr[49] further reports that 30% become pregnant within 1 year after delivery; 40% of those who became pregnant at 1 year were still lactating. Of the lactating women not using contraception, more than half will become pregnant during the first 9 months of lactation. Another view of the statistics, however, indicates that lactation does exert an inhibitory effect on reproductive function. A mother who nurses at least 20 weeks will postpone menstruation 12 weeks and ovulation 18 weeks.

The period of lactational amenorrhea does offer a measure of conception protection for 3 months. The nonlactating woman has a return of her period at 25 days at the earliest, of ovulation at 25 to 35 days, and a 5% chance of regaining fertility prior to 6 weeks postpartum. In a detailed study of 130 women in Chile, Diaz et al.[15] found the cumulative probability of pregnancy at the end of 6 months postpartum in women who were exclusively nursing and amenorrheic to be 1.8%. For exclusively nursing women who had a return of menses, it was 27.2%, and for those partially nursing it was 40.5%.

Perez et al.[38] diagnosed the first postpartum ovulation by endometrial biopsy, basal body temperature, vaginal cytology, and cervical mucus in a group of 200 women in a prospective study. The dates of first ovulation, first menses, and nursing status were analyzed. No woman ovulated before the thirty-sixth day, whether lactating or not. The intensity and length of nursing affected the date when ovulation occurred, according to the researchers. About 78% of the women ovulated prior to the first menses. Twelve pregnancies occurred with first ovulation. Of the 170 women who breastfed, 24 ovulated while completely nursing, 49 while partially nursing, and 97 after weaning (Table 18-1).

Although many investigators continue to evaluate the impact of lactation upon ovulation and menstruation, the fundamental observations remain the same.[2,18,26] Following is a general summation of available data on return of ovulation and menstruation.[49]

    I. Nursing mothers

Earliest possible menstruation: 4 to 6 weeks postpartum (pp)

Most women menstruating: fourth month pp

Return of menstruation: 6 weeks pp—15%

                          12 weeks pp—45%

                          24 weeks pp—85%

Earliest possible ovulation: 6 weeks pp

Return of ovulation: 6 weeks pp—5%

                    12 weeks pp—25%

                    24 weeks pp—65%

First ovular cycle: preceded in about 80% by one or more anovular cycles

Early pp: mainly anovular cycles

Later pp: more often ovular cycles

Ovular cycles: in about 50% of regularly menstruating mothers

  II. Amenorrheic nursing mothers

Endometrium: state of undifferentiation or hypoproliferation

Return of ovulation: 6 weeks pp—2%

                    16 weeks pp—10%

                    After first menstruation—14%

 III. Nonnursing mothers

Earliest possible menstruation: 4 weeks pp

Most women menstruating: third month pp

Return of menstruation: 6 weeks pp—40%

                          12 weeks pp—65%

                          24 weeks pp—90%

Earliest possible ovulation: 3½-5 weeks pp

Ovular cycles: in about 50% with first menstrual period pp

Early pp ovulation: possible occurrence late in the menstrual cycle—shortening of secretory phase and greater tendency toward irregular menses

Return of ovulation: 6 weeks pp—15%

                    12 weeks pp—40%

                    24 weeks pp—75%

 IV. Amenorrheic nonnursing mothers

Return of ovulation: 12 weeks pp—20%

                    16 weeks pp—40%

Data collected in preindustrialized societies show more prolonged lactational amenorrhea, which is probably due to more prolonged total breastfeeding and, to a degree, the relative malnutrition of the mother. Peters et al.[40] indicate that the mean duration of breastfeeding in their study of women in India is 16½ months and of amenorrhea 12 months.

The difference between postpartum and nutritional amenorrhea should be pointed out because true nutritional amenorrhea is predictable on the basis of the height/weight ratio, whereas lactational amenorrhea is hormonal and nutrition has only a trivial effect on postpartum amenorrhea.[17]

Among !Kung hunter-gatherers there are long intervals between births, which has puzzled investigators because the tribes are well nourished, have low fetal wastage, and do not employ contraceptives or prolonged abstinence. The !Kung eat only what they hunt and gather. They have no agriculture. They are lean, spare people. They have late menarche (about 16 years of age), first pregnancy at age 18, and early menopause at about 40, leaving 24 reproductive years during which they produce 4.4 children, which, with some perinatal mortality, exactly replaces their society. This compares with industrial society where productive years begin at 11 and end at 51. Konner and Worthman[28] report that the !Kung have unusual temporal patterns of nursing characterized by highly frequent nursing bouts with short space between nursings. The !Kung nurse several times an hour with only 15 minutes at most between bouts, which last only 15 to 120 seconds each. Serum estradiol and progesterone levels are correspondingly low. Infants are always in the immediate proximity of their mothers until they are weaned, at about 3½ years, during a new sibling's gestation. In Nigeria the effect of duration and frequency of breastfeeding on postpartum amenorrhea is comparable in that Nigerians breastfeed for 16.5 months with a frequency of 4.5 times a day. The mean length of amenorrhea is 12.5 months. Amenorrheic mothers who were lactating had lower levels of serum estradiol and lactic dehydrogenase. There was a significant association of hyperprolactinemia with amenorrhea. The incidence of amenorrhea declined parallel to that of the hyperprolactinemia.[13]

When fertility postpartum during lactation was studied in Edinburgh, suckling was the most important factor inhibiting the return to ovulation.[35] Suckling duration was the first factor to discriminate the mothers who experienced early ovulation. Those mothers who ovulated while breastfeeding had all introduced two or more supplementary feeds per day and had reduced suckling to under six times a day, with 60 minutes or less suckling time per day. The basal prolactin levels were below 600 μ/L. The mothers who did not ovulate until after 40 weeks postpartum breastfed longest, suckled most intensely, maintained night feeds longest, and introduced supplementary feeds most slowly.[23] The prolactin levels remained substantially above 600 μ/L.

In a study of fertility after childbirth and specifically pregnancy while lactating, McNeilly et al.[31] followed 12 breastfeeding women without contraception, eight of whom became pregnant. In all the mothers who became pregnant, there was a significant decrease in suckling frequency and duration. No mother conceived with a suckling frequency of greater than three times per day, although ovulation did occur with suckling four times a day. They conclude that breastfeeding produces reliable lactational amenorrhea even in industrialized countries. There must be five sucklings per day with a total suckling duration of 65 minutes (more than 10 minutes per feed). The authors caution that any reduction of suckling below these limits may indeed result in a return to fertility. (See Tables 18-2 and 18-3.[24])

Another review of the effects of hormonal contraceptives on lactation by Hull[25] concludes that there is a significant number of reports of decrease in milk yield. The

Table 18-2. Ovulation while lactating in longitudinal study

	Ovulated/total mothers	% Ovulated
Ovulated while lactating	13/27	50%
While lactating first ovulation followed by menses	9/27	33%
While lactating first cycle ovulation occurred	9/20	45%
While lactating second cycle or more ovulation occurred	16/23	70%
Postlactation ovulated first cycle	16/23	70%
Postlactation ovulated second cycle or more	26/31	84%

Modified from Howie PN et al: Clin Endocrinol 17:323, 1982.

Table 18-3. Intermenstrual intervals

Mean interval between first days of menstrual bleeding	Days
During lactation	37.0 (± 3.3 SE)
First cycles immediately postlactation	29.8 (± 1.0 SE)
Bottle feeding women	29.5 (± 1.0 SE)

Modified from Howie PN et al: Clin Endocrinol 17:323, 1982.

Table 18-4. Distribution of natural mothering* sample by months of breastfeeding†

Months of breastfeeding	Number of experiences	Percent of total experiences
12	1	3.5
13-16	5	17.2
17-20	7	24.2
21-24	4	13.7
25-28	6	20.7
29-32	3	10.3
33-36	2	6.9
37	1	3.5

From Kippley S: Breast feeding and natural child spacing, New York, 1974, Harper & Row, Publishers, Copyright © 1974 by Sheila K. Kippley, Reprinted by permission of Harper & Row, Publishers.
*Natural mothering includes, among other things, no pacifiers used, no bottles used, no solids or liquids for 5 months, no feeding schedules other than infant's, presence of night feedings, and presence of lying-down nursing (naps, night feedings).
†N = 29 experiences (22 mothers). Mean months of breastfeeding = 22.8; median months of breastfeeding = 23.0.

Table 18-5. Distribution of natural mothering* sample by months of amenorrhea†

Months of amenorrhea	Number of experiences	Percent of total experiences
1-4	2	6.9
5-8	2	6.9
9-12	7	24.1
13-16	9	31.0
17-20	5	17.2
21-24	2	6.9
25-28	1	3.5
29-30	1	3.5

From Kippley S: Breast feeding and natural child spacing, New York, 1974, Harper & Row, Publishers, Copyright © 1974 by Sheila K. Kippley, Reprinted by permission of Harper & Row, Publishers.
*Natural mothering includes, among other things, no pacifiers used, no bottles used, no solids or liquids for 5 months, no feeding schedules other than infant's, presence of night feedings, and presence of lying-down nursing (naps, night feedings).
†N = 29 experiences (22 mothers). Mean months of amenorrhea = 14.6; median months of amenorrhea = 14.0.

description of severe growth failure[17] in the nursling, even leading to "contraceptive marasmus," in Egypt and Tunisia is cause for concern.

A significant distinction should be made between token breastfeeding with early solids and more rigid feeding schedules and the ad lib breastfeeding around the clock with no solids until the infant is 6 months old. The amount and frequency of sucking are closely related to the continued amenorrhea in most women. When a totally breastfed infant sleeps through the night at an early age, requiring no suckling for 6 hours or so at night, the suppressive effect on menses diminishes. It has also been shown that if the infant uses a pacifier rather than receiving nonnutritive sucking at the breast, the suppression of ovulation is diminished (Tables 18-4 and 18-5).

CONTRACEPTION DURING LACTATION
Natural child spacing

Although lactation provides some degree of protection early in the postpartum period, a woman who is seriously concerned about avoiding conception should be informed of her options. If she does not wish to use contraceptives, medications, or devices, she should be instructed in the external signs of ovulation. In most studies of lactation, the initial menses occur prior to the onset of ovulation. The risk of pregnancy during lactational amenorrhea, however, is about 5% unless some effort is made to identify ovulation by basal temperature or cervical secretions.[27]

The sympto-thermal method of fertility awareness during lactation was studied in Canada.[36] A special postpartum chart was designed to record morning temperature, cervical mucus, and other signs of fertility/infertility in relation to dates and postpartum days. The intensity of the breastfeeding was also recorded. There were 54 breastfeeding experiences in 47 women whose ages ranged from 20 to 39. Parity ranged from 1 to 7 with an average of 3.3. The duration of full breastfeeding averaged 3.6 months (range of 3 weeks to 8 months). The duration of breastfeeding ranged from 2 to 28 months with an average of 8.8 months. These mothers found that in general they could predict their fertile times with accuracy while breastfeeding. During times of weaning or change in suckling pattern, special caution was suggested in which the mothers watched for signs of first ovulation.

The effectiveness of periodic abstinence was reviewed for lactating women for *Population Reports*.[39] Long periods of lactational infertility can be identified by either lack of mucus or continuous unchanging mucous flow. As ovulation resumes, irregular mucus patterns occur that are difficult to interpret and therefore require prolonged abstinence. A pregnancy rate with this method was 9.1 per 100 women-years. Because two thirds of the 82 women studied were totally breastfeeding, many of the ensuing postpartum cycles may have been anovulatory or had an inadequate luteal phase, thus helping to keep the pregnancy rate low.

Studies of cervical secretions alone (mucus patterns) during lactation have indicated that the same signs in mucus are reliable during lactation. Charting is carried out in the usual manner and feedings are also recorded. A woman who is following her pattern postpartum should be seen every 2 weeks for guidance until her pattern is well documented. The couple should make careful observations when (1) the infant sleeps through the night, (2) the mother reduces the number of breastfeedings, (3) the infant begins solid foods, (4) the infant begins other liquids or a bottle, or (5) there is illness in either mother or baby. Abstinence is advised until the situation is clear. If there has been no prior ovulation or menstruation when weaning begins, ovulation may occur quite quickly.[9]

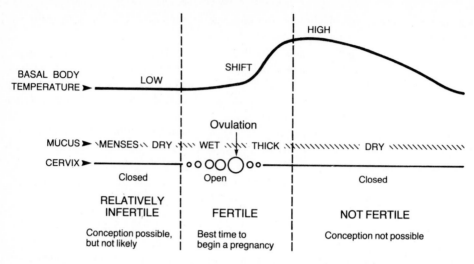

Fig. 18-5.   Temperatures, mucus, and cervical assessment during lactation to identify ovulation. (With permission from National Family Planning of Rochester, New York.)

An illustration of temperature, mucus, and cervical assessments during lactation is given in Fig. 18-5.

Although the contraceptive methods such as barrier methods and "the pill" have a statistically better record in avoiding pregnancy, that is a mute point for the woman for whom these methods are not an option for religious, ethical, moral, or medical grounds.[3] It is important that the clinician therefore be as well informed about natural child spacing as possible so the best advice can be provided. Ideally the woman has used natural family planning before the pregnancy so she is familiar with her own patterns but more urgent that she knows how to check her mucus, her cervix, and her temperature and is not trying to learn about her fertility signs during lactation. Locally based natural family planning programs across the country are gaining experience with lactating women using the ovulation method and are available to assist lactating women. Further information can be obtained from the Office of Natural Family Planning, PO Box 29260, Washington, DC 20017, if no local office is available.

In a carefully designed study conducted in Chile by Perez at the Pontificia Universidad Catolica De Chile Department of Obs/Gyn and members of the faculty at Johns Hopkins University School of Hygiene and Public Health, 419 postpartum women were enrolled in the Natural Family Planning Program and taught the method and how to record their observations.[37] The purpose was to define cervical mucus patterns in relation to time since delivery, time of first bleed, frequency of feeding, introduction of supplements and solid foods, and time of weaning. One hundred ten women with detailed records were selected for critical evaluation of their diaries. To date, 49 have been reviewed and the preliminary observations reported by Barker. Two characteristics of mucus (sensation and observation) were charted each day along with their breastfeeding pattern. Only seven women had used natural family planning previously. No woman menstruated prior to 4 months, when 10% did have first menses. Fifty percent of women detected mucus by the fourth month, and not until the seventh month had 50% had first menses. Mucus was observed about 2 months prior to first menses. As women moved from total breastfeeding to partial and to complete weaning, the duration of mucus episodes increased. Mucus duration approached normal upon weaning.

Oral contraceptives and lactation

The significant issues related to lactation and the use of oral contraceptives are the potentially adverse effects of oral contraceptives on milk production, uterine involution, and growth and development of the breastfed infant. A single case is reported by Curtis[12] of breast enlargement in a breastfed male infant whose mother began taking norethynodrel with ethynylestradiol 3-methyl ether (Enovid) on the third day postpartum. Breast enlargement began on the third week of life. The mother had noted her milk was not as "rich" and started supplements the second week. Nursing was discontinued at about 4 weeks of age and the breasts of the infant returned to normal in 2 to 3 weeks. The additional risks to the mother of thromboembolism, hypertension, and cancer have also been discussed extensively in the literature.

The data available have been well reviewed by Vorherr.[48,49] He summarizes the information by noting that preparations containing 2.5 mg or less of a 19-norprogestogen and 50 μg or less of etinylestradiol or 100 μg or less of mestranol present no hazard to mother or infant. He further points out that milk yield can be decreased with larger doses of combination oral contraceptives containing estrogen and 5 to 10 mg of progestogen/dose. Only two studies of many suggest any variation in the content of the milk (protein, fat, and calcium) due to oral contraceptives.

Toddywalla et al.[47] reported the effect of injectable contraceptives as well as oral combinations on milk production. They found an increase in the protein content of the milk and slight increase in quantity from the group given injection of 150 mg of medroxyprogesterone (Depo-Provera) every 3 months. The group receiving 300 mg of medroxyprogesterone every 6 months showed significant increase in quantity but a decrease in protein, fat, and calcium as compared with controls (who used mechanical means of contraception). The secretion of hormones in human milk is poorly documented, with only a few infants studied in each hormone combination. In all cases a small but measurable amount was found in the milk. Unfortunately, measurements in the infant's serum are not reported.

The impact of the distribution of oral contraceptives on breastfeeding and pregnancy status in rural Haiti indicated that it did not alter breastfeeding patterns.[6] Women began the pills at 8 to 9 months postpartum. Pregnancy prevalence also decreased as a result.

It is the concern of many that use of any hormone combination to suppress ovulation during lactation is contraindicated because of the potential risk to the infant, not only immediately but also in the long-range view. As discussed earlier, there have been reports of enlargement of the breasts in male and female infants when nursed by mothers taking oral contraceptives with higher dosages of estrogen and/or progesterone than are presently used.

No adverse effects on the infant during the ensuing years in bone maturation, genital development, or impaired fertility have been substantiated. Vorherr responds to the reports of such effects in animal studies by pointing out that (1) only small amounts of progesterone reach the infant and the androgenic capabilities are a fraction of those of testosterone, (2) long-range follow-up from the middle 1950s of nursing mothers given up to 20 mg of progestogen/day showed no bone maturation acceleration in infancy nor impairment of ovarian function and fertility in the infants' reproductive years, and (3) the dosages given

Table 18-6. Effects of contraceptive agents on milk yield and infant development

Agent	Milk yield	Effect on infant
Combined estrogen/progestin	Moderate inhibitory effect Shorter breastfeeding Milk concentration un- changed Small amount of steroid in milk	Slower weight gain No long-term effects
Progestin only Mini pill (Micronor, Nory-D)	No effect on volume No effect on duration Small amount of steriod in milk	No effect on weight gain No reported long-term effects

Future products
  Injectable depot midroxy
  Progesterone acetate,
    DMPA, Depo-Provera
    and norethindrone enan-
    thate NET-EN, NORIS-
    TERAT)
	Breastfeeding lasts longer
	? change in milk—protein
	  increased, fat decreased
	Steroid present in milk
		No long-term effects

Norplant® implants	No effect Small amount steroid in milk	Normal growth No long-term effects
Vaginal rings containing nat- ural hormone progesterone	No significant differences	No effect on growth Long-term effects under study

Modified from Winikoff B, Semeraro P, and Zimmerman M: Contraception during breastfeeding, New York, 1987, Population Council Publishers.

the animals in the studies reporting abnormalities were excessive on a comparable weight basis (1 mg in a 6 g newborn rat). It is too early in the history of oral contraceptives to be entirely sure that there is no long-range increase in risk of cancer in the infants so nursed. (See Table 18-6.)

An algorithm for initiating contraceptive treatment is illustrated in Fig 18-6.

Intrauterine devices and other contraceptive methods

Various alternatives to oral contraceptives do exist and have been observed to have different degrees of reliability. The intrauterine devices (IUDs) (95% to 98% effective), cervical caps and diaphragms (85% to 88% effective), condoms (80% to 85% effective), and vaginal suppositories, jellies, or creams (80% effective) have no known contraindication during breastfeeding, since no chemicals are absorbed. The only contraceptive that is 100% effective is abstinence.

A study of 2271 postpartum women who had IUDs inserted between 1976 and 1981 and were followed for 6 to 12 months was reported with careful attention to details of lactation.[10] Data were analyzed separately for IUDs inserted immediately after birth (within 10 minutes of placental expulsion). The results of this analysis indicate that IUD insertion for breastfeeding women would be appropriate either immediately after delivery or later (≥42 days postpartum). When inserted immediately postpartum, the Delta Loop and Delta T were modified by adding projections of chromic sutures, which help the device remain in the uterus. The sutures biodegrade in 6 weeks, leaving a standard device in place. These

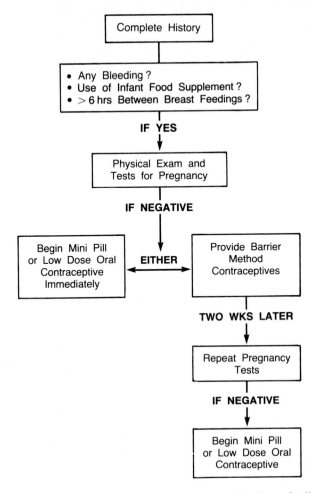

Fig. 18-6. Algorithm for initiating contraceptive treatment in a breastfeeding woman. (Modified from Winikoff B, Semeraro P, and Zimmerman M: Contraception during breastfeeding: a clinician's source book, New York, 1988, The Population Council.

authors report that breastfeeding is not a contraindication to IUD insertion. There is not an increased expulsion rate. Conversely, the presence of an IUD has no adverse effect on lactation. The appropriate time for insertion should be selected to predate anticipated ovulation but guarantee patient compliance.

A group of 32 women hospitalized for uterine perforation necessitating transperitoneal IUD removal and a matched control group of 497 women who had worn IUDs uneventfully were compared.[21] Of the women in the study, 97% were postpartum compared with 68% of the controls. Of the parous study group, 42% were lactating and of the parous controls, 7% were lactating when the IUD was inserted. The risk of perforation was 10 times greater in the lactating than in the nonlactating women, unrelated to time of the insertion postpartum. In another group hospitalized for difficult transcervical IUD removal, the risk was 2.3 times greater for lactating women. The authors recommend caution, not abandonment of the procedure during lactation, because they feel the IUD is the best form of artificial contraception during lactation. Because of problems with the Dacron Shield, IUDs have been generally unavailable in the United States in 1986 and 1987, although in other parts of the world they were still in use. In 1989 a copper T device became available again. The ideal candidate is a woman who wants reversible contraception to space births or limit size of the family, especially parous women with a monogamous relationship, especially if they are breastfeeding.

Many cultures and societies place taboos on sexual intercourse for the nursing mother as an effective means of spacing children. Usually there are no medical contraindications to sexual relationships during lactation. In a study on contraceptive use in the United States, Ford and Labbok reported that among white women 34% were not sexually active in the first month postpartum, 12.5% in the second month, and 4.3% during the third month.[18] Among black women in the survey, 25% were not sexually active the first month, 8.1% the second, and 4.2% the third. Contraceptive use among those sexually active was absent in 16% in the first postpartum month in 12.2% and 13.8% in the second and the third postpartum month among whites. Among blacks, 27.3% used no method the first month, 22.7% and 22.3% the second and third month.

SEX AND THE NURSING MOTHER
Sexual arousal associated with suckling

If one examines the normal adult female in regard to the menstrual cycle, sexual intercourse, pregnancy, childbirth, and lactation, one observes that these events are all influenced by the interaction of the same hormones, not only estrogen, progesterone, testosterone, FSH, and LH but oxytocin and prolactin as well. The breast is known to respond during all these phases, enlarging before menstruation, during pregnancy, before orgasm, and during lactation.[16] The nipples also respond during these phases. Furthermore, it is noted that the uterus contracts during childbirth, orgasm, and lactation. Body temperature rises during ovulation, childbirth, orgasm, and lactation. As pointed out in Chapter 3, oxytocin is a critical element in the let-down reflex during lactation. Oxytocin levels also rise during orgasms and labor, and oxytocin causes the uterus to contract and the nipples to become erect. Newton and Newton[33] report other similarities in women during these events, including sensory perception and emotional reactions. Following are the psychophysiologic similarities between lactation and coitus.[33]

1. The uterus contracts.
2. The nipples become erect.
3. Breast stroking and nipple stimulation occur.
4. The emotions experienced involve skin changes (vascular dilation and raised temperature).
5. Milk let-down (or ejection) reflex can be triggered.
6. The emotions experienced may be closely allied.
7. An accepting attitude toward sexuality may be related to an accepting attitude to breastfeeding (and vice versa).

Given the biologic and hormonal similarities of lactation to the other events in the sexual cycle of the adult female, it is not surprising that some women experience some form of sexual gratification during suckling on certain occasions. It has been reported by Masters and Johnson[30] in a study of 111 parturient women, only 24 of whom breastfed, that there was sexual arousal experienced during suckling on some occasions. The exact incidence of this response is unknown, but it is believed to be uncommon. Nursing mothers may have an element of guilt surrounding these experiences and thus it is underreported. It has been suggested that guilt leads to early weaning in some cases. For some women the breasts are highly erogenous. The handling and manipulation of the breast necessary during lactation by both mother and infant can, in the right circumstances and mood, be stimulating. Clearly the majority of women who enjoy breastfeeding have no feelings or responses to the stimulation of the breast that could be construed as sexual arousal, although they enjoy breastfeeding and the intimacy with their infant that it provides. The erotic response to nursing the infant has no significance in terms of being normal or abnormal. The decline of breastfeeding because of feelings of shame, modesty, embarrassment, and distaste has been reported by Bentovim[5] and interpreted as indicating that breastfeeding is viewed as a forbidden sexual activity. For such women any sexual allusions and excitement accompanying breastfeeding are not permissible and cause shame. Such attitudes are more common in lower social groups and need to be considered in counseling mothers about breastfeeding prepartum or when premature weaning takes place. Major changes in the number of women who breastfeed may not be possible until society can accept the breast in its relationship to nurturing the infant and also as an object of less sexual ambivalence.

The sensuousness of breastfeeding has been the topic of discussion in popular women's magazines as more is written about women and their bodies.[41] For the well-educated, well-read woman who breastfeeds her infant because she intellectually arrives at the decision, such discussions are an avenue of increased knowledge.[42] Others may still be uncomfortable about breastfeeding if it is apt to be "pleasurable." The physician may sense this discomfort in his patient prenatally by her responses to bodily change during pregnancy. Cultural attitudes are an important part of this response and are deeply ingrained in an individual by the time she reaches the age of parenting. Professionals need to be sensitive to the patient and cautious about imposing cultural change on a given patient, while being alert to needs for information and openness.

The sexual activity of the nursing mother

A review of the limited data available on lactating women in the Masters and Johnson study[30] does indicate that in their group of 111 postpartum women, the nursing mothers were more eager than nonnursing mothers to resume sexual relations postpartum. The data were independent of the fear of pregnancy. They report that this interest was apparent 2 to 3 weeks postpartum. Individual reports through a questionnaire reported by Ladas[29] indicated that 30% of nursing mothers believed their sexual relationships were improved and 2.5% believed they were worse postpartum. The individual testimonies of nursing mothers reported by Ladas indicated they had a better feeling about themselves as well as their relationships with their husbands and family in general. In a study of sexual behavior during pregnancy and lactation, Kenney,[26] reported that the desire returned by 4 weeks for most women, long before they felt it was safe. The longer they had been married and the more children, the sooner the interest returned and the sooner they felt it was safe. There was no change in interest or enjoyment upon weaning.

More general observations indicate that although some women may have increased interest in sexual relations while nursing, others may experience no interest at all for 6 months or so. Whether this is due to the saturation of the mother's needs for intimate relationship and stimulus through nursing, general fatigue, or fear of pregnancy is debatable. Sexual stimulus may trigger the ejection reflex, and milk ejection may have a negative effect on some men. A practical solution to spraying milk during lovemaking is feeding the infant or expressing some milk beforehand. The total knowledge of nursing and suckling as a biologic phenomenon will help couples to understand such reactions and thus avoid inappropriate response psychologically. The conflict in some adult men over their role in regard to the nursing mother's breasts is usually a result of guilt or upbringing. There is no need to advise against fondling the lactating breast during lovemaking, although physicians have often imposed rigid restrictions on sexual activity in the lactating woman. There is no scientific basis for such restriction and no difference in the incidence of infection and mastitis associated with such activity. Unusually restrictive protocols are often imposed on patients without medical indication. Bradley[7] recommends, in fact, oral and manual manipulation of the breasts by the husband during both pregnancy and lactation to prevent sore nipples.

It is helpful to discuss with the lactating woman that the hormonal effect on the vagina may be excessive dryness with an increase in dyspareunia. With the abrupt withdrawal of gonadotropins and ovarian hormones and elevation of prolactin at the time of delivery of the infant and placenta, the vaginal epithelium becomes thin and atrophic.[46] Normally the vagina and ectocervix are lined with stratified squamous epithelium, which is multilayered and protective. It is also very responsive to ovarian hormones. The greatest maturation and thickness occur around ovulation in response to peak estrogen secretion. During pregnancy, progesterone inhibits the maturation of the epithelial cells. The vaginal lining retains its thickness, but cells do not fully mature as the effect of progesterone overtakes the effect on the epithelium and cervical mucus of estrogen, both of which are abundant during pregnancy. The lowered ovarian hormones during lactation cause vaginal dryness and lack of cervical mucus as well, leading to discomfort during intercourse. The dryness responds to locally applied lubricants and tends to improve over time. A sudden change may actually reflect ovulation. The breast that is being stimulated by feeding frequently may not be as sensitive during lovemaking. Usually this too is only transient. The physician should perhaps remind the mother that some adjustment to attend to the father's needs may be necessary.

NURSING WHILE PREGNANT AND TANDEM NURSING

Pregnancy can and does occur while lactating. When it does occur it produces a number of questions. There is no need to hastily wean the first infant from the breast, which is often ordered by the physician. It is possible to lactate throughout pregnancy and then to have two infants at the breast postpartum. It is now a sufficiently common event to be called tandem nursing. Obviously the amount of nourishment provided the first infant at the breast depends on his age and other supplements. When the infant at the breast is only a few months old when pregnancy occurs, there is some rationale to continued breastfeeding for the benefit of the infant until it is time to wean to solids and other liquids at 6 months of age or so. This child will be about a year old when the new infant arrives and if still at the breast may have demands in excess of the mother's ability to provide. Concern had been expressed that the older infant will take much of the nourishment needed by the new infant. In some societies it is believed that a suckling infant will "take the spirit" from the newly conceived fetus; thus weaning is mandated once pregnancy is confirmed. The milk produced immediately postpartum by the mother who never stopped nursing appears to be colostrum. The kangaroo has been observed to have a teat for the older offspring with mature milk and a teat for the new offspring who requires significantly different nourishment. Such a provision does not exist for the human. It has been shown by mothers who wish to maintain both infants at the breast that it can be done without any apparent effect on the nourishment of the new infant. Counseling of such a mother should take into account the mother's resources to get adequate rest, nourishment, and psychologic support to withstand the added demand on her, physically and mentally.

If the first child is older and will be well beyond a year of age when the new infant arrives, the need for physical nourishment is minimal and continuation at the breast is more for the security and psychologic benefits. This is referred to as comfort nursing and may continue for several years. (See Chapter 10.) Abrupt weaning should be avoided, and consideration should be given to the impact of separation when the mother is confined during the birth of the new infant. This is an argument for 12-hour hospitalizations for delivery for women who request it. The first few days of colostrum are most vital for the new infant and the supply is not infinite; therefore priorities need to be set as far as the older child is concerned. The new baby should be nursed first.

Many of the changes in child-rearing practices in recent years have increased the freedom and response to human needs. Carried to extremes, instant gratification becomes a right rather than a privilege. Sometimes a mother may need help in seeing that she need not feel guilty if she decides to wean the older child. If it is only an occasional feeding or suckling experience for added security, especially when security is threatened by the arrival of a new infant, it is tolerable in terms of endurance for the mother and she agrees willingly. When, however, continuing nursing becomes a strain or is painful or stressful, she should feel free to stop. When the mother feels real resentment toward the older child who is nursing, Pryor[41] points out that it is time to gently but firmly wean. If such a situation could be anticipated, it is probably easier for the older child to be weaned prior to delivery of the new infant. As with any such decisions to wean, it is best for the physician to work this decision out in frank discussion with the mother (and father, too, if he is available) so that any misgivings, resentment, or feeling of failure can be dealt with openly. Many patients automatically suspect the physician of being antagonistic to breastfeeding if the physician suggests weaning. Even when the reason is purely but urgently medical, discussion should be open and include options and alternatives and their risks. Pryor[41] expresses it succinctly when she says, "Weaning is part of the baby's growing up, but it is sometimes part of the mother's growing up, too."

The dilemma of tandem nursing and weaning the older child has been dealt with in other societies with various manipulations such as painting the breast with pepper or bitter herbs to make it taste terrible. Having the mother leave the child with other caregivers is also done. The provision of love and affection during this difficult adaptation for the child is what makes the difference between a traumatic occasion and a step toward growing up. Equally important is the provision of some opportunity for the mother to express her concerns and doubts during the process to her physician, who should be neither judgmental nor unduly rigid in his medical care plan.

REFERENCES

1. Abdulia K, Elwan S, Salem H, and Shaaban M: Effect of early postpartum use of the contraceptive implants, Norplant®, on the serum levels of immunoglobulins of the mothers and their breastfed infants, Contraception 32:261, 1985.

2. Adnan AM and Bakr SA: Postpartum lactational amenorrhoea as a means of family planning in the Sudan: a study of 500 cases, J Biosoc Sci 15:9, 1983.

3. Barker DC: Use of natural family planning by breastfeeding women. In Shivanandan M, editor: Breastfeeding and natural family planning, Fourth International Symposium on Natural Family Planning, Chevy Chase Md, 1985, KM Associate Publishers.

4. Beling CG, Frandsen VA, and Josimovich JB: Pituitary and ovarian hormone levels during lactation, Acta Endocrinol 155(suppl):40, 1971.

5. Bentovin A: Shame and other anxieties. In Ciba Foundation Symposium no 45, Breastfeeding and the mother, Amsterdam, 1976, Elsevier Scientific Publ. Co.

6. Bordes A, Allman J, and Verly A: The impact on breastfeeding and pregnancy status of household contraceptive distribution in rural Haiti, Am J Public Health 72:835, 1982.

7. Bradley RA: Husband-coached childbirth, New York, 1965, Harper & Row.

8. Brambilla F and Sirtori CM: Gonadotropin-inhibiting factor in pregnancy, lactation and menopause, Am J Obstet Gynecol 109:599, 1971.

9. Brown RE: Breast-feeding and family planning: a review of relationships between breast-feeding and family planning, Am J Clin Nutr 35:162, 1982.

10. Cole LP et al: Effects of breastfeeding on IUD performance, Am J Public Health 73:384, 1983.

11. Committee on Drugs, American Academy of Pediatrics: Breastfeeding and contraception, Pediatrics 68:138, 1981.

12. Curtis EM: Oral-contraceptive feminization of a normal male infant, Obstet Gynecol 23:295, 1964.

13. Delvoye P et al: Serum prolactin, gonadotropins, and estradiol in menstruating and amenorrheic mothers during two years' lactation, Am J Obstet Gynecol 130:635, 1978.

14. Diaz S, Jackanicz T, Herreros C et al: Fertility regulation in nursing women. VIII. Progesterone plasma levels and contraception efficacy of a progesterone-releasing vaginal ring, Contraception 32:603, 1985.

15. Diaz S, Peralta O, Juez G et al: Fertility regulation in nursing women living in an urban setting, J Biosoc Sci 14:329, 1982.

16. Eiger MS and Olds SW: The complete book of breastfeeding, ed 2, New York, 1987, Workman Publishing.

17. Frisch RE and McArthur JW: Difference between postpartum and nutritional amenorrhea, Science 203:921, 1979.

18. Ford K and Labbok M: Contraceptive usage during lactation in the United States: an update, Am J Public Health 77:79, 1987.

19. Gioiosa R: Incidence of pregnancy during lactation in 500 cases, Am J Obstet Gynecol 70:162, 1955.

20. Gray RH, Campbell OM, Zacur HA et al: Postpartum return of ovarian activity in nonbreastfeeding women monitored by urinary assays, J Clin Endocrinol Metab 64:645, 1987.

21. Hartwell S and Latuchi GI: IUD perforation, Obstet Gynecol 61:31, 1983.

22. Heikkila M and Luukkainen T: Duration of breastfeeding and development of children after insertion of a Levonorgestrel-releasing intrauterine contraceptive device, Contraception 25:279, 1982.

23. Howie PW et al: Fertility after childbirth: infant feeding patterns, basal PRL levels, and postpartum ovulation, Clin Endocrinol 17:315, 1982.

24. Howie P, McNeilly A, Houston M et al: Fertility after childbirth: postpartum ovulation and menstruation in bottle and breastfeeding mothers, Clin Endocrinol 17:323, 1982.

25. Hull VJ: The effects of hormonal contraceptives on lactation: current findings, methodological considerations and future priorities, Stud Fam Plann 12:134, 1981.

26. Kenney JA: Sexuality of pregnant and breastfeeding women, Arch Sex Behav 2:215, 1973.

27. Kippley S: Breast feeding and natural child spacing, New York, 1976, Harper & Row.

28. Konner M and Worthman C: Nursing frequency, gonadal function, and birth spacing among !Kung hunter-gatherers, Science 207:788, 1980.

29. Ladas AK: How to help mothers breastfeed: deductions from a survey, Clin Pediatr 9:702, 1970.

30. Masters WH and Johnson VE: Human sexual response, Boston, 1966, Little, Brown & Co.

31. McNeilly AS, Glasier A, Howie PW et al: Fertility after childbirth: pregnancy associated with breastfeeding, Clin Endocrinol 18:167, 1983.

32. McNeilly AS, Glasier A, and Howie PW: Endocrine control of lactational infertility. In Dobbin J, editor: Maternal nutrition and lactational infertility, New York, 1985, Nestle Nutrition, Vevey Raven Press.

33. Newton N and Newton M: Psychologic aspects of lactation, N Engl J Med 277:1179, 1967.

34. Nilsson S, Melbin T, Hofvander Y et al: Long-term follow-up of children breastfed by mothers using oral contraceptives, Contraception 34:443, 1986.

35. Ojofeitimi EO: Effect of duration and frequency of breastfeeding on postpartum amenorrhea, Pediatrics 69:164, 1982.

36. Perez A: Lactational amenorrhea and natural family planning. In Hafez ESE, editor: Human ovulation: mechanisms, prediction, detection, and induction, Amsterdam, 1979, North-Holland Publishing.

37. Perez A: Natural family planning: postpartum period, Int J Fertil 26:219, 1981.

38. Perez A et al: First ovulation after child birth: the effect of breast feeding, Am J Obstet Gynecol 114:1041, 1972.

39. Periodic abstinence: how well do new approaches work, Popul Rep (I):3, Sept. 1981.

40. Peters H, Israel S, and Purshottan S: Lactation period in Indian women: duration of amenorrhea

and vaginal and cervical cytology, Fertil Steril 9:134, 1958.

41. Pryor K: Nursing your baby, New York, 1973, Pocket Books.

42. Riordan J: A practical guide to breastfeeding, St. Louis, 1983, The CV Mosby Co.

43. Sas M, Gellen JJ, Dusitsin N et al: An investigation on the influence of steroidal contraceptives on milk yield and fatty acids in Hungary and Thailand, Contraception 33:159, 1986.

44. Selye H and McKeown T: The effect of mechanical stimulation of the nipples on the ovary and the sexual cycle, Surg Gynecol Obstet 59:856, 1934.

45. Tankeyoon M, Dusitsin N, Chalapati S et al: Effects of hormonal contraceptives on milk volume and infant growth, Contraception 30:505, 1984.

46. Taylor RS: Physiology of the vagina and cervix in breastfeeding women. In Shivanandan M, editor: Breastfeeding and natural family planning, Fourth International Symposium on Natural Family Planning, Chevy Chase Md, 1985, KM Associate Publishers.

47. Toddywalla VS, Joshi L, and Virkar K: Effect of contraceptive steroids on human lactation, Am J Obstet Gynecol 127:245, 1977.

48. Vorherr H: The breast: morphology, physiology and lactation, New York, 1974, Academic Press, Inc.

49. Vorherr H: Human lactation and breast feeding. In Larson BL, editor: Lactation: a comprehensive treatise, New York, 1978, Academic Press, Inc.

50. Winikoff B, Semeraro P, and Zimmerman M: Contraception during breastfeeding: a clinician's handbook, New York, 1988, Population Council Publishers.

51. Zacharias S, Aguilera E, Assenzo JR et al: Effects of hormonal and nonhormonal contraceptives on lactation and incidence of pregnancy, Contraception 33:203, 1986.

52. Zarate A et al: Ovarian refractoriness during lactation in women: effect of gonadotropin stimulation, Am J Obstet Gynecol 112:1130, 1972.

The storage of human milk and cross-nursing

19

The human milk bank has entered another era. The interest in providing human milk for human infants with special needs, especially prematures, has increased, but the concerns regarding donor milk have also escalated. It is the strong conviction of most neonatologists that donor human milk must be pasteurized before use in an infant, and only mother's own milk may be used fresh in a sick neonate. In addition, donors must be carefully screened and women at high risk for certain infection eliminated.

When there are risks of using even mother's own milk for a given baby, the risk/benefit ratio is determined. In a Third World country where the risk of dying in the first year of life if an infant is not breastfed is over 50%, a mother with hepatitis or AIDS should probably breastfeed her infant. In Western countries, the risk of dying in the first year of life if not breastfed is less than 1%; then to risk infection with AIDS or hepatitis is inappropriate. Similarly, the risk/benefit ratio of human milk in a compromised premature when mother's milk may contain the AIDS virus tips against human milk as too risky even for the great benefits nutritionally and immunologically. Because of the effect of heating, cooling, freezing, and storing milk, some of the most valued and precious qualities are diminished or destroyed, thus feeding the milk fresh or at least fresh frozen and not heated preserves most of the constituents. The value of the milk produced by women who deliver prematurely has been discussed in Chapter 14. There are no reported cases of infection acquired from milk provided by a milk bank in compliance with the standards prescribed by the Human Milk Banking Association of North America.

STORING HUMAN MILK

It is often necessary to store milk for infants, especially in the hospital. The storage of human milk involves two types of milk: mother's milk and donor milk. The distinction becomes important in how the milk is stored and how it is prepared for the infant. It is also important because many states have developed codes for donor milk but fortunately have not regulated mother's milk as yet. Certain guidelines are appropriate for each milk.

Milk banks have been in continuous operation for over 50 years. The indications for use of such milk have been alluded to in other chapters but are briefly summarized.

Mother's milk

1. The mother plans to breastfeed the infant ultimately but needs to provide pumped milk until the infant can be put to the breast.
2. The infant requires the special nutritional benefits of human milk (as with those infants who are recovering from intestinal surgery) yet cannot nurse.
3. The infant weighs 1500 g or less and has difficulty digesting and absorbing other milks.

Donor milk

1. The infant is at risk of infection or necrotizing enterocolitis. Although effects are not clearly demonstrated with mature milk, fresh colostrum is held to be especially protective and may be collected from low-risk carefully screened mothers.
2. The physician believes the infant would benefit from the nourishment in human milk because of prematurity, especially if the infant weighs less than 1500 g.
3. The mother is temporarily unable to nourish a breastfed infant completely. It may be that the mother's supply is inadequate when she first puts the infant to the breast after weeks of pumping or when the mother has been ill or hospitalized. Usually these infants are already at home.
4. Pooled samples of donor milk are prepared as a dried preparation for addition to fresh mother's milk to increase the calorie and nutrient value for high-risk premature infants whose requirements exceed those available with unsupplemented human milk.

Structure of a milk bank

Most informal and casual milk banks operating in conjunction with a neonatal intensive care unit (NICU) have disappeared. NICUs may provide a deep freeze for storage of mother's own milk for use in her infant. They store it for feeding of the infant and do not process it at all except to culture random samples for contamination. Most do not permit "donating" milk to other infants except by private arrangement between the two mothers with physician's approval. No feeding is given an infant in the hospital without a physician's order, of course. Smaller public milk banks have phased out since state legislation or local medical practice standards have mandated strict surveillance of samples and pasteurization.

A few large, well-established banks continue to operate in the United States and around the world. A network of these milk banks that meets and shares information is known as the Human Milk Banking Association of North America. The 1988-1989 address is via the president, Maria Teresa Asquith, Director, Mother's Milk Bank, Institute for Medical Research, 2260 Clove Drive, San Jose, CA 95128. There is a similar network in Europe.

The Georgetown University Hospital operates an active breast milk bank near the NICU with full-time staff and a medical director. There are other centers in Canada and the USA. The Mother's Milk Bank (MMB) of the Institute for Medical Research in San Jose, California, was established in 1974. It has a full-time coordinator and a medical director. It provides milk for hundreds of infants and contributes to the fund of knowledge on human milk. Because the milk is provided to patients only by physician's prescription, it is reimbursable by health insurance carriers of California. MMB has developed procedures and policies regarding milk collection, storage, and processing. This is described in detail by Asquith and colleagues and documented with an extensive bibliography.[1] The MMB has prepared and keeps current a comprehensive manual for the organization and operation of a modern human milk bank that is available to health-care facilities by contacting MMB, Institute for Medical Research, San Jose, California.

The Georgetown University Milk Bank continues to make donor milk available after careful donor screening, rigid collection techniques, culturing, and processing (Fig. 19-1). The Hawaii Mother's Milk Bank in Honolulu is another major source of human milk in the United States. The names and addresses of other centers are available from the association.

The state of New York passed an amendment to the public health law in 1980 in which it was declared policy that any and all infants requiring human breast milk be assured access to sufficient quantities of wholesome human breast milk donated by concerned lactating mothers on a continued and systematic basis (see Appendix I for entire law). This law resulted in an addition to the rules and regulations of the hospitals' minimum standards, since it was anticipated that the greatest number of infants requiring human milk would be hospitalized in tertiary neonatal units. The administrative rules and regulations were developed with the consultation of experts in milk banking and neonatal care. Because the items cover all of the considerations known to be necessary to provide the safest and most effective human milk for recipients, the regulations are duplicated in Appendix I for reference. Similarly, the Committee on Medical Aspects of Food Policy[8] in the United Kingdom held a Working Party on Human Milk Banks from 1979 to 1980, publishing a formal report in 1981 as an operational guideline for pediatric departments of hospitals that were setting up milk banks. The consultants included pediatricians, obstetricians, dietitians, nurses, and scientists with special expertise in lactation and human milk. The document is available from Her Majesty's Stationery Office (London Reports on Health and Social Subjects, no. 22). The recommendations for the expansion of the human milk banking system have not gone without challenge from neonatologists who offer sincere concerns for the risk/benefit ratio because alteration during storage and contamination may detract from the value of the original product for the mother's own infant. A series of sobering letters[2,33] appeared in the British medical press following the release of the document cautioning that the cavalier feeding of unsterile unsupplemented breast milk to small premature infants may produce iatrogenic problems.

Qualification of donors

A mother who is willing to donate milk should be healthy and fulfill these qualifications:

1. Normal pregnancy and delivery
2. Serologically negative for syphilis, hepatitis B surface antigen, cytomegalovirus, and HIV
3. No infection, acute or chronic, i.e., not at high risk
4. Not taking medications, smoking, or using excessive alcohol
5. Capable of carrying out sterile technique
6. If donating for other infants, own child is healthy and without jaundice

Pregnancy and delivery should have been relatively uncomplicated. The mother should have a negative VDRL and negative chest x-ray results. Whether donors should be

Georgetown University
Community Human Milk Bank

HUMAN MILK BANKING

How the Human Milk Bank Program Works

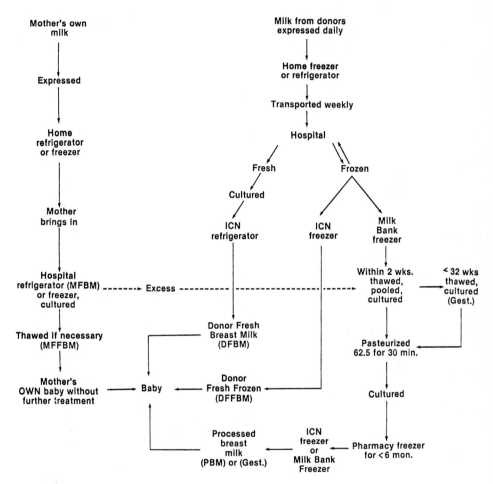

Fig. 19-1.   Flow chart of human milk bank program. (Courtesy Georgetown University Hospital, Washington DC.)

screened for HIV is controversial, as typical donors are considered at low risk and pasteurization kills the virus. Mother should not be taking medications, including birth control pills or any nonprescription medications such as aspirin or acetaminophen. Her infant should be well and should not have had neonatal jaundice. If the mother is donating only for her own infant, the state of the infant's health does not prevent her from donating. Anytime the mother becomes ill she should discard milk from the previous 24-hour period and not save milk until the illness is over and any maternal medications stopped.

Discarding milk during maternal illness is the hardest regulation to which a mother must adhere. The wish to contribute may overshadow the mother's understanding of the risk it poses for an infant receiving such milk. On the East coast in 1977 a mother developed diarrhea and continued to contribute for her own infant as well as others. This was the source of a serious outbreak of *Salmonella* in the nursery, resulting in unnecessary death and illness for many infants. This is one factor that has persuaded some banks not to pay donors for fear of developing a problem similar to that of blood banks, in which paid donors have more hepatitis and other problems than volunteers. The one limiting factor in donating milk, however, is that one has to be lactating. Becoming a professional donor of milk today is highly unlikely. The amount of protein has been noted to be lower after 6 months of lactation; thus it is advisable to limit a given mother's contributions to 6 months or, at most, 8 months postpartum.

Technique for collection

Whether collecting for a mother's own infant or for other uses, it is of prime importance to maintain cleanliness and minimize bacteria in the process of collection. The mother should be instructed in washing her hands and her breasts before handling the equipment or pumping.

There are two major ways of collecting: letting the milk drip while the infant nurses on the other side and pumping or manually expressing the milk.[21,22,49] In general, the latter is preferable. Dripped milk has been found to have lower caloric value and a much higher incidence of contamination. Pumped milk has a higher fat content than dripped or manually expressed milk, and in most individuals the volume is also greater. Any equipment used, such as hand pumps, tubing, and collecting bottles, should be sterile. If an electric pump is used, the parts that come in contact with the milk should be sterile and/or disposable (Fig. 19-2). Many hospitals own an electric pump, or one may be rented from a local rental company.

The hospital or the bank should provide a program of education for the donors. Milk samples should be cultured initially to ensure proper technique and the absence of significant contamination. Then samples should be sent for culture on a random basis. Studies have shown that milk collected at home has a higher contamination rate than that collected while the donor is hospitalized or with equipment maintained by the hospital. Collection at the hospital also avoids the transportation problem.

Many hospitals use the 4-oz sterile water-nursing bottles packaged by formula companies for collections by discarding the water at the time of collection and then filling them with milk. Other programs suggest the use of 50 ml plastic centrifuge tubes,* which are presterilized and have tight-fitting tops. These tubes have the advantage of more appropriate volume and easy measurability and sterility. Whether slightly acid human milk will leach plasticizers from plastic containers when stored in the freezer for weeks or months is unknown. Storage of mature milk in polypropylene containers decreases lysozyme and lactoferrin, whereas polyethylene containers decrease the titer of secretory IgA (see discussion on storage and processing).

The use of most of the modern electric pumps with their disposable tubing and collecting vessels makes mechanical pumping most efficient and cleanest. In addition, the milking action produces more physiologic stimulus to the breast. When a Y-connector is

---

*No. 25330, manufactured by Corning Glass Works.

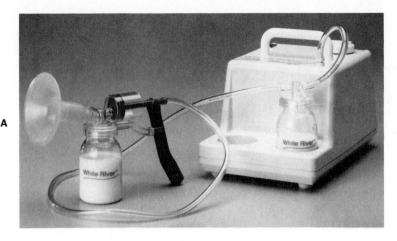

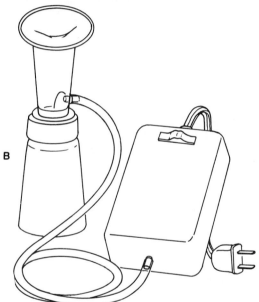

Fig. 19-2. A, White River Electric Breast Pump with milking action. Breast flange is made of Silastin. Milk cannot reverse into motor. Tubing and flange are sterilizable. (Courtesy of White River.) **B,** Purse-sized electric pump. Serviceable for women who are fully lactating.

used and both breasts are pumped simultaneously, overall production is increased and time in pumping is cut in half.

Bank milk collected by manual expression is less likely to be contaminated than that collected by hand pumps, however, including Lloyd B, even when pumps are boiled or placed in electric dishwasher.[31,52] The rubber bulb of the hand pump that resembles a bicycle horn retains milk and bacteria and should not be used. Nesty cups have been associated with the highest level of contamination. The contamination has included coliforms, and gentamicin-resistant gram-negative rods were found when donors used pumps at home.

Contaminated breast milk was the source of *Klebsiella* bacteremia in a neonatal intensive care unit according to Donowitz et al.[12] Unpasteurized human milk from a single donor fed via nasogastric and nasoduodenal tubes to sick newborns was found to be contaminated from the safety overflow bottle and tubing of the electric breast pump maintained in the neonatal intensive care unit. This part of the tubing and equipment should be sterilized or disposed of between collections according to the manufacturer's instructions. Strict attention to sterilization of equipment is imperative. Older electric pumps that do not have a built-in mechanism to prevent milk from getting into the permanent "works" should be discarded, and only pumps with disposable and/or cleanable parts and a safety valve should be used.

The bacteriologic benefit to discarding the first 5 to 10 ml of milk pumped from the breast remains disputed.[7] The MMB requires that their donors follow instruction for discarding the first 5 to 10 ml of milk expressed at each pumping and each breast. When a donor is collecting for long-term storage, this may be appropriate. When a mother is collecting for her own baby and her volume is meager, discarding 10 ml may be counterproductive. This is particularly important initially when early colostrum and milk are less in total volume but high in value to the infant. At home, later, when production is abundant and technique may be less stringent, discarding 2 to 3 ml might be appropriate.

Collection and storage containers

Colostrum was reported by Goldblum et al.[22] to impart greater stability to its components than did mature milk. None of the cellular or humoral immunological factors investigated was diminished when colostrum was stored at 4° C for 24 hours in any of the containers.

The effect of the container on the stability of the constituents of milk was investigated by Garza et al.[20] Pyrex and polypropylene containers were found not to interact with water- and fat-soluble nutrients such as vitamin A, zinc, iron, copper, sodium, and protein nitrogen. Polyethylene bags were found to spill easily, to be harder for mothers to fill without contamination, and to be difficult to handle in the nursery. The containers also leaked and punctured easily, resulting in 60% lower secretory IgA levels because of adherence to the material. It appears that rigid polypropylene plastic containers may have a significant advantage in maintaining the stability of all constituents in human milk collections and may be easier and safer to handle.

Paxson and Cress[41] have reported a significant difference in the survival of the leukocytes when the milk is collected and stored in plastic containers rather than glass, since the cells apparently stick to the glass. The phagocytosis of these cells, however, is not affected by the container. The researchers further demonstrated that varying the osmolarity or protein concentration does not alter the number or the phagocytosis of the cells. Because they believe the main reason for feeding preterm infants human milk is for the protection against infection, they suggest nasogastric feedings instead of nasojejunal feeding (to maintain pH in the acid range; in the small bowel, the pH is 6.5 to 8). The milk is collected in sterile plastic containers and maintained in the refrigerator until it is fed to the infant, avoiding heating, freezing, and alkaline solutions.

Storage and testing of milk samples

Fresh refrigerated unsterilized human milk can be used for 24 hours following collection. Mothers are instructed to bring milk to the nursery within 3 hours if it is to be

Table 19-1. Positive bacterial cultures from 41 breastfeeding mothers

Bacterial groups*	No. (%) of cultures	
	Skin and nipple	Milk
Staphylococcus epidermidis	77 (94)	29 (71)
Streptococcus	17 (21)	6 (15)
Propionibacterium	10 (12)	5 (12)
S. aureus	4 (5)	. . .
Pseudomonas aeruginosa	2 (2)	. . .
Klebsiella pneumoniae	1 (1)	2 (5)

*Two or more organisms were identified in several skin, nipple, and milk cultures.

Table 19-2. Positive rate of breast milk cultures over time

Cultures	Time of refrigeration, h		
	0	48	120
Positive	33	27	11
Negative	8	14	30
TOTAL	41	41	41

From Sosa R and Barness L: Am J Dis Child 141:111, 1987.

used fresh. If it is to be frozen, this should be done immediately at 0° F (-18° C) (standard home freezer) or in top of a refrigerator freezer. The milk stored in the latter should be deep frozen within a week if it is to be stored any length of time. The milk kept at -18° C can be kept for 6 months. Freezing and thawing significantly alter the energy content.

All samples should be labeled with name of donor, date, and time. Milk is stored in the freezer in such a way that the oldest milk is used first, and all milk of a single donor is kept together.

When a hospitalized mother is contributing fresh milk to her own infant, it is usually not cultured, as pumping is usually done with the help of the nursing staff and colostrum seems to be more resistant to contamination. But once a mother has been discharged home and she is producing mature milk, random sample culturing of mother's milk samples every week or two is a mechanism for checking milk-expression technique. Intensive care units have found that random testing improves technique in general.

Since using the fresh milk from the mother to feed a premature is becoming commonplace, it is important to be aware of the bacteria cultured from fresh samples during refrigeration. Samples pumped by hand pump and manually expressed were cultured at zero time and after 48 and 120 hours of refrigeration by Sosa and Barness.[47] Although 8 of 41 samples had no growth, the others had the same bacteria on skin and nipple as appeared in the milk (Table 19-1). Concentration was low and decreased over time (Table 19-2), which is attributed to the bacterial inhibitory factors present in milk and suggests that refrigeration of breast milk that has been carefully collected is a safe method for over 48 hours.

Standards for raw donor human milk

All raw donor milk should be screened microbiologically before use. There are no generally accepted microbiologic criteria for such milk except that no potential pathogens should be present.[6] Such pathogens include *Staphylococcus aureus,* β-hemolytic streptococci, *Pseudomonas* species, *Proteus* species, and *Streptococcus faecalis*. Some milk that cannot be fed raw can be pasteurized.[57]

Other guidelines include the following:

1. A total aerobic mesophilic colony count of less than 2.5×10^6 colony-forming units/ml with a predominance of normal skin flora
2. A count of staphylococci of less than 1×10^5 colony-forming units/ml
3. No enterobacteria

Standards for pasteurization of donor human milk

Milk suitable for pasteurization should meet minimum standards[57]:

1. A total aerobic count that does not exceed 1×10^6 colony-forming units/ml
2. *S. aureus* that does not exceed 1×10^3; there is the risk of feeding heat-treated enterotoxins when *S. aureus* exceeds 1×10^6
3. Presence of organisms defined as being of fecal origin not exceeding 1×10^4
4. Presence of organisms not part of normal flora not exceeding 1×10^7 colony-forming units/L
5. Presence of no unusual organisms such as *P. aeruginosa,* spore-bearing aerobes, or spore-bearing anaerobes

Testing milk for protein, fat, and carbohydrate is not necessary and is costly and time-consuming. A new quick method of analysis has been suggested by Lucas et al.[34] It involves standard hematocrit microtubes and a centrifuge. The percentage of cream or "creamatocrit" is read from the capillary tube. There is a linear relationship to fat and energy content.

$$\text{Fat (g/L)} = \frac{(\text{Creamatocrit [\%]} - 0.59)}{0.146}$$

$$\text{kcal/L} = 290 + (66.8 \times \text{Creamatocrit [\%]})$$

Accuracy is within 10%.

The Research Institute for Health Sciences provides the following formula for calculating the fat and energy content of milk using the measurement of the creamatocrit (%)[45]:

$$\text{Fat (g/L)} = (6.24 \times \text{Creamatocrit [\%]}) - 3.08$$
$$[r = 0.98, 95\% \text{ confidence limit} = \pm 4.39 \text{ g/L}]$$

$$\text{kcal/dl} = (5.57 \times \text{Creamatocrit [\%]}) + 45.13$$
$$[r = 0.92, 95\% \text{ confidence limit} = \pm 12.61 \text{ kcal/dl}]$$

Studies done comparing energy value calculated by creamatocrit with energy value from percentage of carbon, as measured by Manchester Bomb Calorimeter using pooled pasteurized milk samples, were somewhat inaccurate as compared to data obtained by creamatocrit on fresh or fresh frozen samples.

The methodology was validated with further analysis by Lemons et al.,[29] who repeated the studies and confirmed actual measurements of total fat and caloric content. As the protein and lactose content remains relatively constant over time, the variation in fat content is the primary constituent affecting caloric value of the milk. There was no effect of either freezing for up to 2 months or of pasteurization on the creamatocrit. There was no evidence of fat globule degradation during storage that affected the test.

Special cautions while performing this simple test should include the following:
- Use a representative, well-mixed sample.
- Complete a sample of pumping from at least one breast; do not take just a spot sample.
- A well-mixed 24-hour sample can be used.
- Use tube at least three-fourths filled; seal one end.
- Centrifuge for 15 minutes in standard table-top centrifuge.
- Occasional small layer of liquid fat on top (free fatty acids) should not be included.
- Keep tube vertical.
- Make measurement within 1 hour of centrifugation.

The effect of heating and freezing on the various constituents of human milk has been studied by a number of investigators whose data should be considered before deciding how to store milk for special purposes.

Heat treatment

When human milk was pasteurized at 73° C for 30 minutes, there was little IgA, IgG, lactoferrin, lysozyme, and C_3 complement left, and when the temperature was kept at 62.5° C for 30 minutes there was a loss of 23.7% of the lysozyme, 56.8% of the lactoferrin, and 34% of the IgG, but no loss of IgA, according to work done by Evans et al.[16] Similar studies of heat treatments of graded severity were carried out by Ford et al.[17] The findings were similar. Pasteurization at 62.5° C for 30 minutes (Holder method) reduced IgA by 20% and destroyed IgM and lactoferrin. Lysozyme was stable at 62.5° C but destroyed at 100° C, as was lactoperoxidase and the ability to bind folic acid against bacterial uptake. Growth of *Escherichia coli* increased in heated milk. B_{12}-binding capacity declined progressively with increasing temperature of the heat treatment. These data raise the question as to whether any heat treatment might not increase the risk of enteric infection in the infant. Some milk banks have advocated heating when the bacterial count is at a certain level, which may be too cumbersome to be practical. Ford et al.[17] suggest that for batch processing, 62.5° C for 30 minutes may be the method of choice.

The alterations of the lymphocyte and antibody content after processing were studied by Liebhaber et al.[31] They, too, found significant changes with heat, including a decrease in total lymphocyte count and in specific antibody titer to *E. coli*.

Welsh and May[55] discuss anti-infective properties of breast milk and provide two tables (Tables 19-3 and 19-4) to demonstrate the stability of the antibacterial and antiviral properties of human milk.

Short-time low-temperature pasteurization of human milk was reported by Wills et al.[58] using the Oxford Human Milk pasteurizer. Heating at 56.0° C for 15 minutes destroyed over 99% of the inoculated organisms, which included *E. coli*, *S. aureus*, and group B β-hemolytic streptococci. The remaining activity of antimicrobial proteins after different time/temperature treatments is shown in Table 19-5.

High-temperature short-time (HTST) (72° or 87° C up to 15 seconds) treatment of human milk inoculated with endogenous bacteria and cytomegalovirus rendered the milk bacteria free in 5 seconds and CMV free in 15 seconds.[23] Folic acid and vitamins B_1, B_2, B_6, and C were not affected. Bile salt–stimulated lipase was inactivated by these conditions. Lactoferrin and secretory IgA and sIgA antibody activity were stable at 72° C for 15

Table 19-3. Antibacterial factors in breast milk

Factor	Shown in vitro to be active against	Effect of heat
L bifidus growth factor	Enterobacteriaceae, enteric pathogens	Stable to boiling
Secretory IgA	E. coli; E. coli enterotoxin; C. tetani, C. diphtheriae, D. pneumoniae, Salmonella, Shigella	Stable at 56° C for 30 min; some loss (0% to 30%) at 62.5° C for 30 min; destroyed by boiling
C_1-C_9	Effect not known	Destroyed by heating at 56° C for 30 min
Lactoferrin	E. coli; C. albicans	Two thirds destroyed at 62.5° C for 30 min
Lactoperoxidase	Streptococcus; Pseudomonas, E. coli, S. typhimurium	Not known; presumably destroyed by boiling
Lysozyme	E. coli; Salmonella, M. lysodeikticus	Stable at 62.5° C for 30 min; activity reduced 97% by boiling for 15 min
Lipid (unsat'd fatty acid)	S. aureus	Stable to boiling
Milk cells	By phagocytosis: E. coli, C. albicans By sensitized lymphocytes: E. coli	Destroyed by 62.5° C for 30 min

From Welsh JK and May JI: J Pediatr 93:1, 1979.

Table 19-4. Antiviral factors in breast milk

Factor	Shown in vitro to be active against	Effect of heat
Secretory IgA	Polio types 1, 2, 3, coxsackie types A9, B3, B5; ECHO types 6, 9; Semliki Forest virus, Ross River virus, rotavirus	Stable at 56° C for 30 min; some loss (0% to 30%) at 62.5° for 30 min; destroyed by boiling
Lipid (unsat'd fatty acids and monoglycerides)	Herpes simplex; Semliki Forest virus, influenza, dengue, Ross River virus, Murine leukemia virus, Japanese B encephalitis virus	Stable to boiling for 30 min
Nonimmunoglobulin macromolecules	Herpes simplex; vesicular stomatitis virus	Destroyed at 60° C; stable at 56° C for 30 min; destroyed by boiling for 30 min
	Rotavirus	Unknown
Milk cells	Induced interferon active against Sendai virus; Sensitized lymphocytes? Phagocytosis?	Destroyed at 62.5° C for 30 min

From Welsh JK and May JT: J Pediatr 93:1, 1979.

Table 19-5. Influence of pasteurization temperatures on human milk

	% IgA	% Lactoferrin	% Lysozyme
62.5° C	67	27	67
62.5° C 5 min	77	59	96
56.0° C 15 min	90	91	100

Table 19-6. Effect of rapid high-temperature treatment on selected vitamins in human milk

			Time (sec)					
	0		**1**		**3**		**15**	
	$\overline{X} \pm SD$	n	$\overline{X} \pm SD$	n	$\overline{X} \pm SD$	n	$\overline{X} \pm SD$	n
Vitamin B_1, (μg/ml)	0.104 ± 0.013	9						
72°C			0.098 ± 0.005	3	0.091 ± 0.008	3	0.088 ± 0.009	3
87°C			0.084 ± 0.011*	3	0.095 ± 0.027	3	ND	
Vitamin B_2 (μg/ml)	0.724 ± 0.132	9						
72°C			0.75 ± 0.08	3	0.70 ± 0.09	3	0.56 ± 0.07	3
87°C			0.66 ± 0.13†	3	0.72 ± 0.22	3	ND	
Vitamin B_6 (μg/ml)	0.237 ± 0.081	9						
72°C			0.27 ± 0.05	3	0.26 ± 0.025	3	0.22 ± 0.012	3
87°C			0.25 ± 0.07	3	0.26 ± 0.02	3	ND	
Folic acid (μg/ml)	0.106 ± 0.020	9						
72°C			0.089 ± 0.005‡	3*	0.065 ± 0.018	3	0.101 ± 0.012	3
87°C			0.088 ± 0.008	3	0.080 ± 0.023	3	ND	
Vitamin C (μg/ml)	9.2 ± 2.4	9						
72°C			11.2 ± 1.2	3	21.5 ± 3.0*	3	8.7 ± 1.7	3
87°C			16.0 ± 4.9*	3	22.5 ± 13.3	3	ND	

From Goldblum RM, Dill CW, Abrecht TB et al: J Pediatr 104:380, 1984.

n. Number of experiments; *ND,* not done.

*$P<0.07$.

†$P<0.001$.

‡$P<0.04$.

seconds. Lysozyme concentration and enzymatic activity were increased, suggesting to the researchers that lysozyme may be sequestered in the milk (Tables 19-6 and 19-7).

Lyophilization and freezing

The impact of lyophilization was similar to that of heating, showing a decrease in total lymphocyte count and in immunoglobulin concentration and specific antibody titer to *E. coli.* (Lyophilization is the creation of a stable preparation of a biological substance by rapid freezing and dehydration of the frozen product under high vacuum–freeze drying.)

Table 19-7. Effect of rapid high-temperature treatment on immunologic proteins in human milk

	Time (sec)							
	0		**1**		**3**		**15**	
	$\overline{X} \pm SD$	n	$\overline{X} \pm SD$	n	$\overline{X} \pm SD$	n	$\overline{X} \pm SD$	n
Lactoferrin	0.67 ± 0.10	8						
(mg/ml)								
72°C			0.95 ± 0.21	2	0.58 ± 0.2	3	0.83 ± 0.05	3
87°C			0.50 ± 0.02	3	0.50 ± 0.2	3	0.47 ± 0.17	2
Lysozyme	15.0 ± 8.7	8						
(μg/ml)								
72°C			86.0 ± 3.5*	2	78.0 ± 16.0	3†	59.0 ± 7.0*	3
87°C			86.0 ± 9.1*	3	59.0 ± 9.0	3†	36.0 ± 7.7	2
Total IgA	0.37 ± 0.08	8						
(mg/ml)								
72°C			0.37 ± 0.07	2	0.25 ± 0.06	3	0.3 ± 0.04	3
87°C			0.06 ± 0.04*	3	0.04 ± 0.02	3†	0.05 ± 0.03	2
sIgA Ab	10.0 ± 4.8	7						
(recipro-								
cal titer)								
72°C			10.2 ± 12.4	2	10.6 ± 4.8	2	15.0 ± 3.5	3
87°C			<1	3	<1	2	<1	2

From Goldblum RM, Dill CW, Abrecht TB et al: J Pediatr 104:380, 1984.
*$P<0.01$.
†$P<0.05$.

Freezing specimens up to 4 weeks showed no change in IgA or *E. coli* antibody titer, although the lymphocyte count was decreased. The technique involved freezing to −23° C and thawing at 1, 2, 3, and 4 weeks. Although there were cells present after freezing, they showed no viability when tested with the trypan blue stain exclusion method. The storage of human milk at 4° C for 48 hours caused a decrease in the concentration of milk macrophages and neutrophils but not of the lymphocytes, which also maintained their activity, according to work reported by Pittard and Bill.[42] The loss of cells may be desirable if the graft versus host reaction in a premature infant who is possibly immunodeficient is of concern. Evans and associates[16] reported their results with 3-month storage −20° C and of freeze-drying and reconstitution (lyophilization). They found no significant change in lactoferrin, lysozyme, IgA, IgG, and C3 after 3-month freezing but a small loss of IgG after lyophilization (Table 19-8). Whether factors that promote the growth of normal flora in the gut survive treatment was also investigated.[3] These researchers propose that "human milk should be collected in as sterile a manner as possible and deep frozen shortly after collection. If a donor mother maintains a low bacterial count in her milk, then its use unheated should be considered. Pasteurization, if used, should be at minimum temperature capable of adequate bacterial killing (about 62° C for 30 min)."[16]

Nutritional consequences of heat treatment

Initially the focus was on the effect of processing human milk on its unique anti-infective properties,[22,25] but attention has been given to the nutritional consequences as

Table 19-8. Effect of deep freezing (3 mo) at $-20°$ C and lyophilization of human milk proteins (mg/100 ml milk)

	Raw milk (mean ± SE)	Deep frozen milk			Lyophilized milk		
		Mean ± SE	Mean as % raw	P	Mean ± SE	Mean as % raw	P
α_1-Antitrypsin (16 samples)	2.38 ± 0.3	1.98 ± 0.2	83.2	<0.05	2.22 ± 0.3	93.3	>0.1
IgA (8 samples)	9.55 ± 0.84	9.25 ± 0.83	96.9	>0.1	9.33 ± 0.74	97.7	>0.1
IgG (16 samples)	0.42 ± 0.05	0.42 ± 0.04	100	>0.1	0.33 ± 0.04	78.6	<0.05
Lactoferrin (11 samples)	332 ± 71.7	338 ± 57.4	102	>0.1	363 ± 79	109.3	>0.1
Lysozymes (11 samples)	5.1 ± 1.26	4.6 ± 0.67	90.2	>0.1	4.8 ± 1.19	94.1	>0.1
C3 (16 samples)	1.35 ± 0.13	1.26 ± 0.11	93.3	>0.1	1.27 ± 0.13	94.1	>0.1

From Evans TJ et al: Arch Dis Child 53:239, 1978.

well.[44] Storage for 24 hours did not affect vitamin A, zinc, iron, copper, sodium, or protein nitrogen concentrations at 37° C.[50,56] Ascorbic acid levels fell markedly when stored at 37° C and 4° C at 24 and 48 hours. (They remain stable for 4 hours.) Other investigators have found that ascorbic acid levels drop 40% with heating.[20,50]

Levels of unsaturated fatty acids apparently are also affected by heating and cold storage, but the data need clarification. It is anticipated that heating or freezing and thawing are capable of damaging membranes surrounding milk fat globules.[44] The fat globule could then undergo fragmentation and allow greater access of milk lipases to triglycerides.[54] The percentages of polyunsaturated fatty acids, linoleic ($C_{18:2}$) and linolenate ($C_{18:3}$), decreased after both heating and freezing, while monounsaturates and saturated fatty acids were unaffected.[54] When milk is stored at $-11°$ C over 48 hours, there is release of fatty acids progressing over time with an increase in the proportion of free 18:2, 20:4, and other long-chain polyenic acids. There was no measurable lipolysis when milk was stored at $-70°$ C. The higher the temperature and the longer the time, the greater the accumulation of free fatty acids.[28] Other investigators have confirmed this, concluding the lipoprotein lipase and bile salt–stimulated lipase remain fully active at $-20°$ C but not $-70°$ C with or without presence of serum. Berkow et al.[4] recommend therefore that milk be stored at $-70°$ C. Other enzymes were not affected by freezing and storing except lactoperoxidase, which lost activity (Table 19-9).

Because the nourishment of low-birth-weight infants has been the purpose of many bank milks, the ability of preterm infants to utilize treated bank milk is relative. Pasteurization at 62.5° C for 30 minutes was reported not to influence nitrogen absorption or retention in low-birth-weight infants.[44] When raw, pasteurized, and boiled human milks were fed to very low-birth-weight (<1.3 kg) preterm infants in 3 separate consecutive weeks, fat absorption was reduced by one third in the heat-treated group. There was a reduction in the amount of nitrogen retained in the heat-treated group as well, although the absorption was unaffected. The absorption and retention of calcium, phosphorus, and sodium were unaffected by heating or freezing. The mean weight gain was greater by one third when the infants were fed raw human milk.[56]

Table 19-9. Protein N concentrations (mg N/dl)

Storage time (h)	Storage temperature		
	37°C	4°C	−72°C
4	187 ± 8*	181 ± 7*	
24	183 ± 7*,**	178 ± 5*,**	186 ± 8**
48	189 ± 8*	178 ± 5*	

From Garza C, Johnson CA, Harrist R et al: Early Hum Dev 6:295, 1982.
Mean ±1 SM (n = 11).
*Effects due to temperature significant when samples stored at 37 and 4°C are compared (P<0.05, F = 9.3).
**Comparison of storage temperature effects on samples stored only for 24 h not significant (P>0.05, F = 1.4).

Table 19-10. Thermal destruction of milk components (follows first-order reaction kinetics)

	D value at 60°C (sec)	Z values†
IgA	4.9×10^4	5.5°C
Lactoferrin	2.4×10^3	4.7°C
Thiamin	7.7×10^5	28.4°C
Folic acid	1.9×10^4	6.4°C

Adapted from Morgan JN, Toledo RT, Eitenmiller RR et al: J Food Sci 51:348, 1986.
*D value = 90% degradation at 60°C in seconds.
†Z value = Temperature change to alter degradation rate by a factor of 10.

Pasteurization decreased B_{12} by about 50% and folate binding capacity by 10% (Table 19-10). Sterilization (100° C for 20 minutes), on the other hand, had similar effects on B_{12} binding and completely inactivated folate binding.[50] Vitamins A, D, E, B_2, B_6, choline, niacin, and pantothenic acid were barely affected by pasteurization, whereas thiamin was reduced up to 25%, biotin up to 10%, and vitamin C up to 35%. Refrigeration at 4° C to 6° C for 72 hours allows little bacterial growth and causes no change in nutrients or infection-protective properties. Freezing does have a little effect on both and the milk can be kept for months, whereas heating has significant effect and the milk still requires freezing for storage. Experience feeding donated raw milk to newborns has shown no ill effects if carefully monitored according to Björksten et al.[5] Quick freezing and frozen storage do not significantly affect levels of biotin, niacin and folic acid, vitamin E, or the fatty soluble vitamins. Photo-oxidation and absorption by the container or tubing are always a consideration. Vitamin C is reduced by all of these.[19]

Ultrasonic homogenization to prevent fat loss

Pooling specimens of human milk may not result in a milk of uniform fat content after storage. The separation of fat during processing, storage, and administration by continuous nasogastric infusion, whether by gravity flow or continuous mechanical pump, results in significant loss of fat and variation in the milk received (47.4% of fat with slow infusion and 16.8% with fast infusion). Homogenization by ultrasonic treatment was studied by Martinez et al.,[35] who found changes in fat concentration during infusion and loss of fat during administration, due to sticking to container and tubes, were eliminated. Furthermore, the fat-soluble vitamins are preserved. Since 31% of iron, 15% of copper, 12% of zinc, 10% of calcium, and 2% of magnesium sulfate are in the fat fraction of both human and cow milk, preserving the fat is essential to maximizing nutrient intake from human milk, especially in compromised infants. Tube feedings have been noted to reduce vitamins B_2, B_6, A, and C in human milk.

Ultrasonic homogenization was accomplished in this study by subjecting the milk to treatment in a Tekmar Sonic Disruptor TSD-P 250 (Tekmar Co., Cincinnati, Ohio). The homogenization time (2, 4, or 8 minutes) is a function of the volume of milk and intensity of vibration. The procedure should be done in milk in an ice bath.

Viruses in human milk

The dilemma of cytomegalovirus (CMV) is a significant one, since the virus does pass into the milk. In a study of postpartum women, CMV was recovered from the genital tract in 10%, from the urine in 7%, from the saliva in 2%, and from the breast milk in 30%. CMV does persist after storage at 4° C and −20° C in some specimens.[48] It is destroyed at 62° C after 30 minutes.[13] Donor milk should be accepted only from CMV-negative mothers. Mothers who are seropositive may be permitted to provide for their own infants because they have already provided the protection as well.

Hepatitis virus also passes into milk, and donors should therefore be screened and be seronegative. The question of having seropositive women feed their own infants is discussed in Chapter 14.

The AIDS virus has been identified in human milk.[51,59] Most banks require that donors be HIV negative, but since seropositivity may take months to develop, some mechanism for excluding high-risk donors should be in place. Holding all milk samples for several months may not be practical, and pasteurizing all milk may decrease the value of the nutrient. Some AIDS experts are concerned that the threat may seriously alter the future of milk banks.[32] On the other hand, some feel that donors should not be screened. It has been demonstrated that heat treatment kills the virus when milk is inoculated experimentally.[14]

Special considerations

Thawing milk should be done in the refrigerator, and each bottle should be used completely within 24 hours. Defrosting in the microwave oven may lead to separation of layers. Microwaves do decrease vitamin C content but are not known to destroy other factors. The greatest danger of microwaving is that the milk heats and the container does not, so that an infant could be burned or the milk significantly overheated.

Donor milk is at risk for being contaminated with cow's milk by the donor. The California Mother's Milk Bank checks its contributions with a simple test directed at precipitating the casein. They mix 1 ml of donor milk with 1 ml of 8N sulfuric acid and 8 ml water and let it sit at room temperature for 5 hours. If cow's milk is present, it will precipitate.[40]

Financial aspects

Established milk banks have various financial structures. Income can include charges for equipment rental and for processing milk. Certainly the hospital should recover costs of collecting and processing. This should be a reimbursable item of hospital costs. Precedent for this has been set in the United States. Since legislation has been passed by some states mandating the availability of human milk for all babies who need it, there must be reimbursement for it and funds available for its proper handling.

The recommendations from the State of New York (see Appendix I) suggest that the monitoring of standards of a hospital-based bank be absorbed into existing hospital surveillance. Free-standing banks would be monitored by the state and local health departments. Economic analysis indicates that the primary costs would be administrative overhead costs. The human milk supply is considered a donated product. Also acknowledged are staff costs, minimal equipment costs, and laboratory costs as well as costs to the state health department to administer the system. Much consideration is being given to limiting banks to hospital settings, where health professionals and equipment are readily available.

WET NURSING OR CROSS-NURSING

Although feeding an infant by one who is not his mother is an established means of sustaining life, it is uncommon in Western cultures since the 1930s. There are no medical contraindications provided the nursing woman is in good health, is infection-free, and is taking no medications. The chief obstacle is psychologic or social. Actually women who are trying to develop a supply of milk when their own infant cannot nurse because of prematurity or illness would be greatly benefited by having a vigorous normal suckling infant nurse at their breasts. In contemporary society, the term *cross-nursing* has replaced *wet nursing* to disassociate the phenomenon from the negative historical connotations. In cross-nursing the mother continues to breastfeed her own child in addition to the child she takes for a feeding or two per day. The circumstances described in the report by Krantz and Kupper[27] usually involve babysitting arrangements, which may be daily and formal or random and informal. They interviewed three women involved in a mutual agreement for baby-sitting purposes. The mothers were married and well educated. The babies were female and 4 months old. There appeared to be no physical effects on the babies according to the mothers. The behavioral reactions of the babies were "looking puzzled" and being disturbed if the surrogate mother spoke. Some difficulty was noticed in let-down, and all three mothers noted a difference in the way each baby suckled.

Another purpose of cross-nursing is for maternal benefit, wherein an experienced vigorous infant is nursed by a woman whose own baby is unable to give proper stimulus to milk production. This has been done by private arrangement and has not caused any known problems. Usually the normal newborn is younger than 2 months. Cross-nursing has also been used to stimulate lactation in adoptive nursing. In this situation the infants are exchanged to stimulate the adoptive mother's breasts and also to show the adopted infant that milk comes from breasts and how to suckle at the breast.

The hazards to cross-nursing are undocumented but worthy of consideration. The physical problems are the potential for infection, either of mother or of baby, interruption of milk supply for the mother's own baby, and the difference in composition of milk if babies are of different chronologic or conceptual ages. The psychologic hazards could include failure of mother to let-down, refusal of infant to nurse (which does occur when infants are introduced to the phenomenon beyond 4 months of age), and negative impact on siblings and household. The long-range effects are not documented.

Reasonable caution is certainly appropriate, taking care to assure that the cross-nursing mother is healthy and well nourished, without any general or local infection, and not taking any medications or smoking. The infants should probably be close in age and also free of infection, especially thrush. If this were a commercial venture in a public day-care setting, regulations of certification screening for tuberculosis, syphilis, hepatitis, CMV, herpesvirus, HIV, and other infectious agents might be in order. Documents of liability might be required.

Perhaps as breastfeeding knowledge and understanding reach a greater number of professionals and women, such opportunities may be more common. At present it is significant to recognize this as a viable option.

Breast pumping equipment

In this chapter, several types of breast pumping devices have been alluded to around questions of the sterility of milk collected. Additional issues need to be considered, including efficiency, ease of use, potential for breast trauma, availability, and cost. A good pump should be capable of completely emptying the breast and of stimulating production. It should be clean, contamination free, easy to use, and atraumatic.

Hand pumps

The bicycle horn pump has been marketed in drugstores for years without instructions for use or cleaning. At the museum at the Corning Glass Works in Corning, New York there is a glass and rubber hand pump made by Davol circa 1830 AD on display next to glass baby bottles and pewter nipples. The current model is the same, except the glass has been replaced by plastic. The dangers of this pump are legion but can be summarized by saying the milk is contaminated, a squirt of milk can go directly into the bulb, the pump requires constant emptying, and it can be quite traumatic to the nipple, areola, and breast.

Modifications of this style insert a removable collecting bottle in place of the well in the bicycle horn pump. The modification permits feeding the infant directly from the collecting vessel by placing a nipple on it. Milk does not wash back over the breast, and pumping is not interrupted for emptying. The tube and bulb still may harbor bacteria because they are hard to clean. The limitations of the effect of creating a simple vacuum and applying a simple, rigid, sharp-edged flange against the breast are still present. This pump is satisfactory for temporary use, but it takes time to become proficient in its use, and it may never create enough pressure to be effective. Another model (Nurture) with special flexible silicone funnel overcomes these problems and is now available from White River.

The cylindric pumps are two all-plastic cylindric tubes that fit inside one another to create a vacuum. A flange to accommodate the nipple and areola is at top of inner tube, which also has a gasket for tight fit at the other end. The outer tube collects the milk and is adapted for use as a feeding unit when a nipple is screwed on top. The mother creates the vacuum by pulling the outer tube and creates rhythm by pushing the outer tube in and out (Fig. 19-3). It is simple, easy to clean, and the milk is usable. This pump is excellent in hands of an experienced, dextrous mother. There are several manufacturers, and the product differs slightly. Some have a choice of flanges. The Lloyd-B pump has a trigger handle adapted to a flange mechanism that empties into a collection jar the size of a baby-food jar (not a baby bottle). It does have a vacuum relief switch; however, the entire mechanism requires a certain dexterity and a rather large hand to operate. It is portable and also easily cleaned. No parts harbor bacteria.

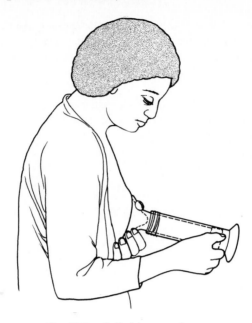

Fig. 19-3. Cylindric pump in use.

Mechanical pumps

Battery-operated pumps are available but in most cases are not sufficiently powerful to stimulate the breast adequately and so are ineffective for women whose infants are not feeding at the breast, such as prematures or infants hospitalized in an NICU. These small hand pumps work for some fully lactating women who need a pump that fits in their purse for use while at work or school. There are also small purse-sized electric pumps that may be effective for the fully lactating woman. They have the advantage over a manually powered hand pump that the electric power frees one hand for the mother to stroke the breast and encourage let-down. If flow is going well, then the hand is free to do other things such as read, telephone, or write, not an insignificant advantage for a busy working breastfeeding woman. The small electric models have a small hole in the flange base that must be closed with a finger to develop the suction as in most hospital suctioning devices. This gives the mother control over the pressure. By rhythmically opening and closing the hole with the finger, the operator can simulate milking action that is very effective in pumping milk. The manufacturers unfortunately do not always point this out. Electric pumps are most efficient as the mechanical effort is applied by the motor and the mother can concentrate on applying the cup to her breast, massaging the breast, and relaxing so that adequate let-down can take place. All electric pumps are not equal, and some guidance is needed to be sure that the mother understands the principles involved. Nursery staff should be familiar with the equipment. The pumps are no challenge to skilled intensive care nursery nurses who are adept at handling complicated electronic equipment.

A pump that cycles pressure instead of maintaining constant negative pressure will be less likely to cause petechiae or internal trauma. Negative pressures should have a governor mechanism to avoid excessive pressures. Mean sucking pressures of most normal full-term infants range from -50 to -155, with a maximum up to -220 mm Hg/in^2. Manufacturers recommend about 200 mm Hg/in^2 to initiate flow in most women.

A careful study by Johnson[26] of over 1000 patients at the University of Texas using a variety of pumps has confirmed some facts about pumps. The amount of negative pressure possible and the control mechanisms were recorded. The findings are summarized in Tables 19-11 and 19-12.

Table 19-11. Electrical pumping devices

Mechanical pump	Advantages	Disadvantages
All mechanical pumps		Expensive Can rent Should be covered by insurance
Egnell/Medela (Fig. 19-6) Rhythmic vacuum Stimulates nursing	Helpful in initiating let-down Simulates rhythm of suckling Disposable tubing and collecting cups	Well serviced by company

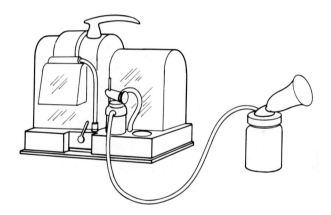

Gomco/Sorenson Adapted from suction apparatus Finger control of T-tube will cycle vacuum	Good visibility Good collection vessel	Poor cup design—painful Continuous negative pressure can run too high Hard to control Not good for long use Noisy

Continued.

Table 19-11. Electrical pumping devices—cont'd

Mechanical pump	Advantages	Disadvantages
White River	Excellent milking action	Becoming more available (see Fig. 19-2)
	Comfortable	
	Portable in compact case	
	Easily cleaned	
	Inexpensive	
	Special Silastin cup	
	Initiates and maintains milk supply	
	Can be rented	
	Disposable tubing	
	Quiet	
	Good backup by company	
Whittlestone Milker	Excellent milking action	Availability
Physiologic milk with breast cups that milk breast	Comfortable	Can be rented
	Initiates and maintains milk supply	

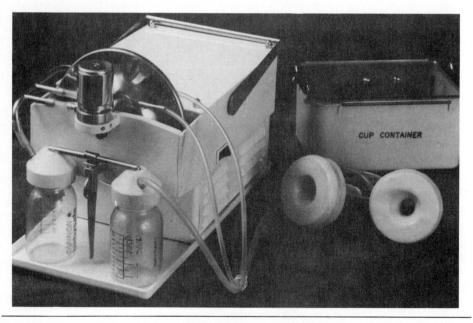

Breast pumps have been identified as the source of infection on a number of occasions.[38] Improvement in design so that there is a safety trap between the collecting vessel and the machine to avoid milk getting into the mechanism is important. In addition, all equipment that comes in contact with milk or the breast should be sterilizable and/or disposable. The well-designed electric pump properly used is probably the best system.

In the hospital, as with all special equipment, it is advisable to select the best

Table 19-12. Hand pumping devices

Hand pump	Advantages	Disadvantages
Bicycle horn pump	Inexpensive Portable	Difficult to clean Bulb retains bacteria Works as vacuum No instructions Can cause trauma Not appropriate for donor milk Milk washes back over nipple Requires constant emptying
Evenflo pump	Inexpensive	Difficult to clean, bulb harbors bacteria even when boiled
White River hand pump	Pliable flange Can feed baby from collecting container	Works well for less experienced mother with good let-down

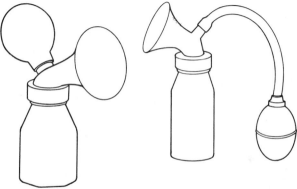

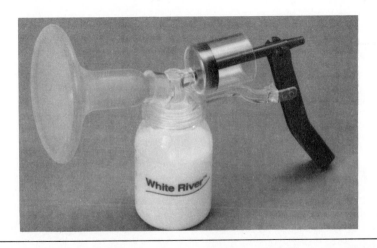

Continued.

Table 19-12. Hand pumping devices—cont'd

Hand pump	Advantages	Disadvantages
Cylindric Two all plastic cylindric tubes that fit inside one another to create vacuum. Inner tube has flange at top ad rubber or nylon gasket	Less expensive than electric Portable Can feed baby from collecting container Easily cleaned and sterilized	Requires some dexterity Works as vacuum with some rhythm Rigid flange

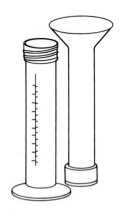

Hand pump	Advantages	Disadvantages
Lloyd B pump Glass flange attached to collecting jar. Trigger handle mechanism creates vacuum; has vacuum relief switch	Less expensive than electric Portable Can be cleaned	Handle difficult to squeeze Hand becomes cramped Awkward Large breast and nipple may hit flange Transfer of milk to feeding unit necessary

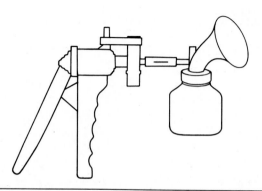

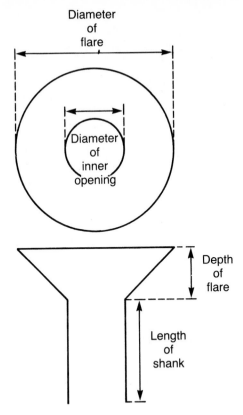

Fig. 19-4. Measurement of nipple cups. (From Johnson CA: Clin Pediatr 22:40, 1983.)

equipment to fill the needs of that hospital and then purchase all one make so that staff learns how to use it properly and can instruct the patient.

Similarly, the equipment should be checked on a routine basis, cleaned, and bacteriologically tested. Accessory equipment (disposable) can be resterilized for the same patient but not for a second patient.

Although attention is usually given to the pressure mechanisms, equally important is the cup that is applied to the breast. The diameter and depth of the flare are fixed for the hand pumps and the Gomco electric pump, but a choice is offered for the Egnell, Medela, White River, and Whittlestone pumps. The nipple should have room to be drawn out, and the flange should be adequate to transmit pressure or milking action to the collecting ampullae under the areola. The hand pumps are too small; however, bigger is not always better, and a mother may find that the smaller model of the two offered may suit her anatomy more physiologically. This feature does not correlate directly with overall size of breast. The ideal range is 68 to 82 mm outer diameter and 35 to 40 mm depth of flare[26] (Fig. 19-4). The White River and the Nurture silicone funnels adapt well to all sizes and shapes because of flexibility.

The relative efficacy of four methods of human milk expression was measured by Green et al.[24] The electric pump (Egnell) enabled mothers to pump significantly more milk with higher fat content in the 10-minute time allotted for the study than did the Lloyd B, the Evenflo hand pump, or manual expression, all three of which were about equal in efficacy.

REFERENCES

1. Asquith MT, Pedrotti PW, Stevenson DK, and Sunshine P: Clinical uses, collection, and banking of human milk, Clin Perinatol 14:173, 1987.
2. Barrie H: Human milk bank, Lancet 1:284, 1982.
3. Beerens H, Romond C, and Neut C: Influence of breastfeeding on the bifid flora of the newborn intestine, Am J Clin Nutr 33:2434, 1980.
4. Berkow SE, Freed LM, Hamosh M et al: Lipases and lipids in human milk: effects of freeze-thawing and storage, Pediatr Res 18:1257, 1984.
5. Björksten B et al: Collecting and banking human milk: to heat or not to heat? Br Med J 281:765, 1980.
6. Carroll L et al: Bacteriological criteria for feeding raw breast-milk to babies on neonatal units, Lancet 2:732, 1979.
7. Carroll L, Osman M, and Davies DP: Does discarding the first few millilitres of breast milk improve the bacteriological quality of bank breast milk, Lancet 2:898, 1979.
8. Committee on Medical Aspects of Food Policy: The collection and storage of human milk, London, 1981, Her Majesty's Stationery Office.
9. Committee on Mother's Milk, America Academy of Pediatrics: Operation of mother's milk bureaus, J Pediatr 23:112, 1943.
10. Committee on Nutrition, American Academy of Pediatrics: Human milk banking, Pediatrics 65:854, 1980.
11. Davidson DC, Poll RA, and Roberts G: Bacteriological monitoring of unheated human milk, Arch Dis Child 54:760, 1979.
12. Donowitz LG et al: Contaminated breast milk: a source of *Klebsiella* bacteremia in a newborn intensive care unit, Rev Infect Dis 3:716, 1981.
13. Dworsky M et al: Persistence of cytomegalovirus in human milk after storage, J Pediatr 101:440, 1982.
14. Eglin RP and Wilkinson AR: HIV infection and pasteurization of breast milk, Lancet 1:1093, 1987.
15. Eidelman AI and Szilagyi G: Patterns of bacterial colonization of human milk, Obstet Gynecol 53:550, 1979.
16. Evans TJ et al: Effect of storage and heat on antimicrobial proteins in huamn milk, Arch Dis Child 53:239, 1978.
17. Ford JE et al: Influence of heat treatment of human milk on some of its protective constituents, J Pediatr 90:29, 1977.
18. Freier S and Faber J: Loss of immune components during the processing of human milk. In Williams AF and Baum J, editors: Human milk banking, New York, 1984, Nestle Nutrition, Vivey/Raven Press.
19. Friend BA, Shahani KM, Long CA et al: The effect of processing and storage on key enzymes, B vitamins, and lipids of mature human milk. I. Evaluation of fresh samples and effects of freezing and frozen storage, Pediatr Res 17:61, 1983.
20. Garza C et al: Effects of methods of collection and storage on nutrients in human milk, Early Hum Dev 6:295, 1982.
21. Gibbs JH et al: Drip breast milk: its composition, collection and pasteurization, Early Hum Dev 1:227, 1977.
22. Goldblum RM et al: Human milk banking. II. Relative stability of immunologic factors in stored colostrum, Acta Paediatr Scand 71:143, 1982.
23. Goldblum RM, Dill CW, Albrecht TB et al: Rapid high-temperature treatment of human milk, J Pediatr 104:380, 1984.
24. Green D et al: The relative efficacy of four methods of human milk expression, Early Hum Dev 6:153, 1982.
25. Hernandez J et al: Effect of storage processes on the bacterial growth-inhibiting activity of human breast milk, Pediatrics 63:597, 1979.
26. Johnson CA: An evaluation of breast pumps currently available on the American market, Clin Pediatr 22:40, 1983.
27. Krantz JZ and Kupper NS: Cross-nursing: wet-nursing in a contemporary context, Pediatrics 67:715, 1981.
28. Lavine M and Clark RM: Changing patterns of free fatty acids in breast milk during storage, J Pediatr Gastroenterol Nutr 6:769, 1987.
29. Lemons JA, Schreiner RL, and Gresham EL: Simple method for determining the caloric and fat content of human milk, Pediatrics 66:626, 1980.
30. Liebhaber M et al: Alterations of lymphocytes and of antibody content of human milk after processing, J Pediatr 91:897, 1977.
31. Liebhaber M et al: Comparison of bacterial contamination with two methods of human milk collection, J Pediatr 92:236, 1978.
32. Lucas A: AIDS and human milk bank closures, Lancet 1:1092, 1987.
33. Lucas A: Human milk banks, Lancet 1:103, 1982.
34. Lucas A et al: Creamatocrit: simple clinical technique for estimating fat concentration and energy value of human milk, Br Med J 1:1018, 1978.
35. Martinez FE, Desai ID, Davidson AGF et al: Ultrasonic homogenization of expressed human milk to prevent fat loss during tube feeding, J Pediatr Gastroenterol Nutr 6:593, 1987.
36. McEnery G and Chattopadhyay B: Human milk bank in a district general hospital, Br Med J 2:794, 1978.

37. Moffatt PA, Lammi-Keefe CJ, Ferris AM, and Jensen RG: Alpha and gamma tocopherols in pooled mature human milk after storage, J Pediatr Gastroenterol Nutr 6:225, 1987.

38. Moloney AC, Quoraishi AH, Parry P et al: A bacteriological examination of breast pumps, J Hosp Infections 9:169, 1987.

39. Morgan JN, Toledo RT, Eitenmiller RR et al: Thermal destruction of immunoglobulin A, lactoferrin, thiamin, and folic acid in human milk, J Food Sci 51:348, 1986.

40. Mother's Milk Unit, California Transplant Bank: Procedures and protocols, San Jose, Calif, 1988, The Mothers' Milk Bank: The Institute for Medical Research.

41. Paxson CL and Cress CC: Survival of human milk leukocytes, J Pediatr 94:61, 1979.

42. Pittard WB and Bill K: Human milk banking: effect of refrigeration on cellular components, Clin Pediatr 20:31, 1981.

43. Reynolds GJ, Lewis-Jones DI, Isherwood DM et al: A simplified system of human milk banking, Early Hum Dev 7:281, 1982.

44. Schmidt E: Effects of varying degrees of heat treatment on milk protein and its nutritional consequences, Acta Paediatr Scand Suppl 296:41, 1982.

45. Silprasert A, Dejsarai W, Keawvichit R, and Amatayakol K: Effect of storage on the creamatocrit and total energy content of human milk, Hum Nutr Clin Nutr: 40C:31, 1986.

46. Smith L, Bickerton J, Pilcher G, and D'Souza SW: Creamatocrit, carbon content, and energy value of pooled banked human milk: implications for feeding preterm infants, Early Hum Dev 11:75, 1985.

47. Sosa R and Barness L: Bacterial growth in refrigerated human milk, Am J Dis Child 141:111, 1987.

48. Stagno S et al: Breast milk and the risk of cytomegalovirus infection, N Engl J Med 302:1073, 1980.

49. Stocks RJ et al: A simple method to improve the energy value of bank human milk, Early Hum Dev 8:175, 1983.

50. Sunshine P, Asquith MT, and Liebhaber M: The effects of collection and processing on various components of human milk. In Frier S and Eidelman AI, editors: Human milk: its biological and social value, Amsterdam, 1980, Excerpta Medica.

51. Thiry I, Sprecher-Goldberger S, Jonckheer T et al: Isolation of AIDS virus from cell-free breast milk of three healthy virus carriers, Lancet 2:891, 1985.

52. Tyson JE et al: Collection methods and contamination of bank milk, Arch Dis Child 57:396, 1982.

53. Van Zoeren-Grobben D, Schrijver J, Van Den Berg H et al: Human milk vitamin content after pasteurization, storage or tube feeding, Arch Dis Child 62:161, 1987.

54. Wardell JM, Hill CM, and D'Souza SW: Effect of pasteurization and of freezing and thawing human milk on its triglyceride content, Acta Paediatr Scand 70:467, 1981.

55. Welsh JK and May JT: Anti-infective properties of breast milk, J Pediatr 94:1, 1979.

56. Williamson S et al: Effect of heat treatment of human milk on absorption of nitrogen, fat, sodium, calcium, and phosphorus by protein infants, Arch Dis Child 53:555, 1978.

57. Williamson S et al: Organization of bank of raw and pasteurized human milk for neonatal intensive care, Br Med J 1:393, 1978.

58. Wills ME et al: Short-time low-temperature pasteurization of human milk, Early Hum Dev 7:71, 1980.

59. Ziegler JB, Johnson RO, Cooper DA et al: Postnatal transmission of AIDS-associated retrovirus from mother to infant, Lancet 1:896, 1985.

The role of mother support groups and community resources

20

$\mathbf{C}$ertain changes in cultural aspects of Western civilization have contributed to the wide-spread use of artificial feedings for human infants as well as to the changing structure of the family. Urbanization has been associated not only with industrialization but also with the separation of generations. This has produced the nuclear family. Nuclear families are smaller, mobile, isolated families often stranded in a large urban population. The young couple and their new infant are totally without personal human resources. That is, there is no one who cares enough to give individual support to the family. There is no one to turn to, share the experience with, and receive advice, encouragement, and support from.

Rites de passage were described by the French author Van Gennep[23] as the ceremonies and rituals that mark special changes in people's lives. The list includes marriage, motherhood, birth, death, circumcision, graduation, ordination, and retirement. In our present culture there is support for most of these events except birth and motherhood. The most critical *rite de passage* in a woman's life, Raphael[17] points out, is when she becomes a mother. Raphael further distinguishes this period of transition with the term *matrescence,* "to emphasize the mother and to focus on her new life-style." Traditional cultures herald a mother giving birth, whereas our culture announces the birth of an infant. The former highlights the mother, the latter the infant. Matrescence is a time of coddling. In preindustrial societies the mother is coddled for some time after birth, having only the responsibility of the infant's care while the mother's needs are met by doulas. Mothering the mother should be part of the postpartum support for a new mother.

A number of other forces added momentum to the bottle feeding trend that began in the 1920s when manufacturers finally were able to mass-produce an inexpensive container and rubber nipple with which to feed infants cheaply. Pediatrics was a new specialty to guard the health of children. The stress was on measuring and calculating. Physicians seemed more secure when they could prescribe nutrition. The rise in the female labor force has also been credited with having an impact on the method of feeding infants, who were no longer brought everywhere with the mother to be nursed but were instead left behind to be bottle fed. The technology of the infant food industry was a continuing influence on nutritional thinking of both medical and lay groups.

Breastfeeding was never totally abandoned. There was always a group of women who prepared themselves for childbirth and read and researched feeding and nutrition and chose to breastfeed.[15] In the middle 1940s Dr. Edith Jackson began the Rooming-In Project in New Haven. Families in New Haven who sought "childbirth without fear" and an opportunity to room-in with their infants usually wished to breastfeed. In the rooming-in unit, breastfeeding was often "contagious" because one mother successfully nursing would encourage others to try. Hospital stays averaged 5 to 7 days, during which time the mother-infant couple was cared for as a pair. About 70% of the patients left the hospital breast-feeding. Students and staff who were exposed to the philosophy of this unit went to many parts of the country, taking with them tremendous commitment to prepared childbirth and nurturing through breastfeeding. The classic article on the management of breastfeeding by Barnes et al.[3] was published as a result of counseling hundreds of nursing mothers. The students of Jackson inoculated many hundreds of hospitals and communities with a zeal for breastfeeding.

DEVELOPMENT OF MOTHER SUPPORT GROUPS

There still remained the need for nuclear families to have access to support and conversation about healthy infants, mothering, and breastfeeding.[5] The La Leche League was developed to meet these needs in Franklin Park, Illinois, in 1956. The original intent was to provide other nursing mothers with information, encouragement, and moral support. There are now thousands of local chapters and a network of state and regional coordinators who all synchronize their activities with the headquarters in Franklin Park. La Leche League's 4,000 groups are in 43 countries, in the United States, Canada, parts of Europe, New Zealand, and Africa, and other parts of the world.[9]

An excellent publication, *The Womanly Art of Breastfeeding*,[9] was prepared by the original group of mothers involved in the La Leche League. The publication was revised for the twenty-fifth anniversary of the organization in 1981 and again in its fifth edition in 1987. La Leche League continues to provide information and updated publications about common questions that arise during lactation. Local groups offer classes to prepare mothers to breastfeed. They help with suggestions about the nitty-gritty details of preparation, nutrition, clothing, and mothering in general. They also provide every mother with a telephone counselor. To be qualified to serve as a consultant to another mother, a member must demonstrate knowledge and expertise in breastfeeding as well as an understanding of how to counsel and render support. "Telephone mothers" do not give medical advice and are instructed to tell a troubled mother to call her own physician for such advice. Interested local physicians provide medical expertise for the group in situations in which a medical opinion is appropriate. The league provides support for mothers to reduce the time the physician needs to spend counseling on the nonmedical aspects of lactation. Most information needed by the new mother is not medical. In the decades that this support system has been in place, no good substitute for this mother-to-mother program has evolved, as a woman needs a true doula.

Similar programs have been developed in 15 other countries. A well-established and respected program in Norway is Ammehjelpen; in Australia, the Nursing Mothers' Association of Australia; and in the United Kingdom, The National Childbirth Trust.

The Breastfeeding Association of South Africa is a nongovernmental, nonprofit vol-untary organization founded in 1978 by South Africans for the express needs of South African women. Their special problems and solutions are well described by Bergh.[4] Support groups for all of life's events, especially those covering health, have become a common feature (there are over 150 parent support groups, for instance). In the field of perinatal care, there are groups for infertile couples, couples who are expecting, those who have experienced pregnancy loss, experienced loss of a premature, loss of a term baby, those who have had a cesarean birth, and so on. The physicians should be aware of the groups' functions in the community and the policies and philosophies they embrace.

The International Childbirth Education Association also provides resources for the new family in many countries. Its program makes preparation and training available for couples during pregnancy and afterward as parents. Its scope embraces the entire childbirth concept, of which breastfeeding is part.

Sociologist Alice Ladas[10] studied women who attended La Leche League preparation classes and compared them to a similar group who attempted to breastfeed but did not have this preparation. She was able to demonstrate clearly that the women who attended such programs had more confidence and seemed to profit by receiving accurate, up-to-date and relevant information as well as receiving individual and group support.[11]

Silverman and Murrow[20] studied league activities and concluded that group dynamics are important and feelings of normalcy are reinforced. The information and experience were shown to be important, but the support from the group had the greatest influence on success in breastfeeding.[22] Meara[14] reports similar observations on league activities in a nonsupportive culture.

A follow-up study of breastfeeding in Oxford was carried out by Sloper et al.[21] In this study it was observed that significantly more mothers went home breastfeeding, mothers nursed longer, and solid foods were started later when support was provided. The authors attribute this shift to the change in advice and support given in the hospital and at home visits.

There are also a few carefully researched and accurate videotapes on the subject of perinatal experiences including breastfeeding (e.g., VIDA's tape, entitled "Baby"). Some done by popular TV personalities reflect only an individual's experience.

COMMUNITY RESOURCES

Most hospitals provide training in preparation for childbirth. Part of the program is about the new infant and how to plan for his care. These programs often serve as the initial stimulus to consider breastfeeding.

Since hospitals have become competitive and are marketing their services, many are developing birthing centers and are trying to capture the attention of the childbearing public with special services. These services often include classes on child rearing, including breastfeeding. The physician would do well to investigate the programs and printed materials distributed by the hospitals where patients deliver. Many pediatricians are coping with the flood of patient information from conflicting sources by printing up an office manual (desk-top printers make this quite feasible). This is especially helpful if the patients are born at more than one hospital or there is more than one lay advocacy group active in the community. Common hospital procedures and policies can influence the success or failure of breastfeeding mothers.[19] (See Table 20-1.)

In a few short decades we have gone from a paucity of support groups and resource literature to an overwhelming flood. Health care books and childbearing and family-rearing advice books are cascading off the press, written by everyone from qualified experts to poorly informed freelance writers. Some are written by health care professionals who have

Table 20-1. Hospital practices that influence breastfeeding initiation

Strongly encouraging	Encouraging	Discouraging	Strongly discouraging
Physical contact:			
• Baby put to breast immediately in delivery room	• Staff sensitivity to cultural norms and expectations of woman	• Scheduled feedings regardless of mother's breastfeeding wishes	• Mother-infant separation at birth
• Baby not taken from mother after delivery			• Mother-infant housed on separate floors in postpartum period
• Woman helped by staff to suckle baby in recovery room			• Mother separated from baby due to bilirubin problem
• Rooming-in, staff help with baby care *in* room, not only in nursery			• No rooming-in policy
Verbal communication:			
• Staff initiates discussion re woman's intention to breastfeed pre- and intrapartum	• Appropriate language skills of staff, teaching how to handle breast engorgement and nipple problem	• Staff instructs woman "to get good night's rest and miss the feed"	• Woman told to "take it easy," "get your rest" . . . impression that breastfeeding is effortful/tiring
• Staff encourages and reinforces breastfeeding immediately on labor and delivery	• Staff's own skills and comfort re: art of breastfeeding and time to teach woman on one-to-one basis	• Strict times allotted for breastfeeding regardless of mother/baby's feeding "cycle"	• Woman told she doesn't "do it right," staff interrupts her efforts; corrects her re positions, etc.
• Staff discusses use of breast pump and realities of separation from baby re breastfeeding			

From Scrimshaw SMC: The cultural context of breastfeeding in the United States, report of the Surgeon General's workshop on breastfeeding and human lactation, 1984, DHHS pub no HRS-D-MC-84-2.
Continued.

Table 20-1. Hospital practices that influence breastfeeding initiation—cont'd

Strongly encouraging	Encouraging	Discouraging	Strongly discouraging
Nonverbal communication:			
• Pictures of woman breastfeeding		• Pictures of woman bottle feeding	• Woman given infant formula kit and infant food literature
	• Literature on breastfeeding in understandable terms		
• Staff (doctors as well as nurses) give reinforcement for breastfeeding (respect; smiles; affirmation)		• Staff interrupts her breastfeeding session for lab tests, etc.	
• Nurse (or any attendant) making mother comfortable and helping to arrange baby at breast for nursing			• Sees official-looking nurses authoritatively caring for babies by bottle feeding (leads to woman's insecurities re own capability of care)
• Woman sees others breastfeeding in hospital	• Closed circuit TV show in hospital on breastfeeding	• Woman doesn't see others breastfeeding	
Experiential:			
• If breastfeeding not *immediately* successful, staff continues to be supportive			
• Previous success with breastfeeding experience in hospital			• Previous failure with breastfeeding experience in hospital

a personal experience in childbearing and write about it. The pediatrician should be familiar with a few good references for parents and provide a list for patients.

The YWCA in most communities provides preparation for childbirth. Its classes usually provide programming that appeals to young and unwed women, a group in need of services rarely provided by other sources.

The Visiting Nurses Association and the public health nurses on the staff of the local county health department are special resources particularly skilled at counseling new mothers with their infants. They can provide valuable information to the physician who is working with an infant who fails to thrive at the breast by witnessing the breastfeeding scene at home.

Many other organizations, local and national in scope, have the perinatal period and the family as their focus. Many of these are also interested in promoting breastfeeding as part of their overall goals.

A model program in Rochester was developed as a cooperative effort among The Home Care Program of the Genesee Region, which was already serving the chronically ill and recently hospitalized population, and health-care providers.[1] The pediatricians, obstetricians, and medical society worked with the home care staff to devise a program of early discharge from the hospital of mothers and their newborns (less than 24 hours postpartum) followed by daily visits by a specially trained perinatal nurse. A homemaker was also provided to take care of the chores and other children. Laboratory services were provided at home. An important focus of the program has been counseling for successful breastfeeding. The regional Blue Cross pays for the service in its regular contract. The target population is the healthy family that wishes to "normalize" its birth experience.

The government has taken an active interest in the promotion of breastfeeding as well. In the goals for national health prepared by a multidisciplinary task force, it is stated that by 1990, 75% of infants leaving the hospital shall be breastfed and at 6 months of age at least 35% will still be breastfeeding.[16] The plan of action to reach these goals has included the development of a Healthy Mothers–Healthy Infants Program. There is also a national committee for the promotion of breastfeeding, which includes representation from major professional organizations of physicians, dietitians, social service workers, nurses, nurse-midwives, and hospital administrators. A major thrust of the national effort has been through the Women, Infants, and Children program (WIC), in which mothers are being encouraged to breastfeed and given nutritional and practical lactation management instruction and support. An instruction manual is available for WIC workers.[6] The Surgeon General conducted a national workshop on breastfeeding and human lactation in Rochester, New York, in June 1984 to develop recommendations for national policy. Publication from the workshop is available from the Government Printing Office in Washington, DC. A follow-up workshop was held in Washington, DC, in 1985 gathering the representatives of the major official national organizations for obstetrics and pediatrics, including the credential organizations for physicians, nurses, nurse-midwives, and dietitians. The organizations responded to a request to have each approve a model statement in support of breastfeeding. This was accomplished by January 1987. The organizations have also undertaken a review of curriculum within their discipline to assure adequate education, training, and accreditation regarding human lactation and breastfeeding for their members. There has been a significant increase in the number of highly skilled and specialized health care professionals available to support breastfeeding.

Issues of rural health have begun to include those surrounding birth and the infant's welfare. Programs are being developed to increase breastfeeding among rural people.

Although the incidence of breastfeeding has increased among well-educated self-motivated middle Americans, the number of impoverished, less well-educated women who breastfeed remains small. Progress is being made, community by community, by dedicated health-care workers, dietitians, and WIC staff. Health professionals often serve as a catalyst in developing such programs but should always be ready to serve as knowledgeable, supportive consultants to the effort of others.[7]

Grants and other incentives provided by public and private sources have enlarged the communications network in states where breastfeeding remains minimal. Groups such as the Healthy Mothers Healthy Babies Program maximize communications between resource programs and offer opportunities to share ideas, logos, publications, and strategies that work. Information about these resources is available from The Healthy Mothers Healthy Babies Coalition.

Lactation centers have been developed in health care facilities such as the program developed by Naylor in San Diego and by Neifert in Denver, Colorado. The purpose of these programs is to provide consultation services for mothers as well as education, training, and information for health-care workers. Efforts have been made to change hospital policy regarding breastfeeding to increase the success rate.[13] A very impressive program was initiated in the Philippines by Relucio-Clavano.[18] She has not only increased the incidence of breastfeeding but has also improved the morbidity from sepsis, diarrhea, and malnutrition.

Lactation consultants

For years, many medical and nursing professionals have served as lactation consultants ready to respond to any colleague's request for knowledge and expertise. With the great national movement to embrace breastfeeding, however, a new type of lactation consultant is evolving from the vast pool of women who have served in local mother-to-mother programs to help others breastfeed. While many of these consultants do have the educational credentials one expects from a consultant, many have no such credentials. The health-care professional needs to see that the lactation resources available in the community are truly of professional quality and background. Counseling is a special skill requiring more than personal experience with the situation.

The International Board of Lactation Consultant Examiners (IBLCE) was developed as a separate organization by the La Leche League International to credential women who wish to counsel about breastfeeding.[8] Those who successfully complete the IBLCE certification process are entitled to use the designation IBCLC (International Board Certified Lactation Consultant) after their names. The IBLCE has defined lactation consultants as "allied health care providers who possess the necessary skills, knowledge, and attitudes to facilitate breastfeeding." These lactation consultants perform as employees in some situations and as independent contractors in states where the medical practice act allows such activity. A lactation consultant should have professional liability insurance coverage.

Lactation counselor as a member of the health-care team

Modern medicine has developed a team approach to the management of many patient populations such as the elderly or the handicapped.* There is a team approach to the

---

*From Lawrence RA: Introduction. In Lauwers J and Woessner C, editors: *Counseling the nursing mother: a reference handbook for health care providers and lay counselors,* Wayne NJ, 1983, Avery Publishing Group, Inc.

management of many categories of diseases such as cancer and diabetes. There is also a health-care team that provides medical service for the family during the perinatal period. This team includes an obstetrician and a pediatrician or a family physician; nurse midwives; nurses working in prenatal care, obstetrics, newborn, and public health; social workers; dietitians; and, when a problem develops, perinatologists, neonatologists, and the skilled team from the perinatal center. These team members are well-educated and extensively trained professionals. Together they have improved the morbidity and mortality rates of childbirth. The long-range prognosis for the intact survival of infants has been significantly improved. Thus medical progress has occurred concomitantly with the isolation of the nuclear family. The result is a medically successful birth to a family emotionally and socially ill prepared to cope. The family is ill prepared to take over when the mother and baby are discharged from the hospital and instantly placed on their own without a transitional period of adjustment with close support and supervision.

The counselor becomes a very important addition to the health-care team, replacing the traditional family support system. The counselor not only needs to know the role as counselor interacting with the family but also must understand how she interfaces with other members of the health-care team. The professional team members are beginning to understand the importance of the counselor and how to work most effectively with her. Some practitioners provide a nurse practitioner whose role is to fill that gap between medical care and family support. The counselor will quickly earn the respect of the health-care team if she communicates openly with them, supports the mother in a positive manner, and encourages a relationship of mutual trust and respect between mother and the team.

The peer counselor will complement the work of the health professionals but should never replace the role of the health-care provider.

Who shall counsel

When one is working closely with people in critical life situations, there are people who make good counselors and there are equally good people who are not appropriate as counselors and should have other jobs in the organization.

Counseling is a profession, and professional counselors are carefully screened, educated, and trained. Therefore, individuals who help mothers breastfeed should be screened, educated, and trained also. They should have some special abilities:

To truly listen
To avoid judgment
To understand other life-styles
To admit it when they do not know
To seek appropriate help from professionals
To recognize incompatibility in a given relationship

In the past few decades, peer counseling has become widespread and has been successful, not only with breastfeeding and childbirth but also with chronic disease such as cystic fibrosis and with devastating illnesses such as cancer. The first thing all these groups have had to acknowledge is that just because one has experienced a life event one is not automatically qualified to counsel others experiencing similar situations.

The candidate must first put one's own experiences into perspective and understand what has motivated one to seek this counseling role. Counseling is an opportunity to help by listening, and being a sympathetic listener is the most important quality. This is not a time to talk about the counselor's pregnancies. The counselor cannot have a personal agenda and press personal views or life-style on the mother being counseled, nor should it be used as a personal platform to promote organizational biases.

The counselor must understand that assuming a place on the health-care team demands time and effort. One must be available at the convenience and need of the client, even when this is inconvenient to the counselor.

The most difficult time for any counselor is when she must recognize that the problem is beyond her expertise. This takes sufficient knowledge of the subject matter to recognize the danger signs of a problem that requires other intervention. More difficult is that it takes the inner strength and courage to admit that one is indeed beyond one's own resources and skills before a little problem becomes a serious medical or psychologic crisis. A timeworn adage of the health-care professional is *First, do no harm.*

Learning to help mothers

The suggestions put forth to guide a counselor in training must be general overall guidelines about attitude and posture. The emphasis is on listening, encouraging a mother to talk, and ultimately helping her to solve her own problem by understanding it. Professional counselors are trained using didactic sessions, role play, and supervisory sessions until skills are developed. Continued reinforcement of philosophy and techniques forms the basis of growth and improvement. The lay counselor should attend counselor training sessions provided by her parent organization and work closely with her supervisor. Sharing counseling situations with others with more experience will give further insight. Returning to the reference materials again and again will bring to light new thoughts that have been read before but not truly assimilated initially because of lack of experience.

Just as there is no substitute for good training, there is no substitute for correct information. Much research is under way in this country and worldwide in the field of human lactation. Working in the arena of breastfeeding counseling mandates continual updating of information. For the past decades this country has experienced a renaissance in the art of breastfeeding. It is only recently that there has been a renaissance in the science of human lactation. The basic reference information about human lactation is available in resource texts. Readers should seek out the original references for a fuller understanding. It is often difficult to sort out the old wives' tales from scientific fact in some of the myriad of lay publications available, so reference material should be selected cautiously. When there is a question of management that requires additional resource material, it is probably a question that should be referred to the mother's physician.

The counselor does not provide medical advice. The counselor can encourage the mother to contact her doctor. When the infant is doing poorly or is sick, the pediatrician should be consulted promptly. The rare condition of failure to thrive while breastfeeding is increasing in frequency, paralleling the increased incidence of breastfeeding. It has serious implications for the infant and for the continuation of breastfeeding unless treatment is initiated promptly by the physician. The physician is powerless to help if not consulted. When the infant's problem is identified and it is prudent to continue breastfeeding, the counselor can be an invaluable asset in supporting and reassuring the mother.

Maternal problems such as mastitis should respond well if treated early, but recurrent mastitis may develop when home remedies are substituted for proper treatment. The role of the counselor in such situations is significant. Encouraging the mother to seek medical care promptly is most important. Reinforcing medical advice will further enhance its effectiveness. For example, if rest is prescribed, the counselor can help the mother to understand how critical rest is to recovery and then help her figure out how she is going to cope at home with family responsibilities and a newborn and still rest.

The question of maternal drugs during lactation is a complex issue that cannot be resolved without a knowledge of pharmacology, maternal and infant metabolism, and the influences of dose, time, age of infant, and pharmacokinetics. Checking a list of drugs that appear in milk is not sufficient. The physician should be consulted. If more data are needed, the regional Poison Control Center can be consulted by the physician. No counselor should assume this responsibility. On the other hand, when a decision has been reached by the physician on the safety of the use of the medication, the counselor can help the mother work through the issues related to her breastfeeding. Perhaps adjustment in dosing and feeding schedule is necessary, and perhaps pumping and discarding the milk is necessary for 24 hours; in any case, managing these lactation modifications can be facilitated by supportive counseling under the direction of the physician.

The role of the counselor is support of the mother. The counselor should work in concert with the medical health-care team, as a team player, not as a competitor or as an adversary, but as a facilitator. The mission of the team is successful lactation, a satisfying mothering experience, and healthy infant. The health-care team will continue to be responsible for the family long after lactation has been discontinued. The confidence and trust developed between the health team and family will be critical to lasting success. The counselor should be remembered as a gentle facilitator and a caring support person who was there through the *rite de passage* of matrescence.

Recommendations of the Academy of Pediatrics

The Academy of Pediatrics[2] has made a statement in support of human milk in 1978.* They have summarized a lengthy presentation with the following:

1. Full-term newborn infants should be breastfed, except if there are specific contraindications or when breastfeeding is unsuccessful.
2. Education about breastfeeding should be provided in schools for all children, and better education about breastfeeding and infant nutrition should be provided in the curriculum of physicians and nurses. Information about breastfeeding should also be presented in public communications media.
3. Prenatal instruction should include both theoretical and practical information about breastfeeding.
4. Attitudes and practices in prenatal clinics and in maternity wards should encourage a climate that favors breastfeeding. The staff should include nurses and other personnel who are not only favorably disposed toward breastfeeding but also knowledgeable and skilled in the art.
5. Consultation between maternity services and agencies committed to breastfeeding should be strengthened.
6. Studies should be conducted on the feasibility of breastfeeding infants at day nurseries adjacent to places of work subsequent to an appropriate leave of absence following the birth of an infant.

---

*Initiated by the Nutrition Committee of the Canadian Paediatric Society, this statement was prepared by both the Committee on Nutrition of the American Academy of Pediatrics and the Nutrition Committee of the Canadian Paediatric Society. Copyright American Academy of Pediatrics, 1978.

REFERENCES

1. Amado A, Lawrence RA, and Roghman K: Perinatal home care: report on a Blue Cross and home care effort, Caring 2:27, 1983.
2. American Academy of Pediatrics, Committee on Nutrition: Stand on breast milk, Pediatrics 62:591, 1978.
3. Barnes GB et al: Management of breast feeding, JAMA 151:192, 1953.
4. Bergh A-M: The role of a nongovernmental organization in breast feeding education, J Nutr Educ 19:117, 1987.
5. Ciba Foundation Symposium no 45, Breast feeding and the mother, Amsterdam, 1976, Elsevier Scientific Publ Co.
6. Food and Nutrition Service, US Dept of Agriculture: Promoting breastfeeding: a guide for health professionals working in the WIC and CSF programs, Washington DC, 1983, US Dept of Agriculture.
7. Gussler J and Bryant C: Helping mothers breastfeed: program strategies for minority communities. Health Action Papers, vol I, Lexington Ky, 1984, Lexington Fayette County Health Department, University of Kentucky Medical Behavioral Sciences Department.
8. International Board of Lactation Consultant Examiners: 2315 Wickersham Cove, Germantown, TN 38138.
9. La Leche League: The womanly art of breastfeeding, ed 5, Franklin Park Ill, 1987, La Leche League International.
10. Ladas AK: How to help mothers breast feed, Clin Pediatr 9:702, 1970.
11. Ladas AK: The less viable option: breast feeding, J Trop Pediatr 18:318, 1972.
12. Lawrence RA: Introduction. In Lauwers J and Woessner C, editors: Counseling the nursing mother: a reference handbook for health care providers and lay counselors, Wayne NJ, 1983, Avery Publishing Group, Inc.
13. Lewis L: Successful breastfeeding programs for low-income, minority mothers, Pub Health Currents 22(1):1, 1982.
14. Meara H: A key to successful breast feeding in a nonsupportive culture, J Nurse Midwife 21:20, 1976.
15. Pryor K: Nursing your baby, New York, 1973, Harper & Row.
16. Public Health Service: Implementation plans for attaining the objectives for the nation, Pub Health Rep 98(suppl): 145, 1983.
17. Raphael D: The tender gift: breast feeding, New York, 1976, Schocken Books.
18. Relucio-Clavano N: The results of a change in hospital practices, Assignment Child 55/56:139, 1981.
19. Scrimshaw SCM: The cultural context of breastfeeding in the United States, Report of the Surgeon General's Workshop on Breastfeeding and Human Lactation, DHHS no HRS-D-MC 84-2, 1984.
20. Silverman PR and Murrow HG: Caregiver during critical role in the normal life cycle, unpublished report, Harvard Medical School.
21. Sloper KS, Elsden E, and Baum JD: Increasing breast feeding in a community, Arch Dis Child 52:700, 1977.
22. Thompson M: The effectiveness of mother to mother help, research on the La Leche League International program, Birth Fam J 3:1, Winter 1976-1977.
23. Van Gennep A: Rites of passage. In Vizedom MB and Caffee GL, translators, London, 1960, Rutledge & Kegan Paul, Publishers.

Composition of human milk

Table A-1. Composition of human colostrum and mature breast milk

Constituent (per 100 ml)		Colostrum 1-5 days	Mature milk >30 days
Energy	kcal	58	70
Total solids	g	12.8	12.0
Lactose	g	5.3	7.3
Total nitrogen	mg	360	171
Protein nitrogen	mg	313	129
NPN	mg	47	42
Total protein	g	2.3	0.9
Casein	mg	140	187
α-Lactalbumin	mg	218	161
Lactoferrin	mg	330	167
IgA	mg	364	142
Amino acids (total)			
Alanine	mg	—	52
Arginine	mg	126	49
Aspartate	mg	—	110
Cystine	mg	—	25
Glutamate	mg	—	196
Glycine	mg	—	27
Histidine	mg	57	31
Isoleucine	mg	121	67
Leucine	mg	221	110
Lysine	mg	163	79
Methionine	mg	33	19
Phenylalanine	mg	105	44
Proline	mg	—	89
Serine	mg	—	54
Threonine	mg	148	58
Tryptophan	mg	52	25
Tyrosine	mg	—	38

Data from multiple references (see Chapter 4).   *Continued.*

Table A-1. Composition of human colostrum and mature breast milk—cont'd

Constituent (per 100 ml)		Colostrum 1-5 days	Mature milk >30 days
Valine	mg	169	90
Taurine (free)	mg	—	8
Urea	mg	10	30
Creatine	mg	—	3.3
Total fat	g	2.9	4.2
Fatty acids (% total fat)			
12:0 tauric		1.8	5.8
14:0 myristic		3.8	8.6
16:0 palmitic		26.2	21.0
18:0 stearic		8.8	8.0
18:1 oleic		36.6	35.5
18:2, n-6 linoleic		6.8	7.2
18:3, n-3 linolenic		—	1.0
C_{20} and C_{22} polyunsaturated		10.2	2.9
Cholesterol	mg	27	16
Vitamins			
Fat soluble			
Vitamin A (retinol equivalents)	μg	89	47
β-Carotene	μg	112	23
Vitamin D	μg	—	0.04
Vitamin E (total tocopherols)	μg	1280	315
Vitamin K	μg	0.23	0.21
Water soluble			
Thiamin	μg	15	16
Riboflavin	μg	25	35
Niacin	μg	75	200
Folic acid	μg	—	5.2
Vitamin B_6	μg	12	28
Biotin	μg	0.1	0.6
Pantothenic acid	μg	183	225
Vitamin B_{12}	ng	200	26
Ascorbic acid	mg	4.4	4.0
Minerals			
Calcium	mg	23	28
Magnesium	mg	3.4	3.0
Sodium	mg	48	15
Potassium	mg	74	58
Chlorine	mg	91	40
Phosphorus	mg	14	15
Sulphur	mg	22	14
Trace elements			
Chromium	ng	—	39
Cobalt	μg	—	1
Copper	μg	46	35
Fluorine	μg	—	7
Iodine	μg	12	7
Iron	μg	45	40
Manganese	μg	—	0.4,1.5
Nickel	μg	—	2
Selenium	μg	—	2.0
Zinc	μg	540	166

Dietary guidance during lactation

General guidelines

1. Follow nutrition guide for regular food plan during pregnancy.
2. Eat a wide variety of foods, including milk and milk products and eggs.
3. If no milk is allowed, use a supplement of 4 μg of vitamin B_{12} daily. If goat and soy milk are used, partial supplementation may be needed.
4. If no milk is taken, also use supplements of 12 mg of calcium and 400 IU of vitamin D daily. Partial supplementation will be necessary if less than four servings of milk and milk products are consumed.
5. Select a variety of plant foods (especially grains, legumes, nuts, and seeds) to obtain "complete" proteins by complementary combinations, as indicated in Table B-1 on p. 508.
6. Use iodized salt.

Table B-1. Vegetarian food guide

	Complementary plant protein combinations	
Food	**Amino acids deficient**	**Complementary protein food combinations**
Grains	Isoleucine Lysine	Rice + legumes Corn + legumes Wheat + legumes Wheat + peanuts + milk Wheat + sesame + soybeans Rice + brewer's yeast
Legumes	Tryptophan Methionine	Legumes + rice Beans + wheat Beans + corn Soybeans + rice + wheat Soybeans + corn + milk Soybeans + wheat + sesame Soybeans + peanuts + sesame Soybeans + peanuts + wheat + rice Soybeans + sesame + wheat
Nuts and seeds	Isoleucine Lysine	Peanuts + sesame + soybeans Sesame + beans Sesame + soybeans + wheat Peanuts + sunflower seeds
Vegetables	Isoleucine Methionine	Lima beans Green beans Brussels sprouts } + Sesame seeds or Cauliflower Brazil nuts or Broccoli mushrooms Greens = millet or rice

Modified from Lappé FM: Diet for a small planet, New York, 1971, Friends of the Earth/Ballantine; from Worthington-Roberts BS and Williams SR: Nutrition in pregnancy and lactation, ed 4, St Louis, 1989, The CV Mosby Co.

Table B-2. Characteristic food choices of ethnic groups

Black	Mexican-American	Japanese	Chinese	Filipino
Protein foods				
Meat	Meat	Meat	Meat	Meat
Beef	Beef	Beef	Pork	Pork
Pork, ham	Pork	Pork	Beef	Beef
Sausage	Lamb	Poultry	Organ meats	Goat
Pig's feet,	Tripe	Chicken	Poultry	Deer
ears, etc.	Sausage	Turkey	Chicken	Rabbit
Bacon	(chorizo)	Fish	Duck	Variety meats
Luncheon	Bologna	Tuna	Fish	Poultry
meats	Bacon	Mackerel	White fish	Chicken
Organ meats	Poultry	Sardines	Shrimp	Fish
Poultry	Chicken	(dried form:	Lobster	Sole
Chicken	Eggs	mezashi)	Oyster	Bonito
Turkey	Legumes	Sea bass	Sardines	Herring
Fish	Pinto beans	Shrimp	Eggs	Tuna
Catfish	Pink beans	Abalone	Legumes	Mackerel
Perch	Garbanzo	Squid	Soybeans	Crab
Red snapper	beans	Octopus	Soybean	Mussels
Tuna	Lentils	Eggs	curd (tofu)	Shrimp
Salmon	Nuts	Legumes	Black beans	Squid
Sardines	Peanuts	Soybean curd	Nuts	Eggs
Shrimp	Peanut butter	(tofu)	Peanuts	Legumes
Eggs		Soybean paste	Almonds	Black beans
Legumes		(miso)	Cashews	Chick peas
Kidney beans		Soybeans		Black-eyed peas
Red beans		Red beans		Lentils
Pinto beans		(azuki)		Mung beans
Black-eyed		Lima beans		Lima beans
peas		Nuts		White kidney
Nuts		Chestnuts		beans
Peanuts		(kuri)		Nuts
Peanut butter				Cashews
				Peanuts
				Pili nuts
Milk and milk products				
Milk	Milk	Milk	Milk	Milk
Fluid	Cheese	Fluid	Flavored	Flavored
Evaporated	Ice cream	Flavored	Whole milk	Evaporated
in coffee		Evaporated	(used in	Cheese
Buttermilk		Condensed	cooking)	Gouda

Modified from Nutrition during pregnancy and lactation, Sacramento Calif., 1975, California Department of Health; from Worthington-Roberts BS and Williams SR: Nutrition in pregnancy and lactation, ed 4, St Louis, 1989, The CV Mosby Co.

Continued.

Table B-2.   Characteristic food choices of ethnic groups—cont'd

Black	Mexican-American	Japanese	Chinese	Filipino
Milk and milk products—cont'd				
Cheese		Cheese	Ice cream	Cheddar
Cheddar		American		
Cottage		Monterey Jack		
Ice cream		Hoop		
		Ice cream		
Grain products				
Rice	Rice	Rice	Rice	Rice
Cornbread	Tortillas	Rice crackers	Noodles	Cooked cereals
Hominy grits	Corn	Noodles	White bread	Farina
Biscuits	Flour	(whole wheat:	Millet	Oatmeal
Muffins	Oatmeal	soba)		Dry cereals
White bread	Dry cereals	Spaghetti		Pastas
Dry cereal	Cornflakes	White bread		Rice noodles
Cooked cereal	Sugared	Oatmeal		Wheat noodles
Macaroni	Noodles	Dry cereal		Macaroni
Spaghetti	Spaghetti			Spaghetti
Crackers	White bread			
	Sweet bread			
	(pan dulce)			
Vegetables				
Broccoli	Avocado	Bamboo shoots	Bamboo shoots	Bamboo shoots
Cabbage	Cabbage	Bok choy	Beans	Beets
Carrots	Carrots	Broccoli	Green	Cabbage
Corn	Chilies	Burdock root	Yellow	Carrots
Green beans	Corn	Cabbage	Bean sprouts	Cauliflower
Greens	Green beans	Carrots	Bok choy	Celery
Mustard	Lettuce	Cauliflower	Broccoli	Chinese celery
Collard	Onion	Celery	Cabbage	Eggplant
Kale	Peas	Cucumbers	Carrots	Endive
Spinach	Potato	Eggplant	Celery	Green beans
Turnip	Prickly pear	Green beans	Chinese cab-	Leeks
Lima beans	cactus leaf	Gourd (kampyo)	bage	Lettuce
Okra	(nopales)	Mushrooms	Corn	Mushrooms
Peas	Spinach	Mustard greens	Cucumbers	Okra
Potato	Sweet potato	Napa cabbage	Eggplant	Onion
Pumpkin	Tomato	Peas	Greens	Peppers
Sweet potato	Zucchini	Peppers	Collard	Potato
Tomato		Radishes (white	Chinese	Pumpkin
Yam		radish: dai-	broccoli	Radishes
		kon; pickled	Mustard	Snow peas
		white: taka-	Kale	Spinach
		wan)	Spinach	Squash
		Snow peas	Leeks	Sweet potato
		Spinach	Lettuce	Tomato
		Squash	Mushrooms	Water chestnuts

Table B-2. Characteristic food choices of ethnic groups—cont'd

Black	Mexican-American	Japanese	Chinese	Filipino
Vegetables—cont'd				
		Sweet potato	Peppers	Watercress
		Taro (Japanese sweet potato)	Potato	Yam
			Scallions	
		Tomato	Snow peas	
		Turnips	Sweet potato	
		Water chestnuts	Taro	
		Yam	Tomato	
			Water chestnuts	
			White radish	
			White turnip	
			Winter melon	
Fruits				
Apple	Apple	Apple	Apple	Apple
Banana	Apricots	Apricots	Banana	Banana
Grapefruit	Banana	Banana	Figs	Grapes
Grapes	Guava	Cherries	Grapes	Guava
Nectarine	Lemon	Grapefruit	Kumquats	Lemon
Orange	Mango	Grapes	Loquats	Lime
Plums	Melons	Lemon	Mango	Mango
Tangerine	Orange	Lime	Melons	Melons
Watermelon	Peach	Melons	Orange	Orange
	Pear	Orange	Peach	Papaya
	Prickly pear	Peach	Pear	Pear
	cactus fruit	Pear	Persimmon	Pineapple
	(tuna)	Persimmon	Pineapple	Plums
	Zapote (sapote)	Pineapple	Plums	Pomegranate
		Pomegranate	Tangerine	Rhubarb
		Plums (dried,		Strawberries
		pickled plums		Tangerine
		called ume-		
		boshi)		
		Strawberries		
		Tangerine		
Other				
Salt pork (fat back)	Salsa (tomato-pepper-onion relish)	Soy sauce	Soy sauce	Soy sauce
		Nori paste (sea-soned rice)	Sweet and sour sauce	Coffee
Carbonated	Chili sauce	Bean thread	Mustard sauce	Tea
beverages	Guacamole	(konyaku)	Ginger	
Fruit drinks	Lard (manteca)	Ginger (shoga;	Plum sauce	
Gravies	Pork cracklings	dried form	Red bean paste	
Coffee	Fruit drinks	called denish-	Black bean	
Iced tea	Kool-aid	oga)	sauce	
	Carbonated	Tea	Oyster sauce	
	beverages	Coffee	Tea	
	Beer		Coffee	
	Coffee			

Continued.

History form for evaluation of infant with failure to thrive

No. _____

Date _____

Slow gaining special history

Mother

Name _____

A. Diet
   1. Do you eat regular meals? _____ How do you rate the kind of food you eat?
      excellent ☐ good ☐ poor ☐
   2. Do you take vitamins? _____ If so, what? _____
      _____
   3. Do you take brewer's yeast? _____
   4. Are you worried about your weight? _____

B. Health
   1. Are you in good health? _____ If not, describe problems _____
      _____
   2. Are you taking any medications? _____ Birth control pills? _____
      Prescriptions? _____ Nonprescription medicines? _____
   3. Have you had any thyroid problems at any time in your life? _____ Are
      thyroid medications being taken now? _____ What kind? _____
      _____
      Dosage _____ Last time you had your blood tested for thy-
      roid _____
   4. Do you have any blood pressure problems? _____

C. Habits
   1. Do you smoke? _____ Which brand? _____
      How many per day? _____
   2. Do you drink coffee? _____ How many cups per day? _____
      Do you drink caffeinated sodas? _____ How many caffeinated sodas per
      day? _____
   3. Do you drink alcohol? _____How much per day? _____
      week? _____ month? _____

D. Nursing
   1. When the infant nurses, do you feel tingling ☐ burning ☐ filling feeling ☐
      leaking on other side ☐ nothing ☐
      other _____
   2. Do you have a quiet environment for nursing? _____ If not, why (describe)?
      (Example, loud music, freeway noise, dogs barking) _____
      _____
   3. Do you own a rocking chair? _____

E. Social environment
   1. Do you have a busy life-style? _____If so, why (name activities)? _____
      _____
      _____
   2. Marriage relationship is good ☐ average ☐ poor ☐
   3. Do you have other children? _____ Ages _____ Breastfed?
      _____ How long? _____
   4. Do you have any source of anxiety or tension? _____ If so, describe _____
      _____

Modified from form developed by Fleiss PM and Frantz KB.   *Continued.*

Slow gaining special history—cont'd

Infant

Name _____ Date of birth _____

1. How often is infant fed? _____
2. Breast milk only? _____ Other? _____
   Does he feed at each breast at each feeding? _____ How long on each breast? _____
3. How long does infant take to finish a feeding? _____ Does infant pause often during feeding? _____
4. Who initiates end of feeding? you ☐ infant ☐
5. How do you rate his sucking? poor ☐ weak ☐ average ☐ strong ☐
6. Is he burping easily? _____ What technique is used? _____
   When is he burped? _____
7. Is a pacifier used? _____ What kind? _____How much usage? _____
8. Number of wet diapers per day _____ Are ultra-absorbent diapers used? _____
9. Number of stools per day _____ consistency _____ color _____
10. Infant is active ☐ average ☐ placid ☐
11. Night sleep pattern: time put to bed _____ Is this on a regular basis? _____
    List awake times _____
12. Is infant healthy? _____ Any problems since birth? _____ If so, what?
    _____
    _____
    Jaundice? _____ How high was the bilirubin level? _____
    Had any medications? _____ If so, what? _____
13. Ever had a urinalysis? _____ When? _____
    Any other test (especially those for slow weight gain)? _____
    If so, what? _____
    Where? _____

Birth history

1. Type of delivery: vaginal ☐ CS ☐ If CS, scheduled ☐ or emergency ☐?
2. Labor: yes ☐ no ☐ Length of time _____
3. Were medications given during labor or delivery? _____ If so, what? _____
   _____
4. Was it a difficult birth? _____ If so, describe problem _____
   _____
5. First time infant put to breast was _____ hr after birth. Did infant take to it easily? _____
6. Where was the birth? Home birth ☐ Hospital with rooming-in ☐ Hospital with infant only in the nursery ☐ Were you separated from infant for any length of time? _____ If so, why? _____
   _____
7. Any medications taken during pregnancy? _____ If so, what? _____
   _____
8. Any medications taken after birth? _____ If so, what? _____
   _____

Family history

1. Have previous infants or relatives with failure to thrive? yes ☐ no ☐
2. Have history of metabolic or malabsorption disease? yes ☐ no ☐
3. Infant has cystic fibrosis? yes ☐ no ☐
4. Infant has milk allergy? yes ☐ no ☐
5. Other _____

Normal serum values for breastfed infants

Table D-1. Serum chemical values of normal breastfed infants*

Concentration/100 ml of serum	Age 28 days			Age 56 days			Age 84 days			Age 112 days		
	N	Mean	SD	N	Mean	SD	N	Mean	SD	N	Mean	SD
Males												
Total protein (g)	22	5.87	0.50	36	5.96	0.42	29	6.16	0.57	51	6.29	0.51
Albumin (g)	22	4.02	0.35	36	4.14	0.34	29	4.27	0.39	51	4.38	0.40
Globulins (g)												
alpha$_1$	22	0.14	0.03	36	0.17	0.03	29	0.18	0.03	51	0.17	0.04
alpha$_2$	22	0.53	0.10	36	0.60	0.11	29	0.74	0.14	51	0.81	0.19
beta	22	0.61	0.11	36	0.67	0.13	29	0.69	0.20	51	0.67	0.11
gamma	22	0.57	0.14	36	0.38	0.09	29	0.28	0.08	51	0.26	0.10
Cholesterol (mg)	21	139	31	32	153	34	25	133	32	47	145	26
Triglycerides (mg)	18	122	36	32	106	57	25	170	76	46	148	57
Urea nitrogen (mg)	43	8.5	3.2	49	6.6	2.1	47	7.0	2.7	51	7.3	4.2
Calcium (mg)	41	10.2	0.8	47	10.3	1.0	42	10.4	0.8	48	10.3	0.8
Phosphorus (mg)	43	6.6	0.7	49	6.4	0.7	47	6.2	0.5	49	6.2	0.7
Alkaline phosphatase†	31	22	6	40	21	8	35	21	8	44	18	7
Magnesium (mg)	40	2.0	0.2	47	2.1	0.2	45		0.2	50	2.2	0.2

Females

Total protein (g)	18	6.04	0.40	27	5.86	0.44	21	6.21	0.57	42	6.31	0.62
Albumin (g)	18	4.07	0.27	27	4.03	0.35	21	4.29	0.37	42	4.36	0.42
Globulins (g)												
alpha₁	18	0.15	0.02	27	0.17	0.04	21	0.17	0.03	42	**0.19**	0.04
alpha₂	18	0.55	0.07	27	0.65	0.12	21	0.74	0.18	42	0.78	0.17
beta	18	0.70	0.18	27	0.63	0.11	21	0.71	0.13	42	0.67	0.16
gamma	18	0.57	0.10	27	0.38	0.10	21	0.30	0.06	42	**0.31**	0.10
Cholesterol (mg)	13	**180**	35	25	157	37	20	**155**	29	40	**165**	36
Triglycerides (mg)	9	**157**	43	24	112	53	18	195	56	38	**170**	52
Urea nitrogen (mg)	37	8.3	2.3	33	6.4	2.2	40	6.4	2.2	42	6.6	3.5
Calcium (mg)	37	10.3	0.8	33	10.3	0.8	40	10.3	0.8	42	10.7	0.7
Phosphorus (mg)	39	6.9	0.8	33	6.4	0.8	40	6.1	0.7	42	6.1	0.7
Alkaline phosphatase	31	19	5	28	17	5	32	17	5	36	17	5
Magnesium (mg)	39	2.0	0.4	32	2.0	0.2	40	2.1	0.2	41	2.1	0.3

From Fomon SJ et al: Acta Paediatr Scand suppl 202:1, 1970.

*Bold figures indicate that value is greater than the corresponding value for infants of the opposite sex and that the difference is statistically significant at the 95% level of confidence.

†King-Armstrong units.

Drugs in breast milk and the effect on the infant

The following list of drugs in Table E-1 is provided to assist the clinician in making judgments about management for specific drugs in an individual mother and her infant. The clinician is referred to Chapter 11 for the discussion of interpretation of risks and benefits. It is also important to point out that the significance of a given blood level would vary with the pH and the binding capacity of the maternal plasma protein, which may differ for various ethnic and racial groups. Furthermore, it is not merely a matter of understanding the pharmacokinetics of a specific drug, but also of understanding the physiology of milk production and finally, most critically, understanding the absorption and excretion of the drug by the newborn, which changes with conceptual and chronologic age.

The drugs have been grouped by their major use to provide an opportunity to compare therapeutic choices and select the medication that is best for both mother and infant. The drugs have also been labeled 1, 2, 3, 4 if they were rated by the Committee on Drugs of the Academy of Pediatrics who has published a list of drugs that transfer into human milk.* When there is no Arabic number, the compound is not included in that list. The committee labeling indicates:

1. Drugs that are contraindicated during breastfeeding
2. Drugs that require temporary cessation of breastfeeding
3. Maternal medication usually compatible with breastfeeding
4. Food and environmental agents: effect on breastfeeding

A classification system for drug information regarding use during pregnancy and breastfeeding has been published by the Swedish catalog of registered specialties (FASS)† to aid in prescribing drugs to women during pregnancy and lactation.‡ The breastfeeding groups are defined as follows:

Group I   Does not enter breast milk

---

*The Committee on Drugs, American Academy of Pediatrics: The transfer of drugs and other chemicals into human breast milk, Pediatrics 72:375, 1983.

†FASS is the abbreviation for "Farmacevtiska Specialiteter i Sverige (Pharmaceutical Specialties of Sweden).

‡Berglund F, Flodh H, Lundsborg P et al: Drug use during pregnancy and breastfeeding, ACTA Obstet Gynecol Scand Suppl 126:1984.

Group II Enters breast milk but is not likely to affect the infant when therapeutic doses are used

Group III Enters breast milk in such quantities that there is a risk of affecting the infant when therapeutic doses are used

Group IV Not known whether it enters breast milk or not

When no Roman numeral appears, FASS did not report the drug.

The classification of the drugs listed are as follows:

The expansion of the drug information resource has been facilitated by the research of Linda R. Friedman, Ph.D.

Table E-1. Relationship of drugs to breast milk and effect on infant

Drug	Ratings		Oral Bioavail. (%)	Peak serum time (hours)	Half-life (hours)	Amount in milk after therapeutic dose	Comments	References
	AAPed.	Scand.						
Analgesics and anti-inflammatory (nonnarcotic)								
Acetaminophen (Datril, Tylenol, Paracetamol)	3	II	88 ± 15		2.0 ± 0.4; increased in neonates	M/P 0.2–1.9; peak milk time 2 h; half-life in milk 2.6 h; 1.85% of maternal oral dose of 1 g; vol. of distrib. 1.0 L/kg	Detoxified in liver; drug and metabolites found in infant's urine; infants handle drug well (see Chapter 11)	7, 31, 49, 109, 251
Antipyrine			Ear drops	0.17	14 ± 8	M/P 1.0, half-life in milk 11.6 ± 5.4 hours; 0.5%–2.4% of maternal dose		32
Aspirin	3	II	68 ± 3	2.25	0.25 ± 0.03	Converted to salicylic acid, which is readily distributed in milk; peak milk time 3 h; M/P 0.03–0.08; infant receives up to 21% of maternal dose; vol. of distrib. 0.15 L/kg	Metabolic acidosis in 16-day-old infant when mother took 650 mg for arthritis every 4 h; caution in early infancy; long history of experience shows complications rare; when mother requires high, continuing level of medication for arthritis, aspirin is drug of choice; mother should increase vitamin C intake, and levels in infant should be monitored as one premature	7, 14, 24, 31, 40, 49, 66, 109, 218, 304

Drug	No.	Category	t½	Time to peak in milk	M/P ratio / milk levels	Comments	References
(continued from previous drug)						infant reported to have 0.085 mg/L in serum when mother took 2.4 g/day (see Chapter 11)	
Aurothioglucose (Solganel)	1		5 ± 1	15 ± 12 days after 1st dose; 27 ± 13 days after 3rd weekly dose; up to 168 days after 11th weekly dose		Gold is excreted into milk, and trace amounts can be recovered in the infant's urine; it is incompatible with nursing.	7, 239, 251
Aurothiomalate (Myochrysine)	1	III	25 ± 5 days		M/P 0.1–0.2; 20% of maternal dose absorbed by infant	Incompatible with nursing	7, 31, 109, 231
Butorphanol (Stadol)	3		2.5 ± 0.5		After oral dose M/P 1.9; after IM M/P 0.7	In 1000 ml of milk, infant gets 4 µg	7, 49, 239, 242
Diclofenac			2		Less than 10 ng/ml	Has 4 active metabolites; their presence in milk is unknown	217, 231
Diflunisal (Dolobid)	100	II	10 ± 2		M/P 0.02–0.07		31, 217, 239
Dipyrone					M/P 1.3; 4 major metabolites in milk; M/P 0.76–1.65 with half-lifes in milk of 2.5–10.85 hours	Excreted in infant's urine; infant's cyanotic crisis stopped when mother stopped taking drug (one case)	256, 333

Continued.

Table E-1.   Relationship of drugs to breast milk and effect on infant—cont'd

Drug	Ratings		Oral Bioavail. (%)	Peak serum time (hours)	Half-life (hours)	Amount in milk after therapeutic dose	Comments	References
	AAPed.	Scand.						
Donnatal (phenobarbital, hyoscyamine sulfate, atropine sulfate, hyoscrine hydrobromide)							Consider for its component parts; can be given to children but can accumulate in neonate	239
Fenoprofen (Nalfon)				2 ± 0.1	3 ± 0.1	M/P 0.017	M/P measured in women given 600 mg every 6 h for 4 d	49, 239, 260
Flufenamic acid (Arlef)	3					0.50 µg/L (mean); maternal plasma level was 50 times that of infant	No apparent effect on infant when maternal dosage was 200 mg, 3 times a day; infant able to excrete via urine	7, 52
Hydroxychloroquine (Plaquenil)						Milk levels ranged from 3.2–10.6 ng/ml when maternal plasma 90–100 ng/ml	In one case, 200 mg bid dose to mother provided 0.0003% in milk	217, 229
Ibuprofen (Advil, Motrin, Rufen)	II		Greater than 80; absorption rate slowed when taken with food	1.5 ± 0.5	2 ± 0.5	M/P 0.01; vol. of distrib. 0.15 L/kg	400 mg bid for 3 weeks; gave unmeasurable amounts; milk levels <0.5 mg/ml up to 8 h after dose	7, 31, 109, 217, 239, 298

Drug							
Indomethacin (Indocin)	3	98	2	4.5 (PDR); 2.4 ± 0.4 (G&G); increased in neonates	M/P greater than 1; vol. of distrib. 0.26 L/kg	Convulsions in breastfed neonate (case report); used to close patent ductus arteriosus; insufficient data as to effect on other vessels; may be nephrotoxic	7, 90, 109, 230
Ketoprofen (Orudis)	II	100 absorbed; greater than 90 available	1.25 ± 0.75	2.6 ± 1.4	Trace amounts; vol. of distrib. 0.11 L/kg		31, 109, 230, 239
Mefenamid acid (Ponstel)	3		3 ± 1	2	M/P 0.23	No apparent effect on infant at therapeutic doses; infant able to excrete via urine	7, 51, 239
Naproxen (Naprosyn, Synaxsyn, Naprosine, Naxen, Proxen)	3	99	1.5 ± 0.5	14 ± 1	M/P 0.01; peak milk time 4 h; 0.26% of dose excreted in infant's urine; vol. of distrib. 0.16 L/kg	Less toxic in adults than some other organic derivatives	7, 31, 49, 109, 139, 239, 258
Noscapine	IV	30	1.5 ± 0.5	2 ± 0.5	M/P 0.15-0.88		31, 225
Oxyphenbutazone (Tandearil)	II			Several days	In milk of 2 of 55 mothers; M/P 0.1-0.8	No known effect	7, 31, 109, 159, 223
Paracetamol (Alvedon)				2.7	500 mg dose; M/P 0.76; less than 0.1% dose	At most 3 µmol/100 ml of milk; no problem	37

Continued.

Table E-1. Relationship of drugs to breast milk and effect on infant—cont'd

Drug	Ratings AAPed.	Ratings Scand.	Oral Bioavail. (%)	Peak serum time (hours)	Half-life (hours)	Amount in milk after therapeutic dose	Comments	References
Pentazocine (Talwin)		IV	1.7	3.6		Not excreted into breast milk	Withdrawal in neonatal period from ingestion during pregnancy	31, 161, 223, 239, 251
Percodan (oxycodone [derived from opiate thebaine], aspirin, phenacetin, caffeine)						Phenacetin M/P 0.37–1.02	Consider for its component parts; in neonatal period sleeplessness and failure to feed, which increase maternal engorgement and neonatal weight loss, have been observed, probably due to oxycodone	239, 326
Phenylbutazone (Butazolidin)	3	II	90 ± 10	2.5 ± 1.4	56 ± 8	M/P 0.13; vol. of distrib. 0.097 L/kg	Drug measured in infant's serum	7, 31, 49, 105, 109, 171, 217, 239
Piroxicam (Feldene)		IV		4 ± 1	58 ± 28	M/P 0.01		31, 230, 239
Propoxyphene (Darvon)	3			2.25 ± 1.4	9 ± 3	M/P 0.50		7, 49, 58, 239

Drug								References
Sulindac (Clinoril)		IV	90	2 when fasting; 3.5 ± 0.5 with food	7.8; sulfide metabolite, 16.4	Not known if excreted into human milk; it is found in rat's milk	Its metabolites are active	31, 217, 239
Suprofen (Suprol)			100; less if taken with food	1.25 ± 0.75	3 ± 1	0.015%–0.03% of maternal dose; peak time in milk 1.5 ± 0.5 hours	Drug does not accumulate in body	238
Tolmetin (Tolectin)			Greater than 90	0.75 ± 0.25	Biphasic; 1.2 ± 0.6 then 6.5 ± 0.5	Peak milk level at 1 h was 0.18 µg/ml; M/P 0.0055	Nonsteroidal anti-inflammatory; weak acid; 99% protein bound; mol wt >200; pK_a 3.5; one case report negligible in milk	49, 109, 217, 239, 244, 262, 270
Anticoagulants Coumarin derivatives								
Dicumarol (bishydroxycoumarin)	3	III	Slow; incomplete	Dose dependent		None measurable	Drug of choice if mother is to continue nursing; if surgery or trauma occurs, monitor prothrombin time; give vitamin K to infant	7, 29, 31, 45, 81, 191, 226, 289
Warfarin (Coumadin, Panwardin)	3	II	100	5 ± 4	37 ± 15	M/P less than 0.2; vol. of distrib. 0.11 L/kg		

Continued.

Table E-1. Relationship of drugs to breast milk and effect on infant—cont'd

Drug	Ratings		Oral Bioavail. (%)	Peak serum time (hours)	Half-life (hours)	Amount in milk after therapeutic dose	Comments	References
	AAPed.	Scand.						
Ethyl biscoumacetate (Tromexan)						M/P 0.013; some milk samples devoid of drug; vol. of distrib. 0.058 L/kg	Hemorrhage around umbilical stump and cephalhematoma reported; prothrombin normal in infants with hemorrhage; vitamin K has no effect; contraindicated while nursing	137, 159
Heparin	I				Dose dependent	Not excreted into breast milk	Heparin is not effective orally	31, 109
Phenindione (Hedulin) (Dindevan)	1						Breast milk a major route of excretion; reports of serious hemorrhage in infant; prothrombin times prolonged in infant; contraindicated while nursing	7, 88, 159
Anticonvulsants and sedatives								
Aminoglutethimide (Cytadren)			100	1.5	12.5 ± 1.6			239
Barbital (Veronal)						8–10 mg/L after 500 mg dose; vol. of distrib. 1.0–1.5	May produce sedation in infant; in general, barbiturates pass into milk	223

Drug						L/kg		
Carbamazepine (Tegretol)	3	II	Greater than 70	4.5 ± 0.5	15 ± 5 multiple doses; 36 ± 5 single dose	M/P 0.4–0.6; carbamazepine 10, 11 epoxide is metabolite; M/P 0.6–1.8; half-life 6.1 ± 0.7 h	but do not sedate infant; watch for symptoms — Animal studies show lack of weight gain, unkempt appearance; infant serum levels 0.4–1.8 µg/ml; levels higher in first few days; estimate infant receives 0.5 mg/kg/d; same risks for idiosyncratic reactions in infant as not dose related	7, 31, 35, 43, 109, 148, 214, 220, 248
Clonazepam (Klonopin)	3	II	98 ± 31	1.5 ± 0.5	23 ± 5 GG 34 ± 16 PDR	M/S 0.33	Only one case reported in 7-day-old who had 2.9 ng/ml in serum	31, 109, 239
Ethosuximide (Zarontin)	3	III	Greater than 90	3 ± 1	45 ± 8	M/P 0.89 ± 0.11; maximum per liter 70 mg	Infants serum range 15–40 µg/ml	7, 31, 109, 162, 165, 251
Glutethimide (Doriden)			Erratic	3.5 ± 2.5	11 ± 1	Mean concentration low after 250 and 500 mg doses; M/P 1		79
Magnesium sulfate (MgSO$_4$)	3					For 24 h after infusion is stopped; M/P 2	Infant receives approximately 6.5 mg/100 ml; calcium levels remain the same; Similac Special Care formula has 8.3 mg/100 ml	7, 77

Continued.

Table E-1. Relationship of drugs to breast milk and effect on infant—cont'd

Drug	Ratings AAPed.	Ratings Scand.	Oral Bioavail. (%)	Peak serum time (hours)	Half-life (hours)	Amount in milk after therapeutic dose	Comments	References
Mephenytoin (Mesantoin) (hydantoin homologue of mephobarbital)					95 (in patients previously exposed to other anticonvulsants)		Detoxified in liver; no information	109, 239
Pentobarbital (Nembutal)		II			32.5 ± 17.5; Dose dependent	0.17 μg/ml detected 19 h after dose of 100 mg daily for 32 d	Depends on liver for detoxification so may accumulate in first week of life until infant able to detoxify; no problem for older infant in usual doses	31, 49, 239
Phenobarbital (Luminal)	3		100 ± 11		99 ± 18	M/P 0.4–0.6; 3 ± 1 mg ingested by infant per day; vol. of distrib. 0.75 L/kg	Sleepiness and decreased sucking possible; on usual analeptic doses infant alert and feeds well; on hypnotic doses infant depressed and hard to rouse	7, 43, 72, 109, 148, 302
Phensuximide (Milontin)	3				8		No specific data	7, 109
Phenytoin (Dilantin)	3	II	98 ± 7	2.25 ± 0.75 (infatabs, suspension);	15 ± 9 (G&G) 24.5 ± 17.5	M/P 0.15–0.55; vol. of distrib. 0.75 L/kg	In premature infants, half-life up to 160 h; full-term, half-life 50 ± 20h;	7, 31, 43, 72, 109,

Drug	No.	Cat.				Comments	References
				8 ± 4 (extended capsule) (PDR)		5–10 days old, half-life 10.5 ± 4.5 h; decreases further over next 2–3 m; no problem should arise if mother's dose is in therapeutic range	148
Primidone (Mysoline)	3	III	92 ± 18	8.0 ± 4.8	M/P 0.4–1.0; half-life in milk 113 h; multiple metabolites: phenobarbitone M/P 0.4–0.6; phenethyl-malondiamide M/P 0.5–1.0	Causes drowsiness and decreased feeds; may cause bleeding due to hypoprothrombinemia; need vitamin K; avoid drug during lactation	7, 31, 43, 109, 111, 148, 214, 220, 223
Sodium bromide (Bromo-Seltzer and across-the-counter sleeping aids)					Up to 6.6 mg/100 ml	Drowsy; decreased crying; rash; decreased feeding	302
Trimethadione (Tridione)				1.25 ± 0.75		No specific data	109
Valproic acid (Depakene)	3	II	100 ± 10	2.5 ± 1.5	14 ± 3 (multiple dose) 9.8 ± 2.6 (single dose) (G&G) 11 ± 5 (PDR)	M/P 0.01–0.16; negligible amounts found in milk	Levels at birth may be higher than mother's; low levels in milk and good clearance in neonate; probably safe if maternal serum levels midrange; poorly absorbed orally by neonate	7, 27, 31, 43, 109, 213, 239

Continued.

Table E-1. Relationship of drugs to breast milk and effect on infant—cont'd

Drug	Ratings AAPed.	Scand.	Oral Bioavail. (%)	Peak serum time (hours)	Half-life (hours)	Amount in milk after therapeutic dose	Comments	References
Antihistaminics						Except where noted, no specific data available; all pass into milk	All of these drugs have anticholinergic action and may suppress lactation; administer after nursing	203
Azatadine (Optimine)				4				239
Brompheniramine (Dimetane)	3	II		3.1 ± 1.1	24.9 ± 9.3			7, 31, 233
Carbinoxamine (Rondec)					15 ± 5			49
Chlorcyclizine		IV			Half-life inactive metabolite norchlorocyclizine about 6 d			31, 233
Chlorpheniramine			Slow, absorption Half-life 0.7 h	4.25 ± 1.75	19 ± 5 adults; 11.25 ± 1.75 children			233
Cinnarizine		IV	Slow absorption	3.25 ± 0.75	3			31, 233

Drug								References
Clemastine (Tavist)	1	II		3.5 ± 1.5	5 ± 1	M/P 0.25–0.5; drug could not be detected in infant's plasma	Drowsiness; irritability	7, 31, 49, 160, 233, 239
Cyclizine (Marezine)		IV				Demethylated to inactive norcyclizine with half-life of 24 h		31, 233, 239
Cyproheptadine (Periactin)		IV		7.5 ± 1.5	16	Completely metabolized, no unchanged drug in plasma (metabolites)		31, 233, 239
Diphenhydramine (Benadryl)	3	II	51 ± 6	2.5	6.35 ± 2.95	Excreted into milk; vol. of distrib. 6.5 L/kg		7, 31, 233, 239
Promethazine (Phenergan)		IV		2.5 ± 0.5	10.5 ± 3.5			31, 233
Ranitidine (Zantac) Histamine (H₂) receptor antagonist			52 ± 11	2.5 ± 0.5	2.45 ± 0.55	Excreted into milk; M/P 1.9 2 h after dose; 2.8 4 h after dose; 6.7 6 h after dose		49, 109, 239, 254
Trimeprazine (Temaril)	3					Detected in low concentrations		7, 49, 223
Tripelennamine (Pyribenzamine)	3					Excreted into bovine milk		7, 49, 223
Triprolidine		IV		2 ± 0.5	5	M/P 0.5–1.2; 0.06%–0.2% of drug excreted into milk		31, 102, 233

Continued.

Table E-1. Relationship of drugs to breast milk and effect on infant—cont'd

Drug	Ratings AAPed.	Ratings Scand.	Oral Bioavail. (%)	Peak serum time (hours)	Half-life (hours)	Amount in milk after therapeutic dose	Comments	References
Anti-infective agents								
Acyclovir (Zovirax)		IV	22.5 ± 7.7 decreases with dose	1.5	2.4 ± 0.7	M/P 0.6–4.1, at 1.5 h after dose; M/P less than 1, but still rising at 3 h; vol. of distrib. 0.7 L/kg	One case reported suggests a facilitated transport mechanism; peak lags in milk to 3–4 h post dose	31, 109, 169
Amantadine (Symmetrel)	3	III		4		Low amount	Vomiting; urinary retention; rash; use with caution	7, 31, 49, 223
Amikacin (Amikin)			Poor	IM 1	2.3 ± 0.4	Low amount; oral absorption bad so ototoxicity not expected	Modification of bowel flora a possible problem	49, 109, 189, 239, 332
ρ-aminosalicylic acid				1.75 ± 0.25	1			223
Amoxicillin		II	93 ± 10	1.5 ± 0.5	1.0 ± 0.1	M/P 0.013–0.043; max. 0.9 mg/L peak at 4+ h; vol. of distrib. 0.41 L/kg	Passes into milk supply slowly; acidic and low fat solubility probably not a problem	31, 109, 144, 251
Ampicillin (Polycillin, Amcil, Omnipen, Penbritin)		II	62 ± 17		1.3 ± 0.2; increased in neonates	M/P 0.17–0.2; max. 1 mg/L; vol. of distrib. 0.28 L/kg	Sensitivity due to repeated exposure, diarrhea, or secondary candidiasis	31, 49, 106, 109, 157, 223, 251, 266, 324

Drug									
Azlocillin (Azlin)			IV; injection	Poor	1.0 ± 0.2; increased in neonate and premature infants			Detected in low concentrations; vol. of distrib. 0.22 L/kg	31, 109, 239
Aztreonam				Poor		IM 1.5		M/P less than 0.01; peak in milk after IM 3 h; peak in milk after IV 4 h	104
Carbenicillin (Pyopen, Geopen)					1.0 ± 0.2; increased in neonates		0.265 µg/ml 1 h after 1 g given	Levels not significant; drug is given to neonate	109, 223
Cephalosporin antibiotics								In general, a small amount is excreted into breast milk; monitor for diarrhea and sensitization; specific data below	144
Cefaclor (Ceclor)		II		Same whether taken with or without food	0.75 ± 0.15 fasting; with food 1.625 ± 0.375	0.75 ± 0.15; serum concentration 50%–75% lower if taken with food			31, 239
Cefadroxil (Duricef, Ultracel)	3	II		Rapid	2.5 ± 0.5	1.5	M/P 0.009–0.02; max. 2.4 mg/L; peak time in milk 5.5 ± 0.5 h for 500 mg dose, 6.5 ± 0.5, for 1 g dose	Levels bactericidal for sensitive organisms	7, 31, 49, 144, 251, 291
Cefamandole (Mandol)		II	Injection		1.25 ± 0.75	IV 0.53; IM 1	M/P 1 h after IV 0.02	Not absorbed orally	31, 49, 239

Continued.

Table E-1. Relationship of drugs to breast milk and effect on infant—cont'd

Drug	Ratings		Oral Bioavail. (%)	Peak serum time (hours)	Half-life (hours)	Amount in milk after therapeutic dose	Comments	References
	AAPed.	Scand.						
Cefazolin (Ancel, Kefzol)	3	II	Injection		1.8 ± 0.4	IV M/P 0.02; IM not detected; peak level in milk 3 h	Not absorbed orally	7, 31, 32, 49, 109, 239, 309, 331
Cefmenoxine		II	Injection			M/S 1.1–1.6; vol. of distrib. 0.12 L/kg	Not absorbed orally	31, 314
Cefonicid (Monocid)		II	Injection		4.4 ± 0.8	M/S 0.002	Not absorbed orally	31, 109, 180
Cefoperazone (Cefobid)		II	Injection		2.1 ± 0.3	0.65 ± 0.25 µg/ml from 1 g IV dose	Not absorbed orally	31, 49, 109, 239
Ceforanide (Precef)		II	Injection	1	2.6 ± 0.5		Not absorbed orally	31, 109, 239
Cefotaxime (Claforan)	3	II	Injection	0.5	1.1 ± 0.2 adults; 4.6 infants less than 1500 mg; 3.4 infants more than 1500 mg	Half-life in milk 2.93 ± 0.55 h; peak milk level 2.5 ± 0.5 h; M/P 0.02–0.16; vol. of distrib. 0.24 L/kg	Not absorbed orally	7, 31, 49, 109, 143, 144, 239
Cefoxitin (Mefoxin)		II	Injection	IM 25 ± 5 minutes	IM 1.08; IV 0.83 ± 0.15	Increased half-life in infants; some moth-	Not absorbed orally	31, 109, 239

					ers excrete drug into milk, some do not	
Ceftazidine (Fortaz, Tazicef)	II	Injection		1.6 ± 0.1	2 g every 8 h × 5 d; peak 1 h 5.2 µg/ml through 3.8 µg/ml 7½ h	Levels higher than most cephalosporins; 80% of dose excreted by newborn in 8 h when given IM; not absorbed orally	31, 39, 239
Ceftizoxime (Cefizox)	II	Injection		1.8 ± 0.7	Less than 0.5 mg/L after 2 g dose		31, 49, 108, 109, 206, 239
Ceftriaxone (Rocephin)	II	Injection		7.25 ± 1.45 adult; 4.45 ± 0.15 children	M/P 0.03–0.04; IV half-life in milk 12.8 h; IM half-life in milk 17.3 h		31, 49, 145, 146, 239
Cefuroxime (Kefurox, Zinacef)	II	Injection		1.7 ± 0.6			31, 109
Cephalexin (Kelfex)	II	90 ± 9	1	0.90 ± 0.18	M/P 0.008–0.14; max. per liter 0.85 mg; peak time 4.5 ± 0.5 h; completely gone by 8 h; vol. of distrib. 0.26 L/kg		31, 49, 109, 144, 239
Cephalothin (Seffin, Keflin)	II	Injection	0.5	0.57 ± 0.32; 65 ± 0.5% excreted by kidneys in first 6 h	Peak milk level 1.5 ± 0.5 h; half-life in milk 2.75 ± 0.45 h		31, 109, 144, 239

Continued.

Table E-1. Relationship of drugs to breast milk and effect on infant—cont'd

Drug	Ratings AAPed.	Ratings Scand.	Oral Bioavail. (%)	Peak serum time (hours)	Half-life (hours)	Amount in milk after therapeutic dose	Comments	References
Cephapirin (Cefadyl)		II	Injection		1.2 ± 0.3	M/P 0.07–0.5; max. amt./L 0.64 mg; peak level in milk 1.5 ± 0.5 h; half-life in milk 2.77 ± 0.23 h	Its major metabolite, desacetyl cephapirin, has antibacterial activity	31, 49, 109, 144, 239, 251
Cephradine (Anspor, Velosef)		II	Greter than 90	1 in fasting state; food in GI tract delays absorption, but total amount absorbed is the same	0.77 ± 0.30; over 90% excreted in 6 h	M/P 0.2		31, 49, 109, 200, 201, 239
Moxalactam (Moxam)		II	IM availability 85 ± 15	1.5 ± 0.5	2.1 ± 0.7	0.5–6.1 mg/ml		31, 109, 198
Chloramphenicol (Chloromycetin)	3	III	82.5 ± 7.5	1	4.0 ± 2	M/P 0.51–0.61; peak in milk 2 ± 1 h	Grey's syndrome; infant does not excrete drug well and small amounts may accumulate; contraindicated; may be tolerated in older infant with mature glycuronide system; possible bone marrow depression	7, 31, 49, 106, 109, 122, 239, 243, 247, 276, 310
Chloroquine	3	II	89 ± 16	2	8.9 ± 3.1 d	M/P 1.96–4.26; metabolite desethyl-	Daily dose of infant 0.55%–0.7% of adult	5, 7, 31, 68, 89,

							M/P / milk level	Comments	References
							chloroquine with M/P 0.54–3.89	dose; can be used to treat child under 6 mo of age who is wholly breastfed	97, 109, 224
Chlortetra-cycline (Aureomycin)	II	Ointment					M/P 0.4		31, 49, 116, 239
Cleocinpe-diatric (Clindamycinpalmitate)				0.75	In children 2 ± 0.10		Appears in breast milk		239
Clindamycin (Cleocin)	3	III	87	0.75	2.7 ± 0.4		Wide differences in milk level among individuals; M/P 0.1–3.0; 3.8 mg max. per L	Caution expressed	7, 31, 109, 239, 251, 283
Cloxacillin (Tegopen)				43 ± 16; delayed if taken with meals	1.25 ± 0.25	0.55 ± 0.07			109, 239
Colistin (Colymycin)							M/P 0.17–0.18	Not absorbed orally	49, 310, 325
Cycloserine (Seromycin)					0.39 ± 0.04		M/P 0.72; 0.6% of adult dose	A 3.5 kg infant would ingest up to 1.7 mg/kg or 11% of usual pediatric dose of 15 mg/kg/d; OK during lactation	133, 280

Continued.

Table E-1. Relationship of drugs to breast milk and effect on infant—cont'd

Drug	Ratings AAPed.	Ratings Scand.	Oral Bioavail. (%)	Peak serum time (hours)	Half-life (hours)	Amount in milk after therapeutic dose	Comments	References
Dapsone			Greater than 95; slowly absorbed	6 ± 2	28 ± 3	M/P 0.22–0.45; max. amt. 14.3% of maternal dose		89, 109, 239
Demeclocycline (Declomycin)						0.2–0.3 mg/500 ml	Not significant in therapeutic doses; can be given to infants	223
Dicloxacillin (Dynapen)			67.5 ± 17.5		0.70 ± 0.07			109
Doxycycline (Doryx)			93	2	16 ± 6	M/P 0.3–0.4		49, 109, 205, 239
Erythromycin (Ilosone, E-Mycin, Erythrocin)	II		35 ± 25	3 (enteric-coated capsule)	1.6 ± 0.7	M/P 0.5	Higher concentrations have been reported in milk than in plasma; should not be given under 1 mo of age if there is any risk of jaundice; dose in milk higher when given IV to mother	31, 49, 106, 125, 223
Ethambutol (Myambutol)	II		77 ± 8	3 ± 1	3.1 ± 0.4	Excreted into milk		31, 109, 239
Gentamicin	3		0			1.2–2.1 M/P; 1 h after 80 mg dose IM milk had 0.16 mg/	Not absorbed from gastrointestinal tract; may change gut flora; drug is	7, 250, 324

Drug		Category		Half-life (h)	Milk concentration / dose	Comments	References
Hydroxy-chloroquine (Plaquenil)	3			L; vol. of distrib. 0.3–0.5 L/kg	M/P 5.5; infant exposed to 2% of maternal dose/d	If chronically used by mother, may cause retinal damage in infant; given to newborns directly; no untoward effects in nursing infants reported	217, 229
Isoniazid (Nydrazid)		II	1.5 ± 0.5	3.1 ± 1.1 (slow acetylator); 1.1 ± 0.1 (fast acetylator)	M/P 1; may be lower in slow acetylators; 0.75%–2.3% of maternal dose; vol. of distrib. 0.67 L/kg	Peak level in milk 3 h; half-life in milk 6 h; major metabolite is acetylisoniazid; it peaks at 5 h with a 13.5 h half-life; drug not detectable in infant's blood but is found in infant's urine	7, 31, 109, 251, 280
Kanamycin (Kantrex)		III	Poor	IM 3 ± 1; IV 1.4 ± 0.6	Peaks in milk at 1 h; M/P 0.33; 0.05% of maternal dose	Infant absorbs little from gastrointestinal tract; infants can be given drug	31, 133, 239, 280
Lincomycin (Lincocin)		III	3 ± 1	5.4 ± 1	M/P 0.13–2.25; max. amt. 2.4 mg/L; 0.25% of mother's daily dose	Not significant in therapeutic doses to affect child	31, 49, 194, 251, 325
Lindane (Kwell, Scabene)		III	7 ± 1		Low conc.		31, 239
Mandelic acid					0.3 g/24 h after dose of 12 g/d	Not significant in therapeutic doses to affect child	223

Continued.

Table E-1. Relationship of drugs to breast milk and effect on infant—cont'd

Drug	Ratings AAPed.	Ratings Scand.	Oral Bioavail. (%)	Peak serum time (hours)	Half-life (hours)	Amount in milk after therapeutic dose	Comments	References
Mebendazole			Minimal				Infants have been given drug directly 100 mg tid for trichuriasis and intestinal parasites	156, 269
Methacycline (Rondomycin)			Poor absorption		16	50–260 µg/100 ml; M/P 0.5	Same precautions as with tetracycline	223, 311
Methenamine (Hexamine)					1		Not significant in therapeutic doses to affect child	223,
Metronidazole (Flagyl)	2	II	99 ± 8		8.5 ± 2.9	M/P 1; mean conc. in infant's plasma 20% of maternal plasma level; vol. of distrib 1.1 L/kg	Contraindicated for infant under 6 mo—may cause neurologic disorders and blood dyscrasia; when single 2 g maternal dose used, withhold breastfeeding; pump and discard milk 24 h, then resume feeding	7, 31, 49, 86, 93, 106, 112, 126, 239
Mezlocillin (Mezlin)		II	Injection	IM 0.75	1.3 ± 0.4	Low conc.		31, 109, 239
Nalidixic acid (Negram)	3	II		1.5 ± 0.5	1.5	M/P 0.08–0.13	Not significant in therapeutic doses beyond neonatal period; hemolytic anemia in an infant	7, 31, 49, 59, 311, 325

Drug							Comment	Reference
Netilmicin (Netromycin)		IV	IM; rapid, complete absorption	0.75 ± 0.25	Adults 2.3 ± 0.7 with long terminal half-life of 37 ± 6; in neonate inversely correlated with body weight; in 6 wks and older, 1.75 ± 0.25	Small	attributed to nalidixic acid in G_6PD deficiency or when mother has renal failure	31, 109, 239
Nitrofurantoin (Furandantin)	3	I	100		39 ± 21 min	Undetectable to 0.5 µg/ml	Not significant in therapeutic doses to affect child except in G_6PD deficiency	7, 31, 306
Novobiocin (Albamycin, Cathomycin)						0.36–0.54 mg/100 ml	Infant can be given drug directly	294
Nystatin (Mycostatin)		I	Negligible			Not absorbed orally	Can be given to infant directly	31, 239, 251
Oxacillin (Prostaphlin)			33	0.55 ± 0.15		Low conc.		49, 109, 159
Penethamate (Leocillin)						24–74 µg/100 ml	Animal study suggests it be avoided	223

Continued.

Table E-1.   Relationship of drugs to breast milk and effect on infant—cont'd

| Drug | Ratings | | Oral Bioavail. (%) | Peak serum time (hours) | Half-life (hours) | Amount in milk after therapeutic dose | Comments | References |
	AAPed.	Scand.						
Penicillin G, benzathine (Bicillin) Penicillin G, potassium Penicillin V (V-cillin K, Veetids)			33 ± 0.5; G absorbed best ½-h before meals or 2–3 h after meal; V may be better absorbed on full rather than empty stomach	0.75 ± 0.25	For equivalent oral dose, plasma concentration of V 2–5 times greater than G	M/P 0.02–0.13 for all types; vol. of distrib. 0.2–0.3 L/kg	Clinical need should supersede possible allergic responses; infant can be given penicillin directly; parents should be told to inform physician that infant has been exposed to penicillin because of potential sensitivity	49, 106, 114, 311
Piperacillin (Pipracil)		II	Injection	0.5 after IM injection	0.93 ± 0.12	Trace	May alter intestinal flora; conc. below any therapeutic or toxic level	23, 31, 109
Povidone-Iodine (Betadine)						M/S 8–25	Absorbed from vaginal mucosa	31, 246
Pyrvinium Pomoate			Negligible			Insoluble in water; unlikely to appear in milk; not absorbed; OK to breastfeed		279
Pyrazinamide			Excellent	Within 2 h	9.4 ± 0.4	In 24 h, 0.5% of adult dose		133

Drug							Effects	References
Pyrimethamine (antimalarial) (Daraprim, Fansidar)	3	II	Excellent	4.75 ± 3.25	105 ± 70	M/P 0.2–0.66; in 1 L/d, over 9-d period, 45.6% of maternal dose will appear in milk	Significant in therapeutic doses when infant is <6 mo old and entirely breastfed; eliminates parasites in breastfed infant	7, 31, 49, 68, 89, 109
Quinine sulfate	3	II	Almost 100	1.5 ± 0.5	11 ± 2 (G&G); 4.5 ± 0.5 (PDR)	M/P 0.14; 0.05% of dose in milk	In therapeutic doses, no affect to child except rare thrombocytopenia	7, 31, 109, 239, 251, 293, 295
Rifampin (Rimactane)	3	II	100	3 ± 1; delayed 1–2 h if taken with food or p-aminosalicylic acid	3.5 ± 0.8	1–3 µg/ml; 0.05% of adult dose in milk per 24 h; vol. of distrib. 1.0 L/kg	No effects reported when used as antituberculosis drug; turns secretions orange; may turn milk orange	7, 31, 49, 109, 133, 310
Sodium fusidate		II				0.02 µg/ml	Not significant in therapeutic doses to affect infant	31, 223
Streptomycin			Poor	1 after IM injection	5.3 ± 2.2	M/P 0.12–1; 0.5% of adult dose in 24 h	Not to be given more than 2 wk; ototoxic and nephrotoxic with long use; given to infants directly	49, 109, 157, 280, 292, 325
Sulfamethoxazole		II	Around 100	2.5 ± 1.5	10.1 ± 4.6	Appears in breast milk	Avoid for first month postpartum as displaces bilirubin	31, 109, 239

Continued.

Table E-1. Relationship of drugs to breast milk and effect on infant—cont'd

Drug	Ratings AAPed.	Scand.	Oral Bioavail. (%)	Peak serum time (hours)	Half-life (hours)	Amount in milk after therapeutic dose	Comments	References
Sulfanilamide						Up to 1.6% of total dose; milk levels persist for several days after mother stops taking drug	Not significant in therapeutic doses; may cause rash or hemolytic anemia; should be avoided for first month postpartum as displaces bilirubin from albumin	2, 49, 118, 157, 177
Sulfapyridine	3			12 (tablets, oral suspension); 18 ± 6 (coated enteric tablets)		M/P 0.09–0.8; max. 15 mg/L	To be avoided; has caused skin rash; found in infant's urine	7, 20, 33, 49, 239
Sulfasalazine (Azulfidine)	3	II		3 (tablets, oral suspension); 6 (coated tablets)		Splits to sulphapyridine and 5-aminosalicylic acid; usually, parent drug not found in milk; rarely, when mother is a slow acetylator, drug is excreted into milk	Risk of recurrent maternal disease outweighs risk to infant unless jaundiced, then postpone until jaundice clears; rare cases of bloody diarrhea have been reported if drug is transferred through milk	7, 20, 31, 47, 49
Sulfathiazole	3					0.5 mg/100 ml after dose of 3 g/d	Not significant in therapeutic doses to affect child after 1 mo of age	7, 157, 177, 223
Sulfisoxazole (Gantrisin)	3		96 ± 14	2.5 ± 1.5	6.6 ± 0.7	M/P 0.06; 0.45% of dose of mother	To be avoided during first month postpartum be-	7, 49, 92, 109,

Drug				Comments	References
				cause of bilirubin albumin-binding displacement; contraindicated in G_6PD deficiency	151, 239, 251
Tetracycline HCl (Achromycin, Panmycin, Sumycin)	3	10.6 ± 1.5	M/P 0.25–1.5	Not enough to treat an infection in an infant; theoretically may cause discoloration of teeth in infant but not detected in the infant's serum; do not give over 10 d or repeatedly	7, 49, 110, 158, 245
Thiamphenicol			3.7 µg/ml after 500 mg dose or 17 mg total dose to infant; levels from multiple doses 2.9 µg/ml for 48 h	Accumulates in newborn; jaundice and Grey's syndrome	243
Ticarcillin (Ticar)	0	IM 0.75 ± 0.25	1.3 ± 0.1	Trace amts.	49, 65, 109, 239
Tinidazole	III	11.4 ± 2.7	M/S 0.62–1.39		31, 98
Tobramycin (Nebcin, Tobrex)	IV Poor	After IM injection 1 ± 0.5	Initially 2.2 ± 0.1; terminal 100 ± 57	After IM injection peak in milk at 4 h; Not absorbed well from GI tract; can be given sparingly to premature or full-term infants less than 1 wk of age	31, 49, 109, 239, 290

Continued.

Table E-1. Relationship of drugs to breast milk and effect on infant—cont'd

Drug	Ratings AAPed.	Ratings Scand.	Oral Bioavail. (%)	Peak serum time (hours)	Half-life (hours)	Amount in milk after therapeutic dose	Comments	References
Trimethoprim (Bactrim, Septra, Trimpex)	3	II	100	2.5 ± 1.5	11 ± 1.4	Milk conc. 1.2–2.4 µg/ml; peak 2–3 h; M/P 1.25	Infants at risk for kernicterus should not be exposed; if child could receive it directly, therapeutically OK	7, 17, 31, 49, 199, 239
Vancomycin (Vancocin)			Poor		5 ± 1	Not known; vol. of distrib. 0.39 L/kg	Poor absorption from GI tract	109, 239
Antineoplastics and antimetabolites								
Allopurinol (Zyloprim, Lopurin)			90	1.5	1.5 ± 0.5	Both drug and its major metabolite are excreted into milk	Alloxanthine, its major metabolite, peaks in plasma at 4.5 h with half-life of 15 h	217
Azathioprine (Imuran)			60 ± 31	1.5 ± 0.5	5 (drug and all metabolites)		Discontinuing breastfeeding recommended, although data is insufficient	109, 203, 239
Busulfan (Myleran)			Slow, almost complete		2.6 ± 0.5		Discontinuing breastfeeding recommended, although data is insufficient	109, 203, 239
Chlorambucil (Leukeran)			100	1	0.95 ± 0.34		Metabolic product, phenylacetic acid mustard, has half-life of 2.4 h; discontinuing breast-	109, 203, 239

Drug						Recommendation	References
Cisplatin (Platinol)	Injection			Initial 0.62 ± 0.2; postdistribution 1.1 ± 0.125	Not found in breast milk	Discontinuing breastfeeding recommended, although data is insufficient	91, 203, 239
Cyclophosphamide (Cytoxan)	1	74 ± 22	4	7.5 ± 4.0	After 500 mg IV, drug found in milk 1, 3, 5, and 6 h after injection	Drug or metabolites can be detected in maternal plasma for up to 72 h; breastfeeding should be terminated prior to medication	7, 109, 203, 239, 321
Cytarabine (Cytosar-U)	Less than 20			2.6 ± 0.6		Discontinuing breastfeeding recommended, although data is insufficient	109, 203, 239
Doxorubicin (Adriamycin)	Injection			36 ± 11	Drug and metabolite appear in breast milk	Discontinuing breastfeeding recommended, although data is insufficient	91, 109, 203, 239
Hydroxyurea (Hydrea)	Greater than 80				6.1 ± 2.3 mg/L		239, 288
Mercaptopurine (Purinethol)	12 ± 7; increased to 60 when first pass metabolism inhibited by allopurinol		Oral 0.90 ± 0.37; IV children 0.35; IV adults 0.78			Discontinuing breastfeeding recommended, although data is insufficient	109, 203, 239

Table E-1. Relationship of drugs to breast milk and effect on infant—cont'd

| Drug | Ratings | | Oral Bioavail. (%) | Peak serum time (hours) | Half-life (hours) | Amount in milk after therapeutic dose | Comments | References |
	AAPed.	Scand.						
Methotrexate			65; lower when doses exceed 80 mg/m²	Oral 1.5 ± 0.5; IV 0.75 ± 0.25	Initially 2, then 7.2 ± 2.1	M/P 0.08; infant would receive 0.26 µg/100 ml; vol. of distrib. 1.0 L/kg	Antimetabolite; discontinuing breastfeeding recommended, although data is insufficient	109, 142, 203, 217, 239
Autonomic drugs								
Acebutolol (Sectral)			37 ± 12	2.5; metabolite diacetolol 3.5	2.7 ± 0.4; metabolite diacetolol 10.5 ± 2.5	M/P 1.9–9.2; metabolite diacetolol M/P 2.3–24.7; vol. of distrib. 1.2 L/kg	In any given milk sample, concentration of active metabolite, diacetolol, greater than that of acebutolol	44, 109, 239
Alprenolol		II	8.6 ± 5.5		2.5 ± 0.6	Vol. of distrib. 3.3 L/kg		31, 109
Amphetamine						M/P 2.8–7.5; vol. of distrib. 0.6 L/kg	Accumulates in milk; urinary excretion of drug is 0.001–0.003 of that of mother	109, 284
Atropine sulfate	3					0.1 mg/100 ml	Hyperthermia, atropine toxicity, infants especially sensitive; also inhibits lactation; infant dose 0.01 mg/kg	7, 223, 255
Baclofen (Lioresal)			Inversely proportional to dose	3.9		0.001% of ingested dose appears in milk over 24 h	Half-life in milk 5.6 h	95, 239

Drug							Comments	References
Carisoprodol (Soma, Rela)						M/P 2–4	Blocks interneuronal activity in descending reticular substance and spinal cord; drowsiness; hypotonia; poor feed	222, 239
Domperidone (Motilium)						M/P 0.25–0.3		131
Ergot derivatives (methylergonovine, ergonovine maleate)							Blocks prolactin secretion by activating dopamine receptors in pituitary; courses of 1–3 d postpartum; no apparent effect on lactation	237
Ergotamine tartrate (Ergostat) (Cafergot = drug + caffeine)	1	III	Slow, incomplete; caffeine increases absorption	2; peak plasma conc. increased by a factor of 2 when taken with caffeine	Disappears quickly from serum—metabolized by liver	Appears in breast milk	Vomiting and diarrhea to weak pulse and unstable blood pressure seen in infants when continued Rx given; short-term therapy for migraine should not exceed 6 mg; drug may inhibit lactation; 0.2 mg postpartum generally tolerated	7, 31, 109, 157, 223, 239, 255
Hyoseyamine (Levsin)		II	100	3.5		Traces	Majority of drug excreted unchanged in 12 h	7, 31, 239
Labetalol (Normodyne)		II	20 ± 5	1.5 ± 0.5	5.2 ± 1.3	0.004% of maternal dose; M/P 0.8–2.6	Drug recovered in some infants, not all	31, 109, 194, 239

Continued.

Table E-1.　Relationship of drugs to breast milk and effect on infant—cont'd

| Drug | Ratings | | Oral Bioavail. (%) | Peak serum time (hours) | Half-life (hours) | Amount in milk after therapeutic dose | Comments | References |
	AAPed.	Scand.						
Mepenzolate bromide (Cantil)		IV	Low				Postganglionic parasympathetic inhibitor used to diminish gastric acidity and decrease spasm of colon	31, 223, 239
Mepindolol						M/P 0.35 at 2 h after a single dose; M/P 0.61 continuous doses for 5 d	Drug detected in serum of 20% of infants; detection limit 1 ng/ml	49, 163
Methocarbamol (Robaxin)						Minimal	Too little in milk to produce effect	223
Metoprolol (Lopressor)		II	38 ± 14		3.2 ± 0.2	M/P 2.5–4.8; infant would receive 20–40 times less than usual adult dose; vol. of distrib. 4.2 L/kg	Amt. of drug in milk collected 1.5–3 h after dosing is less than samples analyzed later in the dosing interval	31, 109, 175, 202, 264
Neostigmine			Less than 100	0.5	1.3 ± 0.8		No known harm to infant	109, 193
Oxprenolol		IV				M/P 0.14–0.49	Max. dose in 500 ml of breast milk is 60 times less than adult dose	31, 275
Pindolol (Visken)		II	64–100	Within 1	3.6 ± 0.6	M/P 1.6		31, 109, 253

Drug						References
Propantheline bromide (Pro-Banthine)	IV	1	1.6	Uncontrolled data indicates no measurable levels	Drug rapidly metabolized in maternal system to inactive metabolite; mother should avoid long-acting preparations, however	31, 223, 292
Pseudoephedrine	III			M/P 2.6–3.3; over 24 h 0.4%–0.6% of maternal dose		31, 102
Pyridostigmine (Mestinon)		14 ± 3	IV 1.9 ± 0.2; Oral 3.7 ± 1.0	M/P 0.36–1.13; infant received 0.1% or less of maternal dose	Drug not detected in infant when maternal dose <300 mg/d	49, 109, 119, 239
Ranitidine			0.38 ± 0.13 injection	M/P 1.9, 2.8, and 6.7 at 2, 4, and 6 h; peak levels 1000–3000 ng/ml	Infant would receive 1 to 3 mg/d	49, 153
Scopolamine (Hyoscine)	II				Usually given as single dose and of no problem to neonate; no data on repeated doses	16, 31
Sytalol	II			M/P 5.4		253
Terbutaline (Bricanyl)	II	15 ± 6; less if taken with meals	16 ± 3 (pill) (G & G); 3.5 ± 0.5 (subcutaneous injection) (PDR)	3.5 ng/ml av. conc. in milk; infant intake up to 0.7% of maternal dose	Infant receives similar amts. regardless of dosing; not detectable in infant plasma	31, 42, 109, 179, 239

Continued.

Table E-1. Relationship of drugs to breast milk and effect on infant—cont'd

Drug	Ratings AAPed.	Ratings Scand.	Oral Bioavail. (%)	Peak serum time (hours)	Half-life (hours)	Amount in milk after therapeutic dose	Comments	References
Timolol (Blocadren)		III	70 ± 20	1.5 ± 0.5	4.1 ± 1.1	M/P 0.59–1.01	When applied as an eye-drop solution, 1.5 h after dose; M/P 6.02	31, 49, 100, 109, 185, 239
Cardiovascular drugs								
Amiodarone (Cordarone)			35 ± 9	5 ± 2	25 ± 12 d	M/P 2.5–9.1; desethylamiodarone, a metabolite, has M/P 0.8–3.8; vol. of distrib. 66 L/kg	Plasma level of infant is about 25% that of mother; drug has approximately 75 mg iodine per 200 mg dose	49, 109, 202, 239, 240
Amrinone (Inocap)			93 ± 12		4.0 ± 1.6	Vol. of distrib. 1.2 L/kg		109
Atenolol (Tenormin) beta-receptor blocking agent	3	II	56 ± 30	3 ± 1	6.3 ± 1.8	M/P 1.3–3.6; not detectable in milk before 4 h; peaks in milk at 8 h	Food decreases absorption of atenolol in adult; infant serum is 10% of mother's serum; no signs of beta-blocker effect in infants	7, 31, 109, 175, 202, 239
Bretylium			23 ± 9		8.9 ± 1.8	Vol. of distrib. 5.9 L/kg		109
Captopril (Capoten)	3	II	65; less if taken with meals	1	1.9 ± 0.5	M/P 0.006; peak level in milk at 4 h	Max. dose to infant 0.002% of maternal dose; no effects seen; probably safest of group	7, 31, 82, 109, 239, 251

Drug							Comments	References
Clofibrate (Atromid)		III	95 ± 10		13 ± 3		Appears in animal milk; not known if it appears in human milk	31, 49, 64, 109
Clonidine (Catapres)		IV	100	12.7 ± 7	8.5 ± 2.0	M/P 1.5–2.0		31, 49, 109, 120, 239
Diazoxide (Proglycem, Hyperstat)		IV	91 ± 5		48 ± 12 (G&G); 28 ± 8.3 (PDR)		Arteriolar dilators and antihypertensive	31, 109, 239
Digoxin (Lanoxicaps)	3	II	70 ± 13		39 ± 13	M/P 0–1.0; vol. of distrib. 7.5 L/kg	Peak level in milk at 4 h 0.07%–0.14% of maternal dose; drug not detected in infant's plasma	7, 31, 32, 49, 62, 103, 109, 172, 181, 251
Diltiazem (Cardizem)			44 ± 10	2.5 ± 0.5	3.2 ± 1.3	M/P 1.0; vol. of distrib. 5.3 L/kg	Peaks in milk at 2.5 ± 0.5 h	109, 239
Disopyramide	3	IV	83 ± 11	2	6.0 ± 1.0	M/P 0.4–0.9; major metabolite has M/P 5.6 ± 2.9	No significant amount of drug found in infant's serum; worst case 1.5 mg/d; metabolite not detected	7, 28, 31, 49, 135, 186, 202
Guanethidine (Ismelin)	3	IV	Individual variation in absorption and metabolism			Small quantity	Not significant in therapeutic doses to affect child	7, 31, 223, 239, 292

Table E-1. Relationship of drugs to breast milk and effect on infant—cont'd

Drug	Ratings		Oral Bioavail. (%)	Peak serum time (hours)	Half-life (hours)	Amount in milk after therapeutic dose	Comments	References
	AAPed.	Scand.						
Hydralazine (Apresoline)	3	II	16 ± 6 (rapid acetylator); 35 ± 4 (slow acetylator)	1.25 ± 0.75		Peak at 2 h of the dose; M/P 1.4; vol. of distrib. 1.5 L/kg	Jaundice; thrombocytopenia; electrolyte disturbances possible	7, 31, 49, 109, 176
Lidocaine			35 ± 11		1.8 ± 0.4; 2 major active metabolites with half-life 2 h and 10 h	Vol. of distrib. 1.1 L/kg		109, 202
Lorcainide			Dose dependent; saturable first pass metabolism; 100 mg dose 2.5 ± 1.5; 200 mg dose 50 ± 15		7.6 ± 2.2; metabolite norlorcainide half-life 27 ± 8		Steady-state ratio norlorcainide/locainide 2.2 ± 0.9	109
Methyldopa (Aldomet)	3	III	25 ± 16		1.8 ± 0.2	Found in breast milk and excreted in infant's urine; 0.1–0.9 mg/ml when maternal dose 750–2000 mg/d	Galactorrhea; affects mother's milk production in large doses; appears in milk in small amounts; no untoward symptoms reported	7, 31, 49, 109, 121, 249, 292

Drug								References
Metoprolol (Lopressor, Seloken) Beta-receptor blocking agent (cardioselective)	3	II	38 ± 14		3.2 ± 0.2 (G&G); 5 ± 2 (PDR)	M/P 2.0–4.8; peak level at 6 h after dose; some subjects had 0	Max. dose to infant estimated to be 0.05 mg/500 ml; infant would get 20–40 times less than usual adult dose	7, 31, 109, 202
Mexiletine (antidysrhythmic) (Mexitil)		II	87 ± 13	2.5 ± 0.5	11.8 ± 4.2	M/P 0.78–2.0; mean 1.45; peak level 960 ng/ml	Possible dose to infant 1.25 mg/d; therapeutic dose 8–10 mg/kg	31, 109, 173, 239, 297
Minoxidil (Loniten)			95	within 1	3.1 ± 0.6 (G&G); 4.2 (PDR)	M/P 0.67–1.0	Rapidly excreted into breast milk; its glucuronide conjugate appears rapidly in mother's plasma but is barely excreted into milk (M/P 0.06) due to low lipid solubility	49, 109, 239, 305
Nadolol (Corgard) Beta-adrenergic receptor blocker	3	II	34 ± 5	3.5 ± 0.5	16 ± 2	M/P 4.6; vol. of distrib. 2.1 L/kg	Infant receives 2%–7% of maternal dose; caution	7, 31, 83, 109, 239
Nifedipine (Procardia)		IV	45 ± 28	0.50	3.4 ± 1.2	Vol. of distrib. 1.2 L/kg		31, 109, 239
Phenoxybenzamine HCl (Dibenzyline)			25 ± 5	12			No data available	109

Continued.

Table E-1. Relationship of drugs to breast milk and effect on infant—cont'd

Drug	Ratings AAPed.	Ratings Scand.	Oral Bioavail. (%)	Peak serum time (hours)	Half-life (hours)	Amount in milk after therapeutic dose	Comments	References
Prazosin (Minipress)			57 ± 10	3	2.9 ± 0.8	Excreted into milk in small amts.; vol. of distrib. 0.60 L/kg		109, 239
Procainamide (Pronestyl)	IV		83 ± 16	1.75 ± 0.25	3.0 ± 0.6	M/P 4.3 ± 2.4; active metabolite N-acetyl procainamide half-life 6.0 ± 0.2, M/P 3.8 ± 1.8	Both absorbed by infant; half-life of drug and metabolite 3–4 times longer in infant	31, 109, 202, 239
Propranolol (Inderal)			36 ± 10	2.5 ± 0.5 (single dose); 3 (maint. dose)	3.9 ± 0.4	M/P 0.2–1.65; peak 2–3 h after dose; infant would get approx. 1% of adult dose in 24 h; half-life of drug in milk 6.5 ± 3.4 h; active metabolites excreted into milk M/P 0.02–0.45	Insignificant amt.; infants reported had no symptoms noted; should watch for hypoglycemia and/or beta-blocking effects; cord blood level needs to be considered regarding accumulation; at 40 mg QID max. to infant is 21 µg/24 h or less than 0.1% of maternal dose	15, 30, 109, 117, 173, 202, 278
Quinidine (Duraquin, Quinaglute)	3	II	75 ± 20	2 (maintained for 12 h)	6.2 ± 1.8	M/P 0.71 ± 0.91	Arrhythmia may occur; may accumulate; milk levels 6.4–8.2 µg/ml when maternal serum 9.0 µg/ml	7, 31, 49, 109, 130, 227, 239
Reserpine (Serpasil)	3	II				M/S 1	May produce galactorrhea, lethargy, diarrhea, or	7, 31, 223,

Drug	Route						References
Verapamil (Calan)	IV	19 ± 12	1.5 ± 0.5	4.8 ± 2.4; with multiple doses there is a greater than 2 times decrease in clearance and prolonged half-life	M/P 0.23–0.94; active metabolite norverapamil M/P 0.25–0.36; vol. of distrib. 4.0 L/kg	Level in infant 2.1 ng/ml; dissipating (less than 1 ng/ml) 38 h; no effect in infant	11, 31, 49, 109, 138, 163, 197, 239

Diagnostic materials and procedures

Drug	Route						References
Barium						Not absorbed	
Iopanoic acid (Telepaque)	3				0.08% of dose	Not sufficient to produce problem in infant in single dose; contains iodine radical	7, 49, 134, 223
Iothalamate				40 min with normal renal function		Water-soluble radiographic contrast media; has been used in newborns IV for angiographic procedures; causes metallic taste (?); flavors milk; may cause transient rejection of milk	244, 312
Metrizamide (Amipaque)	3		6		M/P 1; 0.02% of dose in milk in 44.3 h	High conc. of organically bound iodine (48%); excretion minimal in milk over 2 d (high mol wt)	7, 49, 71, 136

Continued.

Table E-1. Relationship of drugs to breast milk and effect on infant—cont'd

Drug	Ratings AAPed.	Ratings Scand.	Oral Bioavail. (%)	Peak serum time (hours)	Half-life (hours)	Amount in milk after therapeutic dose	Comments	References
Radioactive compounds								
Radioactive sodium	2					0.5%–1.3% of dose/ L; peak at 2 h; detectable for 96 h	Diminished after 24 h; discontinue nursing 24–96 h	7
[⁶⁷Ga] citrate	2						Discontinue nursing until ⁶⁷Ga has cleared, usually 24 h; may have activity 2 wks	7, 159
Iodine isotopes							Iodine concentrated in milk	49, 195, 246
¹²³I					5.8	≤10%	Discontinue feeding for 24–36 h	124
¹²⁵I							Interrupt breastfeeding for 3–4 wks	4
¹³¹I						3% of dose excreted into milk; 1.5% of dose will appear within 4 h; effective half-life 4.0 ± 1.8	Suggest giving infant 60–100 mg KI,* nurse infant, give mother isotope, and discard next 3 milk fractions; another reference advises to discontinue breastfeeding for 36 h if test dosage was used; if therapeutic dose was taken, discontinue for 2 wk	4, 203, 313

^{90}Sr	2	M/P 0.1	Less than in cow's milk; bottle-fed infant doubles stores in 1 mo	7, 320
^{99m}Tc	2	Half-life in milk 3.5 ± 0.5	Kinetics and amt. in milk depend on molecular carrier; feed just before receiving isotope and discard next 3 milk fractions; only first fraction needs to be discarded if using RBC, DTPA, or MDP*	4, 7, 207
Tuberculin test			Tuberculin-sensitive mothers can adoptively immunize their infants through breast milk, and that immunity may last several years	204
X rays			No effect	
Diuretics				
Acetazolamide (Diamox)	2	No specific data available, but probably similar to sulfonamide	Acts as enzyme inhibitor on carbonic anhydrase nonbacteriostatic sulfonamide; observe only for dehydration and electrolyte loss by monitoring urine and turgor	259

*RBC, Red blood cell; DTPA, diethylenetriaminepenta acetic acid; MDP, methylene diphospate; KI, potassium iodide.

Continued.

Table E-1. Relationship of drugs to breast milk and effect on infant—cont'd

| Drug | Ratings | | Oral Bioavail. (%) | Peak serum time (hours) | Half-life (hours) | Amount in milk after therapeutic dose | Comments | References |
	AAPed.	Scand.						
Amiloride (Midamor)		IV		3.5 ± 0.5	7.5 ± 1.5			31, 239
Bendroflu-methiazide	3	IV				Excreted into milk	Suppresses lactation in women who do not wish to breastfeed	7, 31, 71, 239
Chlorothiazide	3	III	Dose dependent; 1 g, 9%; 50 g, 56%		1.5 ± 0.2	Linear relationship between plasma and milk	May suppress lactation in first few mo; less than 1 mg to baby daily; therapeutic dose in neonates 20 mg/kg/d; displaces bilirubin from albumin significantly; requires higher dose in mother	7, 31, 49, 109, 196, 208, 315, 316
Chlorthalidone (Hygroton)	3	III	64 ± 10		44 ± 10	M/P 0.03–0.04; excreted slowly	May suppress lactation in first few mo; maternal dose 50 mg/d; infant receives 180 ng; it is sequestered in RBC so half-life longer in blood than plasma	7, 31, 109, 208
Ethacrynic acid		IV				No data; may impair lactation	Potent competitor for albumin binding sites; however, safe to give directly to neonate in dose of 1 mg/kg	31, 59, 123, 315

Drug							References
Furosemide (sulfamoylanthranilic acid sulfonamide) (Lasix)	I		61 ± 17	1.5 ± 0.15	Not found in breast milk; vol. of distrib. 0.2 L/kg	Drug given to children under medical management; slow plasma clearance in premature infant; displaces bilirubin from albumin	31, 109, 223, 251, 271, 292, 315
Hydrochlorothiazide	(III)		71 ± 15	2.5 ± 0.2	50 mg/d maternal dose; peaked 4 h after dose of 100 ng/ml; mean level 80 ng/ml	Daily dose to infant 0.05 mg; level in infant undetectable (less than 20 ng/ml)	31, 109, 196
Isosorbide (Dilatrate)			22 ± 14	IV 0.34; sublingual 1.0; oral 4.0	Not known if excreted into milk	2 metabolites: 2-mononitrate half-life 2.3 ± 0.8 h; 5-mononitrate half-life 4.8 ± 0.8 h	109, 239
Mercurial diuretics (Dicurin, Thiomerin)			Low—0			In addition to diuretic effect, there is risk of mercury deposition; however, drug not absorbed orally	223
Spironolactone (Aldactone) (Metabolite canrenone)	3	III	Canrenone 3 ± 1	Canrenone has 2 phases: 7.5 ± 4.5 rapid; 54 ± 42 slow	Canrenone appears; M/P 0.5–0.7; only 0.2% of maternal dose appears in milk	Spironolactone rapidly and extensively metabolized to canrenone, which has some activity; acts as antagonist of aldosterone; causes sodium excretion and potassium retention	7, 31, 49, 238, 239

Continued.

Table E-1. Relationship of drugs to breast milk and effect on infant—cont'd

Drug	Ratings AAPed.	Ratings Scand.	Oral Bioavail. (%)	Peak serum time (hours)	Half-life (hours)	Amount in milk after therapeutic dose	Comments	References
Thiazides (Diuril, Enduron, Esdrix, Hydrodiuril, Thi-uretic tab-lets) (See chlorothia-zide)	3					Linear relationship be-tween plasma and milk; in 1 L of milk at 0.1 mg/100 ml there would be 1 mg/d; infant dose is 20 mg/kg/d.	Risk of dehydration and electrolyte imbalance, especially sodium loss, which would require monitoring; watching weight and wet diapers and taking occasional specific gravity of urine and serum sodium would assure status of infant; risk, however, is extremely low; may suppress lactation due to dehydration in mother	3, 59, 316
Triameterene (Dyrenium)			54 ± 12	3	4.2 ± 0.7	Appears in animal milk; not known if appears in human milk	Hydroxytriamterene is ac-tive metabolite; half-life of 3.1 ± 1.2 h	109, 239
Environmental agents								
Aldrin	4					Varies by location	Not a reason to wean from breast; no need to test milk unless inordinate exposure	7, 25
Benzene hexa-chloride (BHC)	4					Varies by location	Not a reason to wean from breast; no need to test milk unless inordinate exposure	7, 25

Substance		Level in milk	Comments	References
Cadmium		3–34 μg/L	Has been found in milk of mothers who smoke	53, 327
Carbon disulfide (volatile solvent)		22–306 μg/L after commercial exposure	Neurovascular and cardiovascular toxin; infant's urine contained 16–71 μg/L; also found on hands and clothing of mothers	55
Chlordane	4	Metabolizes to oxychlordane		7, 265
Chromium		Approx. 0.4 μg/L	Toxicant 5–15 μg/d; half-life in milk 6 ± 1 h for 97%–99% of dose; longer for rest of dose	4, 327
Dichlorodiphenyltrichloroethane (DDT or DDE)	4	Varies by location (gen'l. pop. 70–170 μg/L); M/P 6–7	Not a reason to wean from breast; no need to test milk unless inordinate exposure	7, 257, 327, 329
Dieldrin	4	Varies by location (gen'l. pop. 2–7 μg/L); M/P 6	Also found in permanently mothproofed garments; avoid these; not a reason to wean	7, 25, 265, 327
Heptachlorepoxide	4	Varies by location (gen'l. pop. 2–9 μg/L)	Not a reason to wean from breast; no need to test milk unless inordinate exposure; found in 63% of samples	7, 25, 265, 327

Continued.

Table E-1. Relationship of drugs to breast milk and effect on infant—cont'd

Drug	Ratings AAPed.	Ratings Scand.	Oral Bioavail. (%)	Peak serum time (hours)	Half-life (hours)	Amount in milk after therapeutic dose	Comments	References
Hexachloro-benzene (HCB)	4					Varies by location	Not a reason to wean from breast; no need to test milk unless inordinate exposure; avoid breast-feeding if exposure is heavy and excessive	7, 25
Malathion		IV				Not detected <5 ppb in milk of mothers living where sprayed for 3 mo	Allowable level in cow's milk is 500 ppb	31, 178
Methyl mer-cury	4					500–1000 ng/ml; M/P 0.9; with heavy exposure M/P 8.6	Infant blood level 600 ng/ml in heavy exposure; only in excessive exposure is testing and/or weaning necessary	7, 9, 327
Mirex						Not found in measurable amounts		265
Nitrate						0.023 mM after evening meal	Nitrate is concentrated in saliva but not in milk; high levels cause methemoglobinemia	113
Oxychlordane						Found in 74% of samples of genl. pop.: approx. 3 μg/L	Toxicant 5 μg/L	327
IV Polybromi-nated	4					Varies by location; M/P 3	If mother is at high risk from the environment or	6, 7, 221, 222,

Agent				References
biphenyl (PBB) IV Polychlorinated biphenyl (PCB)		Varies by location; M/P 4–10; positive correlation between conc. in milk and its fat content; the more in mother's milk, the more in infant's tissue	the diet, milk sample should be measured; if level in milk is high, then breastfeeding should be discontinued; those at risk are (1) workers who handle PBB/PCB, (2) individuals who eat game fish from contaminated waters; crash diets mobilize fats and should be avoided, especially if PBB or PCB is present	257, 319
^{90}Sr ^{89}Sr (strontium)		0.1 of that in maternal diet	Cow's milk has 6 times as much as human milk; cow's milk–fed infant doubles amt. in body in 1 mo	286, 320
Tetrachloroethylene (PCE) (cleaning solvent)	4	Depends on exposure; detectable for 2 wks; 1 mg/100 ml when blood was 0.3 mg/100 ml	1 h after exposure at cleaning plant mother had 10 ppm in milk; infant developed severe jaundice	7, 22, 327
Gastrointestinal agents				
Aloin		Low	Occasionally gave symptoms; caused colic and diarrhea in infant	301

Continued.

Table E-1. Relationship of drugs to breast milk and effect on infant—cont'd

Drug	Ratings		Oral Bioavail. (%)	Peak serum time (hours)	Half-life (hours)	Amount in milk after therapeutic dose	Comments	References
	AAPed.	Scand.						
Anthraquinone laxatives (such as dihydroxy-anthraqui-none) (Dorbane and Dorbantyl)						High	Caused colic and diarrhea in infant	128
Calomel						None	None	301
Cascara						Low	Caused colic and diarrhea in infant	49, 223
Diphenoxylate HCl			Tablet 90% of liquid	2	13 ± 1	Metabolite, diphenox-ylic acid, is excreted into milk	Related to narcotic meper-idine	49, 239
Metoclopra-mide (Octamide, Reglan)			80 ± 15.5	1.5 ± 0.5	5.5 ± 0.5	At 2 hours, M/P 1.8; mean amt. in milk is 125 ng/ml	May see sedation and poor feeding in infant	174, 239, 251
Milk of mag-nesia	I					None	No effect	31, 128
Mineral oil						None	No effect	128
Phenol-phthalein	II					Reports differ	Reported to cause symp-toms in some	31, 301
Rhubarb						None	None in syrup form; fresh rhubarb may give symp-	301

			toms of colic and diarrhea	
Saline cathartics		None	No effect	128
Senna		Measurable	17% of infants showed diarrhea and colic	26, 115, 301
Stool softeners and bulk-forming laxatives		None	No effect	128
Suppositories (for constipation)		None	Not absorbed	273
Heavy metals and other elements				
Arsenic		Can be measured for given patient	Can accumulate; check infant's blood level if there is reason to suspect exposure	16
Bromide	4	Appears in milk	Weakness; bromide rash	7, 49, 251, 303
Copper		Appears in milk		16
Fluorine		0–0.35 ppm, depending on local water levels	Supplementation not required if water is treated; when mother received 25 mg Na fluoride (11.25 mg fluoride); breastfed infant had 30 µg/d or 0.2% of dose	239, See Appendix L

Continued.

Table E-1. Relationship of drugs to breast milk and effect on infant—cont'd

Drug	Ratings AAPed.	Ratings Scand.	Oral Bioavail. (%)	Peak serum time (hours)	Half-life (hours)	Amount in milk after therapeutic dose	Comments	References
Iron						Appears in milk		
Lead	4					26–29 µg/L; M/P 1	Nursing contraindicated if maternal serum 40 µg; conflicting reports, breast milk not always cause of lead poisoning in breastfed infant	7, 85, 236, 327
Magnesium							Not sufficient to be toxic	16
Mercury	4						Hazardous to infant	7, 223
Hormones, antithyroid, contraceptives, and steroids								
Betamethasone (Celestone)		II	72		5.6 ± 0.8	Vol. of distrib. 1.4 L/kg		31
Carbimazole (Neo-Mercazole)	3	II			Of methimazole 9.5 ± 3.5	0.47%–16% of dose; peak of methimazole in milk 3 ± 1 h	May cause goiter; sufficient in milk to depress thyroid; methimazole is metabolite that appears in milk; discarding milk produced 2–4 h after taking medication will reduce amt. infant receives	7, 31, 182, 261
Chlormethiazole						0.01–3.23 µg/ml	Drug detected in 3 of 27 blood samples of nursed	251

Drug		Category					Comments	References
Chlorotriani- sene (Tace)	3						Has estrogenic effect, al- though does not change consistency of milk; may have feminizing ef- fect on infant	7
Chlorprop- amide (Diabinese)		IV	Greater than 90	3 ± 1	Acid urine 69 ± 26; basic urine 13 ± 3	Following 500 mg oral dose, amount in milk after 5 h is 5 µg/ml		31, 49, 109, 239
Contraceptives (Oral)							May diminish milk sup- ply and its nitrogen and protein content; no change in compo- sition or volume if progesterone only contraceptive used; Velaquez showed no difference when mothers took noreth- indrone; contracep- tives isolated from in- fant's serum; most significant concern is long-range impact of hormone on young infant, which is not certain; reports of feminization of infant	7, 31, 48, 74, 263, 272, 307
Ethinyl es- tradiol	3	III						
Mestranol		III						
19-Nortes- tosterone								
Norethin- drone (Noriutin)								
Norethy- nodrel (Enovid)	3							
Cortico- tropin		IV					Destroyed in gastroin- testinal tract of infant; no effect	31, 59

Continued.

Table E-1. Relationship of drugs to breast milk and effect on infant—cont'd

Drug	Ratings AAPed.	Ratings Scand.	Oral Bioavail. (%)	Peak serum time (hours)	Half-life (hours)	Amount in milk after therapeutic dose	Comments	References
Cortisone		III			10 ± 2	Appears in breast milk	Animal studies show 50% lower weight than controls and retarded sexual development and exophthalmos	31, 59, 109
Cyclosporine			34 ± 11 variable	3.5	16 ± 8	Appears in breast milk		109, 239
Dexamethasone (Decadron, Hexadrol)		III	78 ± 14		3.0 ± 0.8	Appears in breast milk		31, 109, 239
Dihydrotachysterol (Hytakerol)		IV					May cause hypercalcemia; need monitoring of infant serum and urine calcium	31, 59
Epinephrine (Adrenalin)							Destroyed in GI tract of infant; not absorbed	59
Estrogen	3	III				0.17 μg/100 ml after 1 g	Risks as with oral contraceptives	7, 31, 159
Fluoxymesterone					9.2		Suppresses lactation; masculinizing	223

Drug			Passage into milk	Comments	References
(Halotestin, Ora-Testryl, Ultandren)					
Insulin	0		Does not pass into breast milk	Destroyed in GI tract; not absorbed	59, 239
Liothyronine (Cytomel)	II	95 in 4 h	Minimal amount	Synthetic form of natural thyroid	223, 239
Medroxy-progesterone acetate (Provera)	3	II	Not excreted into milk		223
Methimazole	1	9.5 ± 3.5	M/S 1; peaks at 3 ± 1 h	May cause thyroid dysfunction in infant; discarding milk produced 2–4 h after taking medication will reduce amt. infant receives	49, 75, 109, 261
Phenformin HCl			Minimal	Not sufficient to cause symptoms in infant; does not cause hypoglycemia in normal infants; no case reports available	223
Prednisolone (Pediapred)	Rapid 82 ± 13	2.2 ± 0.5	0.07%–0.23% of maternal dose; peak level at 1 h	Authors believe clinically insignificant amt. found in milk (0.14% of dose)	32, 109, 192, 217
Prednisone	80 ± 11	3.6 ± 0.4; metabolite prednisolone 2.2 ± 0.5	Both drug and metabolite appear M/P 0.05–0.25; M/P increases as maternal serum conc. increases; peak amt. at 2 h	If mother takes a high dose of 80 mg/d, infant gets less than 80 μg/d, which is <10% of infant's endogenous cortisol production	32, 49, 109, 150

Continued.

Table E-1. Relationship of drugs to breast milk and effect on infant—cont'd

Drug	Ratings AAPed.	Ratings Scand.	Oral Bioavail. (%)	Peak serum time (hours)	Half-life (hours)	Amount in milk after therapeutic dose	Comments	References
Pregnanediol						Excreted into milk	Unknown risk as with other female hormones over a long period of time	
Propylthio-uracil	3	II			2	M/P 0.1–0.55; 0.025%–0.077% of maternal dose	Probably safe; risk of goiter and agranulocytosis minimal; with present microtechniques for T_3, T_4, and TSH, close monitoring of infant is possible; compared with agents of this type, propylthiouracil is the most compatible with breastfeeding	7, 31, 49, 109, 147
Thiouracil	1					M/P 3	Contraindicated	323
Thyroid and thyroxine							Does not produce adverse symptoms on long-range follow-up; noted to improve milk supply of hypothyroid mothers; no contraindication	223, 311
Tolbutamide (Orinase)			93 ± 10	3.5 ± 0.5	5.9 ± 1.4	M/P 0.09–0.4; max. amt. 20 mg/L noted after chronic dosing with 500 mg bid	Effect on neonate unknown; could cause hypoglycemia; incompatible with nursing	109, 239, 251

Drug								References
Vasopressin (D DAVP)						Very little	Does not parallel serum levels; less than 1 ng/L	54
Narcotics and anti-addiction drugs								
Cocaine				0.5 intranasal; 100 mg total dose	0.71 ± 0.26	Significant level; no drug or metabolite 36 h after mother's last dose; vol. of distrib. 2.1 L/kg	Cocaine and its metabolite, benzoylecgonine, are found in milk and infant's urine, which is negative by 60 h	63, 109
Codeine	3	II			2.75 ± 0.25	0 to trace after 32 mg every 4 h (6 doses); M/P 0.3–2.5; peaks at 1 h; vol. of distrib. > 5 L/kg	No effect in therapeutic level and transient usage; can accumulate; individual variation; watch for neonatal depression	7, 31, 101, 109, 157, 167, 227
Heroin	3					Significant	Amt. in milk sufficient to cause addiction in infant; 13 of 22 infants had withdrawal; historically, breastfeeding had been used to wean addict's infant; this is no longer recommended	7, 49, 59, 69, 226
LSD (lysergic acid diethylamide)	3		High	Rapid	3 h (175 min); IV dose—not dose dependent; clears body in 24 h		Not measured in milk, but compound is basic and milk is acid; similar to ergot, which appears in milk	109, 244

Continued.

Table E-1. Relationship of drugs to breast milk and effect on infant—cont'd

Drug	Ratings AAPed.	Ratings Scand.	Oral Bioavail. (%)	Peak serum time (hours)	Half-life (hours)	Amount in milk after therapeutic dose	Comments	References
Marijuana (Cannabis)						M/S greater than 1; 105–340 ng/ml plus metabolites	Shown in lab. animals to produce structural changes in nursling's brain cells; impairs DNA and RNA formation; infant at risk of inhaling smoke during feeding when held while smoking; found in infant's urine and stools	57, 67, 78, 209, 210, 211, 212, 235
Meperidine (Demerol)	3		52 ± 3		3.2 ± 0.8 and 7	M/P 1.0–1.4; peak level at 2 h; vol. of distrib. 4.4 L/kg	Marked increase in half-life in neonates	7, 109, 216, 251
Methadone	3	II	92 ± 21		35 ± 12	M/P 0.83; peak level 4 h after dose; results obscured if addict also taking herbal root golden seal; vol. of distrib. 3.8 L/kg	One infant death reported from methadone in milk; breastfeed with caution; abrupt cessation of breastfeeding on methadone may produce signs of opiate withdrawal	7, 31, 41, 49, 164, 277
Morphine	3	II	26.5 ± 6.5		3.0 ± 1.2; elimination half-life in infant's plasma markedly	M/P 0.23 half-h after dose; 5.07 12 h after dose; max. amt. 19 µg/L; vol. of distrib. 3.3 L/kg	Single doses have minimal effect; potential for accumulation; may be addicting to neonate; no longer considered appropriate means of	7, 31, 109, 216, 251

				increased		weaning infant of an addict	
Naloxone	IV	About 2; absorption is 91%, but hepatic first pass metabolism destroys most of drug		1.07 ± 0.20 adults; 3.1 ± 0.5 neonate	Not known if excreted into milk; vol. of distrib. 2.0 L/kg		31, 109, 239
Phencyclidine (PCP)				24–89 h; may take 2 wks to clear maternal system	In one case, 9 d after delivery and more than 42 d after exposure, 3.9 ng/ml; M/P 10 in mouse milk	Infant was not breastfed	152, 219, 274
Triazolam (Halcion)		55	1.3	2.3 ± .04	Not known if excreted into human milk; found in rat milk		109, 239
Zuclopenthixol					M/S 3.4	Amt. in milk is very low	1
Psychotropic and mood-changing drugs							
Alprazolam (Xanax)		Readily absorbed	1.5 ± 0.5	10.6 ± 3.1	Probably excreted into milk		109, 239
Amoxapine 3 (Asendin)	3	100	1.5	8; metabolites active up to 30 h	M/P in 1 patient less than 0.21	Major metabolite is 8-hydroxyamoxepine with half-life of 30 h; M/P 0.37; widely distributed to all tissues	7, 107, 239

Continued.

Table E-1. Relationship of drugs to breast milk and effect on infant—cont'd

Drug	Ratings		Oral Bioavail. (%)	Peak serum time (hours)	Half-life (hours)	Amount in milk after therapeutic dose	Comments	References
	AAPed.	Scand.						
Amphetamine	3						Has caused stimulation in infants with jitteriness, irritability, sleepless- ness; long-acting prepa- rations cumulative	7, 16, 157, 159, 310
Benzodiazepines	Alcohol enhances the effect of this group of drugs; vol. of distrib. >10 L/kg							
Chlordiaz- epoxide HCl (Librium)	3	II	100		10.0 ± 3.4 (G&G) 36 ± 12 (PDR)	Appears in breast milk	Benzodiazepines are de- toxified by glucuronyl system; in first wks of life, may contribute to jaundice; effect on in- fant: hypoventilation, drowsiness, lethargy, weight loss; single doses over 10 mg con- traindicated; accumula- tion in infant possible; symptoms more likely if drug consumed during pregnancy; withdrawal possible; dose greater than 30 mg should be avoided; desmethyldiaz- epam is active metabo- lite of diazepam and pinazepam; it is metab- olized to oxazepam, which has been detected	7, 31, 46, 49, 56, 58, 70, 96, 109, 149, 232, 234, 239
Diazepam (Valium)	3	III	100 ± 14		43 ± 13	M/P 0.2-2.7		
Desmeth- yldiaze- pam	3				62 ± 16	M/P 0.2-2.7		
Oxazepam	3	II	Greater than 90		15.45 ± 9.55	M/P 0.1-0.33; max. amt. 0.001% of ma- ternal dose		
Pinazepam	3					Not found in breast milk		

Drug	Schedule	Oral availability	Peak time	Half-life	Milk	Comments	References
Lorazepam (Ativan)	II	93 ± 10	2		Appears in low conc. in milk	in urine of infants exposed to high doses during lactation. An increased half-life found in neonate	31, 49, 109, 239, 318
Butalbital		Good		35	Appears in milk	Serum levels in infant much lower than therapeutic dose	239
Caffeine	3	100 ± 13		4.9 ± 1.8	M/P 0.48–0.82; about 1% of total dose in breast milk; peak milk level at 1 h; vol. of distrib. 0.6 L/kg	Half-life greater in neonates; irritability; poor sleeping pattern found; excreted slowly; no anticipated adverse reactions in occasional dose	7, 109, 203, 251, 326
Chloral hydrate (Nostec, Somnos)	II		0.75 after rectal dose	Trichloroethanol half-life 6.75 ± 2.75	M/P of drug 0–3; max. amt. 15 µg/ml; M/P of trichloroethanol 0.6–0.8	Trichloroethanol is active metabolite to which effects can be attributed; drug can be given to infant directly	31, 34, 49, 109, 168, 251
Chlorprothixene (Taractan)	IV				M/P 1.2–2.6; infant gets 0.1% of maternal dose	Ratio between the desmethyl metabolite and the drug in maternal plasma is 3.9 ± 2.4 and in milk is 1.6 ± 0.6	31, 188, 239
Dextroamphetamine (Dexedrine)			2 h; 31.2 ± 2 ng/ml	11 ± 0.75	M/P 2.8–7.5	Found in infant's urine	49, 239, 284

Continued.

Table E-1. Relationship of drugs to breast milk and effect on infant—cont'd

| Drug | Ratings | | Oral Bioavail. (%) | Peak serum time (hours) | Half-life (hours) | Amount in milk after therapeutic dose | Comments | References |
	AAPed.	Scand.						
Diethylpropion (Tenuate, Tepanil)						Drug and its metabolites appear in human milk		239
Dyphylline (Lufyllin)	3			0.75	1.95 ± 0.15	M/P 2	Single 5 mg/kg dose produced M/P; milk and serum clearance equivalent	49, 141, 239
Ethanol	3		100		0.24 ± 0.08	M/P 0.9; 1% of maternal dose; peak level in milk 1.5 h; half-life in milk 2.9 h	High amounts of ethanol may suppress lactation; acetaldehyde, a metabolite, is not found in infant, although maternal level rises; activity of alcohol and acetaldehyde dehydrogenase is extremely low in infant so they are more susceptible to alcohol than adults	33, 109, 155, 251
Flurazepam (Dalmane)				0.75 ± 0.25	2.3	Vol. of distrib. 22 L/kg	Active metabolite desalkylflurazepam has half-life of 74 ± 24 h	109, 239
Haloperidol (Haldol)	3	II		70 ± 18	17.9 ± 6.4	M/P 0.6–0.7; 2–5 ng/ml in milk with maternal dose of 12–30 mg/d	A butyrophenone antidepressant; animal studies in nurslings show behavior abnormalities with maternal dose 1 mg/kg; no reported ad-	7, 31, 49, 109, 183, 251, 317

Drug		Route	Absorption	$t_{1/2}$		M/P	verse affects in human nurslings	References
Hydroxyzine (Durrax, Atarax)		IV	Rapidly absorbed	2.0 ± 0.9	20 adults; 7.1 children			31, 233, 239
Lithium carbonate (Eskalith, Lithane, Lithonate)	3	III	100	2 ± 1	22 ± 8	M/P 0.30–1.0; serum level in infant is 10%–50% of mother's	Measurable lithium in infant's serum; infant kidney can clear lithium; however, lithium inhibits adenosine 3',5'-cyclic monophosphate, significant to brain growth; also affects amino acid metabolism; real effects not measurable immediately; report of cyanosis, poor muscle tone, and ECG changes in nursing infant	7, 31, 109, 223, 267, 268, 287, 296, 299, 300
Maprotiline (Ludiomil)		III		12 (9-16 h)	51	M/P 1.0–1.5	A modified tricyclic antidepressant; vol. of distrib. 25 L/kg; pK_a 10.5; 88% protein bound; dry mouth, urinary retention at therapeutic doses	31, 109, 239, 252
Meprobamate (Miltown, Equanil)	3	III			10	M/P 2–4	If therapy continued, infant should be followed closely	7, 10, 31, 223, 239
Methyprylon		IV		1.5 ± 0.5	4		May see sedation and poor feeding in infant	31, 109, 203

Continued.

Table E-1. Relationship of drugs to breast milk and effect on infant—cont'd

Drug	Ratings AAPed.	Ratings Scand.	Oral Bioavail. (%)	Peak serum time (hours)	Half-life (hours)	Amount in milk after therapeutic dose	Comments	References
Monoamine oxidase (MAO) inhibitors (Eutonyl, Nardil)							Inhibits lactation	84
Nicotine	3				2.0 ± 0.7	Range 20–512 ppb; cotinine is a major metabolite of nicotine and can be isolated from infant's urine when smoking women breastfeed or when passive smoking exposure exists; the amount of cotinine in milk is greater than the amount of nicotine	Reported slow initiation of suck and decreased sucking pressure by infant; decreased prolactin and oxytocin response to suckling; fretful and unsettled (carboxyhemoglobin also found in mother and infant)	7, 13, 36, 99, 109, 187, 328, 330
Nortriptyline (Pamelor)	II		51 ± 5		31 ± 13	M/S 0–0.7; excreted into milk in low concentrations	Drug not detected in serum of infant	21, 31, 49, 50, 94, 109
Phenfluridol						Excreted into milk	Animal studies show learning abnormalities in sucklings; this is a potent long-acting oral neuroleptic drug	3, 140

					Amount in milk	Effects	Ref.
Phenothiazines							
Chlorpromazine (Thorazine)	3	II	Vol. of distrib. >30 L/kg 32 ± 19 (single dose); 20 (with repeated doses)	30 ± 7	M/P 0→>1; inconsistent with amts. reported	A galactogogue producing milk in males as well; one report of drowsiness and lethargy when milk contained 92 ng/ml; in most other cases the amount in milk is much less; series of 11 infants whose mothers took avg. 200 mg/d had no effects	7, 18, 19, 31, 38, 49, 109, 322
Fluphenazine (Prolixin)	3					Maternal doses ≤15 mg/d considered safe	19
Mesoridazine (Serentil)	3				Minimal		7, 19, 223
Piperacetazine (Quide)	3				Minimal	Probably no effect	7, 223
Thioridazine (Mellaril)	3	II			Excreted into milk	Drug is less potent in general than other phenothiazines; probably quite safe	7, 31, 56, 223
Trifluoperazine (Stelazine)	3	II			Excreted into milk		7, 31, 239, 251
Prochlorperazine	3	III			Excreted into milk		251

Continued.

Table E-1. Relationship of drugs to breast milk and effect on infant—cont'd

Drug	Ratings AAPed.	Ratings Scand.	Oral Bioavail. (%)	Peak serum time (hours)	Half-life (hours)	Amount in milk after therapeutic dose	Comments	References
Quazepam					32.5 ± 7.5	M/P 4.19; 2 major metabolites: 2-oxoquazepam (half-life 32.5 ± 7.5), M/P 2.02; N-desalkyl-2-oxoquazepam (half-life 72.5 ± 2.5), M/P 0.091	Level of drug and 2-oxo-quazepam decline at same rate in plasma and milk; 0.11% of maternal dose recovered as drug plus metabolites in milk over a 48-h period	129
Secobarbital (seconal sodium)					27.5 ± 12.5	Small amounts excreted into milk		239
Theobromine						M/P 0.82	Max. conc. in milk 7.5 mg/L; reached 2.1–3.3 h after ingesting chocolate	251
Theophylline (Elixophyllin)			96 ± 8		9.0 ± 2.1	M/P 0.7; up to 15% of maternal dose; vol. of distrib. 0.46 L/kg; peak level in milk 2 h	Distributes readily in milk; children under 6 mo of age have extremely low clearance	239, 285
Trazodone			Well absorbed	1 (if on empty stomach; 2 (if taken with food)	Initial 4.5 ± 1.5; final 7.5 ± 2.5	M/P 0.142 ± 0.045; 0.0065% of maternal dose		239, 308
Triazolam (Halcion)			55	1.3	2.3 ± 0.4	Not known if excreted into human milk; found in rat's milk		109, 239

Tricyclic antidepressants

Drug							Comments	Ref.
Amitriptyline HCl (Elavil, Amitril, Endep)	3	III	48 ± 11	4	16 ± 6	M/P 1–1.6; max. amt. 0.15 mg/L; vol. of distrib. 14 L/kg	Active metabolite is nortriptyline; peak serum time 10 h; M/P 0.6; from one case study, no drug detected in infant's urine	7, 21, 31, 49, 50, 239, 241, 251, 324
Desipramine HCl (Norpramin, Pertofrane)	3	II	50		62 ± 16	M/P 0.4–1.2; max. conc. 35 ng/ml; metabolite M/P 1.3–1.6; vol. of distrib. 34 L/kg	Metabolite of imipramine and metabolized into 2-hydroxydesipramine; from study of 1 patient, metabolite/desipramine ratio in maternal plasma is 0.92 ± 0.01 and is 1.1 ± 0.1 in milk; neither drug nor metabolite recovered from infant's urine	7, 31, 49, 109, 281, 282
Doxepin (Adapin, Sinequan)			27 ± 10		17 ± 6	Both drug and metabolite appear in milk. Prefeed M/P 1.08 for drug and 1.02 for metabolite. Postfeed M/P 1.66 for drug and 1.53 for metabolite; 2.2% of maternal dose; vol. of distrib. 20 L/kg	Only metabolite detected in infant's plasma; N-desmethyldoxepin major metabolite; only metabolite detected in infant's plasma	109, 154
Imipramine	3	II				M/P 1; vol. of distrib. 23 L/kg	Desipramine is major metabolite	7, 31, 49, 281

Continued.

Table E-1. Relationship of drugs to breast milk and effect on infant—cont'd

Drug	Ratings AAPed.	Ratings Scand.	Oral Bioavail. (%)	Peak serum time (hours)	Half-life (hours)	Amount in milk after therapeutic dose	Comments	References
Miscellaneous								
Bromocriptine	1					Excreted into milk	Suppresses lactation more effectively than other drugs; 1 case reported of successful lactation while taking 5 mg/d for prolactinoma	49, 166
Bupivacaine (epidural anesthesia) (Marcaine, Sensorcaine)		II	Injection	0.63 ± 0.20	Adults 2.7; neonates 8.1	None identified; limit of measure is less than 0.02 μg/ml; vol. of distrib. 1.05–1.5 L/kg	No symptoms	31, 215, 239
Cimetidine (Tagamet)		III	62 ± 6		1.9 ± 0.3	From one chronic user, M/P 4.6–11.7; max. amt. 6 mg/L	Suppresses gastric acidity and activity; inhibits hepatic metabolism; avoid and seek alternative	31, 109, 203, 251
DPT		IV				Minimal	One case reported: mother breastfed at 3 wks; infant had rapidly decreasing platelets and WBC without affecting mother's levels; does not interfere with immunization schedule	8, 31, 87

Drug						Reference
Enprofylline		1.5		M/P 0.67–0.98; dose for infant is 10% of adult dose	90% of drug is renally excreted by mother	170
Halothane (Fluothane)	II			2 ppm	Nursing mothers who work in environment with halothane should be checked; exposure in operating room while working as an anesthetist; no symptoms in infant	31, 76
Influenza vaccine					A number of antiviral factors are found in human milk; unreported studies indicate flu vaccine no problem and perhaps benefit, especially for infant under 6 mo	61, 190
Isotretinoin (Accutane)		3.2; 2.9 in patients with acne	15 ± 5	Not known if excreted into milk	Major metabolite is 4-oxoisotretinoin; after 6 h, more metabolite than drug in plasma; nursing and taking drug not recommended	239
Poliovirus vaccine	4 IV			Colostrum and early milk may contain antibodies	Live vaccine taken orally; not necessary to withhold nursing before or after dose; no interference at 2, 4, 6, mo of age	31, 73, 80

Continued.

Table E-1. Relationship of drugs to breast milk and effect on infant—cont'd

Drug	Ratings		Oral Bioavail. (%)	Peak serum time (hours)	Half-life (hours)	Amount in milk after therapeutic dose	Comments	References
	AAPed.	Scand.						
Rh antibodies							Destroyed in gastrointestinal tract; not effective orally	157, 159
Smallpox vaccine							Exposure by direct contact; live virus; contraindicated when mother has infant under 1 yr; no longer given to children routinely	8, 60
Rubella virus vaccine	I					Virus may be in milk	Not contraindicated; will not confer passive immunity; mother should not be given vaccine when at risk for pregnancy	8, 31, 60, 127
Thiopentone						M/P 0.391; colostrum/P 0.505		12

REFERENCES

1. Aaes-Jorgensen T, Bjorndal F, and Bartels U: Zuclopenthixol levels in serum and breast milk, Psychopharmacol 90:417, 1986.
2. Adair FL, Hesseltine HC, and Hac LR: Experimental study of the behavior of sulfanilamide, JAMA 111:766, 1938.
3. Ahlenius S, Brown R, and Engel J: Learning deficits in a 4-week-old offspring of nursing mothers treated with neuroleptic drug, penfluridol, Naunyn Schmeidebergs Arch Pharmacol 279:31, 1973.
4. Ahlgren L, Ivarsson S, Johansson L et al: Excretion of radionuclides in human breast milk after the administration of radiopharmaceuticals, J Nucl Med 26:1085, 1985.
5. Akintonwa A, Gbajumo SA, and Biola Mabadeje AF: Placental and milk transfer of chloroquine in humans, Therapeut Drug Monit 10:147, 1988.
6. American Academy of Pediatrics Committee on Environmental Hazards: PCBs in breast milk, Pediatrics 62:407, 1978.
7. American Academy of Pediatrics Committee on Drugs: The transfer of drugs and other chemicals into human breast milk, Pediatrics 72:375, 1983.
8. American College of Obstetrics and Gynecology: Recommendations regarding rubella vaccination for women, ACOG News Jan 1971.
9. Amin-Zaki L et al: Perinatal methylmercury poisoning in Iraq, Am J Dis Child 130:1070, 1976.
10. Ananth J: Side effects in the neonate from psychotropic agents excreted through breast feeding, Am J Psychiatry 135:801, 1978.
11. Andersen HJ: Excretion of verapamil in human milk, Eur J Clin Pharmacol 25:279, 1983.
12. Andersen LW, Quist T, Hertz J, and Mogensen F: Concentrations of thiopentone in mature breast milk and colostrum following an induction dose, Acta Anaesthesiol Scand 31:30, 1987.
13. Anderson AN et al: Suppressed prolactin but normal neurophysin levels in cigarette smoking breastfeeding women, Clin Endocrinol 17:363, 1982.
14. Anderson P: Drugs and breastfeeding: a review, Drug Intell Clin Pharm 11:208, 1977.
15. Anderson P and Salter F: Propranolol therapy during pregnancy and lactation, Am J Cardiol 37:325, 1976.
16. Arena J: Contamination of the ideal food, Nutr Today 5:2, 1970.
17. Arnauld R et al: A study of the passage of trimethoprim into maternal milk, Quest Med 25:959, 1972.
18. Ayd FJ Jr: Children born of mothers treated with chlorpromazine during pregnancy, Clin Med 71:1758, 1964.
19. Ayd F: Excretion of psychotropic drugs in human breast milk, Int Drug Ther News 8:33, 1973.
20. Azad Khan AK and Truelove SC: Placental and mammary transfer of sulphasalazine, Br Med J 2:1553, 1979.
21. Bader TF and Newman K: Amitriptyline in human breast milk and the nursing infant's serum, Am J Psych 137:855, 1980.
22. Bagnell PC and Ellenberger HA: Obstructive jaundice due to a chlorinated hydrocarbon in breast milk, Can Med J 117:1047, 1977.
23. Baier R: Piperacillin in milk, Am Soc Microbiol 1983.
24. Bailey DN, Weilbert RT, and Naylor AJ: A study of salicylate and caffeine excretion in the breast milk of two nursing mothers, J Analyt Tox 6:64, 1982.
25. Bakken A and Seip M: Insecticides in human breast milk, Acta Paediatr Scand 65:535, 1976.
26. Baldwin W: Clinical study of senna administration to nursing mothers: assessment of effects on infant bowel habits, Can Med Assoc J 89:566, 1963.
27. Bardy AH, Granstrom ML, and Hiilesmaa VK: Valproic acid and breastfeeding. In Janz D et al, editors: Epilepsy, pregnancy, and the child, New York, 1982, Raven Press, p 359.
28. Barnett DB, Hudson SA, and McBurney A: Disopyramide and its N-monodesalkyl metabolite in breast milk, Br J Clin Pharmacol 14:310, 1982.
29. Baty JD et al: May mothers taking warfarin breastfeed their infants? Br J Clin Pharmacol 3:969, 1976.
30. Bauer JH et al: Propranolol in human plasma and breast milk, Am J Cardiol 43:860, 1979.
31. Berglund et al: Allocation of drugs to breastfeeding groups, Acta Obstet Gynecol Scand Suppl 126:29, 1984.
32. Berlin CM Jr: The excretion of drugs in human milk. In Schwartz RH and Yaffe SJ, editors: Drugs and chemical risks to the fetus and newborn, New York, 1980, Alan R Liss, Inc, p 115.
33. Berlin CM Jr and Yaffe SJ: Disposition of salicylazosulapyridine (Azulfidine) and metabolites in human breast milk, Dev Pharmacol Ther 1:31, 1980.
34. Bernstine JB, Meyer AE, and Berstine L: Maternal blood and breast milk estimation following the administration of choral hydrate during puerperium, J Obstet Gynaecol Br Emp 63:228, 1956.
35. Bertilsson L and Tomson T: Clinical pharmacokinetics and pharmacological effects of carbamazepine and carbamazepine-10, 11-epoxide, an update, Clin Pharmacolkinet 11:177, 1986.

36. Bisdom W: Alcohol and nicotine poisoning in nurslings, JAMA 109:178, 1937.

37. Bitzen PO et al: Excretion of Paracetamol in human breast milk, Eur J Clin Pharmacol 20:123, 1981.

38. Blacker KH, Weinstein BJ, and Ellman GL: Mother's milk and chlorpromazine, Am J Psychiatry 119:178, 1962.

39. Blanco JD et al: Ceftazidime levels in human breast milk, Antimicrob Agents Chemother 23:479, 1983.

40. Bleyer WA and Breckenridge RT: Studies on the detection of adverse drug reactions in the newborn. II. The effect of prenatal aspirin on newborn hemostasis, JAMA 213:2049, 1970.

41. Blinick G et al: Methadone assays in pregnant women and progeny, Am J Obstet Gynecol 121:617, 1975.

42. Boreus LO et al: Terbutaline in breast milk, Br J Clin Pharmacol 13:731, 1982.

43. Bossi L: Neonatal period including drug disposition in newborns: review of the literature. In Janz D, editor: Epilepsy, pregnancy, and the child, New York, 1982, Raven Press, p 327.

44. Boutroy MJ, Bianchetti G, Dubruc C et al: To nurse when receiving acebutolol: is it dangerous for the neonate? Eur J Clin Nutr 30:737, 1986.

45. Brambel C and Hunter R: Effect of dicumarol on the nursing infant, Am J Obstet Gynecol 59:1153, 1950.

46. Brandt R: Passage of diazepam and desmethyl-diazepam into breast milk, Arzneim Forsch 26:454, 1976.

47. Branski D, Kerem E, Gross-Kieselstein E et al: Bloody diarrhea—a possible complication of sulfasalazine transferred through human breast milk, J Pediatr Gastroenterol Nutr 5:316, 1986.

48. Briggs M and Briggs M: Oral contraceptives and vitamin nutrition, Lancet 1:1436, 1974.

49. Briggs GG, Freeman RK, and Yaffe SJ: Drugs in pregnancy and lactation, ed 2, Baltimore, 1986, Williams & Wilkins Co.

50. Brixen-Rasmussen L, Halgrener J, and Jorgensen A: Amitriptyline and nortriptyline excretion in human breast milk, Psychopharmacology (Berlin) 76:94, 1982.

51. Buchanan R et al: The breast milk excretion of mefenamic acid, Curr Ther Res 10:592, 1968.

52. Buchanan RA et al: The breast milk excretion of flufenamic acid, Curr Ther Res 11:533, 1969.

53. Buchet JP, Roels H, Hubermon G, and Lauwerys R: Placental transfer of lead, mercury, cadmium, and carbon monoxide in women, Envir Res 15:494, 1978.

54. Burrow GN et al: DDAVP treatment of diabetes insipidus during pregnancy and post-partum period, Acta Endocrinol 97:23, 1981.

55. Cai SX and Bao YS: Placenta transfer, secretion into mother's milk of carbon disulphide and the effects on maternal function of female viscose rayon workers, Ind Health 19:15, 1981.

56. Calabrese JR and Gulledge AD: Psychotropics during pregnancy and lactation: a review, Psychosomatics 26:413, 1985.

57. Campbell AMG et al: Cerebral atrophy in young *Cannabis* smokers, Lancet 2:1219, 1971.

58. Catz CS: Diazepam in breast milk, Drug Ther Jan 1973.

59. Catz CS and Giacola G: Drugs and breast milk, Pediatr Clin North Am 19:151, 1972.

60. Center for Disease Control: Recommendations of the Immunization Advisory Committee, rubella prevention, Ann Intern Med 101:505, 1984.

61. Center for Disease Control: Recommendations of the Immunization Practices Advisory Committee, prevention and control of influenza, MMWR 35:317, 1986; MMWR 35:317, 1986b.

62. Chan V, Tse TF, and Wong V: Transfer of digoxin across the placenta and into breast milk, Br J Obstet Gynaecol 85:605, 1978.

63. Chasnoff IJ, Lewis DE, and Squires L: Cocaine intoxication in a breastfed infant, Pediatrics 80:836, 1987.

64. Chhabra S and Kurup CKR: Maternal transport of chlorophenoxyisobutyrate at the fetal and neonatal stages of development, Biochem Pharmacol 27:2063, 1978.

65. Cho N, Nakayama T, Vehara K, and Kunii K: Laboratory and clinical evaluation of ticarcillin in the field of obstetrics and gynecology, Chemotherapy (Tokyo) 25:2911, 1977.

66. Clark JH and Wilson WG: A 16-day-old breastfed infant with metabolic acidosis caused by salicylate, Clin Pediatr 20:53, 1980.

67. Clark L, Hughes R, and Nakashima E: Behavioral effects of marijuana: experimental studies, Arch Gen Psychiatry 23:193, 1970.

68. Clyde D and Shute G: Transfer of pyrimethamine in human milk, J Trop Med Hyg 59:277, 1956.

69. Cobrink RW, Hood T, and Chusid E: The effect of maternal narcotic addiction on the newborn infant, Pediatrics 24:288, 1956.

70. Cole AP and Hailey DM: Diazepam and active metabolite in breast milk and their transfer to the neonate, Arch Dis Child 50:741, 1975.

71. Committee on Drugs, American Academy of Pediatrics: The transfer of drugs and other chemicals into human breast milk, Pediatrics 72:375, 1983.

72. Committee on Drugs, American Academy of Pediatrics: Emergency drug doses for infants and children, Pediatrics 81:462, 1988.

73. Committee on Infectious Disease, American

Academy of Pediatrics: Red book, ed 20, Elk-grove Ill, 1986, American Academy of Pediatrics.

74. Cooke ID, Back DJ, and Shroff NE: Norethisterone concentration in breast milk and infant and maternal plasma during ethynodiol diacetate administration, Contraception 31:611, 1985.

75. Cooper DS: Antithyroid drugs, N Engl J Med 311:1353, 1984.

76. Cote CJ et al: Trace concentrations of halothane in human breast milk, Br J Anaesthesiol 48:541, 1976.

77. Cruikshank DP, Varner MW, and Pitkin RM: Breast milk magnesium and calcium concentrations following magnesium sulfate treatment, Am J Obstet Gynecol 143:685, 1982.

78. Crumpton E and Brill N: Personality factors associated with frequency of marijuana use, Calif Med 115:11, 1971.

79. Curry SH et al: Disposition of glutethimide, Clin Pharmacol Ther 12:849, 1971.

80. Deforest A et al: The effect of breast-feeding on the antibody response of infants to trivalent oral poliovirus vaccine, J Pediatr 83:93, 1973.

81. deSwiet M and Lewis PJ: Excretion of anticoagulants in human milk, N Engl J Med 297:1471, 1977.

82. Devlin RG and Fleiss PMP: Captopril in human blood and breast milk, J Clin Pharmacol 21:110, 1981.

83. Devun RG, Duchin KL, and Fleiss PM: Nadolol in human serum and breast milk, Br J Clin Pharmacol 12:393, 1981.

84. Dickey RP and Stone SC: Drugs that affect the breast and lactation, Clin Obstet Gynecol 18:95, 1975.

85. Dillon H, Wilson D, and Schaffner W: Lead concentrations in human milk, Am J Dis Child 128:491, 1974.

86. Drinkwater P: Metronidazole, Aust NZ J Obstet Gynaecol 27:228, 1987.

87. Durodola JI: Administration of cyclophosphamide during late pregnancy and early lactation: a case report, J Natl Med Assoc 71:165, 1979.

88. Eckstein HB and Jack B: Breast-feeding and anticoagulant therapy, Lancet 1:672, 1970.

89. Edstein MD, Veenendaal JR, Newman K, and Hyslop R: Excretion of chloroquine, dapsone, and pyrimethamine in human milk, Br J Clin Pharmacol 22:733, 1986.

90. Eeg-Olofsson O et al: Convulsions in a breast-fed infant after maternal indomethacin, Lancet 2:215, 1978.

91. Egan PC et al: Doxorubicin and cisplatin excretion into human milk, Can Treat Rpts 69:1387, 1985.

92. Elliott GT and Quinn SI: Sulfisoxazole in human milk, Eur J Pediatr 99:171, 1981.

93. Erickson SH, Oppheim GL, and Smith GH: Metronidazole in breast milk, Obstet Gynecol 57:48, 1981.

94. Erickson SH, Smith GH, and Heidrich F: Tricyclics and breastfeeding, Am J Psychiatry 136:1483, 1979.

95. Eriksson G and Swahn C: Concentrations of baclofen in serum and breast milk from a lactating woman, Scand J Clin Lab Invest 41:185, 1981.

96. Erkkola R and Kanto J: Diazepam and breast-feeding, Lancet 1:1235, 1972.

97. Ette EI, Essien EE, Ogonor JI, and Brown-Awala EA: Chloroquine in human milk, J Clin Pharmacol 27:499, 1987.

98. Evaldson GR, Lindgren S, Nord CE, and Rane AT: Tinidazole milk excretion and pharmacokinetics in lactating women, Br J Clin Pharmacol 19:503, 1985.

99. Ferguson B, Wilson DJ, and Schaffner W: Determination of nicotine concentrations in human milk, Am J Dis Child 130:837, 1976.

100. Fidler J, Smith V, and DeSwiet M: Excretion of oxprenolol and timolol in breast milk, Br J Obstet Gynaecol 90:961, 1983.

101. Findlay JWA et al: Analgesic drugs in breast milk and plasma, Clin Pharmacol Ther 29:625, 1981.

102. Findlay JWA et al: Pseudoephedrine and triprolidine in plasma and breast milk of nursing mothers, Br J Clin Pharmacol 18:901, 1984.

103. Finley JP et al: Digoxin excretion in human milk, J Pediatr 94:339, 1979.

104. Fleiss PM, Richwald GA, and Gordon J: Aztreonam in human serum and breast milk, Br J Clin Pharmacol 19:509, 1985.

105. Fuchs F: Prevention of prematurity, Am J Obstet Gynecol 126:809, 1976.

106. Gaginella TS: Drugs and the nursing mother-infant, US Pharmacol 3:39, 1978.

107. Gelenberg AJ: Amoxapine, a new antidepressant, appears in human milk, J Nerv Ment Dis 167:635, 1979.

108. Gerding DN and Peterson LR: Comparative tissue and extra vascular fluid concentrations of ceftizoxime, J Antimicrob Chemother 10(suppl C):105, 1982.

109. Goodman L and Gilman A, editors: The pharmacological basis of therapeutics, ed 7, New York, 1985, The Macmillan Co.

110. Graf VH and Reimann S: Untersuchungen uber die konzentration von pyrrolidino-methyl-tetracycline in der muttermilch, Dtsch Med Wochenschr 84:1694, 1959.

111. Granstrom ML, Bardy AH, and Hiilesmaa VK: Prolonged feeding difficulties of infants of primidone mothers during neonatal period: prelimi-

nary results from prospective Helsinki study. In Janz D et al, editors: Epilepsy, pregnancy, and the child, New York, 1982, Raven Press, p 357.

112. Gray MS, Kane PO, and Squires S: Further observations on metronidazole (Flagyl), Br J Vener Dis 37:278, 1961.

113. Green LC, Tannenbaum SR, and Fox JG: Nitrate in human and canine milk, N Engl J Med 306:1367, 1982.

114. Greene H, Burkhart B, and Hobby G: Excretion of penicillin in human milk following parturition, Am J Obstet Gynecol 51:732, 1946.

115. Greenhalf JO and Leonard HS: Laxatives in the treatment of constipation in pregnant and breastfeeding mothers, Practitioner 210:259, 1973.

116. Guilbeau JA et al: Aureomycin in obstetrics: therapy and prophylaxis, JAMA 143:520, 1950.

117. Habib A and McCarthy JS: Effects on the neonate of propranolol administered during pregnancy, J Pediatr 91:808, 1977.

118. Hac LR, Adair FL, and Hesseltine HC: Excretion of sulfanilamide and acetylsulfanilamide in human breast milk, Am J Obstet Gynecol 38:57, 1939.

119. Hardell LI, Lindstrom B, Lonnerholm G, and Osterman PO: Pyridostigmine in human breast milk, Br J Clin Pharmacol 14:565, 1982.

120. Hartikainen-Sorri AL, Heikkinen JE, and Koivisto M: Pharmacokinetics of clonidine during pregnancy and nursing, Obstet Gynecol 69:598, 1987.

121. Hauser GJ, Almog S, Tirosh M, and Spirer Z: Effect of alpha-methyldopa excreted in human milk on the breastfed infant, Helv Paediatr Acta 40:83, 1985.

122. Havelka J et al: Excretion of chloramphenicol in human milk, Chemotherapy 13:204, 1968.

123. Healy M: Suppressing lactation with oral diuretics, Lancet 1:1353, 1961.

124. Hedrick WR, DiSimone RN, and Keen RL: Radiation dosimetry from breast milk excretion of radioiodine and pertechnetate, J Nucl Med 27:1569, 1986.

125. Heinonen OP, Slone D, and Shapiro S: Birth defects and drugs in pregnancy, Littleton Mass, 1977, Publishing Sciences Group, p 345.

126. Heisterberg L and Branebjerg PE: Blood and milk concentrations of metronidazole in mothers and infants, J Perinatol Med 11:114, 1983.

127. Herman SJ: Neonatal rubella following maternal immunization, J Pediatr 98:668, 1981.

128. Hervada AR, Feit E, and Sagraves R: Drugs in breast milk, Perinatal Care 2:19, 1978.

129. Hilbert JM, Gural RP, Symchowicz S, and Zampaglione N: Excretion of quazepam into human breast milk, J Clin Pharmacol 24:457, 1984.

130. Hill LM and Malkasion GD: The use of quinidine sulfate throughout pregnancy, Obstet Gynecol 54:366, 1979.

131. Hofmeyr GJ, Van Iddekinge B, and Blott JA: Domperidone: secretion in breast milk and effect on puerperal prolactin levels, Br J Obstet Gynecol 92:141, 1985.

132. Hofmeyr GJ and Sonnendecker EWW: Secretion of the gastrokinetic agent cisapride in human milk, Eur J Clin Pharmacol 30:735, 1986.

133. Holdiness MR: Clinical pharmacokinetics of the antituberculosis drugs, Clin Pharmacokin 9:511, 1984.

134. Holmdahl KH: Cholecystography during lactation, Acta Radiol 45:305, 1956.

135. Hoppu K, Neuvonen PJ, and Korte T: Disopyramide and breastfeeding, Br J Clin Pharmacol 21:553, 1986.

136. Ilett KF, Hackett LP, Paterson JW, and McCormick CC: Excretion of metrizamide in milk, Br J Radiol 54:537, 1981.

137. Illingworth RS and Finch E: Ethyl biscoumacetate (Tromexan) in human milk, J Obstet Gynecol Br Empire 66:487, 1959.

138. Inoue H, Unno N, Ou MC et al: Level of verapamil in human milk, Eur J Clin Pharmacol 26:657, 1984.

139. Jamali F, Tam YK, and Stevens RD: Naproxen excretion in breast milk and its uptake by suckling infant, Drug Intell Clin Pharmacol 16:475 (abstract), 1982.

140. Janssen PAJ, Niemegeers CJE, and Schellekens KHL: The pharmacology of penfluridol (R1634), a new potent and orally long-acting neuroleptic drug, Eur J Pharmacol 11:139, 1970.

141. Jarbor CH et al: Dyphylline elimination kinetics in lactating women: blood-to-milk transfer, J Clin Pharmacol 21:405, 1981.

142. Johns DG et al: Secretion of methotrexate into human milk, Am J Obstet Gynecol 112:978, 1972.

143. Kafetzis DA et al: Transfer of cefotaxime in human milk and from mother to foetus, J Antimicrob Chemother 6(suppl A):135, 1980.

144. Kafetzis DA et al: Passage of cephalosporins and amoxicillin into the breastmilk, Acta Paediatr Scand 70:825, 1981.

145. Kafetzis DA et al: Ceftriaxone distribution between maternal blood and fetal blood and tissues at parturition and between blood and milk postpartum, Antimicrob Agents Chemother 23:870, 1983.

146. Kafetzis DA et al: Placental and breast milk transfer of ceftriaxone (C). In Proceedings of the 22nd Interscience Conference on Antimicrobial Agents and Chemotherapy, New York, 1983, Academic Press, p 155.

147. Kampmann JP et al: Propylthiouracil in human milk, Lancet 1:736, 1980.

148. Kaneko S et al: The problems of antiepileptic medication in the neonatal period: is breast feeding advisable? In Janz D et al, editors: Epilepsy,

pregnancy, and the child, New York, 1982, Raven Press, p 343.

149. Kanta JH: Use of benzodiazepines during pregnancy, labor, and lactation, with particular reference to pharmacokinetic considerations, Drugs 23:354, 1982.

150. Katz FH and Duncan BR: Entry of prednisone into human milk, N Engl J Med 293:1154, 1975.

151. Kauffman RE, O'Brien C, and Gilford P: Sulfisoxazole secretion into human milk, J Pediatr 97:839, 1980.

152. Kaufman KR et al: PCP in amniotic fluid and breast milk: case report, J Clin Psychiatry 44:269, 1983.

153. Kearns A, McConnal RF, Trang JM et al: Appearance of ranitidine in breast milk following multiple dosing, Clin Pharmacol 4:322, 1985.

154. Kemp J, Ilett KF, Booth J, and Hackett LP: Excretion of doxepin and N-desmethyldoxepin in human milk, Br J Clin Pharmacol 20:497, 1985.

155. Kesaniemi YA: Ethanol and acetaldehyde in the milk and peripheral blood of lactating women after ethanol administration, J Obstet Gynaecol Br Commonw 81:84, 1974.

156. Keystone JS and Murdoch JK: Diagnosis and treatment drugs five years later, Mebendazole, Ann Intern Med 91:582, 1979.

157. Knowles JA: Excretion of drugs in milk—a review, J Pediatr 66:1068, 1965.

158. Knowles JA: Drugs in milk, Pediatr Curr 21:28, 1972.

159. Knowles JA: Breast milk: a source of more than nutrition for the neonate, Clin Toxicol 7:69, 1974.

160. Kok THHG et al: Drowsiness due to clemastine transmitted in breast milk, Lancet 1:915, 1982.

161. Kopelman AE: Fetal addiction to pentazocine, Pediatrics 55:888, 1975.

162. Koup JR, Rose JQ, and Cohen ME: Ethosuximide pharmacokinetics in pregnant patient and her newborn, Epilepsia 19:535, 1978.

163. Krause W, Stoppelli I, Milia S, and Rainer E: Transfer of mepindolol to newborns by breastfeeding mothers after single and repeated daily doses, Eur J Clin Pharmacol 22:53, 1982.

164. Kreek MJ et al: Analysis of methadone and other drugs in maternal and neonatal body fluids, Am J Drug Alcohol Abuse 1:409, 1974.

165. Kuhnz W, Koch S, Jakob S et al: Ethosuximide in epileptic women during pregnancy and lactation period: placental transfer, serum concentrations in nursed infants and clinical status, Br J Clin Pharmacol 18:671, 1984.

166. Kulski JK, Hartmann PE, Martin JD, and Smith M: Effects of bromocriptine mesylate on the composition of the mammary secretion in non-breastfeeding women, Obstet Gynecol 52:38, 1978.

167. Kwit NT and Hatcher RA: Excretion of drugs in milk, Am J Dis Child 49:900, 1935.

168. Lacey J: Dichloralphenazone and breast milk, Br Med J 4:684, 1971.

169. Lau RJ, Emery MG, and Galinsky RE: Unexpected accumulation of acyclovin in breast milk with estimation of infant exposure, Obstet Gynecol 69:468, 1987.

170. Laursen LC, Borga O, Ljungholm K, and Weeke B: Transfer of enprofylline into breast milk, Ther Drug Monitor 10:150, 1988.

171. Levin DL: Effects of inhibition of prostaglandin synthesis on fetal development, oxygenation, and the fetal circulation, Semin Perinatol 4:35, 1980.

172. Levy M, Granit L, and Laufer N: Excretion of drugs in human milk, N Engl J Med 297:798, 1977.

173. Lewis AM et al: Mexiletine in human blood and breast milk. Postgrad Med J 57:546, 1981.

174. Lewis PJ, Devenish C, and Kahn C: Controlled trial of metoclopramide in the initiation of breast-feeding, Br J Clin Pharmacol 9:217, 1980.

175. Liedholm H et al: Accumulation of atenolol and metoprolol in human breast milk. Eur J Clin Pharmacol 20:229, 1981.

176. Liedholm H et al: Transplacental passage and breast milk concentrations of hydralazine, Eur J Clin Pharmacol 21:417, 1982.

177. Lien EJ, Kuwabara J, and Koda RT: Diffusion of drugs into prostatic fluid and milk, Drug Intell Clin Pharm 8:470, 1974.

178. Lönnerdal B and Asquity MT: Malathion not detected in breast milk of women living in aerial spraying areas, N Engl J Med 307:439, 1982.

179. Lönnerholm G and Lindström B: Terbutaline excretion into breast milk, Br J Clin Pharmacol 13:729, 1982.

180. Lou MA, Wu YH, Jacob LS, and Pitkin DH: Penetration of cefonicid into human breast milk and various body fluids and tissues, Rev Infect Dis 6(suppl 4):S816, 1984.

181. Loughman PM: Digoxin excretion in human breast milk, J Pediatr 92:1019, 1978.

182. Low LCK, Lang J, and Alexander WD: Excretion of carbinazole and prophylthiouracil in breast milk. Lancet 2:1011, 1979.

183. Lundberg P: Abnormal otogeny in young rabbits after chronic administration of haloperidol to the nursing mothers, Brain Res 40:395, 1972.

184. Lunnell NO, Kulas J, and Rane A: Transfer of labetalol into amniotic fluid and breast milk in lactating women, Eur J Clin Pharmacol 28:597, 1985.

185. Lustgarten JS and Podos SM: Topical timolol and the nursing mother, Arch Ophthalmol 101:1381, 1983.

186. MacKintosh D and Buchanan N: Excretion of

disopyramide in human breast milk, Br J Clin Pharmacol 19:856, 1985.

187. Martin DC, Martin JC, and Streissguth AP: Sucking frequency and amplitude in newborns as a function of maternal drinking and smoking. Current Alcohol 5:359, 1978.

188. Matheson I, Evang A, Fredricson Overo K, and Syversen G: Presence of chlorprothixene and its metabolites in breast milk, Eur J Clin Pharmacol 27:611, 1984.

189. Matsuda C et al: A study of amikcacin in the obstretics field, Jpn J Antibio 27:633, 1974.

190. May HT: Antimicrobial properties and microbial contaminants of breast milk: an update, Aust Paediatr 20:265, 1984.

191. McKenna R, Cole ER, and Vasen U: Is warfarin sodium contraindicated in the lactating mother, J Pediatr 103, 325, 1983.

192. McKenzie SA, Selley JA, and Agnew JE: Secretion of prednisolone into breast milk. Arch Dis Child 50:894, 1975.

193. McNall P and Jafarnia M: Management of myasthenia gravis in the obstetrical patient, Am J Obstet Gynecol 92:518, 1965.

194. Medina A, Fiske N, Hjelt-Harvey I et al: Absorption, diffusion, and excretion of a new antibiotic, lincomycin, Antimicrob Agents Chemother, p 189, 1963.

195. Mehta PS, Mehta SJ, and Vorherr H: Congenital iodide goiter and hypothyroidism: a review, Obstet Gynecol Surv 38:237, 1983.

196. Miller ME, Cohn RD, and Burghart PH: Hydrochlorothiazide disposition in a mother and her breastfed infant. J Pediatr 101:789, 1982.

197. Miller MR, Withers R, Bhamra R, and Holt DW: Verapamil and breast-feeding, Eur J Clin Pharmacol 30:125, 1986.

198. Miller RD, Keegna KA, Thrupp LD, and Brann J: Human breast milk concentration of moxalactam, Am J Obstet Gynecol 148:348, 1984.

199. Miller RD and Slater AJ: The passage of trimethoprim/sulphamethoxazole into breast milk and its significance. In Daikos GK, editor: Progress in Chemotherapy, Proceedings of the 8th International Congress of Chemotherapy, Athens, 1973 and 1974, Hellenic Society for Chemotherapy, p 687.

200. Mischler TW et al: Presence of cephradine in body fluids of lactating and pregnant women, Clin Pharmacol Ther 15:214, 1974.

201. Mischler TW et al: Cephradine and epicillin in body fluids of lactating and pregnant women, J Reprod Med 21:130, 1978.

202. Mitani GM, Steinberg I, Lien EJ et al: The pharmacokinetics of antiarrhythmic agents in pregnancy and lactation, Clin Pharmacokin 12:253, 1987.

203. Mofenson HC and Caraccio TR: Drugs, breast milk, and infants, Pediatr Pharmacol Toxic News 6:47, 1987.

204. Mohr JA: The possible induction and/or acquisition of cellular hypersensitivity associated with ingestion of colostrum. J Pediatr 82:1062, 1973.

205. Morganti G, Ceccarelli G, and Ciaffi EG: Comparative concentrations of tetracycline antibiotic in serum and maternal milk, Antibiotica 6:216, 1968.

206. Motomura R et al: Basic and clinical studies of ceftizoxime in obstetrics and gynecology, Chemotherapy (Tokyo) 28(suppl 5):888, 1980.

207. Mountford PJ and Coakley AJ: Breast milk radioactivity following injection of ^{99}Tc^m-pertechnetate and ^{99}Tc^m-glucoheptonate, Nucl Med Comm 8:839, 1987.

208. Mulley BA et al: Placental transfer of chlorthalidone and its elimination in maternal milk, Eur J Clin Pharmacol 13:129, 1978.

209. Nahas G: Inhibition of cellular mediated immunity in marihuana smokers, Science 183:419, 1974.

210. Nahas G: Marihuana: toxicity, tolerance, and therapeutic efficacy, Drug Ther p 33, Jan 1974.

211. Nahas G: Marihuana, JAMA 233:79, 1975.

212. Nahas G and Paton W editors: Marihuana: chemistry, biochemistry and cellular effects, New York, 1976, Springer-Verlag New York, Inc.

213. Nau H et al: Valproic acid and its metabolites: placental transfer, neonatal pharmacokinetics, transfer via mother's milk and clinical status in neonates of epileptic mothers, J Pharmacol Exp Ther 219:768, 1981.

214. Nau H et al: Anticonvulsants during pregnancy and lactation, Clin Pharmacokinet 7:508, 1982.

215. Naulty JS et al: Bupivacaine in breast milk following epidural anesthesia for vaginal delivery. Reg Anaesth 8:44,1983.

216. Naumberg EG and Meny RG: Breast milk opioids and neonatal apnea, Am J Dis Child 142:11, 1988.

217. Needs CJ and Brooks PM: Antirheumatic medication during lactation, Br J Rheumat 24:291, 1985.

218. Needs CJ and Brooks PM: Clinical pharmacokinetics of the salicylates, Clin Pharmacokin 10:164, 1985.

219. Nicholas JM, Lipshitz J, and Schreiber EC: Phencyclidine: its transfer across the placenta as well as into breast milk, Am J Obstet Gynecol 143:143, 1982.

220. Niebyl JR et al: Carbamazepine in levels in pregnancy and lactation, Obstet Gynecol 53:139, 1979.

221. Niessen KH, Ramolla J, Binder M et al: Chlorinated hydrocarbons in adipose tissue of infants

and toddlers: inventory and studies on their association with intake of mothers' milk, Eur J Pediatr 142:238, 1984.

222. Noren K: Changes in the levels of organochlorine pesticides, polychlorinated biphenyls, dibenzo-*p*-dioxins and dibenzofurans in human milk from Stockholm, 1972–1985. Chemosphere 17:39, 1988.

223. O'Brien T: Excretion of drugs in human milk, Am J Hosp Pharmacol 31:844, 1974.

224. Ogunbona FA, Onyeji CO, Bolaji OO, and Torimiro SEA: Excretion of chloroquine and desethylchloroquine in human milk, Br J Clin Pharmacol 23:473, 1987.

225. Olsson B, Bolme P, Dahlstrom B, and Marcus C: Excretion of noscapine in human breast milk, Eur J Clin Pharmacol 30:213, 1986.

226. Orme ML et al: May mothers given warfarin breast-feed their infants? Br Med J 1:1564, 1977.

227. Oseid BJ: Breast feeding and infant health, Clin Obstet Gynecol 18:149, 1975.

228. Ost L, Wettrell G, Bjorkhem I, and Rane A: Prednisolone excretion in human milk, J Pediatr 106:1008, 1985.

229. Ostensen M, Brown ND, Chiag PK et al: Hydroxychloroquine in human breast milk, Eur J Clin Pharmacol 28:357, 1985.

230. Ostensen M and Husby G: Antirheumatic drug treatment during pregnancy and lactation, Scand J Rheumatol 14:1, 1985.

231. Ostensen M, Skavdal K, Myklebust G et al: Excretion of gold into human breast milk, Eur J Clin Pharmacol 31:251, 1986.

232. Pacifici GM et al: Placental transfer of pinazepam and its metabolite N-desmethyldiazepam in women at term, Eur J Clin Pharmacol 27:307, 1984.

233. Paton DM and Webster DR: Clinical pharmacokinetics of H1-receptor antagonists (the antihistamines), Clin Pharmacokin 10:477, 1985.

234. Patrick MJ. Tilstone WJ, and Reavey P: Diazepam and breast feeding, Lancet 1(7740):542, 1972.

235. Perez-Reyes M and Wall ME: Presence of Δ^9 tetrahydrocannabinol in human milk, N Engl J Med 307:819, 1982.

236. Perkins K and Oski F: Elevated blood lead in a 6-month old breast-fed infant: the role of newsprint logs, Pediatrics 57:426, 1976.

237. Peterson RG and Bowes WA: Drugs, toxins and environmental agents in breast milk. In Neville MC and Neifert MR, editors: Lactation, New York, 1983, Plenum Press.

238. Phelps DL and Karim A: Spironolactone: relationship between concentrations of dethioacetylated metabolite in human serum and milk, J Pharm Sci 66:1203, 1977.

239. Physicians Desk Reference, Oradell NY, 1987, Medical Economics Co.

240. Pitcher D et al: Amiodarone in pregnancy, Lancet 1:597, 1983.

241. Pittard WB and O'Neal W Jr: Amitriptyline excretion in human milk, J Clin Psychopharmacol 6:383, 1986.

242. Pittman KA et al: Human perinatal distribution of butorphanol, Am J Obstet Gynecol 138:797, 1980.

243. Plomb TA, Thiery M, and Maes RAA: The passage of thiamphenicol and chloramphenicol into human milk after single and repeated oral administration. Vet Hum Toxicol 25:3, 1983.

244. Poisondex: Rocky Mountain Drug Consultation Center, 1989, Denver Colo (available through Regional Poison Control Centers).

245. Posner AC, Prigot A, and Konicoff MG: Further observations on the use of tetracycline hydrochloride in prophylaxis and treatment of obstetric infections. In Antibiotics annual, New York, 1954-1955, Medical Encyclopedia, Inc, p 594.

246. Postellon DC and Aronow R: Iodine in mother's milk, JAMA 247:463, 1982.

247. Prochazka J, Havelka J, and Hejzlar M: Excretion of chloramphenicol by human milk, Casleck Cesk 103:378, 1964.

248. Pynnönen S and Sillanpää M: Carbamazepine and mother's milk, Lancet 2:563, 1975.

249. Redman C: Fetal outcome in trial of antihypertensive treatment in pregnancy, Lancet 2:753, 1976.

250. Remmington JS and Klein JO: Infectious diseases of the fetus and newborn infant, Philadelphia, 1976, WB Saunders Co.

251. Reisner SH, Eisenberg NH, Stahl B, and Hauser GJ: Maternal medications and breast-feeding, Dev Pharmacol Ther 6:285, 1983.

252. Reiss W: The relevance of blood level determinations during the evaluation of maprotiline in man. In Research and clinical investigation in depression, Northampton England, 1980, Cambridge Medical Publications, p 19.

253. Riant P, Urien S, Albengres E et al: High plasma protein binding as a parameter in the selection of beta blockers for lactating women, Biochem Pharmacol 35:4579, 1986.

254. Riley AJ, Crowley P, and Harrison C: Transfer of ranitidine to biological fluids: milk and semen. In Misiewicz JJ and Wormsley KG, editors: Proceedings of the 22nd International Symposium on Ranitidine, Oxford, 1981, Medicine Publishing Foundation, p 78.

255. Rivera-Calimlim L: Drugs in breast milk, Drug Ther 8(12):20, 1977.

256. Rizzoni G and Furlanut M: Cyanotic crises in a breastfed infant from mother taking dipyrone, Hum Toxicol 3:505, 1984.

257. Rogan WJ, Bagniewska A, and Damstra T: Pollutants in breast milk, N Engl J Med 302:1450, 1980.

258. Roth S: Anti-inflammatories: exploring new options, Curr Prescrib p 46, May 1976.

259. Rothermal P and Faber M: Drugs in breast-milk: a consumer's guide, Birth Fam J 2:76, 1975.

260. Rubin A et al: A profile of the physiological disposition and gastrointestinal effects of fenoprofen in man, Curr Med Res Opin 2:529, 1974.

261. Rylance GW, Woods CG, Donnelly MC et al: Carbimazole and breastfeeding, Lancet 1:928, 1987.

262. Sagraves R, Waller ES, and Goehrs HR: Tolmetin in breast milk, Drug Intell Clin Pharmacol 19:55, 1985.

263. Sahlberg BL: The characterization of sulphated metabolites of norethindrone in human milk after oral administration of contraceptive steroids, J Steroid Biochem 26:481, 1987.

264. Sandstrom B and Regardb GG: Metoprolol excretion in breast milk, Br J Clin Pharmacol 9:518, 1980.

265. Savage EP et al: National study of chlorinated hydrocarbon insecticide residues in human milk USA, Am J Epidemiol 113:413, 1981.

266. Savage R: Drugs and breast milk, J Hum Nutr 31:459, 1977.

267. Schou M and Amdisen A: Lithium and pregnancy. III. Lithium ingestion by children breastfed by women on lithium treatment, Br Med J 2:138, 1973.

268. Schvehla TJ, Faust LJ, Herjanic M, and Muniz CE: Lithium therapy for affective disorders, AFP 36:169, 1987.

269. Scragg JN, and Proctor EM: Mebendazole in the treatment of severe symptomatic trichuriasis in children, Am J Trop Med 26:198, 1977.

270. Seagraves R, Waller ES, and Goehrs HR: Tolmetin in breast milk, Drug Intell Clin Pharmacol 19:55, 1985.

271. Shankaran S and Poland RL: The displacement of bilirubin from albumin by fluoresmide, J Pediatr 90:642, 1977.

272. Shikary ZK et al: Transfer of levonorgestel (LNG) administered through different drug delivery systems from the maternal circulation into the newborn infant's circulation via breast milk, Contraception 31:611, 1985.

273. Shore M: Drugs can be dangerous during pregnancy and lactation, Can Pharmacol J 103:8, 1970.

274. Sioris LU and Krenzelok E: Phencyclidine intoxication: a literature review, Am J Hosp Pharmacol 35:1362, 1978.

275. Sioufi A et al: Oxprenolol placental transfer, plasma concentrations in newborns and passage into breast milk, Br J Clin Pharmacol 18:453, 1984.

276. Smadel JE et al: Chloramphenicol (Chloromycetin) in the treatment of tsutsugamushi disease (scrub typhus), J Clin Invest 28:1196, 1949.

277. Smialek JE, Monforte JR, Aronow R, and Spitz WU: Methadone deaths in children—a continuing problem, JAMA 238:2516, 1977.

278. Smith MT et al: Propranolol, propranodol glucuronide and naphthoxylactic acid in breast milk and plasma, Ther Drug Monit 5:87, 1983.

279. Smith TC et al: Absorption of pyrvinium pamoate, Clin Pharmacol Ther 19:802, 1976.

280. Snider DE and Powell KE: Should women taking antituberculosis drugs breastfeed? Arch Intern Med 144:589, 1984.

281. Sovner R and Orsulak PJ: Excretion of imipramine and desipramine in human breast milk, Am J Psychiatry 136:451, 1979.

282. Stancer HC and Reed KL: Desipramine and 2-hydroxydesipramine in human breast milk and the nursing infant's serum, Am J Psychiatry 143:1597, 1986.

283. Steen B and Rane A: Clindamycin passage into human milk, Br J Clin Pharmacol 13:661, 1982.

284. Steiner E, Villen T, Hallberg M, and Rane A: Amphetamine secretion in breast milk, Eur J Clin Pharmacol 27:123, 1984.

285. Stirt JA and Sullivan SF: Aminophylline, Anesth Analg 60:587, 1981.

286. Straub C and Murthy G: A comparison of Sr^{90} component and cow's milk, Pediatrics 36:732, 1965.

287. Sykes P, Quarrie J and Alexander F: Lithium carbonate and breast-feeding, Br Med J 2:1299, 1976.

288. Sylvester RK et al: Excretion of hydroxyurea into milk, Cancer 60:2177, 1987.

289. Syversen GB and Ratkje SK: Drug distribution within human milk phases, J Pharmaceut Sci 74:1071, 1985.

290. Takase Z: Laboratory and clinical studies on tobramycin in the field of obstetrics and gynecology, Chemotherapy (Tokyo) 23:1402, 1975.

291. Takase Z, Shirafuji H, and Uchida M: Experimental and clinical studies of cefadroxil in the treatment of infections in the field of obstetrics and gynecology, Chemotherapy (Tokyo) 28 (suppl 2):424, 1980.

292. Takyi BE: Excretion of drugs in human milk, J Hosp Pharmacol 28:317, 1970.

293. Terwilliger WG and Hatcher RA: The elimination of morphine and quinine in human milk, Surg Gynecol Obstet 58:823, 1934.

294. Texeira GC and Scott RB: Further clinical and laboratory studies with novobiocin. II, Novobiocin concentration in the blood of newborn infants and in the breast milk of lactating mothers, Antibiot Med 5:577, 1958.

295. The medical letter on drugs and therapeutics update, Drugs in breast milk 21:21, 1979.

296. Thiels C: Pharmacotherapy of psychiatric disorder in pregnancy and breastfeeding: a review, Pharmacopsychiatr 20:133, 1987.

297. Timmis AD, Jackson G and Holt DW: Mexiletine for control of ventricular dysrhythmias in pregnancy, Lancet 2:647, 1980.

298. Townsend RJ, Benedetti TJ, Erickson S et al: Excretion of ibuprofen into breast milk, Am J Obstet Gynecol 149:184, 1984.

299. Tunnessen W and Hertz C: Toxic effects of lithium in newborn infants: a commentary, J Pediatr 81:804, 1972.

300. Tupin JP and Hopkin JT: Lithium for mood disturbances, Rational Drug Ther 12(9):1, 1978.

301. Tyson RM, Shrader EA, and Periman HH: Drugs transmitted through breast milk. I. Laxatives, J Pediatr 12:824, 1937.

302. Tyson RM, Shrader EA, and Perlman HH: Drugs transmitted through breast milk. II. Barbiturates, J Pediatr 13:86, 1938.

303. Tyson RM, Shrader EA, and Perlman HH: Drugs transmitted through breast milk. III. Bromides, J Pediatr 13:91, 1938.

304. Unsworth J, d'Assis-Fonseca A, Beswick DT, and Blake DF: Serum salicylate levels in a breastfed infant, Ann Rhematol Dis 46:638, 1987.

305. Valdivieso A, Valdes G, Spiro TE, and Westerman RL: Minoxidil in breast milk, Ann Intern Med 102:135, 1985.

306. Varsano L, Fischl J, and Tikvah P: The excretion of orally ingested nitrofurant in human milk (letters), J Pediatr 82:886, 1973.

307. Velázquez JG et al: Effecto de al administracion oral diaria de 0.350 mg. de noretindrona en la lactancia y en la composicion de le leche, Ginecol Obstet Mex 40:31, 1976.

308. Verbeeck RV, Ross SG, and McKenna EA: Excretion of trazodone in breast milk, Br J Clin Pharmacol 22:367, 1986.

309. Von Kobyletzki D et al: Pharmacokinetic studies with cefazolin in obstetrics and gynecology, Infection 2(suppl):60, 1974.

310. Vorherr H: Drug excretion in breast milk, Postgrad Med 56(4):97, 1974.

311. Vorherr H: Drug excretion in breast milk, Senologia 1:27, 1976.

312. Wade A: The extra pharmacopocia. In Martindale W, editor: Squire's companion, 27, London, 1977, The Pharmaceutical Press.

313. Weaver JC, Kamm ML, and Dobson RL: Excretion of radioiodine in human milk, JAMA 173:872, 1960.

314. Weissenbacher ER et al: Clinical results and concentrations of cefmenoxime in serum, amniotic fluid, mother's milk, and umbilical cord, Am J Med 77(suppl 6A):11, 1984.

315. Wennberg RP, Rasmussen LF, and Ahlfors CE: Displacement of bilirubin from human albumin by three diuretics, J Pediatr 90:647, 1977.

316. Werthmann MN and Krees S: Excretion of chlorothiazide in breast milk, J Pediatr 81:781, 1972.

317. Whalley LJ, Blain PG, and Prime JK: Haloperidol secreted in breast milk, Br Med J 282:1746, 1981.

318. Whitelaw AGL, Cummings AJ, and McFadyen IR: Effect of maternal lorazepam on the neonate, Br Med J 282:1106, 1981.

319. Wickizer TM and Brillant LB: Testing for polychlorinated biphenyls in human milk, Pediatrics 68:411, 1981.

320. Widdowson EM et al: Absorption, excretion and retention of strontium by breast-fed and bottle-fed babies, Lancet 2:941, 1960.

321. Wiernik PH and Duncan JH: Cyclophosphamide in human milk, Lancet 1:912-1971.

322. Wiles DH, Orr MW, and Kooakowska T: Chlorpromazine levels in plasma and milk of nursing mothers, Br J Clin Pharmacol 5:272, 1978.

323. Williams RH, Kay GH, and Jandorf BJ: Thiouracil: its absorption, disturbance and excretion, J Clin Invest 23:613, 1944.

324. Wilson JT et al: Drug excretion in human breast milk: principles, pharmacokinetics and projected consequences, Clin Pharmacol Ther 5:1, 1980.

325. Wilson JT: Milk/plasma ratios and contraindicated drugs. In Wilson JT, editor: Drugs in breast milk, Balgowlah Aust, 1981, ADIS Press.

326. Wilson JT, Brown RD, Hinson JL, and Dailey JW: Pharmacokinetic pitfalls in the estimation of the breast milk/plasma ratio for drugs, Ann Rev Pharmacol Toxicol 25:667, 1985.

327. Wolff MS: Occupationally derived chemicals in breast milk, Am J Ind Med 4:259, 1983.

328. Woodward A, Grgurinovich N, and Ryan P: Breast feeding and smoking hygiene: major influences on cotinine in urine of smokers' infants, J Epidemiol Comm Health 40:309, 1986.

329. Wurster CF: DDT in mother's milk, ICEA News, vol 9, Nov-Dec 1970.

330. Yaffe SJ and Waletsky LR: Drugs and chemicals in breast milk. In Waletsky LR, editor. Symposium on human lactation, DHEW pub no 79-5107, Arlington, Va, 1976.

331. Yoshioka H et al: Transfer of cefazolin into human milk, J Pediatr 94:151, 1979.

332. Yuasa M: A study of amikacin in obstetrics and gynecology, Jpn J Antibiot 27:377, 1974.

333. Zylber-Katz E, Linder N, Granit L, and Levy M: Excretion of dipyrone metabolites in human breast milk, Eur J Clin Pharmacol 30:359, 1986.

The Lact-Aid Nursing Trainer System

Lact-Aid is made up of four parts: (1) the body with permanently attached nursing tube, (2) the clamp ring, (3) the extension tube, and (4) the presterilized Lact-Aid bag with 4 oz capacity.

For convenience in filling and assembling Lact-Aid, a bag hanger and funnel have been specially designed. Six T-shaped end tabs provide easy attachment to the nursing bra.

The filled Lact-Aid is attached to the nursing bra or neck cord between the breasts and is positioned so that the supplement cannot siphon out. The presterilized bag is attached to the body by the clamp ring. The infant suckles the tip of the nursing tube and the nipple of the breast at the same time. As the infant nurses, supplement is drawn from the bottom of the presterilized bag by the extension tube attached to the bottom of the body. This keeps the infant from swallowing any air that might be trapped in the top of the bag. The body has an orifice designed to provide the best rate of flow, slower than milk flows from the breast, but fast enough to keep from overtiring the infant. The nursing tube carries the

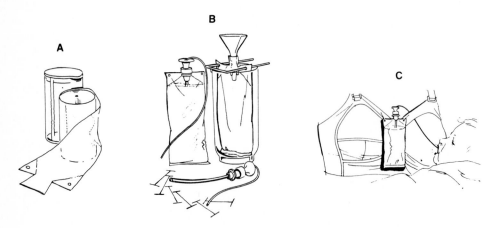

Fig. F-1. **A,** Presterilized, disposable bags have 4-oz capacity. **B,** Lact-Aid System includes detailed instruction booklet plus accessories for filling, cleaning, and use. **C,** Filled Nursing Trainer may be attached directly to the nursing bra as shown or suspended by the Neck Cord as depicted in Fig. 17-4. (From Avery JL: Lact-Aid Nursing Trainer instruction book, Athens, Tenn, 1983 revised ed, Lact-Aid International, Inc.)

supplement to the infant's mouth. It is clear, very soft, and flexible and will not cause the infant's mouth or the nipple any discomfort.

When the infant is put to the breast, the flow of supplement rewards his nursing efforts. This provides a pleasant incentive for the infant to continue nursing, which in turn provides the breasts with suckling stimulation to build up the milk supply. The Lact-Aid is small enough, even when it contains the full 4 oz capacity of supplement, to enable one to nurse discreetly without it showing. It is valuable in adoptive nursing* and in failure to thrive (see Chapters 12 and 17).

---

*Avery JL: A brief discussion of adoptive-nursing: an introduction to the topic, revised ed, Athens Tenn, 1983, Lact-Aid International, Inc. Avery JL: Induced lactation: a guide for counseling and management, Denver, 1973, JL Avery.

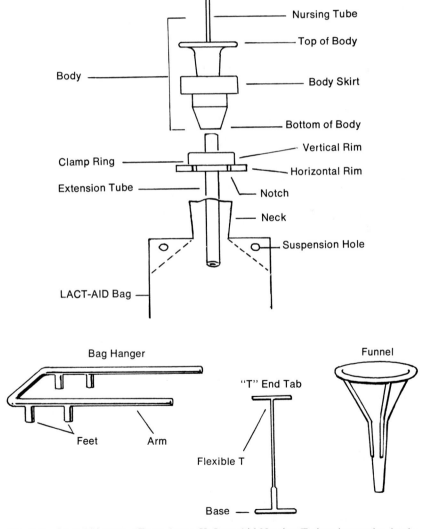

Fig. F-2. Lact-Aid parts. (From Avery JJ: Lact-Aid Nursing Trainer instruction book, Athens, Tenn, 1983 revised ed, Lact-Aid International, Inc.)

Organizations interested in supporting and providing materials for breastfeeding

Government Agencies

Food and Nutrition Information Center
National Agricultural Library Building, Room 304
Beltsville, MD 20705
Tel: (301) 344-3719

The center serves the information needs of people interested in human nutrition, nutrition education, food service management, consumer education, and food technology. It acquires and lends books, journal articles, and audiovisual materials dealing with these areas of concern, including breastfeeding research and education.

International Nutrition Communication Service
Education Development Center
55 Chapel Street
Newton, MA 02160
Tel: (617) 969-7100

Funded by the U.S. Agency for International Development, the service provides support and assistance in designing, implementing, and evaluating nutrition training projects in Third World countries. It has also published the *Nutrition Training Manual Catalogue,* which contains reviews of 116 training manuals. The manuals focus on nutrition in developing countries. Breastfeeding training manuals are included.

National Health Information Clearinghouse
PO Box 1133
Washington, DC 20013
Tel: (703) 522-2590 (Metro-D.C. area)
     (800) 336-4797 (outside Metro-D.C. area)

They help the public locate health information by identifying health information resources. Health questions are referred to appropriate health agencies that, in turn, respond directly to inquirers.

World Health Organization Publications Center, USA
49 Sheridan Avenue
Albany, NY 12210
Tel: (518) 436-9686

Publications available include a statement on infant and young child feeding, a breastfeeding guide for use by community health workers, and a study on patterns of breastfeeding.

Private Educational and Support Organizations

Birth and Life Bookstore, Inc.
PO Box 70625
Seattle, WA 98107
Tel: (206) 789-4444

They make available a large selection of books and pamphlets on breastfeeding, childbirth, and parenting for mothers and health professionals. A 24-page newsletter (published quarterly), *Imprint,* is available free to customers. It contains a review of new publications and a catalog of publications that are currently available. A sample newsletter can be obtained on request.

Clearinghouse on Infant Feeding and Maternal
   Nutrition
American Public Health Association
1015 Fifteenth Street, NW
Washington, DC 20005
Tel: (202) 789-5712

They serve as a resource primarily for health professionals who work in Third World countries. They also respond to domestic requests as time and staffing permit. They have a large collection of materials of all types on breastfeeding. They make available bibliographies and lists of resources on a variety of topics, and refer inquiries to appropriate sources for information.

Health Education Associates
211 S. Easton Rd.
Glenside, PA 19038
Tel: (215) 659-1149

They make available inexpensive pamphlets and other materials as teaching aids on breastfeeding. They sponsor training programs for breastfeeding counseling and promotion techniques.

International Childbirth Education Association
PO Box 20048
Minneapolis, MN 55420
Tel: (800) 328-4815 (outside Minnesota)
    (800) 752-4249 (Minnesota residents)

They have a catalog, *Bookmarks,* that has a large selection of books and inexpensive pamphlets on breastfeeding, childbirth, and parenting. They publish *ICEA News,* with news about childbirth, prenatal, and parenting issues; and *ICEA Review,* which provides in-depth review of current perinatal issues. They also have a resource committee on breastfeeding.

Lact-Aid International, Inc.
PO Box 1066
Athens, TN 80206
Hotline-(615) 744-9090

They formerly published a quarterly journal, *Keeping Abreast, Journal of Human Nurturing.* They make available back issues of the journal and reprints of selected articles. They also produce and market the Lact-Aid Nursing Trainer, and specialize in giving information and consultation on specific breastfeeding situations. These situations include prematurity, relactation, adoptive nursing, and failure to thrive.

La Leche League International, Inc.
9616 Minneapolis Avenue
Franklin Park, IL 60131
Tel: (312) 455-7730

La Leche League International Canadian Supply Depot
Box 39
Williamsburg, Ontario, Canada KOC 2HO

The publications catalog includes a large variety and broad scope of materials for mothers and health professionals to use in promoting and supporting breastfeeding. There is also a directory of League area coordinators by state and foreign country. The coordinators can give information about local support groups.

Nursing Mothers Counsel, Inc.
PO Box 50063
Palo Alto, CA 94303
Tel: (408) 272-1448

They make available a variety of publications on breastfeeding for mothers and health professionals.

WELLSTART$_{SM}$ San Diego Lactation Program
PO Box 87549
4062 First Avenue
San Diego, CA 92138
Helpline (619) 295-5193

WELLSTART, The San Diego Lactation Program is a private, nonprofit organization devoted to health promotion for infants, young children, and their families with special emphasis on breastfeeding and lactation. Wellstart provides individual patient and professional consultations; Helpline, a telephone consultation service; and intensive national and international training sessions in lactation management for physician-nurse teams.

Other Support Groups

Ammehejelpen
Postboks 15
Holmen, Oslo 3, Norway

Arbeitsgruppe and Dritte Welt
Postbach 1007
Bern 300, Switzerland

Association for Improvement of Maternity Services
61 Dartmouth Park Road
London NW 5, United Kingdom

Baby Foods Action Group
103 Gower Street
London WC1E 6AW, United Kingdom

Center for Science in the Public Interest
1779 Church Street, NW
Washington, DC 20036

National Childbirth Trust
Breast-feeding Promotion Group
9 Queensborough Terrace
London W2 3TB, United Kingdom

Nursing Mothers' Association of Australia
99 Burwood Road
Hawthorn, Victoria, Australia 3122

Nursing Mothers Counsel Inc.
PO Box 50063
Palo Alto, CA 94303

Parents Centres of Australia
148 Hereford Street
Forest Lodge, NSW, Australia 2229

War on Want
467 Caledonian Road
London N.7, United Kingdom

Telephone Information Service for Professionals

Breastfeeding and Human Lactation Study Center
University of Rochester School of Medicine and
Dentistry
Box 777
Rochester, NY 14642
(716)-275-0088

Manual expression of breast milk

The health care professional should be familiar with the technique of manual expression and be able to diagnose improper technique.

EXPRESSION OF BREAST MILK

All breastfeeding women should be familiar with the basic technique of manual expression of milk from the breast, and ideally this technique is acquired before discharge from the hospital with the assistance of the nursery or postpartum nursing staff.

The reasons to express milk are many but include:
1. Initiating flow to assist the infant to grasp the breast properly;
2. Early in lactation when the infant is premature or ill;
3. To relieve engorgement;
4. To remove milk when it is not possible to nurse the infant at a given feeding;
5. To maintain lactation when infant cannot be fed;
6. To pump and save milk for feeding infant at another time;
7. Contributing to a milk bank;
8. Pumping and discarding milk while temporarily on a specific medication.

Manual expression is appropriate to initiate the flow before applying a hand pump or an electric pump. Not many women can manually pump large volumes over time without mechanical assistance.

Step 1. Always *wash hands* before handling the breast.

Step 2. Breast massage: whether planning to manually express or mechanically pump, preparing the breast for ejecting the milk facilitates the process. The release of oxytocin and the ejection reflex are stimulated by external stimuli, the baby's cry, a picture of the baby, or gentle handling of the breast. Prolactin release and milk production are stimulated by "sucking" stimulation.

After mother finds a comfortable position to sit and is comfortable and relaxed, the breast is exposed and gently stroked with the fingertips from periphery to areola (see Fig. H-1). As this stroking is intensified, one should avoid slipping the hand across skin and irritating tissues. Gently massage. A warm washcloth soak is also helpful in initiating flow through the ducts. Gentle fingertip massage around all quadrants should follow and be repeated several times during extended mechanical pumping. It should not leave red marks or hurt.

Modified from Chele Marmet and The Lactation Institute and Breastfeeding Clinic, 16161 Ventura Blvd., Suite 223, Encino, CA 91436.

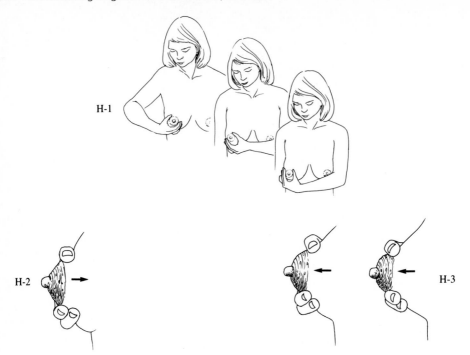

Step 3. Position hands on the breast—usually placing the fingers below and thumb on top is natural for most women. One hand placed above and one hand placed below the areola may be easier when the hand is small compared to breast size. The target area is beyond the ampullae, which are the collecting areas of the main ducts that radiate out from the nipple to the areola. The ampullae are about 3 cm from the nipple base, which may not be at the edge of the areola. Press toward the chest wall and then compress the thumb and fingers together (see Fig. H-2). Continue to compress the breast while moving the hand away from the chest wall in a "milking" action toward the nipple (see Fig. H-3). (Avoid pulling, squeezing, or rubbing motions.) Perform this motion in a repeated rhythmical manner at a comfortable but not abrasive rate. Infant sucking does not involve movement (stroking) of the tongue along the elongated areola and nipple, but an undulating motion of the tongue itself. Simulating that motion is the goal of manual expression. This action is similar to a peristaltic motion. The hand should be rotated around the breast to massage and stroke all quadrants, including the periphery and the axillae.

Use one or both hands to find the most productive grasp. Preventing trauma is essential, thus avoid squeezing, rubbing, or pulling the breast tissue. Every mother develops her own natural pattern, thus rigid adherence to methods may be counter productive. Effectiveness is measured by the comfortable release of milk.

Total emptying of the breast will require 20 to 30 minutes of manual stimulation. Warm compresses, hot showers, or suspending the breast in a bowl of warm water may help, especially if there is engorgement or mastitis. Leaning over and gently shaking the breast may help stimulate flow. Manual expression while leaning over may help empty the lower quadrants.

Legislation regarding human milk

AVAILABILITY OF HUMAN MILK
State of New York

AN ACT to amend the public health law, in relation to the availability of human breast milk for infant consumption

The People of the State of New York, represented in Senate and Assembly, do enact as follows:

Section 1. Legislative findings. The legislature hereby finds and declares that human breast milk, the preferred food for all infants, provides a superior, well tolerated nutritional source because of its unique components. It contains substances, lacking in other forms of infant nutrition, which help control infection and aid in preventing infant disease. For premature infants or those with a low birth weight or infants who are allergic to cow's milk and infant formulas, human breast milk is essential.

It shall be the declared policy of the state of New York that any and all infants requiring human breast milk be assured access to sufficient quantities of wholesome human breast milk, donated by concerned lactating mothers on a continual and systematic basis. The availability of such a supply of human breast milk should be made known to the public so that health providers and families of infants with particular need for human breast milk will be aware of its accessibility.

§2. The public health law is amended by adding a new section twenty-five hundred five to read as follows:

§2505. Human breast milk; collection, storage, and distribution; general powers of the commissioner. The commissioner is hereby empowered to:

(a) adopt regulations and guidelines including, but not limited to donor standards, methods of collection, and standards for storage, and distribution of human breast milk;

(b) conduct educational activities to inform the public and health care providers of the availability of human breast milk for infants determined to require such milk and to inform potential donors of the opportunities for proper donation;

(c) establish rules and regulations to effectuate the provisions of this section.

§3. This act shall take effect immediately.

From Office of Health Systems Management, Bureau of Standards Development, New York State Department of Health, Empire State Plaza, Albany NY, 1984.

NEW YORK STATE CODE: HUMAN MILK BANKS
Chapter II
Administrative rules and regulations
Subchapter G
Maternal and child health
Part 68
Human milk banks
(Statutory authority: Public health law § 2505)

Subchapter G of Chapter II is hereby amended to add a new Part 68 to read as follows:

Sec.	Sec.
68.1 Definitions	68.6 Collection and storage of human milk
68.2 Permit to operate a human milk bank	68.7 Processing of human milk
68.3 Governing responsibility	68.8 Distribution of human milk
68.4 Medical direction	68.9 Records to be maintained
68.5 Qualifications of donors	

68.1 Definitions. As used in this Part:

(a) Human milk bank shall mean an organized service which has been issued a permit to operate by the Commissioner and exists for the selection of donors and for the collection, processing, storage or distribution of human milk for infants other than the donor's own infant.

(b) Donor shall mean a lactating woman who voluntarily contributes milk to a human milk bank for infants other than her own and who does not receive remuneration for human milk.

(c) Single donor milk shall mean the accumulation of milk from one donor.

(d) Multiple donor human milk shall mean the accumulation of human milk from more than one donor.

(e) Collection of human milk shall mean the expression of milk from the breast, placing of the milk into a container and storage of the milk.

(f) Transfer station shall mean the location between the donor site and the milk bank where containers of human milk are held temporarily.

(g) Processing of human milk shall mean the testing of collected human milk for bacterial, and when indicated for viral and/or environmental contamination, and the treatment of milk to reduce or eliminate contaminants.

68.2 Permit to operate a human milk bank.

(a) A valid permit issued by the Commissioner of Health is required for lawful operation of a human milk bank.

(b) A permit will be issued subject to the human milk bank being established, maintained and operated in compliance with this Part.

(c) An applicant for a permit to operate a human milk bank shall submit to the department:

    (1) justification for establishment of the service and plan for coordination with other human milk banks;

    (3) proposed budget for operation of the milk bank;

    (3) the name of the person in charge of the milk bank;

    (4) the name of the medical director;

    (5) selection criteria for donor participation;

(6) procedures for testing human milk and criteria for determining acceptability of milk for infant consumption; and

(7) the education program for potential donors.

(d) A human milk bank shall allow admission to a representative of the Commissioner for the purpose of inspecting premises, procedures, equipment, or records to determine compliance with the standards in this section.

68.3 Governing responsibility. The holder of the permit of the milk bank shall ensure the development and implementation of policies for the operation of the human milk bank, the appointment of a medical director and the designation of the person to be in charge.

68.4 Medical direction.

(a) Medical direction shall be provided by a physician who is licensed and currently registered with the New York State Education Department and who is eligible for board certification in pediatrics.

(b) The medical director shall monitor the medical efficacy of the program and shall, as a minimum, develop:

(1) medical criteria for donor participation;

(2) quality standards for milk; and

(3) a policy for priority distribution of human milk when the demand exceeds the supply.

68.5 Qualifications of donor.

(a) The milk bank shall initially screen and periodically assess the donor for conditions that may adversely affect the quality of milk or impair the donor's health to include but not be limited to:

(1) use of medications, tobacco, alcohol and other substances in quantities likely to be harmful if transmitted through human milk to a recipient;

(2) systemic chronic diseases;

(3) acute and chronic infectious diseases;

(4) emotional and/or behavioral problems;

(5) history of jaundice in own infant after one week of age;

(6) sources of exposures which may be associated with environmental contaminants;

(7) length of postpartum period; and

(8) ability to follow directions.

(b) There shall be evidence that the donor has been tested for presence of hepatitis B surface antigen (HB$_s$Ag) and has been found negative.

(c) The milk bank shall obtain informed signed consent from the donor to participate in the milk bank program.

(d) The milk bank shall provide a program of education for donors which shall include, but not be limited to:

(1) purpose of the milk bank and donor responsibilities;

(2) policies and procedures concerning operation of the milk bank;

(3) procedures for collecting and storing milk;

(4) problems, diseases and medications or other substances contraindicating use of milk;

(5) diet and nutrition; and

(6) breast care and common problems associated with breast feeding.

68.6 Collection and storage of human milk.

(a) The milk bank shall supply presterilized, leak proof containers and container seals to the human milk donor.

(b) The human milk bank shall educate and monitor each donor in collection procedures to include but not be limited to:

(1) cleansing hands and breasts according to currently acceptable techniques;

(2) use of sterilized containers and container seals and method for sterilization of breast pump or other equipment, if used; and

(3) procedures for home storage of collected human milk.

(c) Human milk shall be stored at 45°F (7.2°C) or below for no more than 48 hours after expression; frozen milk shall be stored at 0°F (−18°C) or below for no more than 90 days.

(d) The container shall be identified by a tag affixed to it which shall show the donor's identification number, the date and the hours the milk was expressed. When frozen human milk is held at a transfer station this tag shall also show the identification of the station, time of receipt and of departure.

(e) Human milk shall be transported so that it is protected from contamination, thawing and refreezing and maintained at 45°F (7.2°C) or lower if liquid, 0°F (−18°C) or lower if frozen.

(f) Transfer stations shall not handle liquid milk and when human milk is stored at a transfer station it shall be received in the frozen state, protected from contamination, thawing and refreezing and be stored at 0°F (−18°C) or below.

(g) The physical facilities of the human milk bank minimize the potential for contamination by:

(1) locating the human milk bank in a distinct identifiable area and providing a separate refrigerator and freezer for human milk; and

(2) equipping refrigerators and freezers with a recording thermometer which shall be calibrated against a certified thermometer at least four times a year and which shall be either visually or mechanically monitored for fluctuations in temperature which affect the quality of the milk.

68.7 Processing of human milk.

(a) Policies, procedures and criteria shall be developed and submitted for review and approval by the Department for:

(1) routine bacteriological testing of donated human milk;

(2) virology testing when indicated;

(3) testing for those environmental contaminants to which the donor is likely to have been exposed because of diet, residence or other factors when a judgment is made to include such a donor in the program;

(4) random sample testing of donated milk for adulteration; and

(5) microbiological monitoring to assure the effectiveness of pasteurization.

(b) The human milk bank shall make arrangements with an approved laboratory to perform the required tests.

68.8 Distribution of human milk.

(a) The human milk bank shall distribute human milk to infants regardless of whether the infant is hospitalized or is in another setting according to the pre-established priority distribution.

(b) The human milk bank shall make known the availability of human milk to the public so that health providers and families of infants with particular need for human milk will be aware of its availability.

68.9 Records to be maintained.

(a) An individual file of each donor shall be maintained and shall include but not be limited to:

    (1) findings from the medical history;

    (2) results of tests for diseases transmissible through human milk;

    (3) a consent form signed by the donor which informs the donor of her obligations and of any risks involved;

    (4) documentation of instructions given to the donor for preserving the wholesomeness of donated milk; and

    (5) a record of any donor illness reported to the milk bank during participation in the program.

(b) Records of milk donations filed by donor identification number to include but not be limited to:

    (1) information from the identification tag affixed at the time of collection showing date and hour of collection and, if applicable, the identification of the transfer station with recorded times of receipt and departure;

    (2) results of all tests performed;

    (3) the date of pasteurization, if applicable; and

    (4) the date the milk was distributed or used, and if applicable, identifying information regarding milk accumulated from multiple donors.

(c) Records of information about recipients to include but not be limited to:

    (1) infant's age, birth weight and/or weight history and diagnosis which indicated the medical need for human milk;

    (2) the dates the service began and terminated;

    (3) identification of all milk given to the recipients;

    (4) documentation that the risks of consumption by and infant of donated milk have been disclosed to persons legally responsible for the infant.

(a)(10)(i)

    The hospital with the advice of the maternity staff, shall formulate a program of instruction and provide assistance as needed for maternity patients in the fundamentals of [normal] infant care, post pregnancy care and family planning.

    (ii) Each maternity patient shall be given the opportunity and the right to breast feed her infant unless there is a medical contradiction which is made known to such patient.

        (a) Assistance shall be provided as needed to facilitate breast feeding.

        (b) An educational program shall include the nutritional and physiological benefits of human milk, care of breasts, common problems associated with breast feeding, and the sanitary procedures to follow in collecting and storing human milk. The educational program shall also include problems, diseases and medications or other substances contraindicating breast feeding.

    (b)(21) Human milk bank shall mean an organized service which has been approved by the commissioner through a construction application to the State Hospital Review and Planning Council and exists for the selection of donors and for the collection, processing, storage or distribution of human milk for infants other than the donor's own infant.

    (22) Human milk donor shall mean a lactating woman who voluntarily contributes milk to a human milk bank for infants other than her own and who meets the qualifications defined in Section 68.5 of Part 68 of Chapter II of this Title, Administrative Rules and Regulations. A human milk donor shall not receive remuneration for human milk.

(c)(3) (vi) *(a)* The preparation, handling and storage of human milk, infant formula ingredients and equipment shall be carried out in accordance with written procedures, copies of which shall be filed with the full-time health officer and kept in the 'formula room'. Such procedures and any changes or amendments thereto shall be subject to the approval of the full-time health officer.

    (vii) *(a)* A hospital that is approved to operate a human milk bank shall conform to the provisions of Part 68 of Chapter II of this Title, Administrative Rules and Regulations.

    (b) A hospital that does not routinely collect, store or distribute donated human milk and does require donated human milk for a specific infant does not require approval to operate a human milk bank but shall conform to Sections 68.5, 68.6, 68.7 and 68.8 of Part 68 of Chapter II of this Title, Administrative Rules and Regulations.

NEW YORK STATE CODE IN SUPPORT OF BREASTFEEDING (ADDED 1984)
Chapter V
Subchapter A
Article 2
Part 405
Hospitals—minimum standards
(Statutory authority: Public health law § 2803)
405.8 Maternal, child health and newborn services

    (10)(i) The hospital, with the advice of the maternity staff, shall formulate a program of instruction and provide assistance for each maternity patient(s) in the fundamentals of (normal) infant care including infant feeding choice and techniques, post-pregnancy care and family planning.

    (ii) The hospital shall provide instruction and assistance to each maternity patient who has chosen to breast-feed and shall provide information on the advantages and disadvantages of breast-feeding to women who are undecided as to the feeding method for their infants. As a minimum:

    (a) the hospital shall designate at least one person who is thoroughly trained in breast-feeding physiology and management to be responsible for ensuring the implementation of an effective breast-feeding program; and

    (b) policies and procedures shall be developed to assist the mother to breast-feed which shall include but not be limited to:

        (1) prohibition of the applicaiton of standing orders for antilactation drugs;

        (2) placement of the infant for breast-feeding immediately following delivery, unless contraindicated;

        (3) restriction of the infant's supplemental feedings to those indicated by the medical condition of the infant or of the mother;

(4) provision for the infant to be fed on demand; and

(c) assurance that an educational program has been given as soon after admission as possible which shall include but not be limited to:

(1) the nutritional and physiological aspects of human milk;

(2) the normal process for establishing lactation, including care of breasts, common problems associated with breast-feeding and frequency of feeding;

(3) dietary requirements for breast-feeding;

(4) diseases and medication or other substances which may have an effect on breast-feeding;

(5) sanitary procedures to follow in collecting and storing human milk; and

(6) sources for advice and information available to the mother following discharge.

Vitamin and mineral supplement needs in normal children in the United States

American Academy of Pediatrics—Committee on Nutrition

GUIDELINES FOR SUPPLEMENTATION

Table J-1 summarizes the following guidelines for the use of supplements in healthy infants and children. The indications for vitamin K and fluoride are discussed in the text only.

Newborn infants

Vitamin K administration to all newborn infants is effective as a prophylaxis against hemorrhagic disease of the newborn. This 1961 recommendation was strongly reaffirmed in 1971 to prevent or minimize the postnatal decline of the vitamin K-dependent coagulation factors (II, VII, IX, and X). Vitamin K_1 is considered the vitamin derivative of choice in a single, intramuscular dose of 0.5 to 1 mg or an oral dose of 1.0 to 2.0 mg. In rare instances, the dose may have to be repeated after about four to seven days.

Breast-fed infants

The renewed emphasis on human milk as an ideal food has raised the question whether breast-fed infants require any vitamin or mineral supplements prior to the introduction of solid foods. This subject bears further discussion, particularly with respect to the most sidely used supplements: vitamins A, C, D, and E, iron and fluoride.

From American Academy of Pediatrics Committee on Nutrition: Pediatrics 66:1015, 1980. Copyright American Academy of Pediatrics 1980.

Table J-1. Guidelines for use of supplements in healthy infants and children*

| Child | Multivitamin-multimineral | Vitamins | | | Minerals |
		D	E	Folate	Iron
Term infants					
Breast-fed	0	±	0	0	±†
Formula-fed	0	0	0	0	0
Preterm infants					
Breast-fed‡	+‡	+	±§	±‡	+
Formula-fed‡	+‡	+	±§	±‡	+†
Older infants (after 6 mo)					
Normal	0	0	0	0	±†
High-risk‖	+	0	0	0	±
Children					
Normal	0	0	0	0	0
High-risk	+	0	0	0	0
Pregnant teenager					
Normal	±	0	0	±	+
High-risk¶	+	0	0	+	+

*Symbols indicate: +, that a supplement is usually indicated, ±, that it is possibly or sometimes indicated, 0, that it is not usually indicated. Vitamin K for newborn infants and fluoride in areas where there is insufficient fluoride in the water supply are not shown.

†Iron-fortified formula and/or infant cereal is a more convenient and reliable source of iron than a supplement.

‡Multivitamin supplement (plus added folate) is needed primarily when calorie intake is below approximately 300 kcal/day or when the infant weighs 2.5 kg; vitamin D should be supplied at least until 6 months of age in breast-fed infants. Iron should be started by 2 months of age (see text).

§Vitamin E should be in a form that is well absorbed by small, premature infants. If this form of vitamin E is approved for use in formulas, it need not be given separately to formula-fed infants. Infants fed breast milk are less susceptible to vitamin E deficiency.

‖Multivitamin-multimineral preparation (including iron) is preferred to use of iron alone.

¶Multivitamin-multimineral preparation (including iron and folate) is preferred to use of iron alone or iron and folate alone.

Rickets is uncommon in the breast-fed term infant, despite the fact that human breast milk appears to contain small amounts of vitamin D (ie, about 22 IU/liter). One possible explanation is that the vitamin D in breast milk is in the form of an easily absorbed sulfate analogue, but this needs to be confirmed. The antirachitic properties of breast milk seem to be adequate for the normal term infant of a well nourished mother. However, if the mother's vitamin D nutrition has been inadequate and if the infant does not benefit from adequate ultraviolet light (due to dark skin color and/or little exposure to light) supplements of 400 IU of vitamin D daily may be indicated.

Vitamin A deficiency rarely occurs in breast-fed infants. Historically, vitamin A supplementation was coupled with vitamin D supplementation because both were provided by cod liver oil. Currently there is little reason to provide vitamin A supplements; thus, there would be no harm in omitting vitamin A from supplements designed to provide vitamin D for infants who are breast-fed. Similarly there is not evidence that supplementation with vitamin E is needed for the normal breast-fed term infant.

Vitamin B_{12} deficiency has been reported in breast-fed infants of strict vegetarian mothers, but this is relatively rare in North America. The recent report of a 6-month-old infant of a vegan mother with severe megaloblastic anemia and coma is a reminder that the maternal diet strongly influences the concentration of certain water-soluble vitamins in breast milk. Thiamin deficiency can also occur in breast-fed infants of thiamin-deficient mothers, but this situation is virtually restricted to infants in developing countries. In the United States, the rare breast-fed infants of mothers who are themselves malnourished should receive multivitamin supplements.

Iron deficiency rarely develops before 4 to 6 months of age in breast-fed infants because neonatal iron stores can supply the major portion of iron needs during this period. Although breast milk may contain little more than 0.3 mg iron per liter, about half of this iron is absorbed in contrast to the much smaller proportion that is assimilated from other foods. This iron helps to delay the depletion of neonatal iron stores, but other sources of iron are required in midinfancy. In normal, breast-fed term infants, the addition to the diet of iron-fortified cereal after 6 months of age probably is desirable to supply adequate amounts of iron.

The supplementation of fluoride in the diet of a healthy breast-fed infant is no longer recommended by the Academy of Pediatrics. Evidence supports the contention that there is adequate fluoride in human milk, and fluorosis from excessive amounts is a concern.

The Committee on Nutrition* stated in 1986 "It may not be necessary to give fluoride supplements to breastfed infants who are living in an area where water is adequately fluoridated."

Formula-fed term infants

Infants consuming adequate amounts of commercial cow's milk formulas which are in keeping with the recommendations of the Committee do not need vitamin and mineral supplementation in the first six months of life. They do not require supplements during the latter part of the first year if formula continues to be used in appropriate combination with solid foods. After 4 months of age, iron-fortified formula and/or iron-fortified cereal are convenient sources of iron and are preferable to the use of iron supplements. If powdered or concentrated formula is used, fluoride supplements should be administered only if the community water contains less than 0.3 ppm of fluoride. Ready-to-use formulas are now manufactured with water low in fluoride, and recommendations for fluoride supplementation should be individualized by the pediatrician to provide a total of 0.5 g per day.

Vitamin K deficiency is seen occasionally in infants. It is usually associated with diarrhea and especially with the administration of antibiotics, through a decrease in the synthesis of vitamin K by the intestinal microflora. In the past, the feeding of soy or other non-milk-based formulas was associated with vitamin K deficiency, which was related in part to the type of oil used in the formula. In 1976, the Committee recommended that all infant formulas, particularly non-milk-based formulas, be required to contain an appropriate level of vitamin K.

Preterm infants

The needs of preterm infants for certain nutrients are proportionately greater than those of term infants because of the increased demands of a more rapid rate of growth and less complete intestinal absorption.

---

*From the Committee on Nutrition, American Academy of Pediatrics: Fluoride supplementation, Pediatrics 77:758-761, 1986. If the water supply contains less than 0.3 ppm of fluoride, the infant can be supplemented with 0.25 mg fluoride daily.

During the first weeks of life (prior to consumption of about 300 kcal per day or reaching a body weight of 2.5 kg), a multivitamin supplement that provides the equivalent of the RDAs for term infants should be supplied. The components of this supplement should ideally include vitamin E in a form well absorbed by preterm infants, such as *d*-α-tocopheryl polyethylene glycol 1000 succinate. Folic acid deficiency has been reported in preterm infants, and folic acid should be included in the regimen. Folic acid is not in liquid multivitamin-multimineral mixes because of its lack of stability. However, because the period of administration will generally be in a hospital, folate can be added to a multivitamin preparation in the hospital pharmacy in a concentration to provide 0.1 mg (the US RDA) per daily dose. The shelf life should be limited to one month, and the label should read "shake well" because folate will gradually precipitate. Iron supplementation is best delayed until after the first few weeks of life because extra iron may predispose to anemia when there is insufficient absorption of vitamin E. Neonatal iron stores are still abundant, and iron needs for erythropoiesis are relatively small during the physiologic postnatal decline in hemoglobin concentration.

After several weeks of age, when the infant is consuming more than 300 kcal/day or when the body weight exceeds 2.5 kg, a multivitamin supplement is no longer needed, but it is a convenient method for providing the few specific nutrients that still may be required. These include vitamin D, iron, and possibly folic acid.

There have been sporadic reports of rickets, particularly in breast-fed premature infants. This probably results from the low phosphorus content of breast milk, which has only 150 mg/liter in contrast to about 450 mg/liter in formulas. The condition is also correctable with phosphate supplementation. However, there is also evidence that vitamin D supplementation is helpful. Iron is required at a level of 2 mg/kg/day starting by 2 months of age because neonatal iron stores may become depleted earlier than in term infants—before it is appropriate to supply iron in the form of fortified solid foods. Iron-fortified formula also supplies sufficient iron for the prevention of iron deficiency in preterm infants.

Prenatal dietary prophylaxis of atopic disease

In addition to heredity, the prophylaxis of allergic disease in the potentially allergic child involves four major considerations:

1. The possibility of intrauterine sensitization
2. The nutrition of the newborn infant with particular respect to the fact that human breast milk is the best and only natural food
3. The role of secretory immunoglobulin A (sIgA)
4. The fact that food ingested by the nursing mother may pass through with the breast milk and be immunologically capable of sensitizing a potentially allergic infant or of causing a reaction in a previously sensitized infant

Because specific food allergies occasionally appear to be inherited, the pregnant mother of a potentially allergic child should exclude from her diet not only those foods to which she is allergic but also those foods to which other members of the immediate family are sensitive. Overindulgence in any particular food (pica) is to be avoided, particularly the peanut, which is a rather common offender.

An absolute indication for a strict dietary regimen is the presence in the immediate family of significant asthma or atopic dermatitis. If the prospective mother is sensitive to milk, she should be on a milk-free diet. All of the protein required by the mother may be obtained from beef and other meats and soybean. Adequate vitamins should be supplied, bearing in mind that some of the synthetic coloring, of which tartrazine (FD&C yellow no. 5) is the most common offender, as well as some artificial flavoring materials may cause problems. This coloring is no longer permitted unless so labeled by law. Adequate calcium should be supplied and is least expensive when obtained as calcium carbonate powder, reagent quality, one-half teaspoon (0.4 g calcium) per day during pregnancy and two-thirds teaspoon (0.5 g calcium) per day during lactation. There are many calcium preparations available.

If there is no milk allergy in the immediate family a pint of milk (500 ml) daily, boiled 10 minutes, or the same amount of half evaporated milk and half water may be

From Glaser J, Dreyfuss EM, and Logan J: Prenatal dietary prophylaxis of atopic disease. In Kelley VC, editor: Practice of pediatrics, vol 2, Hagerstown Md, 1976, Harper & Row, Publishers, Inc.

given. In these preparations, bovine γ-globulin, the most heat labile of the milk allergens, followed closely by bovine serum albumin, is rendered immunologically inactive. As a result, milk-allergic individuals sensitive only to these proteins are the only milk-allergic individuals who can tolerate boiled or evaporated milk.

One of the least allergenic substitutes for cow's milk is soybean milk. The preparations designed primarily for infants are rather tasty to adults and may be used as desired. Detailed instructions for their use may be obtained from the manufacturers. Soy products are readily available.

The superheated proprietary milks have been shown to be only somewhat more allergenic than soybean milk. If soybean milk is objectionable, it is reasonable to substitute these milks, not to exceed 1½ pints a day. Enfamil, Similac, and SMA are some of the preparations readily obtained at drug stores and supermarkets.

Glossary

acinus The tube leading to the smallest lobule of a compound gland; it is characterized by a narrow lumen.

adipose tissue *See* panniculus adiposus.

afferent Conducting inward to, or toward, the center of an organ, gland, or other structure or area. Applies to sensory nerves, arteries, and lymph vessels.

alveolus A glandular acinus or terminal portion of the alveolar gland where milk is secreted and stored, 0.12 mm in diameter. From 10 to 100 alveoli, or tubulosaccular secretory units, make up a lobulus.

apocrine A term descriptive of a gland cell that loses part of its protoplasmic substance.

Apt test A test, named after its developer, performed on fresh blood to distinguish between adult and fetal hemoglobin. The blood is suspended in saline, an equal amount of 10% NaOH is added and mixed; adult hemoglobin turns brown, while fetal hemoglobin remains red. A control of known adult blood should also be done.

arborization Development of a branched appearance.

areola mammae Areola. The pigmented area surrounding the papilla mammae, or nipple.

autophagic vacuole Autophagosome. A membrane-bound body within a cell containing degenerating cell organelles.

BALT Bronchus-associated immunocompetent lymphoid tissue, to which the mammary gland may act as an extension. *See* GALT and MALT.

basal lamina The layer of material, 50 to 80 nm thick, that lies adjacent to the plasma membrane of the basal surfaces of epithelial cells. It contains collagen and certain carbohydrates. It is often called the basement membrane.

casein A derivative of caseinogen. The fraction of milk protein that forms the tough curd.

colostrum The first milk. It is a yellow sticky fluid secreted during the first few days postpartum, which provides nutrition and protection against infectious disease. It contains more protein, less sugar, and much less fat than mature breast milk.

columnar secretory cell A type of secretory cell in the shape of a hexagonal prism, which appears rectangular when sectioned across the long axis, the length being considerably greater than the width.

Coopers' ligaments Triangularly shaped ligaments stretching between the mammary gland, the skin, the retinacula cutis, the pectineal ligament, and the chorda obliqua. These underlie the breasts.

corpus mammae The mammary gland; breast mass after freeing breast from deep attachments and removal of skin, subcutaneous connective tissue, and fat.

creamatocrit Measurement for estimating the fat content and, therefore, the caloric content of a milk sample. A microhematocrit tube is filled with milk (usually a mix of foremilk and hind milk) and spun in a microcentrifuge for 15 minutes. The layer of fat is measured as one measures a blood hematocrit.

cross-nursing The breastfeeding by a lactating woman of a baby who is not her own, usually temporarily, in the role of a child-care arrangement.

cuboidal secretory cell A secretory cell whose height and breadth are of similar size.

cytosol Cell fluid.

doula An individual who surrounds, interacts with, and aids the mother at any time within the period that includes pregnancy, birth, and lactation. She may be a relative, friend, or neighbor and is usually but not necessarily female. One who gives psychologic encouragement and physical assistance to a new mother.

efferent Carrying impulses away from a nerve center.

ejection reflex A reflex initiated by the suckling of the infant at the breast, which triggers the pituitary gland to release oxytocin into the bloodstream. The oxytocin causes the myoepithelial cells to contract and eject the milk from the collecting ductules. (Also called letdown reflex or draught.)

engorgement The swelling and distention of the breasts, usually in the early days of initiation of lactation, due to vascular dilation as well as the arrival of the early milk.

eosinophil A granular leukocyte possessing large conspicuous granules in the cytoplasm and containing a bilobed nucleus.

foremilk The first milk obtained at the onset of suckling or expression. Contains less fat than later milk of that feeding (i.e., the hind milk).

galactocele A cystic tumor in the ducts of the breast, which contains a milky fluid.

galactagogue A material or action that stimulates the production of milk.

galactopoiesis The development of milk in the mammary gland. The maintenance of established lactation.

galactorrhea Abnormal or inappropriate lactation.

galactose ($C_6H_{12}O_6$) A simple sugar that is a component of the disaccharide lactose, or milk sugar.

galactosemia A congenital metabolic disorder in which there is an inability to metabolize galactose because of a deficiency of the enzyme galactose-1-phosphate uridyltransferase. It causes failure to thrive, hepatomegaly, and splenomegaly.

GALT Gut-associated lymphoid tissue to which the mammary gland may act as an extension. *See* BALT and MALT.

Golgi apparatus A specialized region of the cytoplasm, often close to the nucleus, that is composed of flattened cisternae, numerous vesicles, and some larger vacuoles. In secretory cells it is concerned with packaging the secretory product. It is also probably concerned with the secretion of polysaccharides in some cells, but its full range of functions has not yet been elucidated.

heterophagic vacuole Heterophagosome. A membrane-bound body within a cell, containing ingested material.

hind milk Milk obtained later during nursing period, that is, the end of the feeding. This milk is usually high in fat and probably controls appetite.

homocystinuria A rare inborn error of amino acid metabolism characterized by mental deficiency, epilepsy, dislocation of the lens, growth disturbance, thromboses, and defective hair growth.

hyperadenia The existence of mammary tissue without nipples.

hypermastia The existence of accessory mammary glands.

hyperthelia The existence of abundant, more or less developed, nipples without accompanying mammary tissue.

immunoglobulin Protein fraction of globulin, which has been demonstrated to have immunologic properties. Immunoglobulins include IgA, IgG, and IgM—factors in breast milk that protect against infection.

induced lactation Process by which a nonpuerperal female (or male) is stimulated to lactate.

lactiferous ducts The main ducts of the mammary gland, which number from 15 to 30 and open onto the nipple. They carry milk to the nipple.

lactiferous sinuses Dilations on the lactiferous ducts at the base of the nipple.

Lactobacillus bifidus Organism of the intestinal tract of breastfed infants.

lactocele Cystic tumor of the breast due to the dilation and obstruction of a milk duct usually filled with milk.

lactoferrin An iron-binding protein of external secretions, including human milk. It inhibits the growth of iron-dependent microorganisms in the gut.

lactogenesis Initiation of milk secretion.

let-down reflex *See* ejection reflex.

lobulus A subunit of the parenchymal structure of the breast made up of 10 to 100 alveoli, or tubulosaccular secretory units. From 20 to 40 lobuli make up a lobus.

lobus A subunit of the parenchymal structure of the breast made up of 20 to 40 lobuli. From 15 to 25 lobi are arranged like the spokes of a wheel with the nipple as the central point.

lymphocyte A mature leukocyte derived through the intermediate stage of lymphoblast from the reticuloendothelium found in lymphatic tissue.

MALT Mucosal-associated lymphoid tissue, which includes gut, lung, mammary gland, salivary and lacrimal glands, and genital tract. There is traffic of cells between secretory sites. Immunization at one site may be an effective means of producing immunity at distant sites. *See* GALT and BALT.

mamilla The nipple; any teatlike structure.

mammogenesis Growth of the mammary gland.

mastitis Inflammation of the breast, including cellulitis, and occasionally abscess formation.

matrescence The state of becoming a mother or motherhood as a new event in an individual's life.

megaloblastic anemia Defective red blood cell formation due to megaloblastic hyperplasia of the marrow; there are often megaloblasts, or primitive nucleated red cells in the peripheral blood.

merocrine Pertaining to the type of secretion in which the active cell remains intact while forming and discharging the secretory product.

mesencephalon The midbrain.

methylmalonic aciduria The condition of the urine being acidic from an accumulation of methylmalonic acid due to an inborn error of metabolism.

milk fever A syndrome of fever and general malaise associated with early engorgement of the breasts or with sudden weaning from the breast.

mitogen A substance capable of stimulating cells to enter mitosis.

Montgomery glands Small prominences, sebaceous glands in the areola of the breast, which become more marked in pregnancy. They number 20 to 24 and secrete a fluid that lubricates the nipple area.

Morgagni's tubercle Small sinuses into which the miniature ducts of the Montgomery glands open in the epidermis of the areola.

myoephithelial cell An epithelial cell, usually lying around a glandular acinus, in which part of the cytoplasm has contractile properties, serving to empty the sinus of its secretion.

nonnutritive sucking The act of suckling the breast with little or no secretion of milk. Infant may suckle when distressed or to be calmed or quieted.

nonpuerperal lactation The production of milk in a woman who has not given birth.

nucleotides Compounds derived from nucleic acid by hydrolysis and consisting of phosphoric acid combined with a sugar and a purine or pyrimidine derivative. The milk nucleotides are secreted from glandular epithelial cells.

opsonic Belonging to or characterized by opsonin, a substance in mammalian blood having the power to render microorganisms and blood cells more easily absorbed by phagocytes.

oxytocin An octapeptide synthesized in the cell bodies of neurons located mainly in the paraventricular nucleus and in smaller amounts in the supraoptic nucleus of the hypothalamus. Oxytocin stimulates the ejection reflex by stimulation of the myoepithelial cells in the mammary gland.

panniculus adiposus Adipose tissue. The superficial fascia, which contains fatty pellicles.

papilla mammae Mamilla. The nipple of the breast.

perinatal Around birth. The time from conception through birth, delivery, lactation, and at least 28 days postpartum.

plasma cell Cell derived from the B cell series, which manufactures and secretes antibodies.

prolactin A hormone present in both male and female and at all ages. During pregnancy it stimulates and prepares the mammary alveolar epithelium for secretory activity. During lactation it stimulates synthesis and secretion of milk. At other ages and in the male it interacts with other steroids.

rachitic Relating to, characterized by, or affected with rickets.

relactation Process by which a woman who has given birth but did not initially breastfeed is stimulated to lactate (also applies to reinstituting lactation after it has been discontinued).

squamous epithelium A sheet of flattened, scalelike epithelium adhering edge to edge.

stroma The connective tissue basis or framework of an organ.

subependymal matrix The layer beneath the ependyma, the layer of ciliated epithelium that lines the central canal of the spinal cord and the ventricles of the brain.

switch nursing Putting the infant to one breast for a short time, usually 5 minutes, moving the infant to the other breast for 5 minutes, and then moving the infant back to the first side in an effort to improve milk production.

tail of Spense The axillary tail of the breast.

transitional milk The milk produced early in the postpartum period as the colostrum diminishes and the mature milk develops.

tubuloalveolar Having both tubular and alveolar qualities.

tubulosaccular Having both tubular and saccular character.

turgescence The swelling up of a part. The unusual turgid feeling resulting from swelling with fluid.

whey protein Protein remaining when the curds of casein have been removed. The mixture of proteins present is complex and includes β-lactoglobulin and α-lactalbumin and enzymes.

witch's milk Product of neonatal galactorrhea due to absorption of placental prolactin.

Index

A

A and D ointment, cracked nipple treated with, 197
Abscess, mastitis complicated with, 211
Accutane; *see* Isotretinoin
Acebutolol in breast milk, infant affected by, 548t
Acetaminophen
  in breast milk, infant affected by, 263, 269, 520t
  engorgement pain treated with, 193
Acetazolamine in breast milk, infant affected by, 559t
Acetone, in diabetic mother, 397
Acetylsalicylic acid in breast milk, infant affected by, 264, 269
Achromycin; *see* Tetracycline HCL
Acid(s), level of; *see also* Names of specific acids
  in colostrum, 78
  in human milk, 226-228
Acidosis
  bilirubin deposition in brain affected by, 353
  in small-for-gestational-age infant, 337
Acquired immune deficiency syndrome
  breastfeeding and, 167-168
  screening for, in milk donors, 483
  transmission of, through milk, 142
Acrodermatitis enteropathica, breastfeeding infant with, 348-349
ACTH; *see* Adrenocorticotropic hormone
Acute lactation failure, causes of, 20
Acute puerperal mammary adenitis, 208
Acute puerperal mammary cellulitis, 208
Acyclovir in breast milk, infant affected by, 532t
Adapin; *see* Doxepin
Adenoma, pituitary, galactorrhea associated with, 393
Adipose tissue, impact of pregnancy on, 229
Adrenal gland, mammary growth affected by, 49
Adrenal hyperplasia, breastfeeding infant with, 351
Adrenocorticotropic hormone, mammary growth affected by, 49
Adriamycin; *see* Doxorubicin
Advil; *see* Ibuprofen
Agent Orange, presence of, in breast milk, 280
AIDS; *see* Acquired immune deficiency syndrome

AIDS-related complex, breastfeeding and, 167-168
α-lactalbumin, lactose synthesis and, 67
Alanine, level of, in human milk, 85t, 505t
Albamycin; *see* Novobiocin
Albumin
  level of
    during weaning, 248
    in premature infant, 353
  normal serum values for, in infant, 516-517t
Alcohol
  colic treated with, 214
  effect of, on nipple and areola, 183
  poor milk production due to, 296
Aldactone; *see* Spironolactone
Aldomet; *see* Methyldopa
Aldrin in breast milk, 279
  infant affected by, 562t
Alkaline phosphatase, normal serum values for, in infant, 516-517t
Allergy(ies)
  breastfeeding and, 24
  colic and, 215
  cow's milk associated with, 420, 423-434
  immunologic aspects of, 425-426
  protection against, in milk, 144-145
Allopurinol in breast milk, infant affected by, 546t
Aloin in breast milk, infant affected by, 565t
Alprazolam in breast milk, infant affected by, 575t
Alprenolol in breast milk, infant affected by, 54t
Aluminum in human milk, 99
Alvedon; *see* Paracetamol
Alveolar cell
  functional components of, 65
  permeability of, 69
Alveolar duct(s), microscopic anatomy of, 44
Alveolar gland, description of, 33
Alveoli
  description of, 33
  growth of, progesterone and, 48
  lactation and, 45
  microscopic anatomy of, 44

Cleocin; *see* Clindamycin

Cleocinpediatric in breast milk, infant affected by, 537t

Clindamycin in breast milk, infant affected by, 537t

Clinoril; *see* Sulindac

Clofibrate in breast milk, infant affected by, 553t

Clonazepam in breast milk, infant affected by, 527t

Clonidine in breast milk, infant affected by, 553t

Clorazepate in breast milk, infant affected by, 279

Clostridium botulinum, 345

Cloxacillin in breast milk, infant affected by, 537t

Cylcloserine in breast milk, infant affected by, 537t

Coach, role of father as, 159

Cobalt, level of, in human milk, 506t

Cocaine in breast milk, infant affected by, 573t

Code for Infant Feeding of the World Health Organization, 2

Codeine
    in breast milk, infant affected by, 269, 573t
    engorgement pain treated with, 193

Coffee, caffeine from, in breast milk, 272

Coitus, lactation and, 462

Cola drink, caffeine from, in breast milk, 272

Colchicine, lactation failure due to, 300

Cold, milk-ejection reflex inhibited by, 200

Colic, 213-215
    definition of, 213
    maternal diet as cause of, 241

Colistin in breast milk, infant affected by, 537t

Colitis
    in breastfed infant, 343
    cow's milk associated with, 344-345
    treatment of, and breastfeeding, 271
    ulcerative, breastfeeding and treatment of, 405-406

Colon, disorders of, breastfeeding infant with, 364-365

Colostomy, imperforate anus treated with, 365-366

Colostral bodies of Donne, 121

Colostrum
    antibodies in, 119
    antioxidant properties of, 144
    biochemistry of, 75-78
    carnitine content in, 90
    cellular components of, 120-126
    concentration of minerials in, 93t
    diastase level in, 108
    distribution of T cells in, 124
    enzyme levels in, 107
    IgA in, 126, 127
        respiratory illness and, 346
    IgM in, 127
    immunoglobulins in, 88, 126
    immunologically active components in, 120t
    lactoferrin in, 126, 136
    polymorphonuclear leukocytes in, 122
    for premature infant, value of, 328
    production of, during pregnancy, 45, 49

Colostrum—cont'd
    vitamin content of, 101t

Colymycin; *see* Colistin

Comedomastitis, causes of, 411

Comfort nursing, definition of, 247

Commercial discharge pack, duration of breastfeeding and, 19-20

Committee on Drugs of the American Academy of Pediatrics, 256

Committee on Nutrition of the Academy of Pediatrics, 240

Committee on Recommended Dietary Allowances of Food and Nutrition Board, 236

Community resources, support from, for breastfeeding mother, 496-500

Computerized axillary tomography, breast cancer diagnosed with, 163

Congenital aganglionic megacolon, 364

Containers for milk collection, 473-474

Contamination during milk collection, 473

Contraception
    breastfeeding as form of, 451, 453-454, 455
    during lactation, 457-462

Contraceptive
    milk production affected by, 460t
    oral
        in breast milk, infant affected by, 569t
        lactation and, 459-460

Cooper's ligament, 39
    effect of engorgement on, 193

Copper
    accumulation of, in preterm infant, 323t
    in breast milk, infant affected by, 567t
    impact of maternal diet supplement on, 235
    level of
        in colostrum, 93t
        in human milk, 93t, 98, 506t
    premature infant's requirement for, 325

Cordarone; *see* Amiodarone

Corgard; *see* Nadolol; Nadolol

Corpus mammae, 33-34
    innervation of, 42
    parenchyma, 33
    stroma, 33

Corticotropin in breast milk, infant affected by, 569t

Cortisone
    in breast milk, infant affected by, 570t
    cracked nipple treated with, 197

Corzide; *see* Nadolol

Coumadin; *see* Warfarin

Coumarin
    in breast milk, infant affected by, 525t
    effects of, 274

Counseling
    for breastfeeding mother, 500-501
    for working mother, 314

Counselor, lactation, 500-502